Basic
Dysrhythmias

Interpretation & Management

Visit our website at www.mosby.com

Basic Dysrhythmias

Interpretation & Management

ROBERT J. HUSZAR, MD

Former Medical Director
Emergency Medical Services
New York State Department of Health
Albany, New York

THIRD EDITION

with **481** *illustrations*

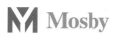 Mosby

A Harcourt Health Sciences Company

St. Louis   London   Philadelphia   Sydney   Toronto

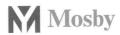

A Harcourt Health Sciences Company

Editor in Chief: Andrew Allen
Executive Editor: Claire Merrick
Developmental Editor: Laura Bayless
Project Manager: Pat Joiner
Production Editor: Karen M. Rehwinkel
Book Design Manager: Gail Morey Hudson
Cover Designer: Teresa Breckwoldt

THIRD EDITION

Mosby, Inc.
A Harcourt Health Sciences Company
11830 Westline Industrial Drive
St. Louis, Missouri 63146

Printed in the United States of America

Library of Congress Cataloging-in-Publication Data

Huszar, Robert J.
   Basic dysrhythmias : interpretation and management / Robert J. Huszar.--3rd ed.
      p. ; cm.
   Includes index.
   ISBN 0-323-01244-2
      1. Arrhythmia. I. Title
   [DNLM: 1. Arrhythmia--diagnosis. 2. Arrhythmia--therapy. 3. Electrocardiography. 4. Heart Conduction System. WG 330 H972b 2001]
   RC685.A65 H89 2001
   616.1'28--dc21

                                                                    2001030945

01   02   03   04   05   GW/KPT   9   8   7   6   5   4   3   2   1

*This book is dedicated
to my wife,*
Jean

Preface

Basic Dysrhythmias: Interpretation and Management, third edition is designed, as were the first and second editions, to help medical, nursing, and paramedical personnel (physicians, nurses, residents, interns, medical students, paramedics, emergency medical technicians, cardiology technicians, and other allied health personnel) acquire the skills to analyze, identify, and manage common arrhythmias.

The chapters dealing with the analysis, identification, and management of the arrhythmias have been extensively updated based on the following:

◆ The 2000 National Conference on Standards and Guidelines for Cardiopulmonary Resuscitation (CPR) and Emergency Cardiac Care (ECC)

◆ Ryan TJ et al: ACC/AHA guidelines for the management of patients with acute myocardial infarction: a report of the American College of Cardiology/American Heart Association Task Force on Practice Guidelines (Committee on Management of Acute Myocardial Infarction), *J Am Coll Cardiol* 28:1328-1428, 1996 (1999 update available at *www.acc.org*).

The terminology relating to the arrhythmias has been updated and the management scrupulously edited and revised to conform as closely as possible to that recommended by the 2000 Advanced Cardiac Life Support (ACLS) guidelines. In addition, treatment algorithms and summaries have been developed to aid in the logical approach to the management of the arrhythmias. The treatment algorithms that relate to the arrhythmias presented in any given chapter are included in that chapter. Tables summarizing the typical diagnostic ECG features of sinus node, atrial, junctional, and ventricular arrhythmias and of AV blocks have also been included.

In recognition of the urgent need to reduce the time between the onset of acute myocardial infarction (MI) and the initiation of treatment to achieve reperfusion of the obstructed coronary artery, several new chapters have been added to help achieve this goal. These include a chapter on the signs and symptoms of acute MI and a chapter on its management, including a set of treatment algorithms, based on the above guidelines. In addition, acute coronary syndromes and the phases of thrombus formation and lysis are reviewed to help in the understanding of the rationale behind the management of acute MI.

Other new subjects covered in the third edition include accessory conduction pathways and associated preexcitation syndromes; ECG patterns typical of early repolarization, hypothermia, and accessory conduction pathways; and right ventricular MI. The glossary has been updated to reflect the new material.

I wish to acknowledge with gratitude the expertise of the following reviewers for their recommendations and assistance in developing the third edition of this book:

Robert Carter, NREMT-P
Paramedic, Baltimore City Fire Department;
Instructor, EMS Training Committee,
Affiliate Faculty,
Hopkins Outreach for Pediatric Education,
The Johns Hopkins Children's Center,
Baltimore, Maryland

Robert Cook, EMT-P, EMD, I/C
Paramedic Supervisor,
Hamilton Hospital,
Webster City, Iowa

Glen A. Hoffman, NREMT-P
Ketchikan Fire Department,
Ketchikan, Alaska

Andrew W. Stern, NREMT-P, MPA, MA
Town Colonie Emergency Services,
Colonie, New York

Ronald D. Taylor, EMT-P
Clinical Development and Special Projects
  Coordinator,
City of Austin EMS,
Austin, Texas

Glen Treankler, EMT-P, EMS-I, ACLS-I, ERT; BS, MA
Center Point Volunteer Ambulance Service,
Center Point, Iowa

My continuing appreciation goes out to *Robert Elling, Timothy Frank, Kevin B. Kraus, Mikel Rothenburg, Judith Ruple,* and *Andrew W. Stern* for their work on the previous editions of this text.

In addition, I would like to thank *Laura Bayless,* Developmental Editor; *Karen Rehwinkel,* Senior Production Editor; and *Claire Merrick,* Acquisitions Editor at Harcourt Health Sciences for their assistance.

Robert J. Huszar

A Note to the Reader

The author and publisher have made every attempt to check dosages and advanced life support content for accuracy. The care procedures presented here represent accepted practices in the United States. They are not offered as a standard of care. Advanced life support level emergency care is performed under the authority of a licensed physician. It is the reader's responsibility to know and follow local care protocols as provided by his or her medical advisors. It is also the reader's responsibility to stay informed of emergency care procedure changes, including the most recent guidelines set forth by the American Heart Association and printed in their textbooks.

Contents

Appendices

Glossary, 508

Basic
Dysrhythmias
Interpretation & Management

1 Anatomy and Physiology of the Heart

CHAPTER OBJECTIVES

Upon completion of all or part of this chapter, you should be able to complete the following objectives:

1. Name and identify the following anatomical features of the heart on an anatomical drawing:
   The four chambers of the heart
   The two main septa of the heart
   The three layers of the ventricular walls
   The base and apex of the heart
2. Name and identify the layers of the pericardium and its major space or cavity.
3. Define the right heart and left heart and the primary function of each with respect to the pulmonary and systemic circulations.
4. Name and locate on an anatomical drawing the following major structures of the circulatory system: the aorta, the pulmonary artery, the superior and inferior vena cavae, the coronary sinus, the pulmonary veins, and the four heart valves.
5. Define (a) atrial systole and diastole and (b) ventricular systole and diastole.
6. Name and identify the parts of the electrical conduction system of the heart.
7. Name the two basic kinds of cardiac cells and give their function.

8. List and define the three major types of accessory conduction pathways, including their location, conduction capabilities, and potential for disrupting normal cardiac function.
9. Name and define the four properties of cardiac cells.
10. Describe a resting, polarized cardiac cell and a depolarized cardiac cell.
11. Define the following:
    Depolarization process
    Repolarization process
    Threshold potential
12. Name and locate on a schematic of a cardiac action potential the five phases of a cardiac potential.
13. Define and locate on an ECG the following:
    Absolute refractory period
    Relative refractory period
    Vulnerable period of repolarization
    Supernormal period
14. Explain the rationale behind the property of automaticity (spontaneous depolarization) and how the slope of phase-4 depolarization relates to the rate of impulse formation.
15. Define (a) dominant and latent pacemaker cells and (b) nonpacemaker cells.

ANATOMY AND PHYSIOLOGY OF THE HEART

Anatomy of the Heart

The heart, whose sole purpose is to circulate blood through the circulatory system (the blood vessels of the body), consists of four hollow chambers (Figure 1-1). The upper two chambers, the *right and left atria,* are thin-walled; the lower two chambers, the *right and left ventricles,* are thick-walled and muscular. The two atria form the base of the heart; the ventricles form the apex of the heart.

The walls of the ventricles are composed of three layers of tissue: the innermost thin layer is called the *endocardium;* the middle thick, muscular layer, the *myocardium;* and the outermost thin layer, the *epicardium.* The myocardium is further divided into the *subendocardial area,* the inner half of the myocardium, and the *subepicardial area,* the outer half of the myocardium. The walls of the left ventricle are more muscular and about three times thicker than those of the right ventricle. The atrial walls are also composed of three layers of tissue, like those of the ventricles, but the middle muscular layer is much thinner.

Enclosing the heart is the *pericardium,* which consists of an outer tough, fibrous sac, the *fibrous pericardium,* and an inner, two-layered, fluid-secreting membrane, the *serous pericardium* (Figure 1-2). The outer, fibrous pericardium comes in direct contact with the covering of the lung, the *pleura.* The inner layer of the serous pericardium, the *visceral pericardium,* or, as it is more commonly known, the *epicardium,* covers the heart itself, and the outer layer, the *parietal pericardium,* lines the fibrous pericardium. Between the two layers of the serous pericardium is the *pericardial space* or *cavity.* It contains up to 50 ml of fluid, the *pericardial fluid,* which helps to lubricate the movements of the heart within the pericardium.

Inferiorly, the pericardium is attached to the center of the diaphragm; anteriorly it is attached to the sternum, and posteriorly to the esophagus, trachea, and main bronchi. In this way, the pericardium anchors the heart to the chest and prevents it from shifting about.

The *interatrial septum* (a thin membranous wall) separates the two atria, and a thicker, more muscular wall, the *interventricular septum,* separates the two ventricles. The two septa, in effect, divide the heart into two pumping systems, the *right heart* and *left heart,* each one consisting of an atrium and a ventricle.

Circulation of the Blood Through the Heart

The right heart pumps blood into the pulmonary circulation (the blood vessels within the lungs and those carrying blood to and from the lungs). The left heart pumps blood into the systemic circulation (the blood vessels in the rest of the body and those carrying blood to and from the body). The systemic circulation includes the coronary circulation, which supplies the heart through the coronary arteries.

The right atrium receives unoxygenated blood from the body via two of the body's largest veins (the superior vena cava and inferior vena cava) and from the heart itself by way of the coronary sinus (Figure 1-3). The blood is delivered to the right ventricle through the tricuspid valve. The right ventricle then pumps the unoxygenated blood through the pulmonic valve and into the lungs via the pulmonary artery. In the lungs, the blood picks up oxygen and releases excess carbon dioxide.

The left atrium receives the newly oxygenated blood from the lungs via the pulmonary veins and delivers it to the left ventricle through the mitral valve. The left ventricle then pumps the oxygenated blood out through the aortic valve and into the aorta, the largest artery in the body. From the aorta, the blood is distributed throughout the body, including

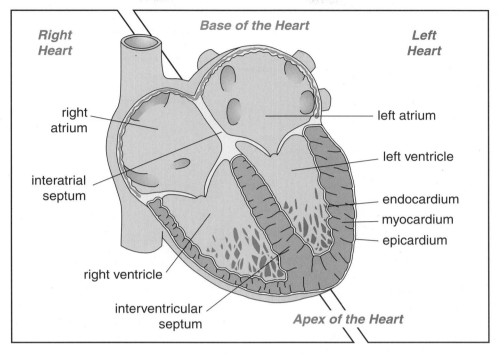

Figure 1-1   Anatomy of the heart.

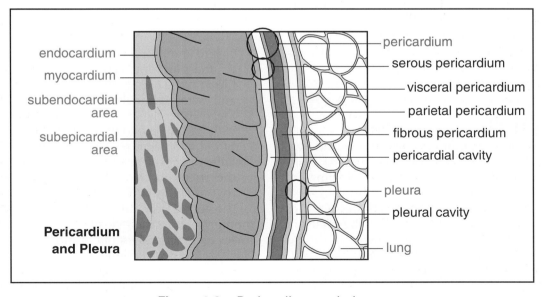

Figure 1-2   Pericardium and pleura.

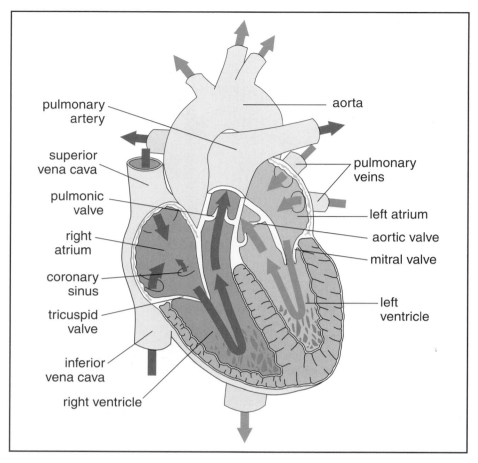

Figure 1-3 Circulation through the heart.

the heart, where the blood releases oxygen to the cells and collects carbon dioxide from them.

Atrial and Ventricular Diastole and Systole

The heart performs its pumping action over and over in a rhythmic sequence as follows (Figure 1-4):

1. First, the atria relax (atrial diastole), allowing the blood to pour in from the body and lungs.
2. As the atria fill with blood, the atrial pressure rises above that in the ventricles, forcing the tricuspid and mitral valves to open and allowing the blood to empty rapidly into the relaxed ventricles.
3. Then, the atria contract (atrial systole), filling the ventricles to capacity. After the contraction of the atria, the pressures in the atria and ventricles equalize and the tricuspid and mitral valves begin to close.
4. Then, the ventricles contract vigorously, causing the ventricular pressure to rise sharply. As the tri-

cuspid and mitral valves close completely, the aortic and pulmonic valves snap open, allowing the blood to be ejected forcefully into the pulmonary and systemic circulations.

5. Meanwhile, the atria are again relaxing and filling with blood. As soon as the ventricles empty of blood and begin to relax, the ventricular pressure falls, the aortic and pulmonic valves shut tightly, the tricuspid and mitral valves open, and the rhythmic cardiac sequence begins anew.

The period from the opening of the aortic and pulmonic valves to their closing, during which the ventricles contract and empty of blood, is called *ventricular systole*. The following period from the closure of the aortic and pulmonic valves to their reopening, during which the ventricles relax and fill with blood, is called *ventricular diastole*. The sequence of one ventricular systole followed by a ventricular diastole is called a *cardiac cycle*, commonly defined as the period from the beginning of one heart beat to the beginning of the next.

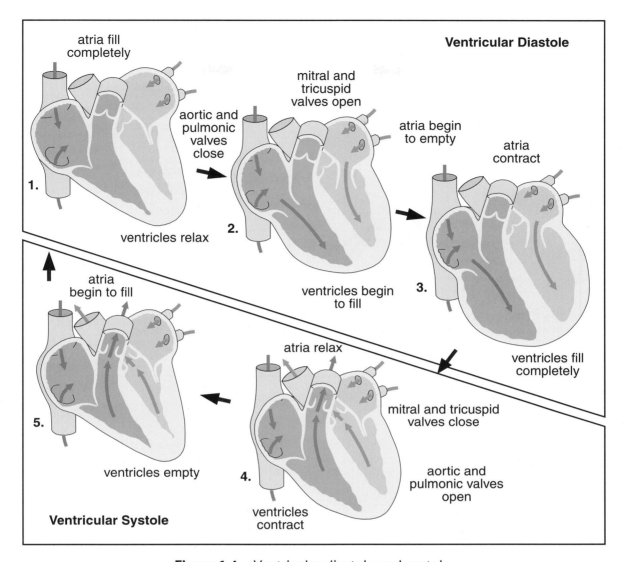

Ventricular Diastole

atria fill completely

mitral and tricuspid valves open

aortic and pulmonic valves close

atria begin to empty

atria contract

ventricles relax

1. **2.** ventricles begin to fill **3.** ventricles fill completely

atria begin to fill

atria relax

ventricles empty

mitral and tricuspid valves close

aortic and pulmonic valves open

5. **4.** ventricles contract

Ventricular Systole

Figure 1-4 Ventricular diastole and systole.

Notes

_____

_____

_____

_____

_____

_____

_____

_____

_____

ELECTRICAL CONDUCTION SYSTEM OF THE HEART

The electrical conduction system of the heart (Figure 1-5) is composed of the following structures:
- The sinoatrial (SA) node
- The internodal conduction tracts and the interatrial conduction tract (Bachmann's bundle)
- The atrioventricular (AV) junction, consisting of the AV node and bundle of His
- The right bundle branch and left bundle branch and its left anterior and posterior fascicles
- The Purkinje network

The prime function of the electrical conduction system of the heart is to transmit minute electrical impulses from the SA node (where they are normally

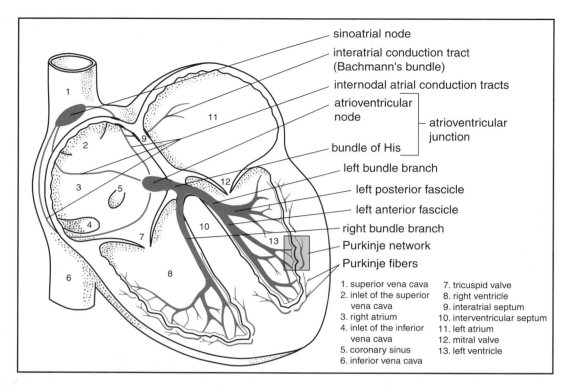

Figure 1-5   Electrical conduction system.

generated) to the atria and ventricles, causing them to contract (Figure 1-6).

The SA node lies in the wall of the right atrium near the inlet of the superior vena cava. It consists of pacemaker cells that generate electrical impulses automatically and regularly.

The three internodal conduction tracts (the anterior, middle, and posterior internodal tracts), running through the walls of the right atrium between the SA node and the AV node, conduct the electrical impulses rapidly from the SA node to the AV node in about 0.03 second. The interatrial conduction tract (Bachmann's bundle), a branch of the anterior internodal tract, extends across the atria, conducting the electrical impulses from the SA node to the left atrium.

The AV node, the proximal part of the AV junction, lies partly in the right side of the interatrial septum in front of the opening of the coronary sinus and partly in the upper part of the interventricular septum above the base of the tricuspid valve. The AV node consists of three regions:

◆ The small, upper atrionodal region, located between the lower part of the atria and the nodal region
◆ The middle, nodal region, the major large central area of the AV node where the electrical impulses

are slowed down in their progression from the atria to the ventricles
◆ The small, lower nodal-His region, located between the nodal region and the bundle of His

The atrionodal and nodal-His regions contain pacemaker cells (described later in the chapter), whereas the nodal region does not. The primary function of the AV node is to channel the electrical impulses from the atria to the bundle of His while slowing their progression so that they arrive at the ventricles in an orderly and timely way. A ring of fibrous tissue insulates the remainder of the atria from the ventricles, preventing electrical impulses from entering the ventricles except through the AV node, unless there are accessory conduction pathways as described later.

The electrical impulses slow as they travel through the AV node, taking about 0.06 to 0.12 second to reach the bundle of His. The delay is such that the atria can contract and empty and the ventricles can fill before they (the ventricles) are stimulated to contract.

The bundle of His, the distal part of the AV junction, lies in the upper part of the interventricular septum, connecting the AV node with the two bundle branches. Once the electrical impulses enter the bundle of His, they travel more rapidly on their way to the bundle branches, taking 0.03 to 0.05 second.

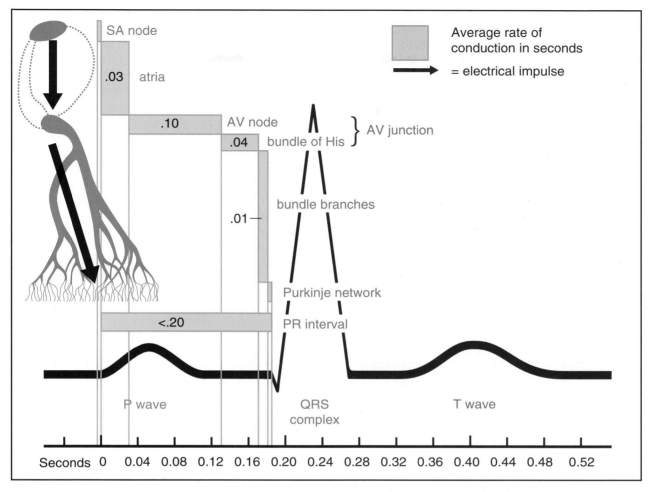

Figure 1-6   The average rate of conduction of the electrical impulse through various parts of the electrical conduction system.

The right bundle branch and the left common bundle branch arise from the bundle of His, straddle the interventricular septum, and continue down both sides of the septum. The left common bundle branch further divides into two major divisions: the left anterior fascicle and the left posterior fascicle.

The bundle branches and their fascicles subdivide into smaller and smaller branches, the smallest ones connecting with the Purkinje network, an intricate web of tiny Purkinje fibers spread widely throughout the ventricles beneath the endocardium. The ends of the Purkinje fibers finally terminate at the myocardial cells. The bundle of His, the right and left bundle branches, and the Purkinje network are also known as the *His-Purkinje system* of the ventricles. Pacemaker cells are located throughout the His-Purkinje system.

The electrical impulses travel very rapidly to the Purkinje network through the bundle branches in less than 0.01 second. All in all, it normally takes the electrical impulses less than 0.2 second on the aver-age to travel from the SA node to the Purkinje network in the ventricles.

Accessory Conduction Pathways

Several distinct electrical conduction pathways have been found in the heart that conduct electrical impulses from the atria to the ventricles more directly, bypassing the AV node, the bundle of His, or both. These accessory conduction pathways (Figure 1-7) activate the ventricles earlier than they would be if the electrical impulses traveled down the electrical conduction system normally. Terms used to identify this premature depolarization of the ventricles via accessory conduction pathways are *ventricular preexcitation* and *preexcitation syndrome.*

The most common of these accessory conduction pathways are the accessory AV pathways (or connections), which conduct the electrical impulses from the atria directly to the ventricles. Less commonly, other accessory conduction pathways conduct the electrical impulses from the atria to the bundle of His (the atrio-His fibers or tracts) and from the AV node and bundle of His to the ventricles (the nodoventricular and fasciculoventricular fibers, respectively). These pathways can not only conduct electrical impulses forward (anterograde), but most of them can conduct the impulses backward (retrograde) as well, setting up the mechanism for reentry tachyarrhythmias.

◆ ACCESSORY ATRIOVENTRICULAR PATHWAYS

Accessory AV pathways (also known as the *bundles of Kent*) consist of bundles of conductive myocardial fibers bridging the fibrous layer insulating the atria

from the ventricles. The accessory AV pathways have been found in the following locations:

◆ Between the posterior free wall of the left atrium and that of the left ventricle (type A Wolff-Parkinson-White [WPW] conduction pathway)
◆ Between the posterior atrial and ventricular walls in the septal region (posteroseptal WPW conduction pathway)
◆ Between the anterior free wall of the right atrium and that of the right ventricle (type B WPW conduction pathway)

These accessory AV pathways are responsible for accessory AV pathway conduction, also known as the *Wolff-Parkinson-White (WPW) conduction*, resulting in abnormally wide QRS complexes, the classic form of ventricular preexcitation. When this type of AV conduction is associated with a paroxysmal supraventricular tachycardia with normal QRS com-

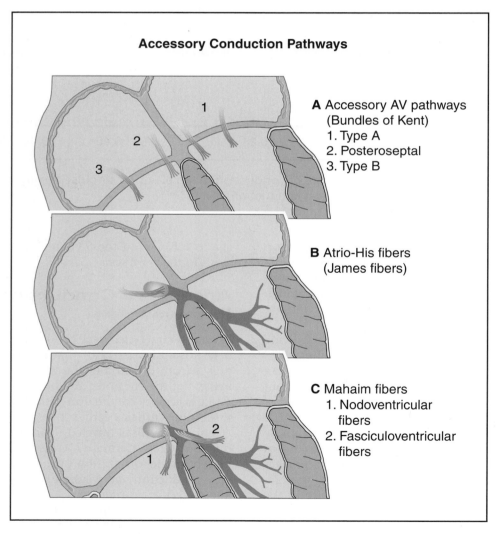

Figure 1-7   Accessory conduction pathways.

plexes, it is known as the *Wolff-Parkinson-White (WPW) syndrome.*

◆ ATRIO-HIS FIBERS

The atrio-His fibers, an accessory conduction pathway also known as the *James fibers,* connect the atria with the lowermost part of the AV node near the origin of the bundle of His, bypassing the AV node. This form of anomalous AV conduction is classified as *atrio-His preexcitation.*

◆ NODOVENTRICULAR/ FASCICULOVENTRICULAR FIBERS

The nodoventricular and fasciculoventricular fibers (also known as the *Mahaim fibers*) are accessory conduction pathways that provide bypass channels between the AV junction and the ventricles in the following locations:

- ◆ Between the lower part of the AV node and the right ventricle (the nodoventricular fibers)
- ◆ Between the bundle of His and the ventricles (the fasciculoventricular fibers)

CARDIAC CELLS

The heart is composed of cylindrical cardiac cells (Figure 1-8) that partially divide at their ends into two or more branches. These connect with the branches of adjacent cells, forming a branching and anastomosing network of cells called a *syncytium.* At the junctions where the branches join together are specialized cellular membranes not found in any other cells—the *intercalated disks.* These membranes contain areas of low electrical resistance called "gap junctions" that permit very rapid conduction of electrical impulses from one cell to another. The ability of cardiac cells to conduct electrical impulses is called the *property of conductivity.*

Cardiac cells are enclosed in a semipermeable cell membrane that allows certain charged chemical particles (ions), such as sodium, potassium, and calcium ions, to flow in and out of the cells, making the contraction and relaxation of the heart and the generation and conduction of electrical impulses possible.

There are two basic kinds of cardiac cells in the heart—the myocardial (or "working") cells and the specialized cells of the electrical conduction system of the heart. The myocardial cells form the thin muscular layer of the atrial wall and the much thicker

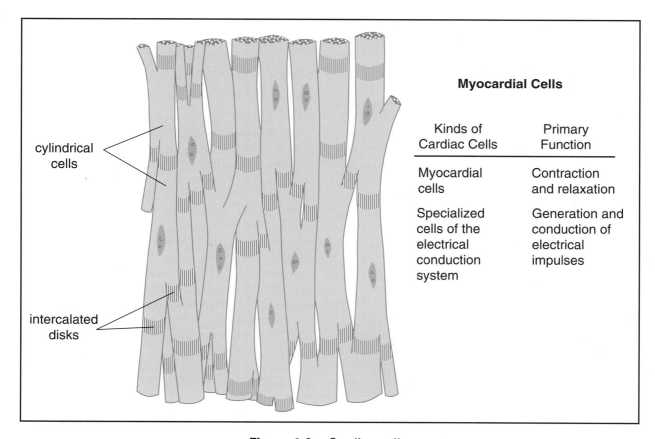

Myocardial Cells	
Kinds of Cardiac Cells	Primary Function
Myocardial cells	Contraction and relaxation
Specialized cells of the electrical conduction system	Generation and conduction of electrical impulses

cylindrical cells

intercalated disks

Figure 1-8 Cardiac cells.

muscular layer of the ventricular wall—the myocardium. These cells contain numerous thin myofibrils that consist of contractile protein filaments called *actin* and *myosin*. The myofibrils give the myocardial cells the property of contractility (i.e., the ability to shorten and return to their original length when stimulated by an electrical impulse).

The force of myocardial contractility increases in response to certain drugs (e.g., digitalis, sympathomimetics) and physiologic conditions (e.g., increased venous return to the heart, exercise, emotion, hypovolemia, anemia). In contrast, other drugs (e.g., procainamide, quinidine, β-blockers, potassium) and pathophysiologic conditions (e.g., shock, hypocalcemia, hypothyroidism) decrease the force of myocardial contractility.

The specialized cells of the electrical conduction system do not contain myofibrils and therefore cannot contract. They do, however, contain more gap junctions than do myocardial cells, permitting them to conduct electrical impulses extremely rapidly (at least six times faster than do myocardial cells). Certain of the specialized cells of the electrical conduction system—the pacemaker cells—are also capable of generating electrical impulses spontaneously, unlike myocardial cells, which cannot do so normally. This capability, the property of automaticity, will be discussed in greater detail later in this chapter.

ELECTROPHYSIOLOGY OF THE HEART

Cardiac cells are capable of generating and conducting electrical impulses that are responsible for the contraction and relaxation of myocardial cells. These electrical impulses are the result of brief but rapid flow of positively charged ions (primarily sodium and potassium ions and, to a lesser extent, calcium ions) back and forth across the cardiac cell membrane. The difference in the concentration of such ions across the cell membrane at any given instant is called the electrical potential (or voltage) and is measured in millivolts (mV).

Resting State of the Cardiac Cell

When a myocardial cell is in the resting state, a high concentration of positively charged sodium ions (Na+) (cations) is present outside the cell. At the same time, a high concentration of negatively charged ions (especially organic phosphate ions, organic sulfate ions, and protein ions) (anions) mixed in with a smaller concentration of positively charged potassium ions (K+) is present inside the cell, making the interior of the cell electrically negative with reference to its positive exterior.

Under these conditions, a negative electrical potential exists across the cell membrane. This is made possible by the cell membrane being impermeable to (1) positively charged sodium ions outside the cell membrane during the resting state and (2) negatively charged phosphate, sulfate, and protein ions inside the cell at all times (Figure 1-9). When a cell membrane is impermeable to an ion, it does not permit the free flow of that ion across it.

The resting cardiac cell can be depicted as having a layer of positive ions surrounding the cell membrane and an equal number of negative ions lining the inside of the cell membrane directly opposite each positive ion. When the ions are so aligned, the resting cell is called *polarized*.

The electrical potential across the membrane of a resting cardiac cell is called the *resting membrane potential*. The resting membrane potential in atrial and ventricular myocardial cells and the specialized cells of the electrical conduction system (except those of the SA and AV nodes) is normally −90 mV. It is somewhat less in the SA and AV nodal cells, −70 mV. In summary, a negative (−) membrane potential indicates that the concentration of positive ions outside the cell is greater than that inside the cell; a positive (+) membrane potential indicates the opposite, that there are more positive ions inside the cell than outside.

Depolarization and Repolarization

When stimulated by an electrical impulse, the membrane of a polarized myocardial cell becomes permeable to positively charged sodium ions, allowing sodium to flow into the cell. This causes the interior of the cell to become less negative with respect to its exterior.

When the membrane potential drops to about −65 mV (−60 to −70 mV) from its resting potential of −90 mV, large pores in the membrane (the fast sodium channels) momentarily open. These channels facilitate the rapid, free flow of sodium across the cell membrane, resulting in a sudden large influx of positively charged sodium ions into the cell. This causes the interior of the cell to become rapidly positive. The moment the concentration of positively charged ions within the cell reaches that outside the cell, the membrane potential becomes 0 mV and the myocardial cell is "depolarized." The influx of positively charged sodium ions continues, resulting in a transient rise in the membrane potential to about +20 to +30 mV (the so-called "overshoot"). The

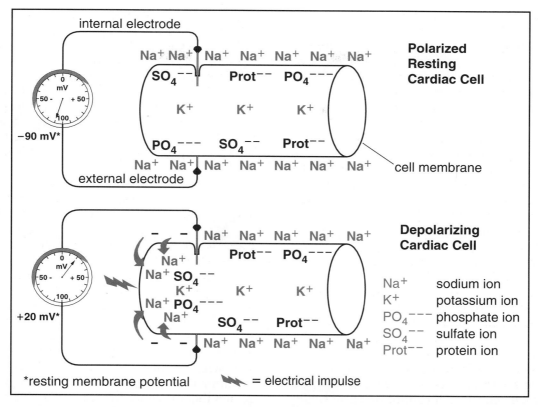

Figure 1-9 Membrane potentials of polarized and depolarized cardiac cells.

process by which the cell's resting, polarized state is reversed is called *depolarization* (Figure 1-10).

The fast sodium channels are typically found in the myocardial cells and the specialized cells of the electrical conduction system other than those of the SA and AV nodes. The cells of the SA and AV nodes, on the other hand, have slow calcium-sodium channels that open when the membrane potential drops to about −50 mV. They permit the entry of positively charged calcium and sodium ions into the cells during depolarization at a slow and gradual rate. The result is a slower rate of depolarization as compared with the depolarization of cardiac cells with fast sodium channels.

As soon as a cardiac cell depolarizes, positively charged potassium ions flow out of the cell, initiating a process by which the cell returns to its resting, polarized state. This process, called *repolarization* (see Figure 1-10), involves a complex exchange of sodium, calcium, and potassium ions across the cell membrane. It must be noted here that the electrical potential external to a resting cardiac cell is more positive than that external to a polarized cardiac cell. This difference in electrical potential between the resting, polarized cardiac cells and the depolarized

cells is the basis of the electric current generated during depolarization and repolarization and detected and displayed as the electrocardiogram (ECG), described later.

Depolarization of one cardiac cell acts as an electrical impulse (or stimulus) on adjacent cells and causes them to depolarize. The propagation of the electrical impulse from cell to cell produces a wave of depolarization that can be measured as an electric current flowing in the direction of depolarization. As the cells repolarize, another electric current is produced that is similar to, but opposite in direction to the first one. The direction of flow and magnitude of the electric currents generated by depolarization and repolarization of the myocardial cells of the atria and ventricles can be detected by surface electrodes and recorded as the ECG. Depolarization of the myocardial cells produces the P waves and QRS complexes (which include the Q, R, and S waves), and repolarization of the cells results in the T waves in the ECG.

Threshold Potential

A cardiac cell need not be repolarized completely to its resting, polarized state (that is, −90 mV or −60

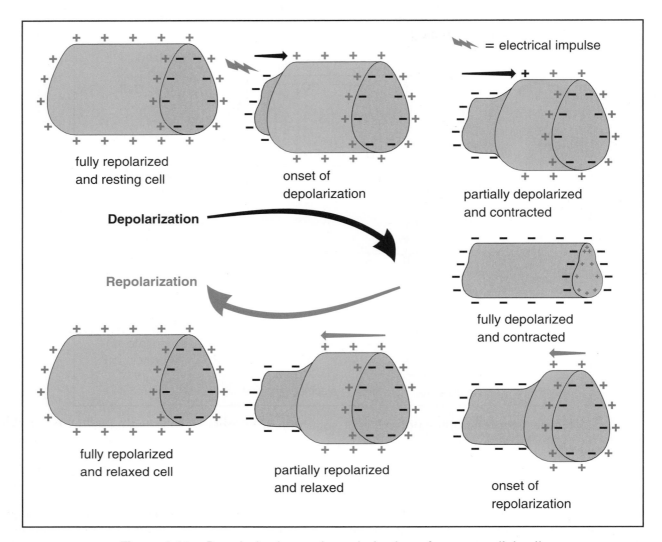

Figure 1-10 Depolarization and repolarization of a myocardial cell.

mV, as the case may be) before it can be stimulated to depolarize again. The cells of the SA and AV nodes can be depolarized when they have been repolarized to about −30 to −40 mV. The rest of the cells of the electrical conduction system of the heart and the myocardial cells can be depolarized when they have been repolarized to about −60 to −70 mV. The level to which a cell must be repolarized before it can be depolarized again is called the *threshold potential.*

It is important to note that a cardiac cell cannot generate or conduct an electrical impulse or be stimulated to contract until it has been repolarized to its threshold potential.

Cardiac Action Potential

A cardiac action potential is a schematic representation of the changes in the membrane potential of a cardiac cell during depolarization and repolarization

(Figure 1-11). The cardiac action potential is divided into five phases—phase 0 to phase 4. The following are the five phases of the cardiac action potential of a typical myocardial cell.

◆ **Phase 0.** Phase 0 (depolarization phase) is the sharp, tall upstroke of the action potential during which the cell membrane reaches the threshold potential, triggering the fast sodium channels to open momentarily and permit the rapid entry of sodium into the cell. As the positively charged ions flow into the cell, the interior of the cell becomes electrically positive to about +20 mV to +30 mV with respect to its exterior. During the upstroke, the cell depolarizes and begins to contract.

◆ **Phase 1.** During phase 1 (early rapid repolarization phase), the fast sodium channels close, terminating the rapid flow of sodium into the cell, followed by a loss of potassium from the cell. The net result is a decrease in the number of positive elec-

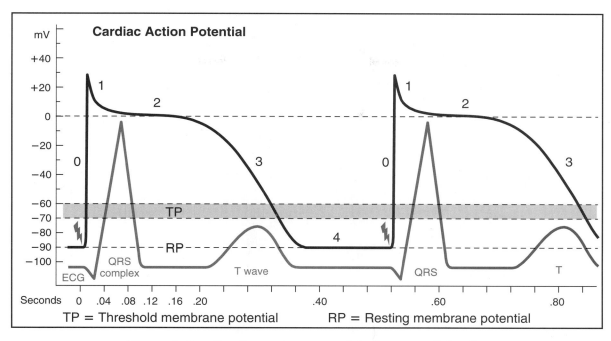

Figure 1-11   Cardiac action potential of myocardial cells.

trical charges within the cell and a drop in the membrane potential to about 0 mV.

◆ **Phase 2.** Phase 2 is the prolonged phase of slow repolarization (plateau phase) of the action potential of the myocardial cell, allowing it to finish contracting and begin relaxing. During phase 2, the membrane potential remains about 0 mV because of a very slow rate of repolarization. In a complicated exchange of ions across the cell membrane, calcium slowly enters the cell through the slow calcium channels as potassium continues to leave the cell and sodium enters it slowly.

◆ **Phase 3.** Phase 3 is the terminal phase of rapid repolarization, during which the inside of the cell becomes markedly negative and the membrane potential once again returns to about −90 mV, its resting level. This is caused primarily by the flow of potassium from the cell. Repolarization is complete by the end of phase 3.

◆ **Phase 4.** At the onset of phase 4 (the period between action potentials), the membrane has returned to its resting potential and the inside of the cell is once again negative (−90 mV) with respect to the outside. But there is still an excess of sodium in the cell and an excess of potassium outside. At this point, a mechanism known as the *sodium-potassium pump* is activated, transporting the excess sodium out of the cell and potassium back in. Because of this mechanism and the impermeability of the cell membrane to sodium during phase 4,

the myocardial cell normally maintains a stable membrane potential between action potentials.

Refractory and Supernormal Periods

The time between the onset of depolarization and the end of repolarization is customarily divided into periods during which the cardiac cells can or cannot be stimulated to depolarize. These are the refractory periods (absolute and relative) and the supernormal period (Figure 1-12).

The refractory period of cardiac cells (e.g., those of the ventricles) begins with the onset of phase 0 of the cardiac action potential and ends just before the end of phase 3. On the ECG, it extends from the onset of the QRS complex to about the end of the T wave.

The refractory period is further divided into the absolute and relative refractory periods. The absolute refractory period (ARP) begins with the onset of phase 0 and ends midway through phase 3 at about the peak of the T wave, occupying over two thirds of the refractory period. During this period, the cardiac cells, having completely depolarized, are in the process of repolarizing. Because they have not repolarized to their threshold potential, the cardiac cells cannot be stimulated to depolarize. In other words, myocardial cells cannot contract, and the cells of the electrical conduction system cannot conduct an electrical impulse during the absolute refractory period.

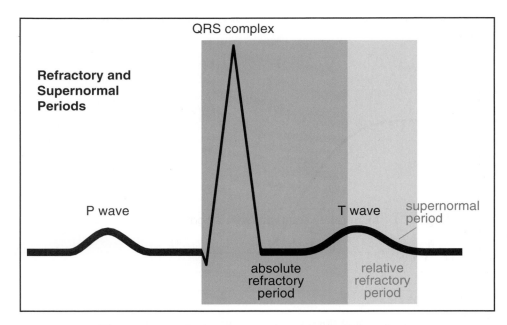

Figure 1-12 Refractory and supernormal periods.

The relative refractory period (RRP) extends through most of the second half of phase 3, corresponding to the downslope of the T wave. During this period, the cardiac cells, having repolarized to their threshold potential, can be stimulated to depolarize if the stimulus is strong enough. This period is also called the *vulnerable period of repolarization.*

During a short portion of phase 3 near the end of the T wave, just before the cells return to their resting potential, a stimulus weaker than is normally required can depolarize cardiac cells. This portion of repolarization is called the *supernormal period.*

Excitability and Automaticity

The capability of a resting, polarized cardiac cell to depolarize in response to an electrical stimulus is called the *property of excitability.* All cardiac cells have this property.

The capability of a cardiac cell to depolarize spontaneously during phase 4—to reach threshold potential and to depolarize completely without being externally stimulated—is called the *property of automaticity.* (This could also be called the *property of self-excitation.*)

Spontaneous depolarization depends on the ability of the cell membrane to become permeable to sodium during phase 4, thus allowing a steady leakage of sodium ions into the cell. This causes the resting membrane potential to become progressively less negative. As soon as the threshold potential is reached, rapid depolarization of the cell (phase 0) occurs.

The rate of spontaneous depolarization is dependent on the slope of phase 4 depolarization (Figure 1-13). The steeper the slope of phase 4 depolarization, the faster is the rate of spontaneous depolarization and the rate of impulse formation (the firing rate). The flatter the slope is, the slower the firing rate.

Certain of the specialized cells in the electrical conduction system normally have the property of automaticity. These cells, the pacemaker cells, are located in the SA node, in some areas of the internodal atrial conduction tracts and AV node, and throughout the bundle of His, bundle branches, and Purkinje network. The pacemaker cells of the SA node, having the fastest firing rate, are normally the dominant (or primary) pacemaker cells of the heart. The pacemaker cells in the rest of the electrical conduction system hold the property of automaticity in reserve should the SA node fail to function properly or electrical impulses fail to reach them for any reason, such as a disruption in the electrical conduction system. For this reason, these pacemaker cells are called *latent* (or *subsidiary* or *escape*) *pacemaker cells.* Myocardial cells, which do not normally have the capability to depolarize spontaneously during phase 4, are called *nonpacemaker cells.*

Increase in sympathetic activity and administration of catecholamines increase the slope of phase 4 depolarization, resulting in an increase in the automaticity of the pacemaker cells and their firing rate. On the other hand, an increase in parasympathetic activity and administration of such drugs as lidocaine, procainamide, and quinidine decrease the slope of phase 4 depolarization, causing a decrease in

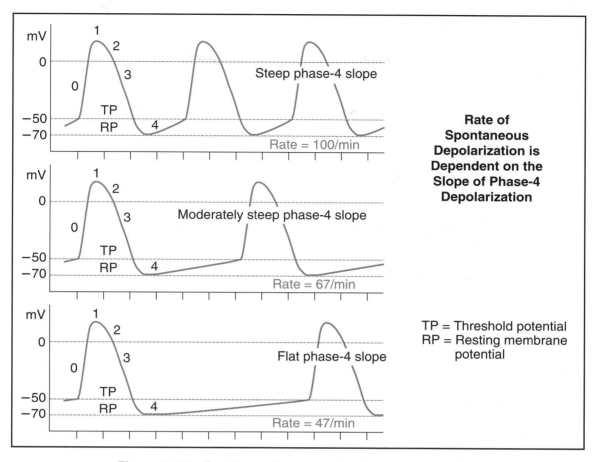

Figure 1-13 Cardiac action potential of pacemaker cells.

the automaticity and firing rate of the pacemaker cells.

Dominant and Escape Pacemakers of the Heart

Normally, the pacemaker cells with the fastest firing rate control the heart rate at any given time. Each time these pacemaker cells generate an electrical impulse the slower-firing latent pacemaker cells are depolarized before they can do so spontaneously. This phenomenon is called *overdrive suppression*.

The SA node is normally the dominant and primary pacemaker of the heart (Figure 1-14) because it possesses the highest level of automaticity; that is, its rate of automatic firing (60 to 100 times per minute) is normally greater than that of the latent pacemaker cells.

If the SA node fails to generate electrical impulses at its normal rate or stops functioning entirely, or if the conduction of the electrical impulses is blocked for any reason (e.g., in the AV node), latent pacemaker cells in the AV junction will usually assume the role of pacemaker of the heart but at a slower rate

(40 to 60 times per minute). Such a pacemaker is called an *escape pacemaker*. If the AV junction is unable to take over as the pacemaker because of disease, an escape pacemaker in the electrical conduction system below the AV junction in the ventricles (i.e., in the bundle branches or Purkinje network) may take over at a still slower rate (less than 40 times per minute). In general, the farther the escape pacemaker is from the SA node, the slower it generates electrical impulses.

The rate at which the SA node or an escape pacemaker normally generates electrical impulses is called the *pacemaker's inherent firing rate*. A beat or a series of beats arising from an escape pacemaker is called an *escape beat* or *rhythm* and is identified according to its site of origin (e.g., junctional, ventricular).

Mechanisms of Abnormal Electrical Impulse Formation

Under certain circumstances, cardiac cells in any part of the heart, whether they are latent pacemaker cells or nonpacemaker, myocardial cells, may take on the

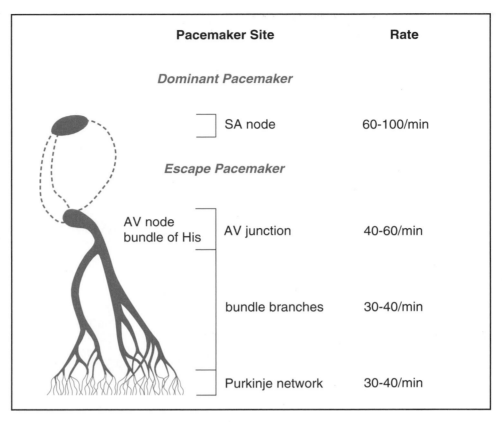

Pacemaker Site	Rate
Dominant Pacemaker	
SA node	60-100/min
Escape Pacemaker	
AV junction	40-60/min
bundle branches	30-40/min
Purkinje network	30-40/min

AV node
bundle of His

Figure 1-14   Dominant and escape pacemakers.

role of a pacemaker and start generating extraneous electrical impulses. Such pacemakers are called *ectopic pacemakers*. The result can be abnormal ectopic beats and rhythms, such as premature contractions, tachycardias, flutters, and fibrillations. These arrhythmias are identified according to the location of the ectopic pacemaker (e.g., atrial, junctional, ventricular). The three basic mechanisms that are responsible for ectopic beats and rhythms (ectopy) are (1) enhanced automaticity, (2) reentry, and (3) triggered activity.

> ### AUTHOR'S NOTE
>
> The term *arrhythmia*, meaning an absence of rhythm, is used in this book by preference instead of the more accurate term *dysrhythmia*, meaning abnormality in rhythm. This choice was dictated by the fact that most medical editors prefer the term *arrhythmia*. The terms, however, can be used interchangeably.

◆ ENHANCED AUTOMATICITY

Enhanced automaticity is an abnormal condition of latent pacemaker cells in which their firing rate is in-

creased beyond their inherent rate. This occurs when the cell membrane becomes abnormally permeable to sodium during phase 4. The result is an abnormally high leakage of sodium ions into the cells and, consequently, a sharp rise in the phase-4 slope of spontaneous depolarization. Even myocardial cells that do not ordinarily possess automaticity (nonpacemaker cells) may acquire this property under certain conditions and depolarize spontaneously. Enhanced automaticity can cause atrial, junctional, and ventricular ectopic beats and rhythms.

Common causes of enhanced automaticity are an increase in catecholamines, digitalis toxicity, and administration of atropine. In addition, hypoxia, hypercapnia, myocardial ischemia or infarction, stretching of the heart, hypokalemia, hypocalcemia, and heating or cooling of the heart may also cause enhanced automaticity.

◆ REENTRY

Reentry is a condition in which the progression of an electrical impulse is delayed or blocked (or both) (Figure 1-15, *A-B*) in one or more segments of the electrical conduction system while being conducted normally through the rest of the conduction system.

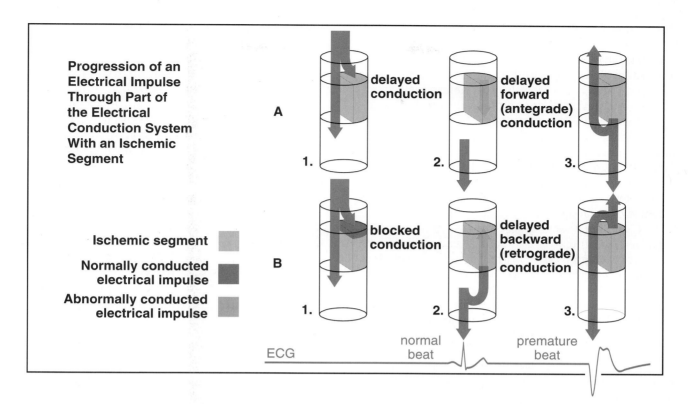

Progression of an Electrical Impulse Through Part of the Electrical Conduction System With an Ischemic Segment

Ischemic segment

Normally conducted electrical impulse

Abnormally conducted electrical impulse

A

1. delayed conduction
2. delayed forward (antegrade) conduction
3.

B

1. blocked conduction
2. delayed backward (retrograde) conduction
3.

ECG   normal beat   premature beat

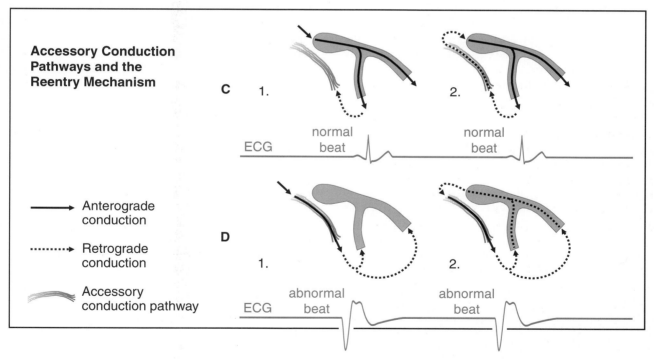

Accessory Conduction Pathways and the Reentry Mechanism

C   1.   2.

ECG   normal beat   normal beat

Anterograde conduction

Retrograde conduction

Accessory conduction pathway

D   1.   2.

ECG   abnormal beat   abnormal beat

Figure 1-15   Examples of reentry mechanism. **A,** Delayed conduction. **B,** Blocked and delayed conduction. **C,** Anterograde conduction through the electrical conduction system. **D,** Retrograde conduction through the electrical conduction system.

This results in delayed antegrade or retrograde conduction of electrical impulses into adjacent cardiac cells that have just been depolarized by the normally conducted electrical impulse. If these cardiac cells have repolarized sufficiently, the delayed electrical impulse depolarizes them prematurely, producing ectopic beats and rhythms. Myocardial ischemia and hyperkalemia are the two most common causes of delay or block in the conduction of an electrical impulse through the electrical conduction system responsible for the reentry mechanism.

Another cause of the reentry mechanism is the presence of an accessory conduction pathway (Figure 1-15, *C-D*), such as the accessory AV pathways located between the atria and ventricles described earlier in this chapter. After normal antegrade progression of an electrical impulse through the electrical conduction system and depolarization of the cardiac cells, the electrical impulse enters the accessory conduction pathway and progresses retrogradely to reenter the proximal end of the electrical conduction system much sooner than the next expected normal electrical impulse. The electrical impulse is then conducted anterogradely as before, causing depolarization of the cardiac cells prematurely. Thus a reentry circuit is set up that can result in the conduction of a rapid series of electrical impulses through the electrical conduction system and a tachyarrhythmia. The electrical impulse can also progress anterogradely through the accessory conduction pathway and retrogradely through the electrical conduction system.

The reentry mechanism can result in the abnormal generation of single or repetitive electrical impulses in the atria, AV junction, bundle branches, and Purkinje network. This produces atrial, junctional, or ventricular ectopic beats and rhythms, such as atrial, junctional, and ventricular tachycardias. Such reentry tachycardias typically start and stop abruptly. If the delay in the conduction of the electrical impulse through the reentry circuit responsible for ectopic beats is constant for each conduction cycle, the abnormal beat will always follow the normal one at exactly the same interval of time. This is called *fixed coupling* and *bigeminal rhythm,* or simply *bigeminy.*

◆ TRIGGERED ACTIVITY

Triggered activity is an abnormal condition of latent pacemaker and myocardial cells (nonpacemaker cells) in which the cells may depolarize more than once after stimulation by a single electrical impulse. The level of membrane action potential spontaneously increases after the first depolarization until it reaches threshold potential, causing the cells to depolarize, once or repeatedly. This phenomenon, called *afterdepolarization,* can occur almost immediately after depolarization in phase 3 (early afterdepolarization [EAD]) or later in phase 4 (delayed afterdepolarization [DAD]).

Triggered activity can result in atrial or ventricular ectopic beats occurring singly, in groups of two (paired or coupled beats), or in bursts of three or more beats (paroxysms of beats or tachycardia).

Common causes of triggered activity, like those of enhanced automaticity, include an increase in catecholamines, digitalis toxicity, hypoxia, myocardial ischemia or injury, and stretching or cooling of the heart.

Notes

_____

_____

_____

NERVOUS CONTROL OF THE HEART

The heart is under constant control of the autonomic nervous system, which includes the sympathetic (adrenergic) and parasympathetic (cholinergic or vagal) nervous systems (Figure 1-16), each producing opposite effects when stimulated. These two systems work together to cause changes in cardiac output (by regulating the heart rate and stroke volume) and blood pressure.

Nervous control of the heart originates in two separate nerve centers located in the medulla oblongata, a part of the brainstem. One is the cardioaccelerator center, a part of the sympathetic nervous system; the other is the cardioinhibitor center, a part of the parasympathetic nervous system. Impulses from the cardioaccelerator center reach the electrical conduction system of the heart and the atria and ventricles by way of the sympathetic nerves. Impulses from the cardioinhibitor center innervate the SA node, atria, and AV junction and to a small extent the ventricles by way of the right and left vagus nerves.

Another important cardioinhibitor (parasympathetic) nerve center is the carotid sinus, a slight dilatation of the common carotid artery, located at the point where it branches into the internal and external carotid arteries. It contains sensory nerve endings important in the regulation of blood pressure and heart rate.

As the blood requirements of the body change, multiple sensors in the body relay impulses to the cardioinhibitor and cardioaccelerator centers for analysis. From here, the sympathetic and parasympathetic nerves transmit the appropriate impulses to the electrical conduction system of the heart and the

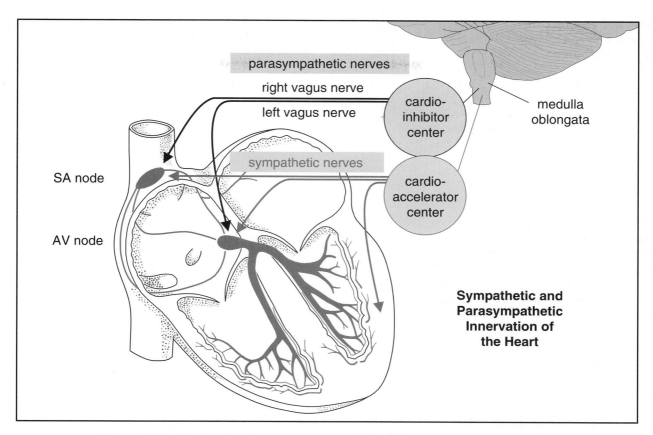

parasympathetic nerves

right vagus nerve

left vagus nerve

cardio-
inhibitor
center

medulla
oblongata

sympathetic nerves

cardio-
accelerator
center

SA node

AV node

**Sympathetic and
Parasympathetic
Innervation of
the Heart**

Figure 1-16 Sympathetic and parasympathetic innervation of the heart.

atrial and ventricular myocardium, where they influence the automaticity, excitability, conductivity, and contractility of the heart's cardiac cells.

Stimulation of the sympathetic nervous system produces the following adrenergic effects on the cardiovascular system:

◆ An increase in the firing rate of the SA node and escape and ectopic pacemakers throughout the heart by increasing their automaticity and excitability
◆ An increase in the conductivity of electrical impulses through the atria and ventricles, especially through the AV node
◆ An increase in the force of atrial and ventricular contractions

The result is an increase in heart rate, cardiac output, and blood pressure. This is accomplished by direct stimulation of the cardiac cells and indirectly by the secretion of catecholamines, such as epinephrine (adrenaline), and their effect on the cardiac cells.

Stimulation of the parasympathetic nervous system produces the following cholinergic (vagal) effects on the cardiovascular system:

◆ A decrease in the firing rate of the SA node and escape and ectopic pacemakers in the atria and AV junction by decreasing their automaticity and excitability

◆ A slowing of conduction of electrical impulses through the AV node

The result is a decrease in heart rate, cardiac output, and blood pressure and, sometimes, an AV block.

The following maneuvers and bodily functions stimulate the parasympathetic nervous system:

◆ Pressure on the carotid sinus
◆ The Valsalva maneuver (the action of straining against a closed glottis or taking a deep breath while in a head-down tilt position)
◆ Straining to move the bowels
◆ Distention of the urinary bladder

Nausea, vomiting, bronchial spasm, sweating, faintness, and hypersalivation are examples of excessive parasympathetic activity. The drug atropine, a parasympathetic blocking agent, effectively blocks parasympathetic activity.

Notes

_____

_____

_____

CHAPTER REVIEW QUESTIONS

1. The visceral pericardium, the inner layer of the serous pericardium, which covers the heart itself, is more commonly called the:
   A. myocardium
   B. epicardium
   C. endocardium
   D. pericardium

2. The _____ side of the heart pumps blood into the _____ circulation, while the _____ side of the heart pumps blood into the _____ circulation.
   A. right, systemic: left, pulmonic
   B. left, pulmonary: right, systemic
   C. right, pulmonary: left, systemic
   D. left, systemic: right, pulmonic

3. The right ventricle pumps unoxygenated blood through the _____ valve and into the lungs through the _____ artery.
   A. pulmonic: pulmonary
   B. mitral: tricuspid
   C. aortic: mitral
   D. tricuspid: pulmonary

4. The period of relaxation and filling of the ventricles with blood is called:
   A. atrial diastole
   B. ventricular systole
   C. ventricular diastole
   D. atrial systole

5. Which structure is not a component of the electrical conduction system?
   A. Purkinje network
   B. coronary sinus
   C. right bundle branch
   D. sinoatrial node

6. Which structure is not an accessory conduction pathway?
   A. accessory AV pathway
   B. atrio-His fibers
   C. bundle of His
   D. nodoventricular fibers

7. The ability of cardiac cells to conduct electrical impulses is called the property of:
   A. conductivity
   B. automaticity
   C. self-excitation
   D. contractility

8. In the resting state a myocardial cell has a high concentration of _____ charged _____ ions present outside the cell.
   A. negatively: sodium
   B. positively: potassium
   C. negatively: potassium
   D. positively: sodium

9. Cardiac cells cannot be stimulated to depolarize during the:
   A. relative refractory period
   B. absolute refractory period
   C. supernormal period
   D. downstroke of the T wave

10. The normal and dominant pacemaker of the heart is the _____.
    A. Purkinje fibers
    B. AV node
    C. SA node
    D. Bundle of His

11. A condition in which the progression of an electrical impulse is delayed or blocked in one or more segments of the electrical conduction system while being conducted normally through the rest of the electrical conduction system, resulting in a delayed or retrograde conduction of electrical impulses into the adjacent cardiac cells is called:
    A. automaticity
    B. reentry
    C. bigeminy
    D. triggered activity

CHAPTER 2

The Electrocardiogram: Basic Concepts and Lead Monitoring

CHAPTER OBJECTIVES

Upon completion of all or part of this chapter, you should be able to complete the following objectives:

1. Explain what the electrocardiogram (ECG) represents.
2. Identify the measurements of time and distance as represented by the dark and light vertical and horizontal lines on an ECG grid.
3. Name and identify the components of the ECG, including the waves, complexes, segments, and intervals.
4. List at least four causes of artifacts in the ECG.
5. Define an ECG lead, a bipolar lead, and a unipolar lead.
6. Describe how monitoring leads I and II are obtained.
7. Describe the sequence and direction of normal ventricular depolarization and its relation to the QRS complex in lead II.
8. Explain what a monitoring lead MCL_1 is, under what circumstances it is useful, and how it is obtained.
9. Describe how monitoring lead MCL_6 is obtained.

BASIC ECG CONCEPTS

Electrical Basis of the ECG

The *electrocardiogram (ECG)* is a graphic record of the changes in magnitude and direction of the electrical activity (Figure 2-1), or more specifically, the electric current generated by the wave of depolarization that progresses through the atria and ventricles (the P wave and QRS complex) followed by the wave of repolarization of the atria and ventricles (the Ta wave and T wave) in the opposite direction. This electrical activity is readily detected by electrodes attached to the skin. But neither the electrical activity that results from the generation and transmission of electrical impulses responsible for triggering the depolarization (the electrical impulses are too feeble to be detected by skin electrodes) nor the subsequent mechanical contractions and relaxations of the atria and ventricles (which do not generate electrical activity) appear in the ECG.

ECG Paper

The paper used in recording ECGs has a grid to permit the measurement of time in seconds (sec) and

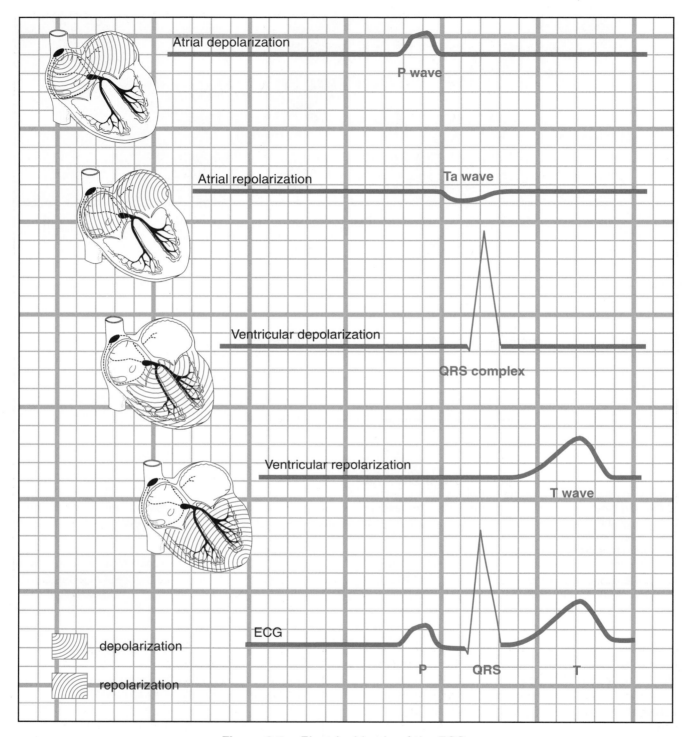

Figure 2-1   Electrical basis of the ECG.

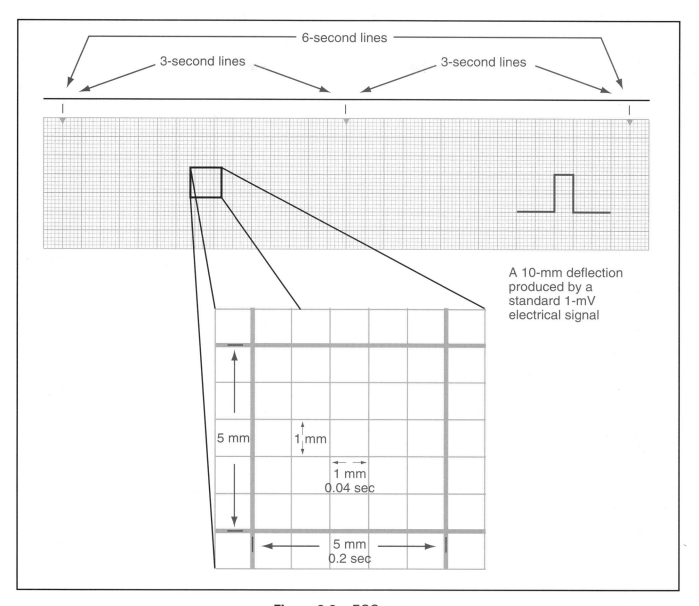

Figure 2-2   ECG paper.

distance in millimeters (mm) along the horizontal lines and voltage (amplitude) in millimeters (mm) along the vertical lines (Figure 2-2).

The grid consists of intersecting dark and light vertical and horizontal lines that form large and small squares. The distance between the vertical lines depends on the paper speed at the time of the ECG recording (i.e., 25 mm or 50 mm per second).

When the ECG is recorded at the standard paper speed of 25 mm/sec, the measurements between the vertical and horizontal lines are as follows:

◆ The dark vertical lines are 0.20 second (5 mm) apart
◆ The light vertical lines are 0.04 second (1 mm) apart

◆ The dark horizontal lines are 5 mm apart
◆ The light horizontal lines are 1 mm apart
◆ One large square is 5 × 5 mm
◆ One small square is 1 × 1 mm

Conventionally, the sensitivity of the ECG machine is adjusted (i.e., calibrated, or standardized) so that a 1-millivolt (mV) electrical signal produces a 10-mm deflection (two large squares) on the ECG.

Printed along one edge of the ECG paper, usually the upper one, are regularly spaced short, vertical lines (or small arrowheads) denoting intervals of time (time lines). Usually, the lines are spaced 15 large squares apart (75 mm, or about 3 inches apart). When the ECG is recorded at the standard paper speed of 25 mm/sec, the vertical lines are 3 seconds apart, and every third vertical line is 6 seconds apart. Some ECG papers have the time lines spaced every five large squares apart (25 mm, or about 1 inch apart) so they are 1 second apart at the standard paper speed.

Components of the ECG

After the electric current generated by depolarization and repolarization of the atria and ventricles is detected by electrodes, it is amplified, displayed on an oscilloscope, and recorded on ECG paper as waves and complexes (Figure 2-3).

The electric current generated by atrial depolarization is recorded as the *P wave*, and that generated by ventricular depolarization is recorded as the *Q, R,* and *S waves*—the *QRS complex*. Atrial repolarization is recorded as the *atrial T wave (Ta)*, and ventricular repolarization as the *ventricular T wave*, or simply the *T wave*. Because atrial repolarization normally occurs during ventricular depolarization, the atrial T wave is buried or hidden in the QRS complex.

In a normal cardiac cycle, the P wave occurs first, followed by the QRS complex and then the T wave.

The sections of the ECG between the waves and complexes are called *segments* and *intervals:* the PR

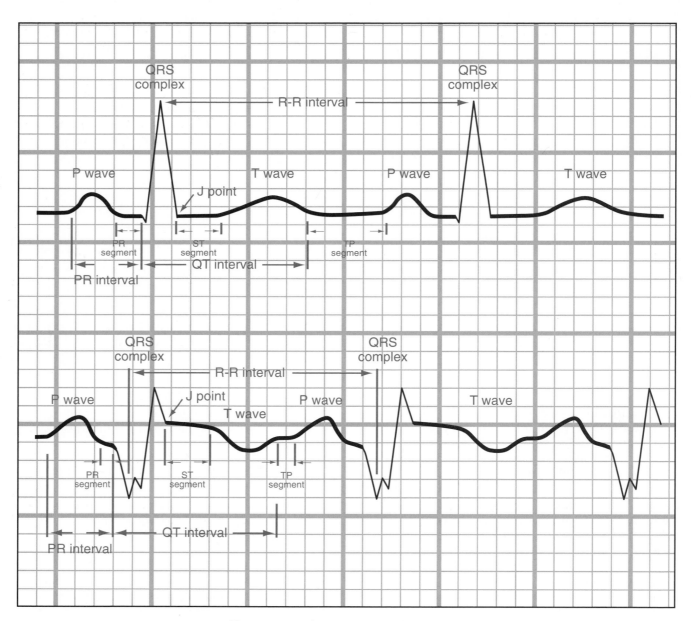

Figure 2-3   Components of the ECG.

segment, the ST segment, the TP segment, the PR interval, the QT interval, and the R-R interval. Intervals include waves and complexes, whereas segments do not. The point at which the QRS complex becomes the ST segment is called the "J point."

When electrical activity of the heart is not being detected, the ECG is a straight, flat line—the *isoelectric line,* or *baseline.*

Artifacts

Abnormal waves and spikes in an ECG that result from sources other than the electrical activity of the heart and interfere with or distort the components of the ECG are called *artifacts.* The causes of artifacts include muscle tremor, alternating current (AC) interference, poor electrode contact with the skin, interference related to biotelemetry, and external chest compression.

Muscle tremor (Figure 2-4) can occur in tense or nervous patients or those shivering from cold and it can give the ECG a finely or coarsely jagged appearance.

AC interference (Figure 2-5) can occur when an improperly grounded, AC-operated ECG machine is used, or when an ECG is obtained near high tension wires, transformers, or electric appliances. This results in a thick baseline composed of 60-cycle waves.

Loose electrodes, or electrodes that are in poor electrical contact with the skin (Figure 2-6) because of insufficient or dried electrode paste or jelly, can cause multiple, sharp spikes and waves in the ECG. Loose connecting wires can also cause similar artifacts. In addition, any extraneous matter on the skin, such as blood, vomitus, sweat, and hair can result in poor electrode contact and the appearance of artifacts.

Biotelemetry-related interference (Figure 2-7) that occurs when ECG signals are poorly received over a biotelemetry system can result in sharp spikes and waves and a jagged appearance of the ECG. Such interference can occur when the ECG transmitter's power is low because of weak batteries or when the ECG transmitter is used in the outer fringes of the reception area of the base station receiver.

External chest compressions (Figure 2-8) during cardiopulmonary resuscitation (CPR) cause regularly spaced, wide, upright waves synchronous with the downward compressions of the chest. It must be emphasized that such waves do not indicate that the chest compressions are producing adequate cardiac output and circulation.

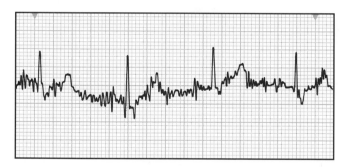

Figure 2-4   Muscle tremor.

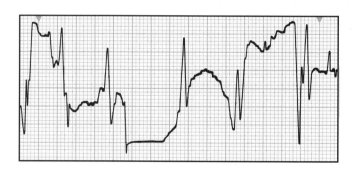

Figure 2-6   Loose electrodes.

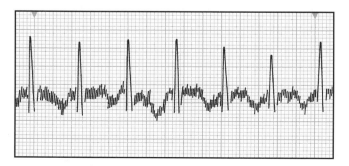

Figure 2-5   AC interference.

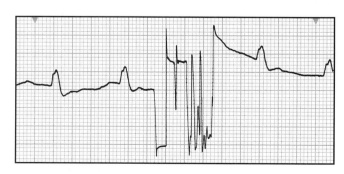

Figure 2-7   Biotelemetry.

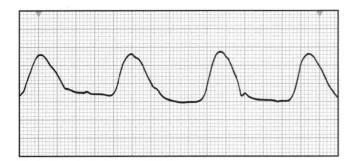

Figure 2-8　External chest compression.

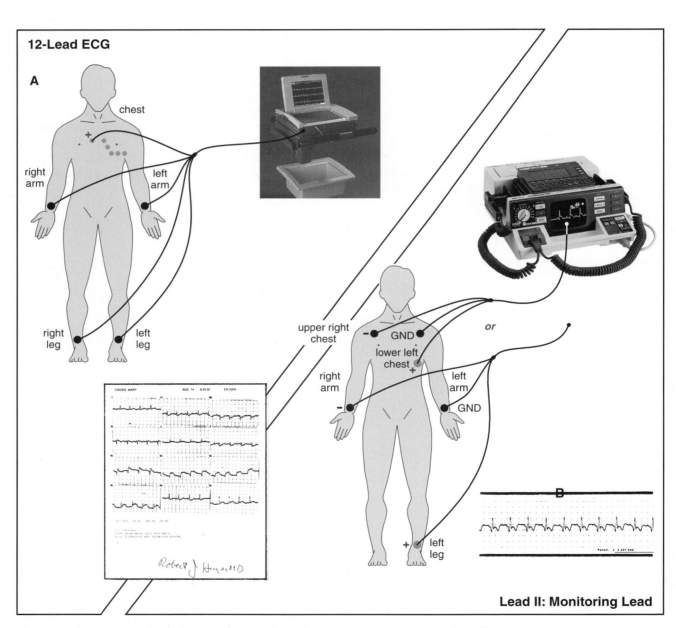

Figure 2-9　**A,** 12-lead ECG. **B,** Lead II: monitoring lead. (**A,** Photo courtesy GE Marquette Medical Systems. **B,** Photo courtesy Laerdahl Medical Corporation.)

ECG LEADS

The Basics of ECG Leads

An ECG is obtained by using electrodes (usually designated as either negative or positive) attached to the skin that detect the electric current generated by the depolarization and repolarization of the heart. The placement of the positive electrodes on specified areas of the body (the right or left arm, the left leg, or one of several locations on the anterior chest wall) determines what view of the heart's electrical activity is obtained. Each view is called a "lead." There are 12 leads in the standard ECG (Figures 2-9, *A* and 2-10), providing a detailed analysis of the heart's electrical activity.

A 12-lead ECG consists of the following:

◆ Three standard (bipolar) limb leads (leads I, II, and III)
◆ Three augmented (unipolar) leads (leads aVR, aVL, and aVF)
◆ Six precordial (unipolar) leads (V₁, V₂, V₃, V₄, V₅, and V₆)

The term *bipolar* means that two electrodes, one positive and the other negative, are used to obtain the ECG. Thus a bipolar lead represents the difference in electrical potential (or voltage) between two electrodes. A *unipolar lead*, on the other hand, measures the electrical potential between a positive electrode and a *central terminal (CT)* created electronically within the circuitry of the ECG machine by combining the electric currents obtained from electrodes at-

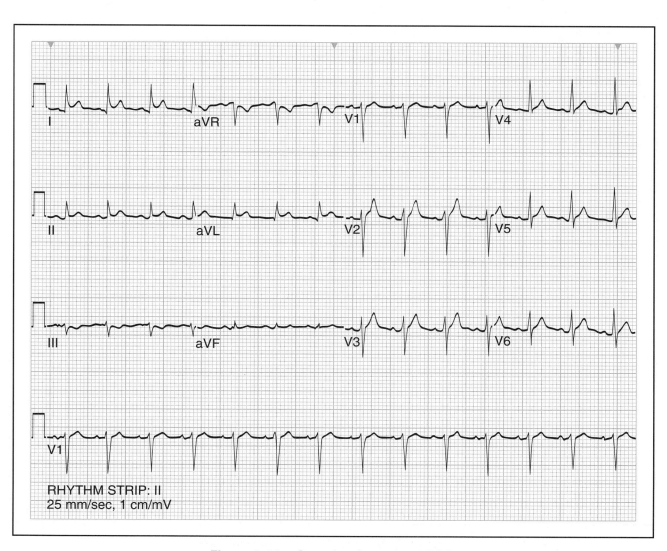

Figure 2-10   Sample of a 12-lead ECG.

tached to the right and left arms and left leg. The electrical potential of the central terminal is essentially zero.

The 12-lead ECG is used to diagnose myocardial infarction (MI) and ischemia, bundle branch blocks, and most miscellaneous ECG changes (described later) and to help in the differentiation between certain tachycardias (i.e., supraventricular versus ventricular). Although the 12-lead ECG is used primarily in the hospital setting, its use is becoming more frequent in the prehospital phase of emergency cardiac care to identify and diagnose acute MI to facilitate triage and/or initiate advanced cardiac life support, including the administration of antiplatelet and thrombolytic therapy. The 12-lead ECG is discussed in detail in Chapter 11.

When monitoring the heart solely for arrhythmias, a single bipolar ECG lead, such as the standard (bipolar) limb lead II (Figure 2-9, *B*), or its equivalent, is commonly used, especially in the prehospital phase of emergency cardiac care. Another commonly used bipolar monitoring lead is lead MCL_1, particularly in the monitoring of arrhythmias in the hospital. Bipolar leads less frequently utilized for monitoring include leads MCL_6, I, and III.

Monitoring Lead II

Lead II is obtained by attaching the negative electrode to the right arm and the positive electrode to the left leg (Figure 2-11). Lead II can also be obtained by attaching the negative electrode to the upper right anterior chest wall below the right clavicle and the positive electrode to the lower left anterior chest wall over the apex of the heart (usually in the fifth left intercostal space in the midclavicular line). However, such electrode placement may cause baseline movement and artifacts because of the respiratory chest movements. To eliminate or reduce electrical interference ("noise") in the ECG when using lead II for monitoring, a third, electrically neutral electrode (or ground electrode) is commonly attached to the upper left chest, to an extremity (the left arm or right leg), or, for that matter, to any part of the body.

When an electric current flows toward the positive electrode of a lead, a *positive* (upright) deflection is recorded on the ECG. Conversely, a *negative* (downward) deflection is recorded when an electric current flows away from the positive electrode. If the positive ECG electrode is attached to the left leg, all of the electric currents generated in the heart that flow toward the left leg will be recorded as positive (upright) deflections; those that flow away from the left leg will

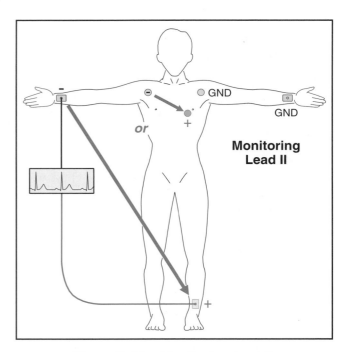

Figure 2-11   Monitoring lead II.

be recorded as negative (downward) deflections (Figure 2-12).

It should be noted here that because normal depolarization of the atria and ventricles generally progresses from the right upper chest downward toward the left leg, the electric currents generated during normal depolarization of the heart will, for the most part, flow toward the left leg and be recorded as two positive (upright) deflections—a positive P wave (atrial depolarization) and a large positive R wave (ventricular depolarization)—in lead II.

The relationship between the depolarization and repolarization of the atria and ventricles and the P wave, QRS complex, and the T wave (Figure 2-13) is as follows:

◆ **P wave.** Depolarization of the atria normally begins near the SA node and then proceeds downward and to the left, producing a positive P wave.

◆ **QRS complex.** Depolarization of the ventricles usually starts with the depolarization of the relatively thin interventricular septum from left to right resulting in a small negative (inverted) deflection—the Q wave. This is immediately followed by the depolarization of the large left ventricle from right to left, which overshadows the almost simultaneous left-to-right depolarization of the smaller right ventricle, resulting in a large R wave. In addition, depending on the position of

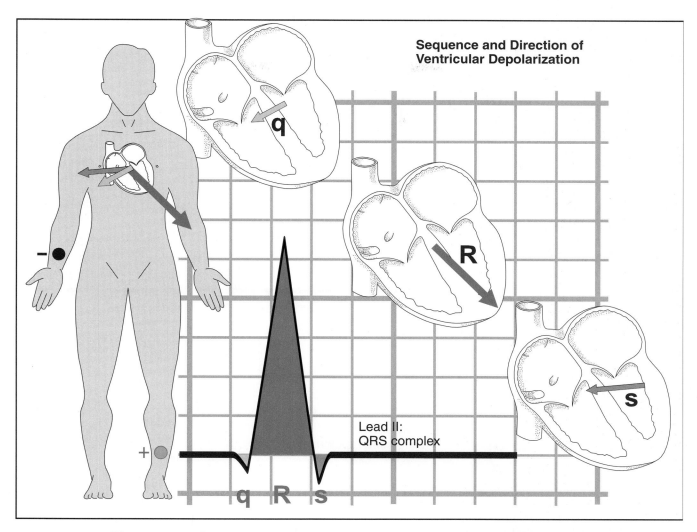

Figure 2-12   Sequence and direction of normal ventricular depolarization and the QRS complex in lead II.

the heart in the chest, the size of the ventricles, and the rotation of the heart, depolarization of the base of the left ventricle from left to right produces a small negative (inverted) deflection after the R wave—the S wave.

◆ **T wave.** Finally, as the ventricles repolarize from left to right, the T wave is produced.

AUTHOR'S NOTE

The ECG components and strips shown in this book are depicted as they would appear in lead II unless otherwise noted.

Monitoring Leads I and III

The two other bipolar leads, leads I and III, are also used for ECG monitoring (Figure 2-14). The placement of the electrodes for these leads is as follows:

◆ **Lead I.** Lead I is obtained by attaching the negative electrode to the right arm, the positive electrode to the left arm, and the ground electrode to the right leg. Lead I can also be obtained by attaching the negative electrode to the upper right anterior chest wall below the right clavicle and the positive electrode to the upper left anterior chest wall below the left clavicle. The ground electrode is attached to the right lower chest wall.

◆ **Lead III.** Lead III is obtained by attaching the negative electrode to the left arm, the positive electrode to the left leg, and the ground electrode to

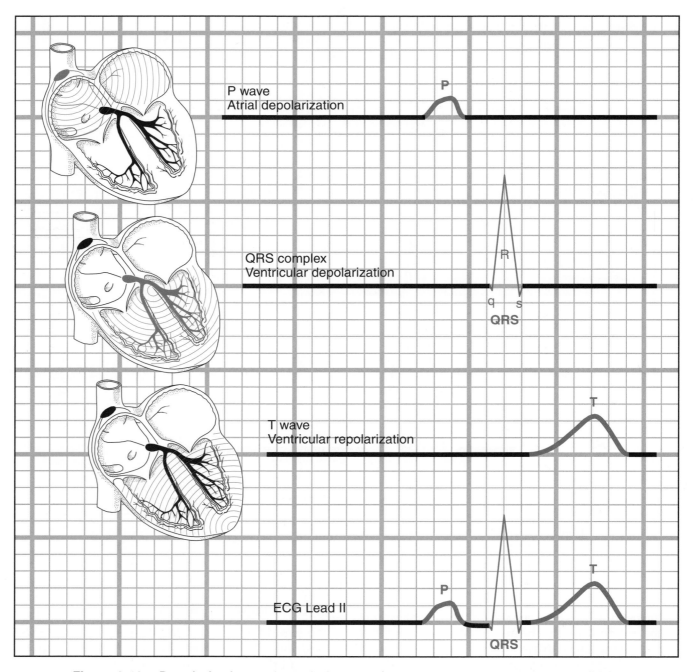

Figure 2-13 Depolarization and repolarization of the atria and ventricles and the ECG.

the right leg. Lead III can also be obtained by attaching the negative electrode to the upper left anterior chest wall below the left clavicle and the positive electrode to the lower left anterior chest wall at the intersection of the fifth intercostal space and the midclavicular line. The ground electrode is attached to the right lower chest wall.

Leads I and III in normal hearts may or may not resemble lead II because of the normal variations in the mean QRS axis (the average direction of ventricular depolarization), which affects the direction of the QRS deflection in these three leads. This is discussed in Chapters 11 and 12.

Monitoring Lead MCL₁

Lead MCL_1 is a bipolar lead similar to lead V_1 of the 12-lead ECG (Figure 2-15). It is obtained by attach-

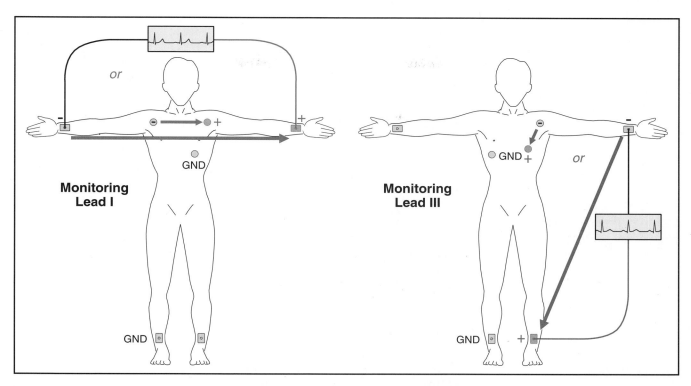

Figure 2-14 Monitoring leads I and III.

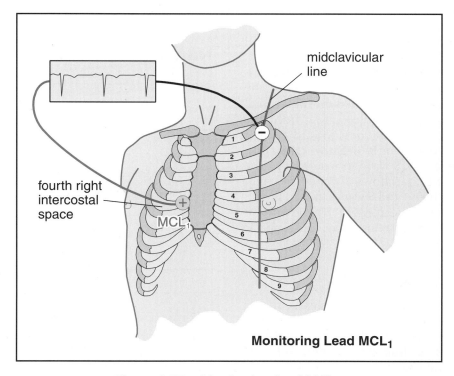

Figure 2-15 Monitoring lead MCL$_1$.

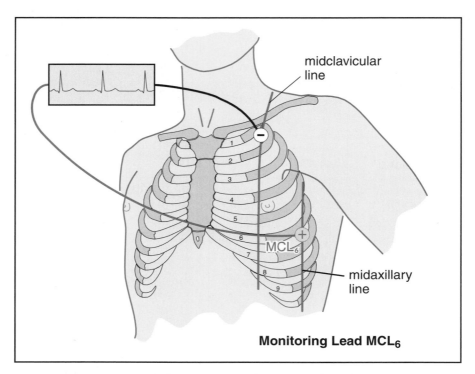

midclavicular line

midaxillary line

Monitoring Lead MCL$_6$

Figure 2-16   Monitoring lead MCL$_6$.

ing the positive electrode to the right side of the anterior chest in the fourth intercostal space just right of the sternum and the negative electrode to the left chest in the midclavicular line below the clavicle. Lead MCL$_1$ is helpful in identifying the origin of certain arrhythmias with wide QRS complexes. This will be discussed later in the book.

Unlike in lead II in which a predominantly positive QRS complex with a large R wave is normally present, the electric current generated during normal ventricular depolarization will flow away from the positive electrode on the right chest toward the left leg, producing a predominantly negative QRS complex with a large negative S wave in lead MCL$_1$. The small electric current that flows toward the right shoulder, producing the Q and S waves in lead II, will produce small R waves in lead MCL$_1$. The P wave in lead MCL$_1$ may be positive, negative, or biphasic (partly positive and partly negative).

Monitoring Lead MCL$_6$

Lead MCL$_6$, a bipolar lead that resembles V$_6$ of the 12-lead ECG, is obtained by attaching the positive electrode to the left chest in the sixth intercostal space in the midaxillary line and the negative electrode in the midclavicular line below the clavicle on the same side (Figure 2-16). The P waves, QRS com-

plexes, and T waves are similar to those in lead II when the ECG is normal, but in certain heart conditions (e.g., acute MI, bundle branch block) the QRS complexes and T waves are usually dissimilar.

Notes

_____
_____
_____
_____
_____
_____
_____
_____
_____
_____
_____
_____
_____
_____

CHAPTER REVIEW QUESTIONS

1. The electrocardiogram (ECG) is a record of the electrical activity generated by:
   A. the transmission of electrical impulses responsible for initiating depolarization of the atria and ventricles
   B. the mechanical contraction and relaxation of the atria and ventricles
   C. the depolarization and repolarization of the atria and ventricles
   D. all of the above

2. When an ECG is recorded at the standard paper speed of 25 mm/sec, the dark vertical lines are _____ second apart and the light vertical lines are _____ second apart.
   A. 5: 1
   B. 20: 4
   C. .20: .4
   D. .20: .04

3. The sensitivity of the ECG machine is calibrated so that a _____ electrical signal produces a _____ deflection on the ECG.
   A. 0.5 mV: 1-mm
   B. 1 mV: 10-mm
   C. 5 mV: 10-mm
   D. 10 mV: 5-mm

4. The electric current generated by ventricular depolarization is recorded as the:
   A. P wave
   B. QRS complex
   C. atrial T wave (Ta)
   D. T wave

5. The electric current generated by ventricular repolarization is recorded as the:
   A. P wave
   B. QRS complex
   C. atrial T wave (Ta)
   D. T wave

6. The part of the ECG when electrical activity of the heart is not being detected is:
   A. referred to as the isoelectric line
   B. referred to as the baseline
   C. a straight flat line
   D. all of the above

7. Causes of artifacts on an ECG tracing include:
   A. muscle tremor
   B. poor electrode contact with the skin
   C. external chest compression
   D. all of the above

8. An ECG lead composed of a single positive electrode and a zero reference point, the central terminal, is called a:
   A. unipolar lead
   B. multifocal lead
   C. bipolar lead
   D. MCL_1 lead

9. An example of a unipolar lead would be:
   A. aVL
   B. V_3
   C. both of the above
   D. none of the above

10. Monitoring lead II is obtained by attaching the negative electrode to the _____ and the positive electrode to the _____.
    A. left arm: left leg
    B. right arm: left leg
    C. right arm: left arm
    D. right arm: left upper chest

11. If the positive electrode is attached to the left leg or lower left anterior chest, all of the electric currents generated in the heart that flow toward the positive electrode will be recorded as a _____ (_____) deflection.
    A. positive (inverted)
    B. negative (upright)
    C. positive (upright)
    D. negative (inverted)

12. Monitoring lead MCL_1 is obtained by attaching the positive electrode:
    A. to the right side of the anterior chest in the fourth intercostal space next to the sternum
    B. to the middle of the sternum at the level of the fourth intercostal space
    C. to the left side of the sternum in the fourth intercostal space
    D. to the left chest below the clavicle

CHAPTER 3

Components of the Electrocardiogram

CHAPTER OUTLINE

Waves
  P Wave
  QRS Complex
  T Wave
  U Wave
Intervals
  PR Interval
  QT Interval
  R-R Interval

Segments
  ST Segment
  PR Segment
  TP Segment

CHAPTER OBJECTIVES

Upon completion of all or part of this chapter, you should be able to complete the following objectives:

1. Define the following components of the electrocardiogram:

P wave	QT interval
QRS complex	R-R interval
T wave	ST segment
U wave	PR segment
PR interval	TP segment

2. Name and identify the components of the ECG, including the waves, complexes, segments, and intervals in an ECG.
3. Give the characteristics, description, and significance of the following waves and complexes:

Normal P wave	Abnormal QRS complex
Abnormal P wave	Normal T wave
Ectopic P wave	Abnormal T wave
Normal QRS complex	U wave

4. Give the characteristics, description, and significance of the following intervals and segments:

Normal PR interval	Normal ST segment
Abnormal PR interval	Abnormal ST segment
QT interval	PR segment
R-R interval	TP segment

5. Define the following:
  P pulmonale
  P mitrale
  Retrograde conduction
  J point
  Prime ('); double prime ('')
  Notch in the R or S wave
  Ventricular activation time (VAT)
  Incomplete bundle branch block
  Complete bundle branch block
  Supraventricular arrhythmia
  Aberrant ventricular conduction (aberrancy)
  Ventricular preexcitation
  Delta wave
  Ectopy
  QT_c
  Torsade de pointes

WAVES

P Wave

> **KEY DEFINITION**
>
> *A* **P wave** *represents depolarization of the right and left atria. There are three types of P wave:*
> - *Normal sinus P wave*
> - *Abnormal sinus P wave*
> - *Ectopic P wave*

◆ NORMAL SINUS P WAVE

Characteristics

Pacemaker site. The pacemaker site is the sinoatrial (SA) node.

Relationship to cardiac anatomy and physiology. A normal sinus P wave (Figure 3-1) represents normal depolarization of the atria. Depolarization of the atria begins near the SA node and progresses across the atria from right to left and downward. The first part of the normal sinus P wave represents depolarization of the right atrium; the second part represents depolarization of the left atrium. During the P wave, the electrical impulse progresses from the SA node through the internodal atrial conduction tracts and most of the atrioventricular (AV) node. The P wave normally occurs during ventricular diastole.

Description

Onset and end. The onset of the P wave is identified as the first abrupt or gradual deviation from the baseline. The point where the wave flattens out to return to the baseline, joining with the PR segment, marks the end of the P wave.

Direction. The direction is positive (upright) in lead II.

Duration. The duration is 0.10 second or less.

Amplitude. The amplitude is 0.5 to 2.5 mm in lead II. The normal P wave is rarely over 2 mm high.

Shape. The shape is smooth and rounded.

P wave-QRS complex relationship. A QRS complex normally follows each sinus P wave, but in certain arrhythmias, such as AV blocks (see Chapter 9), a QRS complex may not follow each sinus P wave.

PR interval. The PR interval may be normal (0.12 to 0.20 second) or abnormal (greater than 0.20 second or less than 0.12 second).

Significance

A normal sinus P wave indicates that the electrical impulse responsible for the P wave originated in the SA node and that normal depolarization of the right and left atria has occurred.

Notes

_____

_____

_____

_____

◆ ABNORMAL SINUS P WAVE

Characteristics

Pacemaker site. The pacemaker site is the SA node.

Relationship to cardiac anatomy and physiology. An abnormal sinus P wave (Figure 3-2) represents depolarization of altered, damaged, or abnormal atria. Increased right atrial pressure and right atrial dilatation and hypertrophy (right atrial overload)—as found in chronic obstructive pulmonary disease, status asthmaticus, acute pulmonary embolism, and acute pulmonary edema—may result in tall and symmetrically peaked P waves (P pulmonale). Abnormally tall P waves may also occur in sinus tachycardia (see Chapter 5).

Increased left atrial pressure and left atrial dilatation and hypertrophy (left atrial overload)—as found in systemic hypertension, mitral and aortic valvular disease, acute myocardial infarction (MI), and pulmonary edema secondary to left heart failure—may cause wide, notched P waves (P mitrale). Such P waves may also result from a delay or block of the progression of electrical impulses through the interatrial conduction tract between the right and left atria.

Biphasic P waves occur in both right and left atrial dilatation and hypertrophy. These waves, typically present in leads V_1 and V_2, have an initial positive deflection (right atrial depolarization) followed by a negative deflection (left atrial depolarization). Biphasic P waves are described in Chapter 14.

Description

Onset and end. The onset and end of the abnormal sinus P wave are the same as those of a normal P wave.

Direction. The direction is positive (upright) in lead II.

Duration. The duration may be normal (0.10 second or less) or greater than 0.10 second.

Amplitude. The amplitude may be normal (0.5 to 2.5 mm) or greater than 2.5 mm in lead II. By definition, a P pulmonale is 2.5 mm or greater in amplitude.

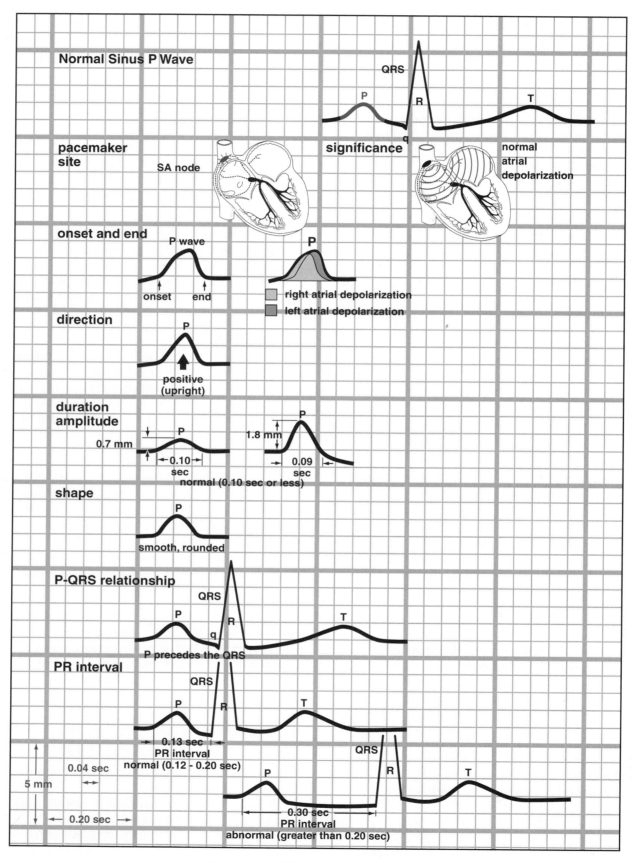

Figure 3-1   Normal sinus P wave.

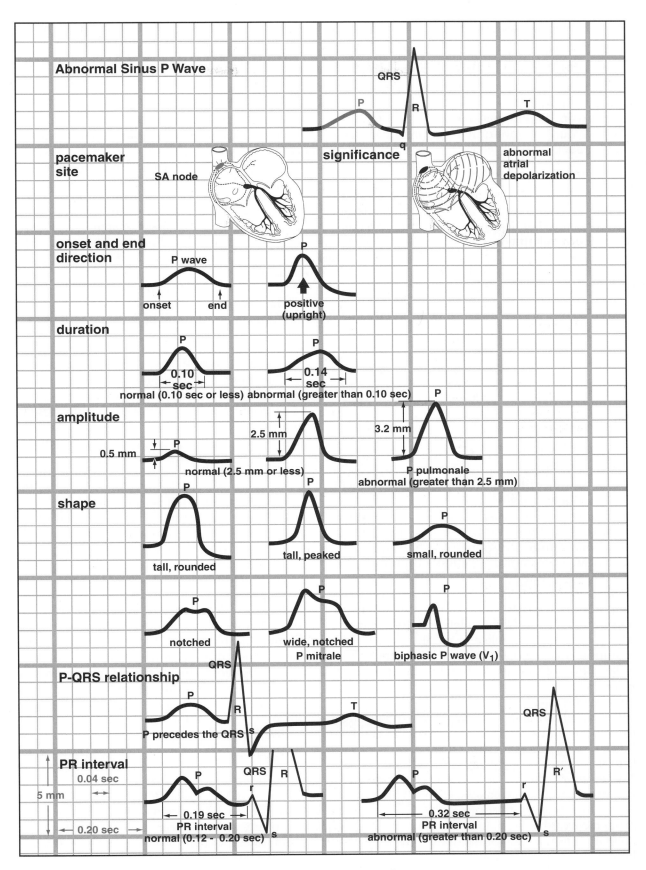

Figure 3-2   Abnormal sinus P wave.

Shape. The abnormal sinus P wave may be tall and symmetrically peaked or may be wide and notched in lead II. It may be biphasic in leads V_1 and V_2.

P wave-QRS complex relationship. The P wave-QRS complex relationship is the same as that of a normal sinus P wave.

PR interval. The PR interval may be normal (0.12 to 0.20 second) or abnormal (greater than 0.20 second or less than 0.12 second).

Significance

An abnormal sinus P wave indicates that the electrical impulse responsible for the P wave originated in the SA node and that depolarization of altered, damaged, or abnormal atria has occurred.

Notes

_____

_____

_____

_____

◆ ECTOPIC P WAVE (P PRIME OR P')

Characteristics

Pacemaker site. The pacemaker site is an ectopic pacemaker in the atria outside of the SA node or in the AV junction or ventricles.

Relationship to cardiac anatomy and physiology. An ectopic P wave (P') (Figure 3-3) represents atrial depolarization occurring in an abnormal direction or sequence or both, depending on the ectopic pacemaker's location.

◆ If the ectopic pacemaker is in the upper or middle right atrium, depolarization of the atria occurs in a normal direction (right to left and downward)

◆ If the ectopic pacemaker is in the lower right atrium near the AV node or in the left atrium, depolarization of the atria occurs in a retrograde direction (left to right and upward)

◆ If the ectopic pacemaker is in the AV junction or ventricles, the electrical impulse travels upward through the AV junction into the atria (retrograde conduction), causing retrograde atrial depolarization

Ectopic P waves occur in various atrial, junctional, and ventricular arrhythmias, including the following:

◆ Wandering atrial pacemaker
◆ Premature atrial contractions
◆ Atrial tachycardia
◆ Premature junctional contractions
◆ Junctional escape rhythm
◆ Nonparoxysmal junctional tachycardia
◆ Paroxysmal supraventricular tachycardia
◆ Premature ventricular contractions (occasionally)

See Chapters 6, 7, and 8, as appropriate, for details.

Description

Onset and end. The onset and end of the abnormal ectopic P wave are the same as those of a normal P wave.

Direction. The ectopic P wave may be either positive (upright) or negative (inverted) in lead II if the ectopic pacemaker is in the atria. The P' wave is always negative (inverted) in lead II if the ectopic pacemaker is in the AV junction or ventricles. Generally, if the ectopic pacemaker is in the upper part of the right atrium, the P' wave is positive, resembling a normal sinus P wave.

If the ectopic pacemaker is in the middle of the right atrium, the P' wave is less positive (upright) than one arising in the upper right atrium. If the ectopic pacemaker is in the lower right atrium near the AV node or in the left atrium or in the AV junction or the ventricles, the P' wave is negative (inverted).

Duration. The duration may be normal (0.10 second or less) or greater then 0.10 second.

Amplitude. The amplitude is usually less than 2.5 mm in lead II, but it may be greater.

Shape. The ectopic P wave may be smooth and rounded, peaked, or slightly notched.

P' Wave-QRS complex relationship. The ectopic P wave may precede, be buried in, or follow the QRS complex with which it is associated.

◆ If the ectopic pacemaker is in any part of the atria or in the upper part of the AV junction, the P' wave generally precedes the QRS complex

◆ If the ectopic pacemaker is in the lower part of the AV junction or in the ventricles, the P' wave may occur either during or after the QRS complex

If the P' wave occurs during the QRS complex, it is buried in the QRS complex and is said to be hidden or invisible. If it follows the QRS complex, it becomes superimposed on the succeeding ST segment and/or T wave, distorting them. The ectopic P wave may also be superimposed on the preceding T wave, resulting in a T wave that differs in amplitude and shape from the other T waves not so affected.

P'R interval. The P'R (or RP') interval varies depending on the location of the ectopic pacemaker.

◆ If the ectopic pacemaker is in the upper or middle right atrium, the P'R interval is generally normal (0.12 to 0.20 second).

◆ If the ectopic pacemaker is in the lower right atrium, close to the AV node, in the left atrium, or in the upper part of the AV junction, the ectopic P wave usually precedes the QRS complex with a P'R interval of less than 0.12 second.

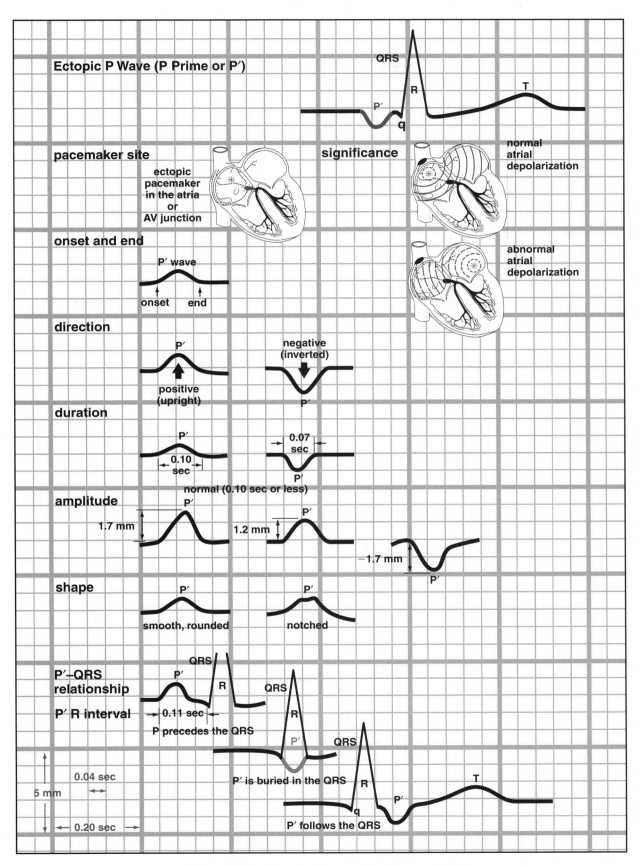

Figure 3-3 Ectopic P wave (P prime or P').

◆ If the ectopic pacemaker is in the lower part of the AV junction or in the ventricles, the ectopic P wave may be buried in the QRS complex or follow it. In the latter case, the interval between the end of the QRS complex and the onset of the P' is called the *RP' interval.* It is usually less than 0.21 second.

Significance

An ectopic P wave indicates that the electrical impulse responsible for the ectopic P wave originated in part of the atria outside the SA node or in the AV junction or ventricles and that depolarization of the right and left atria has occurred in an abnormal direction or sequence or both.

Notes

_____

_____

_____

_____

QRS Complex

> **KEY DEFINITION**
>
> *A QRS complex represents depolarization of the right and left ventricles. There are two types of QRS complex:*
> ◆ *Normal QRS complex*
> ◆ *Abnormal QRS complex*

◆ NORMAL QRS COMPLEX

Characteristics

Pacemaker site. The pacemaker site of the electrical impulse responsible for a normal QRS complex is the SA node or an ectopic or escape pacemaker in the atria or AV junction.

Relationship to cardiac anatomy and physiology. A normal QRS complex (Figure 3-4) represents normal depolarization of the ventricles. Depolarization begins in the left side of the interventricular septum near the AV junction and progresses across the interventricular septum from left to right. Then, beginning at the endocardial surface of the ventricles, depolarization progresses through the ventricular walls to the epicardial surface.

The first short part of the QRS complex, usually the Q wave, represents depolarization of the interventricular septum; the rest of the QRS complex represents the simultaneous depolarization of the right

and left ventricles. Because the left ventricle is larger than the right ventricle and has more muscle mass, the QRS complex represents, for the most part, depolarization of the left ventricle.

The electrical impulse that causes normal ventricular depolarization originates above the ventricles in the SA node or an ectopic or escape pacemaker in the atria or AV junction and has normal conduction down the right and left bundle branches to the Purkinje network. Also a relatively normal-appearing QRS complex may originate in an ectopic or escape pacemaker in the proximal left bundle branch. The QRS complex precedes ventricular systole.

Description

Onset and end. The onset of the QRS complex is identified as the point where the first wave of the complex just begins to deviate, abruptly or gradually, from the baseline. The end of the QRS complex is the point where the last wave of the complex begins to flatten out (sharply or gradually) at, above, or below the baseline. This point, the junction between the QRS complex and the ST segment, is called the *junction* or *J point.*

Components. The QRS complex consists of one or more of the following: positive (upright) deflections called *R waves* and negative (inverted) deflections called *Q, S,* and *QS waves.* The characteristics of the waves that make up the QRS complex in lead II are as follows:

◆ **Q wave:** The Q wave is the first negative deflection in the QRS complex not preceded by an R wave.

◆ **R wave:** The R wave is the first positive deflection in the QRS complex. Subsequent positive deflections that extend above the baseline are called *R prime (R'), R double prime (R''),* and so forth.

◆ **S wave:** The S wave is the first negative deflection that extends below the baseline in the QRS complex after R wave. Subsequent negative deflections are called *S prime (S'), S double prime (S''),* and so forth.

◆ **QS wave:** A QS wave is a QRS complex that consists entirely of a single, large negative deflection.

◆ **Notch:** A notch in the R wave is a negative deflection that does not extend below the baseline; a notch in the S wave is a positive deflection that does not extend above the baseline.

> **KEY POINT**
>
> Although there may be only one Q wave, there can be more than one R and S wave in the QRS complex.

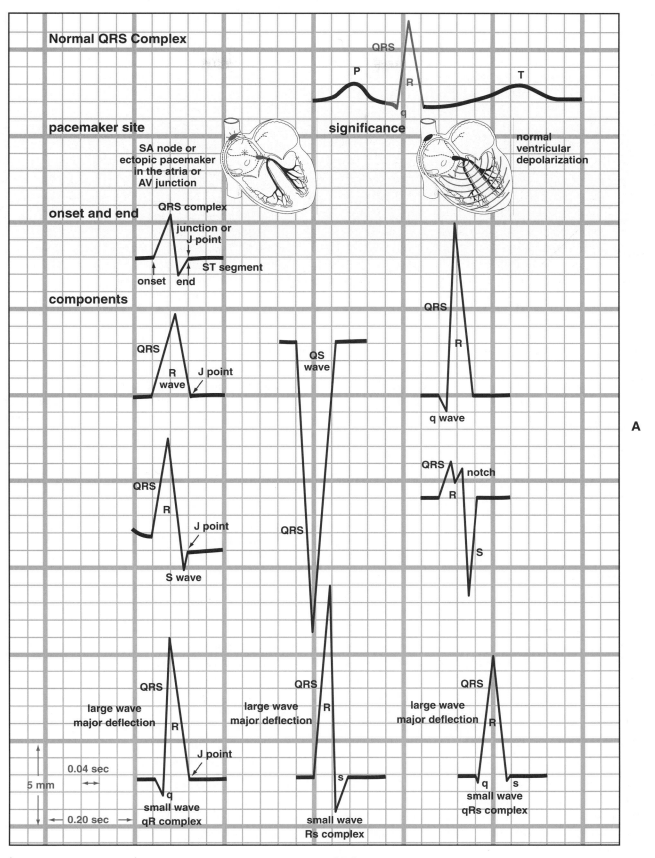

Figure 3-4 Normal QRS complex.

Continued

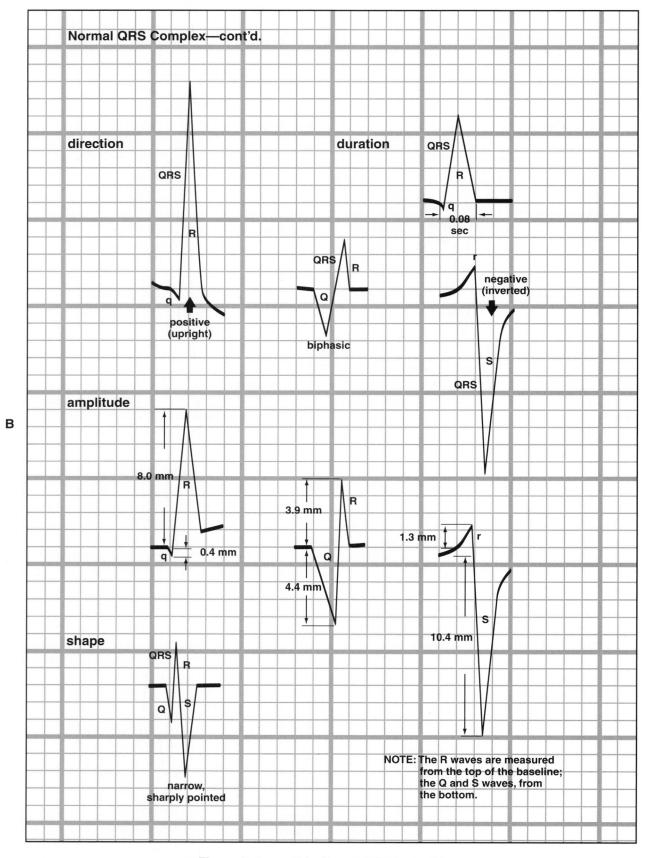

Figure 3-4, cont'd   Normal QRS complex.

The waves comprising the QRS complex are usually identified by upper or lower case letters, depending on the relative size of the waves. The large waves that form the major deflections are identified by upper case letters (QS, R, S). The smaller waves that are less than half of the amplitude of the major deflections are identified by lower case letters (q, r, s). Thus the ventricular depolarization complex can be described more accurately by using upper and lower case letters assigned to the waves (e.g., qR, Rs, qRs).

Direction. The direction of the QRS complex may be predominantly positive (upright), predominantly negative (inverted), or equiphasic (equally positive and equally negative). A predominantly positive QRS complex, for example, has more area encompassed by the R wave, the major deflection, than is encompassed by the Q and S waves.

Duration. The duration of the normal QRS complex is 0.10 second or less (0.06 to 0.10 second) in adults and 0.08 second or less in children. The QRS complex is measured from the onset of the Q or R wave to the end of the last wave of the complex or the J point. The duration of the Q wave does not normally exceed 0.04 second. The time from the onset of the QRS complex to the peak of the R wave is the ventricular activation time (VAT). The VAT represents the time taken for the depolarization of the interventricular septum plus depolarization of the ventricle from the endocardium to the epicardium under the facing lead. The upper limit of the normal VAT is 0.05 seconds.

Amplitude. The amplitude of the R or S wave in the QRS complex in lead II may vary from 1 to 2 mm to 15 mm or more. The normal Q wave is less than 25% of the height of the succeeding R wave.

Shape. The waves in the QRS complex are generally narrow and sharply pointed.

Significance

A normal QRS complex indicates that the electrical impulse responsible for the QRS complex has originated in the SA node or an ectopic or escape pacemaker in the atria or AV junction and has progressed normally from the bundle of His to the Purkinje network through the right and left bundle branches and that normal depolarization of the right and left ventricles has occurred.

Notes

_____

_____

_____

_____

◆ ABNORMAL QRS COMPLEX

Characteristics

Pacemaker site. The pacemaker site of the electrical impulse responsible for an abnormal QRS complex is the SA node or an ectopic or escape pacemaker in the atria, AV junction, bundle branches, Purkinje network, or ventricular myocardium.

Relationship to cardiac anatomy and physiology. An abnormal QRS complex (Figure 3-5) represents abnormal depolarization of the ventricles. This may result from any one of the following:
◆ Intraventricular conduction disturbance (such as a bundle branch block)
◆ Aberrant ventricular conduction
◆ Ventricular preexcitation
◆ An electrical impulse originating in a ventricular ectopic or escape pacemaker
◆ Ventricular pacing by a cardiac pacemaker

Intraventricular conduction disturbance occurs most commonly as a right or left bundle branch block and to a lesser extent as a nonspecific, diffuse intraventricular conduction defect (IVCD) seen in MI, fibrosis, and hypertrophy; electrolyte imbalance, such as hypokalemia and hyperkalemia; and excessive administration of such cardiac drugs as quinidine, procainamide, and flecainide. Bundle branch block results from partial or complete block in conduction of the electrical impulse from the bundle of His to the Purkinje network through the right or left bundle branch while conduction continues uninterrupted through the unaffected bundle branch (see Chapter 13). A block in one bundle branch causes the ventricle on that side to be depolarized later than the other.

For example, in complete right bundle branch block depolarization of the right ventricle is delayed because of a block in conduction through the right bundle branch. This results in an abnormal QRS complex—one that is greater than 0.12 second in duration and appears bizarre (i.e., abnormal in size and shape).

On the other hand, in complete left bundle branch block, the block is in the left bundle branch and, therefore, depolarization of the left ventricle is delayed, also resulting in an abnormal QRS complex.

In partial or incomplete bundle branch block, conduction of the electrical impulse is only partially blocked, resulting in less of a delay in depolarization of the ventricle on the side of the block than in complete bundle branch block. Consequently, the QRS complex is greater than 0.10 second but less than 0.12 second in duration, and it often appears normal.

Complete and incomplete bundle branch block may be present in normal sinus rhythm and in any supraventricular arrhythmia (i.e., any arrhythmia arising above the ventricles in the SA node, atria, or

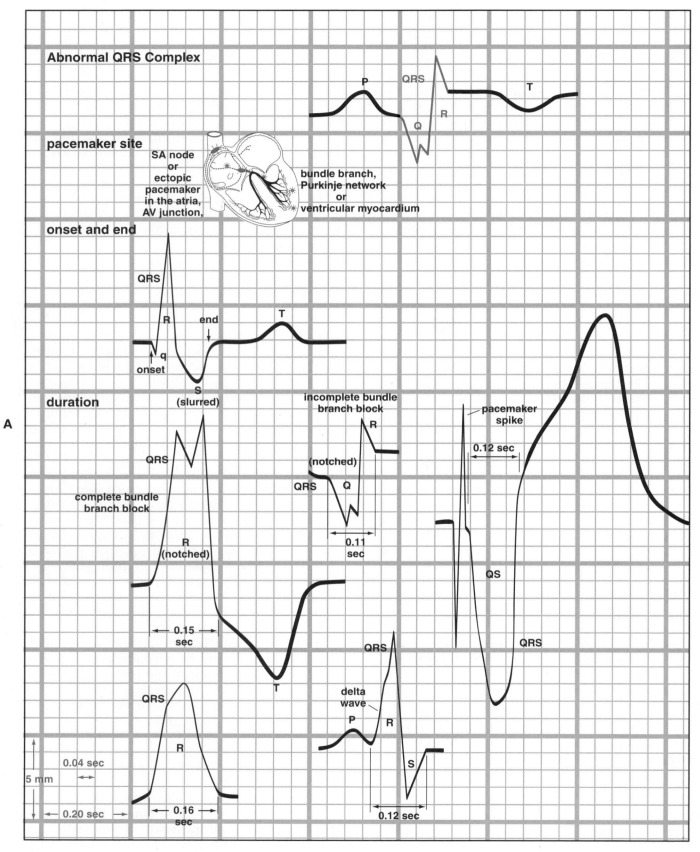

Figure 3-5 Abnormal QRS complex.

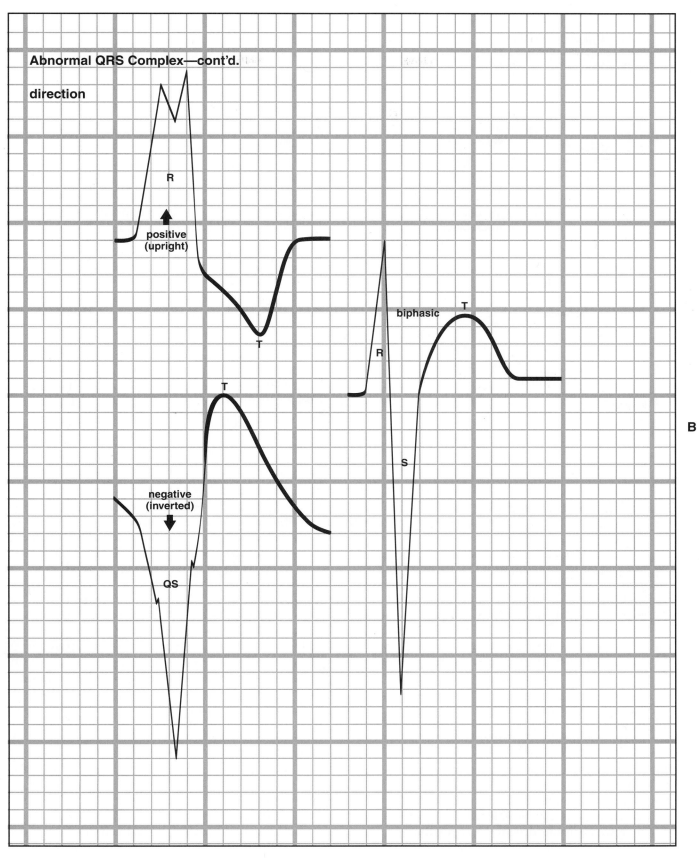

Abnormal QRS Complex—cont'd.

direction

R

positive
(upright)

T

T

negative
(inverted)

QS

biphasic

R

T

S

B

Figure 3-5 cont'd   Abnormal QRS complex.

Continued

C

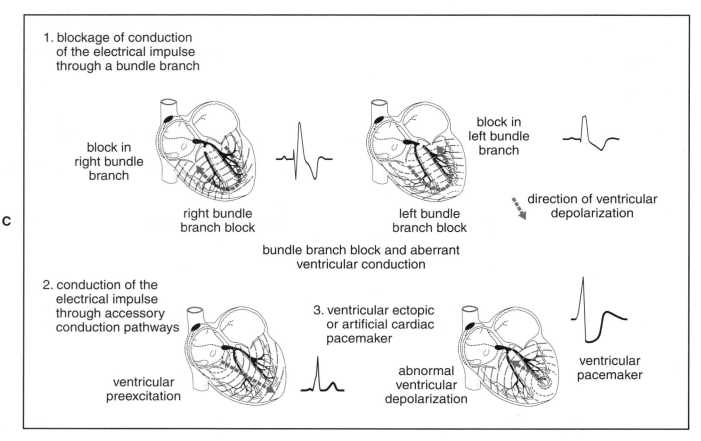

1. blockage of conduction of the electrical impulse through a bundle branch

block in right bundle branch

right bundle branch block

block in left bundle branch

left bundle branch block

direction of ventricular depolarization

bundle branch block and aberrant ventricular conduction

2. conduction of the electrical impulse through accessory conduction pathways

ventricular preexcitation

3. ventricular ectopic or artificial cardiac pacemaker

abnormal ventricular depolarization

ventricular pacemaker

Figure 3-5, cont'd Abnormal QRS complex.

AV junction). Certain supraventricular arrhythmias with bundle branch block may mimic ventricular arrhythmias.

Aberrant ventricular conduction (or, simply, *aberrancy*) is a transient inability of the right or left bundle branch to conduct an electrical impulse normally. This may occur when an electrical impulse arrives at the bundle branch while it is still refractory after conducting a previous electrical impulse, as in premature contractions and tachycardias. This results in an abnormal QRS complex that often resembles an incomplete or complete bundle branch block.

Aberrant ventricular conduction may occur in the following supraventricular arrhythmias, resulting in arrhythmias that mimic ventricular arrhythmias (see Chapter 8):
◆ Premature atrial and junctional contractions
◆ Atrial tachycardia
◆ Atrial flutter and fibrillation
◆ Nonparoxysmal junctional tachycardia
◆ Paroxysmal supraventricular tachycardia

Ventricular preexcitation is the premature depolarization of the ventricles associated with one of the following abnormal accessory conduction pathways described in Chapter 1:
◆ The accessory AV pathways (also known as the *bundles of Kent*) run between the atria and ventricles, bypassing the AV junction
◆ The nodoventricular/fasciculoventricular fibers (also known as the *Mahaim fibers*) extend from the AV junction to the ventricles, bypassing the bundle of His

These anomalous conduction tracts bypass the AV junction or bundle of His, allowing the electrical impulses to initiate depolarization of the ventricles earlier than usual. This results in an abnormally wide QRS complex of greater than 0.10 second that characteristically has an abnormal slurring, and sometimes notching, at its onset—the delta wave. The abnormal shape and width of the QRS complex is the result of the fusion of the abnormal premature depolarization of the ventricle—the delta wave—with the normal depolarization of the rest of the ventricles.

The PR interval is usually less than 0.12 second when ventricular preexcitation is the result of an accessory AV pathway, and it is usually normal when nodoventricular/fasciculoventricular fibers are the

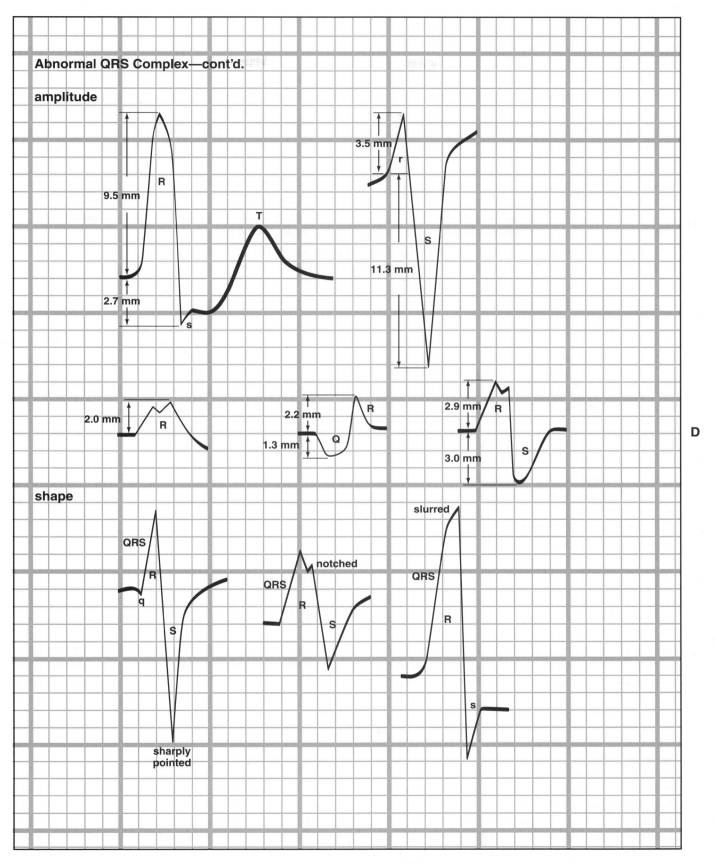

Figure 3-5, cont'd   Abnormal QRS complex.

cause. When the PR interval is less than 0.12 second and the QRS complex is abnormally wide and demonstrates a delta wave, the ECG pattern is often termed the *Wolff-Parkinson-White (WPW) pattern,* or *preexcitation.*

When episodes of paroxysmal supraventricular tachycardia with normal QRS complexes occur in the presence of a WPW pattern during sinus or atrial rhythms, the ECG findings are called the *WPW syndrome.* Supraventricular tachycardia and atrial flutter and fibrillation with ventricular preexcitation may resemble ventricular tachycardia (see Chapter 8).

An electrical impulse originating in an ectopic or escape pacemaker in the bundle branches, Purkinje network, or myocardium of one of the ventricles depolarizes that ventricle earlier than the other. The result is an abnormal QRS complex that is greater than 0.12 second in duration and appears bizarre. Such QRS complexes typically occur in ventricular arrhythmias such as accelerated idioventricular rhythm, ventricular escape rhythm, ventricular tachycardia, and premature ventricular contractions (see Chapter 8). The occurrence of ventricular ectopic beats or rhythms is often referred to as *ventricular ectopy.*

Cardiac pacemaker-induced QRS complexes are generally 0.12 second or greater in width and appear bizarre. Preceding each pacemaker-induced QRS complex is a narrow deflection, often biphasic, called the *pacemaker spike* (see Chapter 9).

Description

Onset and end. The onset and end of the abnormal QRS complex are the same as those of a normal QRS complex.

Direction. The direction of the abnormal QRS complex may be predominantly positive (upright), predominantly negative (inverted), or equiphasic (equally positive and equally negative).

Duration. The duration of the abnormal QRS complex is greater than 0.10 second. If a bundle branch block is present and the duration of the QRS complex is between 0.10 and 0.12 second, the bundle branch block is called *incomplete.* If the duration of the QRS complex is greater than 0.12 second, the bundle branch block is called *complete.* In ventricular preexcitation, the duration of the QRS complex is 0.11 second or greater.

The duration of a QRS complex caused by an electrical impulse originating in an ectopic or escape pacemaker in the Purkinje network or ventricular myocardium is always greater than 0.12 second; typically, it is 0.16 second or greater. However, if the electrical impulse originates in a bundle branch, the duration of the QRS complex may be only slightly greater than 0.10 second and appear normal.

Amplitude. The amplitude of the waves in the abnormal QRS complex varies from 1 to 2 mm to 20 mm or more.

Shape. An abnormal QRS complex varies widely in shape, from one that appears quite normal—narrow and sharply pointed (as in incomplete bundle branch block)—to one that is wide and bizarre, slurred and notched (as in complete bundle branch block and ventricular arrhythmias). In ventricular preexcitation the QRS complex is wider than normal at the base because of an initial slurring or bulging of the upstroke of the R wave (or of the downstroke of the S wave, as the case may be)—the delta wave.

Significance

An abnormal QRS complex indicates that abnormal depolarization of the ventricles has occurred because of one of the following:

◆ A block in the progression of the electrical impulse from the bundle of His to the Purkinje network through the right or left bundle branch (bundle branch block and aberrant ventricular conduction)
◆ The progression of the electrical impulse from the atria to the ventricles through an abnormal accessory conduction pathway (ventricular preexcitation)
◆ The origination of the electrical impulse responsible for the ventricular depolarization in a ventricular ectopic or escape pacemaker
◆ The excitation of the ventricles by a cardiac pacemaker

Notes

_____

_____

_____

T Wave

> **KEY DEFINITION**
>
> **A T wave *represents ventricular repolarization. There are two types of T wave:***
> ◆ ***Normal T wave***
> ◆ ***Abnormal T wave***

◆ NORMAL T WAVE

Characteristics

Relationship to cardiac anatomy and physiology. A normal T wave (Figure 3-6) represents normal repolarization of the ventricles. Normal repolarization begins at the epicardial surface of the ventricles and progresses inwardly through the ventricular walls to the endocardial surface. The T wave occurs during the last part of ventricular systole.

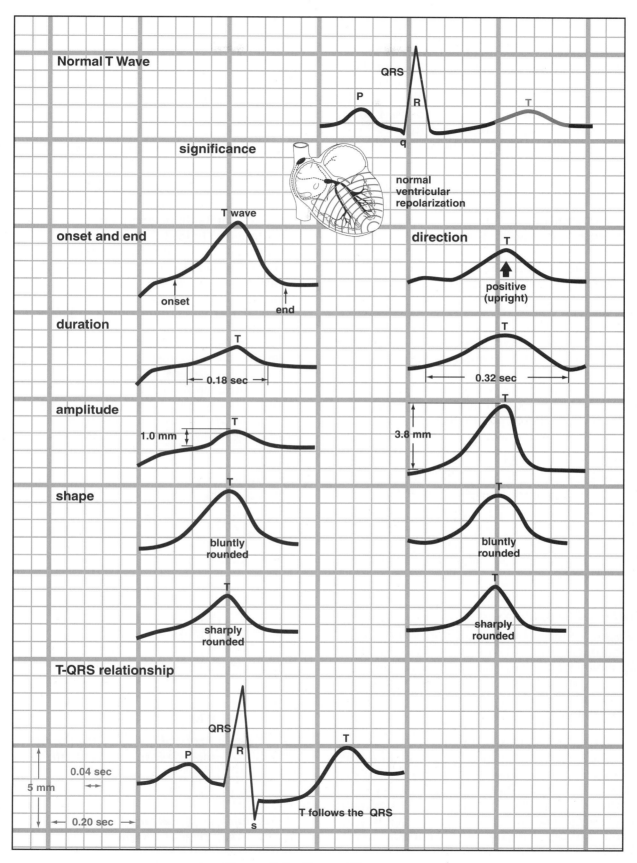

Figure 3-6   Normal T wave.

Description

Onset and end. The onset of the T wave is identified as the first abrupt or gradual deviation from the ST segment (or the point where the slope of the ST segment appears to become abruptly or gradually steeper). If the ST segment is absent, the T wave begins at the end of the QRS complex (or the J point). The point where the T wave returns to the baseline marks the end of the T wave. In the absence of an ST segment, the T wave is sometimes called the *ST-T wave.* Often the onset and end of the T wave are difficult to determine with certainty.

Direction. The direction of the normal T wave is positive (upright) in lead II.

Duration. The duration is 0.10 to 0.25 second or greater.

Amplitude. The amplitude is less than 5 mm.

Shape. The normal T wave is sharply or bluntly rounded and slightly asymmetrical. Ordinarily, the first, upward part of the T wave is longer than the second, downward part.

T Wave-QRS complex relationship. The T wave always follows the QRS complex.

Significance

A normal T wave preceded by a normal ST segment indicates that normal repolarization of the right and left ventricles has occurred.

Notes

_____

_____

_____

_____

◆ ABNORMAL T WAVE

Characteristics

Relationship to cardiac anatomy and physiology. An abnormal T wave (Figure 3-7) represents abnormal ventricular repolarization. Abnormal repolarization may begin at either the epicardial or endo- cardial surface of the ventricles. When abnormal repolarization begins at the epicardial surface of the ventricles, it progresses inwardly through the ventricular walls to the endocardial surface, as it normally does, but at a slower rate, producing an abnormally tall, upright T wave in lead II. When it begins at the endocardial surface of the ventricles, it progresses outwardly through the ventricular walls to the epicardial surface, producing a negative T wave in lead II.

Abnormal ventricular repolarization may occur in the following:

◆ Myocardial ischemia, acute MI, myocarditis, pericarditis, and ventricular enlargement (hypertrophy)

◆ Abnormal depolarization of the ventricles (as in bundle branch block and ectopic ventricular arrhythmias)

◆ Electrolyte imbalance (e.g., excess serum potassium) and administration of certain cardiac drugs (e.g., quinidine, procainamide)

◆ Athletes and persons who are hyperventilating

Description

Onset and end. The onset and end of an abnormal T wave are the same as those of a normal T wave.

Direction. The abnormal T wave may be positive (upright) and abnormally tall or low, negative (inverted), or biphasic (partially positive and partially negative) in lead II. The abnormal T wave may or may not be in the same direction as that of the QRS complex. The T wave after an abnormal QRS complex is almost always opposite in direction to it, being abnormally wide and tall or deeply inverted.

Duration. The duration is 0.10 to 0.25 second or greater.

Amplitude. The amplitude varies.

Shape. The abnormal T wave may be rounded, blunt, sharply peaked, wide, or notched. Normal T waves with superimposed P waves (T/P waves) can resemble abnormal peaked, wide, and notched T waves.

T Wave-QRS complex relationship. The abnormal T wave always follows the QRS complex.

Significance

An abnormal T wave indicates that abnormal repolarization of the ventricles has occurred.

Notes

_____

_____

_____

_____

U Wave

> **KEY DEFINITION**
>
> A U wave *probably represents the final stage of repolarization of the ventricles.*

Characteristics

Relationship to cardiac anatomy and physiology. A U wave (Figure 3-8) probably represents repolarization of a small segment of the ventricles (such as the papillary muscles or ventricular septum) after most of the right and left ventricles have been repo-

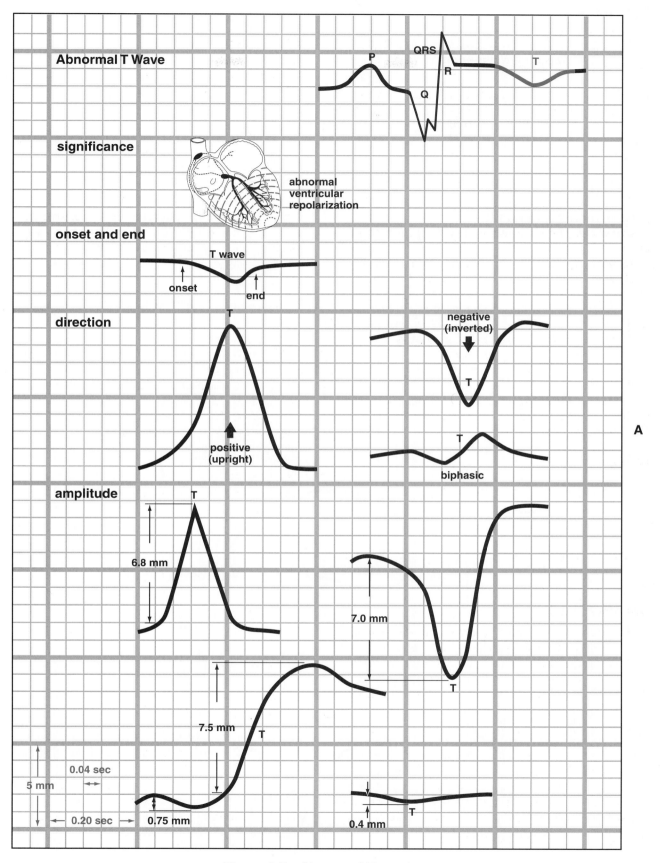

Figure 3-7   Abnormal T wave.

Continued

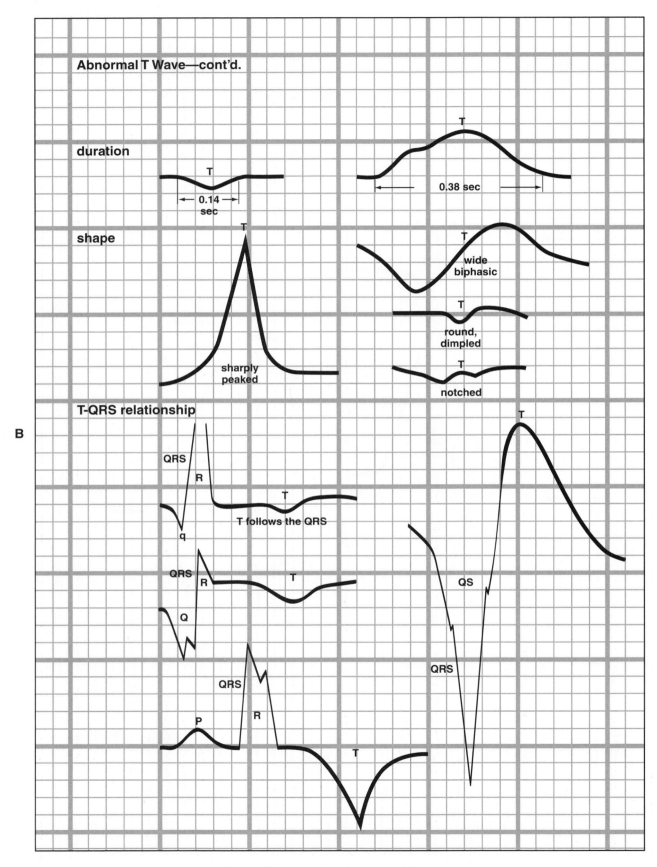

Figure 3-7, cont'd Abnormal T wave.

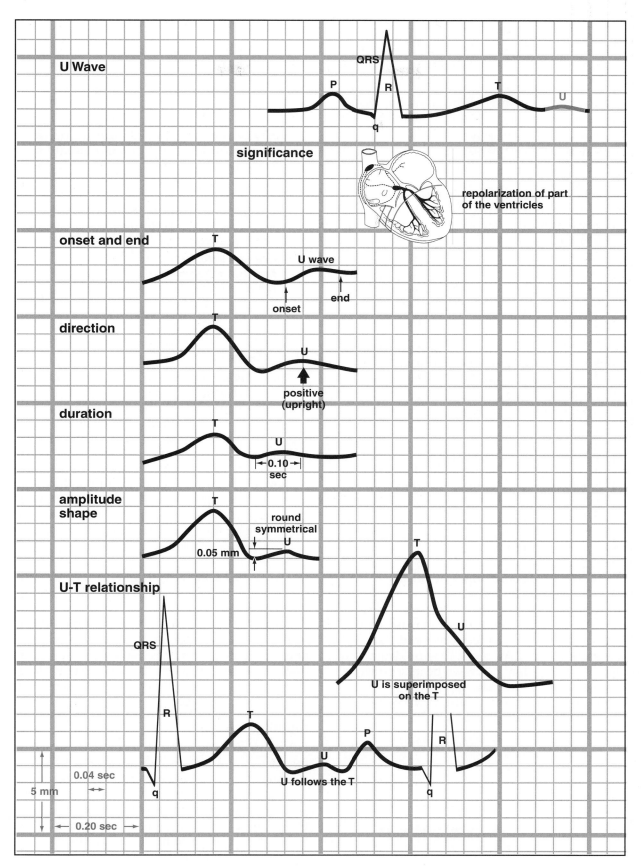

Figure 3-8 U wave.

larized. Although uncommon and not easily identified, the U wave can best be seen when the heart rate is slow.

Description

Onset and end. The onset of the U wave is identified as the first abrupt or gradual deviation from the baseline or the downward slope of the T wave. The point where the U wave returns to the baseline or downward slope of the T wave marks the end of the U wave.

Direction. The direction of a normal U wave is positive (upright), the same as that of the preceding normal T wave in lead II. An abnormal U wave may be positive (upright), flat, or negative (inverted).

Duration. The duration is not determined routinely.

Amplitude. The amplitude of a normal U wave is usually less than 2 mm and always smaller than that of the preceding T wave in lead II. A U wave taller than 2 mm is considered to be abnormal.

Shape. The U wave is rounded and symmetrical.

U Wave relationship to other waves. The U wave always follows the peak of the T wave and occurs before the next P wave.

Significance

A U wave indicates that repolarization of the ventricles has occurred. Small U waves of less than 2 mm are a normal finding. Abnormally tall U waves of over 2 mm in height may be present in the following:

◆ Hypokalemia
◆ Cardiomyopathy
◆ Left ventricular hypertrophy
◆ Excessive administration of digitalis, quinidine, and procainamide

A large U wave may sometimes be mistaken for a P wave. If a P wave is absent, as in a junctional rhythm, and a large U wave is present, a sinus rhythm with a first-degree AV block may be mistakenly diagnosed. If both a large P wave and a large U wave are present, a 2:1 AV block may be diagnosed incorrectly. The fact that a U wave bears a constant relationship to the T wave and not to the P wave or QRS complex helps to identify the U wave and differentiate it from a P wave.

Notes

_____

_____

_____

_____

_____

INTERVALS

PR Interval

KEY DEFINITION

A PR interval (Figure 3-9) represents the time of progression of the electrical impulse from the SA node, an ectopic pacemaker in the atria, or an ectopic or escape pacemaker in the AV junction, through the entire electrical conduction system of the heart to the ventricular myocardium, including the depolarization of the atria. There are two types of PR interval:
◆ *Normal PR interval*
◆ *Abnormal PR interval*

◆ NORMAL PR INTERVAL

Characteristics

Relationship to cardiac anatomy and physiology. A normal PR interval represents the time from the onset of atrial depolarization to the onset of ventricular depolarization during which the electrical impulse progresses normally from the SA node or an ectopic pacemaker in the atria adjacent to the SA node, through the internodal atrial conduction tracts, AV junction, bundle branches, and Purkinje network to the ventricular myocardium. The PR interval includes a P wave and the short, usually flat (isoelectric) segment, the PR segment that follows it.

Description

Onset and end. The PR interval begins with the onset of the P wave and ends with the onset of the QRS complex.

Duration. The duration of the normal PR interval is 0.12 to 0.20 second and is dependent on the heart rate. When the heart rate is fast, the PR interval is normally shorter than when the heart rate is slow (Example: heart rate 120, PR interval 0.16 second; heart rate 60, PR interval 0.20 second).

Significance

A normal PR interval indicates that the electrical impulse originated in the SA node or an ectopic pacemaker in the adjacent atria and has progressed normally through the electrical conduction system of the heart to the ventricular myocardium. The major significance of a normal PR interval is that the electrical impulse has been conducted through the AV node and bundle of His normally and without delay.

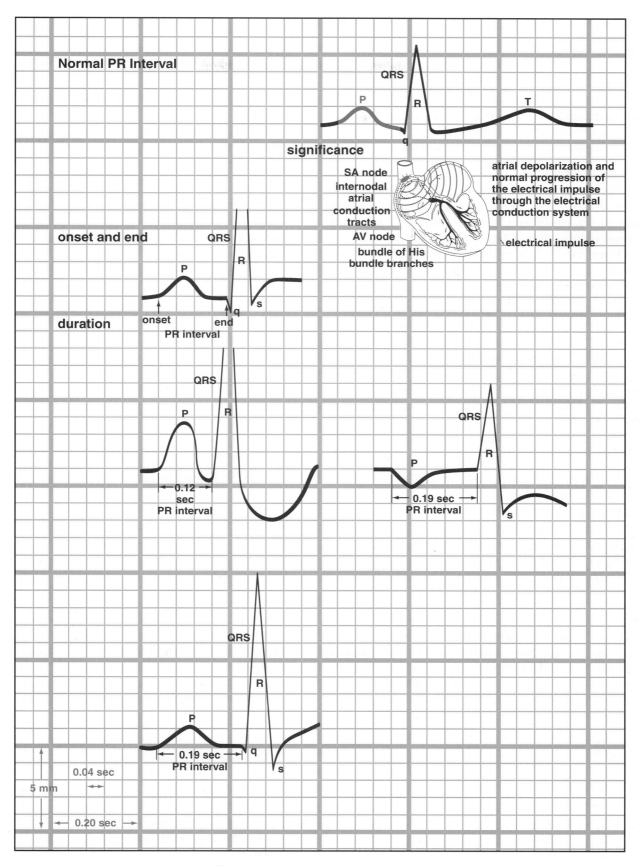

Figure 3-9   Normal PR interval.

Notes

_____

_____

_____

_____

◆ ABNORMAL PR INTERVAL

Characteristics

Relationship to cardiac anatomy and physiology. A PR interval greater than 0.20 second (Figure 3-10) represents delayed progression of the electrical impulse through the AV node, bundle of His, or, rarely, the bundle branches. The P wave associated with a prolonged PR interval may be normal or abnormal. A PR interval less than 0.12 second is commonly present when the electrical impulse originates in an ectopic pacemaker in the atria close to the AV node or in an ectopic or escape pacemaker in the AV junction. Negative (inverted) P waves in lead II are commonly associated with abnormally short PR intervals.

A PR interval less than 0.12 second also occurs when the electrical impulse progresses from the atria to the ventricles through one of several accessory conduction pathways, which bypass the entire AV junction or just the AV node itself, depolarizing the ventricles earlier than usual. These anomalous conduction pathways include the following:

◆ **Accessory AV pathways (bundles of Kent):** These abnormal AV conduction pathways that run from the atria to the ventricles bypass the AV junction, causing _ventricular preexcitation._ In this AV conduction anomaly, the short PR interval is commonly followed by a wide, abnormally shaped QRS complex with a delta wave (the slurring and sometimes notching at the onset of the QRS complex). This type of abnormal AV conduction is also called _WPW preexcitation._

◆ **Atrio-His fibers (James fibers):** This accessory conduction pathway, which extends from the atria to the lowermost part of the AV node near the onset of the bundle of His, bypassing the AV node, results in a short PR interval followed by a normal QRS complex. This anomalous AV conduction is called _atrio-His preexcitation._

The P waves in these AV conduction anomalies are usually positive (upright) in lead II.

Description

Onset and end. The onset and end of the abnormal PR interval are the same as those of a normal PR interval.

Duration. The duration of the abnormal PR interval may be greater than 0.20 second or less than 0.12 second.

Significance

An abnormally prolonged PR interval indicates that a delay of progression of the electrical impulse through the AV node, bundle of His, or, rarely, the bundle branches is present. An abnormally short PR interval indicates one of the following:

◆ That the electrical impulse originated in an ectopic pacemaker in the atria near the AV node or in an ectopic or escape pacemaker in the AV junction

◆ That the electrical impulse originated in the SA node or atria and progressed through one of several abnormal accessory conduction pathways that bypass the entire AV junction or just the AV node

Notes

_____

_____

_____

_____

QT Interval

> **KEY DEFINITION**
>
> **A QT interval _represents the time between the onset of depolarization and the termination of repolarization of the ventricles._**

Characteristics

Relationship to cardiac anatomy and physiology. The QT interval (Figure 3-11) represents the refractory period of the ventricles during which they depolarize and repolarize. An abnormally prolonged QT interval, one that exceeds the average QT interval for any given heart rate by 10% represents a slowing in the repolarization of the ventricles. Abnormally prolonged QT intervals may occur in the following:

◆ Pericarditis, acute myocarditis, acute MI, left ventricular hypertrophy, and hypothermia

◆ Bradyarrhythmias (e.g., marked sinus bradycardia, third-degree AV block with slow ventricular escape rhythm)

◆ Electrolyte imbalance (hypokalemia and hypocalcemia) and liquid protein diets

◆ Excess of certain drugs (quinidine, procainamide, disopyramide, amiodarone, phenothiazines, and tricyclic antidepressants)

◆ Central nervous system disorders (e.g., cerebrovascular accident, subarachnoid hemorrhage, and intracranial trauma)

◆ Without a known cause (idiopathic)

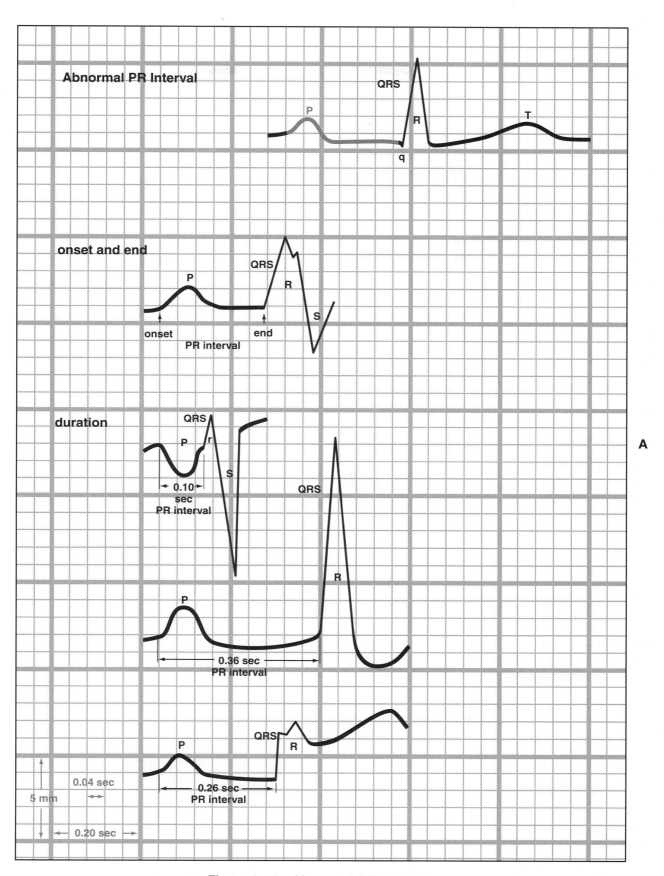

Figure 3-10 Abnormal PR interval.

Continued

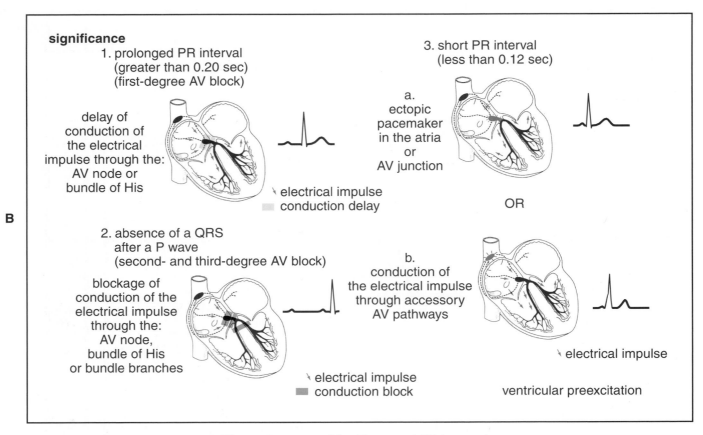

B

significance

1. prolonged PR interval
(greater than 0.20 sec)
(first-degree AV block)

delay of
conduction of
the electrical
impulse through the:
AV node or
bundle of His

↘ electrical impulse
▨ conduction delay

2. absence of a QRS
after a P wave
(second- and third-degree AV block)

blockage of
conduction of the
electrical impulse
through the:
AV node,
bundle of His
or bundle branches

↘ electrical impulse
▨ conduction block

3. short PR interval
(less than 0.12 sec)

a.
ectopic
pacemaker
in the atria
or
AV junction

OR

b.
conduction of
the electrical impulse
through accessory
AV pathways

↘ electrical impulse

ventricular preexcitation

Figure 3-10, cont'd   Abnormal PR interval.

An abnormally short QT interval, one that is less than the average QT interval for any given heart rate by 10%, represents an increase in the rate of repolarization of the ventricles. This occurs in digitalis therapy and hypercalcemia.

Description

Onset and end. The onset of the QT interval is identified as the point where the first wave of the QRS complex just begins to deviate, abruptly or gradually, from the baseline. The end of the QT interval is the point where the T wave returns to the baseline.

Duration. The duration of the QT interval is dependent on the heart rate, being somewhat less then half of the preceding R-R interval. In general, a QT interval less than half the R-R interval is normal, one that is greater than half is abnormal, and one that is about half is "borderline." When the heart rate is fast, the QT interval is shorter than when the heart rate is slow (e.g., heart rate 120, QT interval about 0.29 second; heart rate 60, QT interval about 0.39 second). The QT intervals may be equal or unequal in duration depending on the underlying rhythm. The average duration of the QT interval normally expected at a given heart rate, the corrected QT interval (or QTc), and the normal range of 10% above and 10% below the average value are shown in Table 3-1. Regardless of heart rate, a QT interval of greater than 0.45 seconds is considered abnormal.

> ### KEY POINT
>
> The determination of the QT interval should be made in the lead where the T wave is most prominent and not deformed by a U wave and should not include the U wave. Furthermore, the measurement of the QT interval assumes that the duration of the QRS complex is normal, with an average value of 0.08 second. If the QRS is widened beyond 0.08 second for any reason, the excess widening beyond 0.08 second must be subtracted from the actual measurement to obtain the correct QT interval.

Significance

A QT interval represents the time between the onset of ventricular depolarization and the end of ventric-

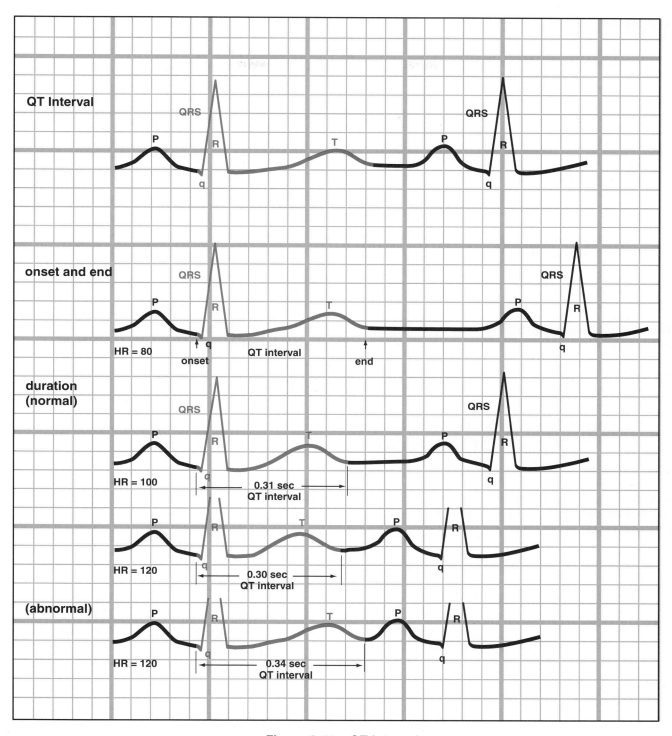

Figure 3-11   QT interval.

ular repolarization, the refractory period of the ventricles. A prolonged QT interval indicates slowing of ventricular repolarization. The most common causes of this include the following:

◆ Electrolyte imbalance (hypokalemia and hypocalcemia)

◆ Drug therapy (quinidine, procainamide, disopyramide, amiodarone, phenothiazines, and tricyclic antidepressants)

◆ Pericarditis

◆ Acute myocarditis

◆ Acute MI

TABLE

3-1 QT$_c$ Intervals

Heart Rate/min	R-R Interval (sec)	QT$_c$ (sec) and Normal Range
40	1.5	0.46 (0.41-0.51)
50	1.2	0.42 (0.38-0.46)
60	1.0	0.39 (0.35-0.43)
70	0.86	0.37 (0.33-0.41)
80	0.75	0.35 (0.32-0.39)
90	0.67	0.33 (0.30-0.36)
100	0.60	0.31 (0.28-0.34)
120	0.50	0.29 (0.26-0.32)
150	0.40	0.25 (0.23-0.28)
180	0.33	0.23 (0.21-0.25)
200	0.30	0.22 (0.20-0.24)

◆ Left ventricular hypertrophy
◆ Hypothermia

The prolongation of the QT interval after administration of excessive amounts of such antiarrhythmic agents as quinidine, procainamide, and disopyramide may provoke the appearance of torsade de pointes, an ominous, potentially lethal form of ventricular tachycardia. In this regard, a QT interval greater than 0.50 seconds, regardless of heart rate, is considered potentially hazardous.

A decrease in the QT interval indicates an increase in the rate of repolarization of the ventricles. The most common causes of this are digitalis therapy and hypercalcemia.

Notes

_____

_____

_____

_____

_____

_____

R-R Interval

KEY DEFINITION

An R-R interval *represents the time between two successive ventricular depolarizations.*

Characteristics

Relationship to cardiac anatomy and physiology. An R-R interval (Figure 3-12) normally represents one cardiac cycle during which the atria and ventricles contract and relax once.

Description

Onset and end. The onset of the R-R interval is generally considered to be the peak of one R wave; the end, the peak of the succeeding R wave.

Duration. The duration is dependent on the heart rate. When the heart rate is fast, the R-R interval is shorter than when the heart rate is slow (e.g., heart rate 120, R-R interval 0.50 second; heart rate 60, R-R interval 1.0 second). The R-R intervals may be equal or unequal in duration, depending on the underlying rhythm. Examples of unequal rhythms include the following:

◆ A regular rhythm interspersed with premature atrial, junctional, and ventricular premature beats
◆ Sinus arrest and SA exit block
◆ Atrial fibrillation
◆ Second-degree AV blocks

Significance

An R-R interval represents the time between two successive ventricular depolarizations.

Notes

_____

_____

_____

_____

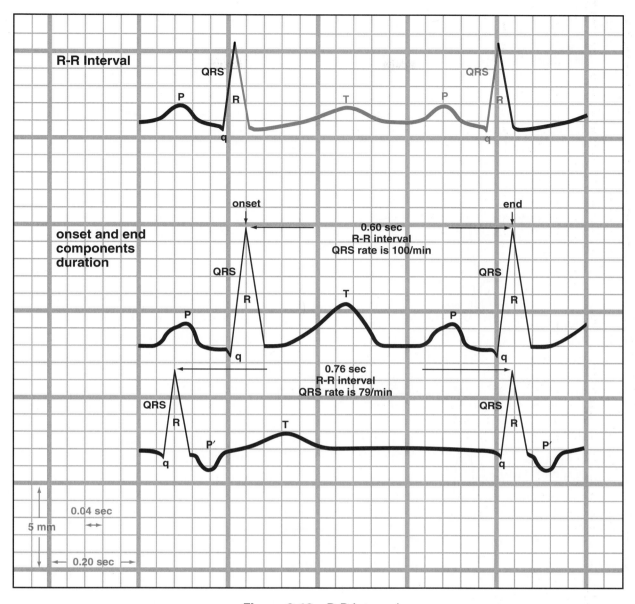

Figure 3-12 R-R interval.

SEGMENTS

ST Segment

> **KEY DEFINITION**
>
> *An ST segment represents the early part of repolarization of the right and left ventricles. There are two types of ST segment:*
> - *Normal ST segment*
> - *Abnormal ST segment*

◆ NORMAL ST SEGMENT

Characteristics

Relationship to cardiac anatomy and physiology. The ST segment (Figure 3-13) represents the early part of ventricular repolarization.

Description

Onset and end. The ST segment begins with the end of the QRS complex and ends with the onset of the T wave. The junction between the QRS complex and the ST segment is called the *junction* or *J point.*

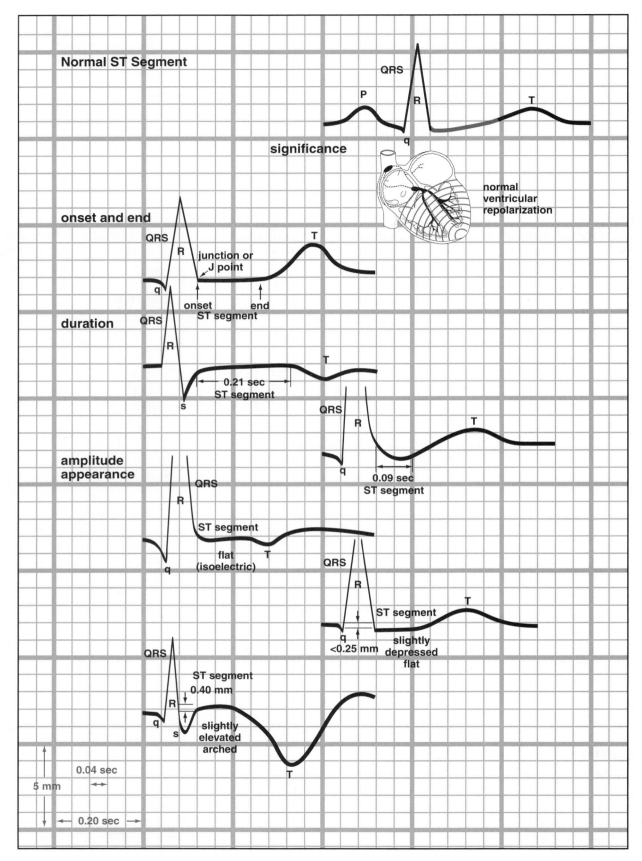

Figure 3-13 Normal ST segment.

Duration. The duration is 0.20 second or less and is dependent on the heart rate. When the heart rate is fast, the ST segment is shorter than when the heart rate is slow.

Amplitude. Normally, the ST segment is flat (isoelectric). However, it may be slightly elevated or depressed and still be normal if it is elevated or depressed by less than 1.0 mm, 0.04 second (1 small square) after the J point of the QRS complex. The TP segment is normally used as a baseline reference for the determination of the amplitude of the ST segment. However, if the TP segment is absent because of a very rapid heart rate, the PR segment is used instead.

Appearance. If slightly elevated, the ST segment may be flat, concave, or arched. If slightly depressed, the ST segment may be flat, upsloping, or downsloping.

Significance

A normal ST segment followed by a normal T wave indicates that normal repolarization of the right and left ventricles has occurred.

Notes

_____

_____

_____

_____

_____

◆ ABNORMAL ST SEGMENT

Characteristics

Relationship to cardiac anatomy and physiology. An abnormal ST segment (Figure 3-14) signifies abnormal ventricular repolarization, a common consequence of myocardial ischemia and injury. It is also present in ventricular fibrosis or aneurysm, pericarditis, left ventricular enlargement (hypertrophy), administration of digitalis, and various other conditions noted.

Description

Onset and end. The onset and end of the abnormal ST segment are the same as those of a normal ST segment.

Duration. The duration is 0.20 second or less.

Amplitude. An ST segment is abnormal when it is elevated or depressed 1.0 mm or more 0.04 second (1 small square) after the J point of the QRS complex.

Appearance. If elevated, the ST segment may be flat, concave, or arched. If depressed, the ST segment may be flat, upsloping, or downsloping.

Significance

An abnormal ST segment indicates that abnormal ventricular repolarization has occurred. Common causes of ST segment elevation include the following:
- ◆ Acute Q-wave MI (transmural myocardial ischemia and injury)
- ◆ Prinzmetal's angina (severe transmural myocardial ischemia from coronary artery spasm)
- ◆ Ventricular aneurysm
- ◆ Acute pericarditis
- ◆ Early repolarization pattern (a form of myocardial repolarization seen in normal healthy people that produces ST segment elevation closely mimicking that of acute MI)
- ◆ Left ventricular hypertrophy and left bundle branch block (leads V_1-V_3)
- ◆ Hyperkalemia (leads V_1-V_2)
- ◆ Hypothermia (along with the J wave and Osborne wave)

Common causes of ST segment depression include the following:
- ◆ Acute non-Q-wave MI (subendocardial myocardial ischemia and injury)
- ◆ Angina pectoris (subendocardial myocardial ischemia)
- ◆ Reciprocal ECG changes in acute Q-wave MI
- ◆ Right and left ventricular hypertrophy ("strain" pattern)
- ◆ Right and left bundle branch block
- ◆ Digitalis effect
- ◆ Hypokalemia

Notes

_____

_____

_____

_____

PR Segment

> ### KEY DEFINITION
>
> *A* PR segment *represents the time of progression of the electrical impulse from the AV node through the bundle of His, bundle branches, and Purkinje network to the ventricular myocardium.*

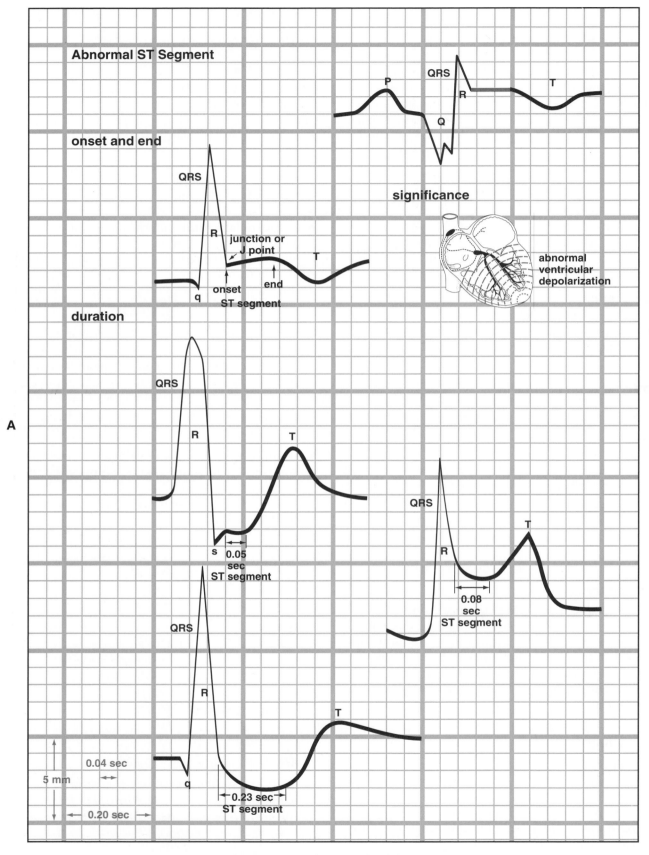

Figure 3-14 Abnormal ST segment.

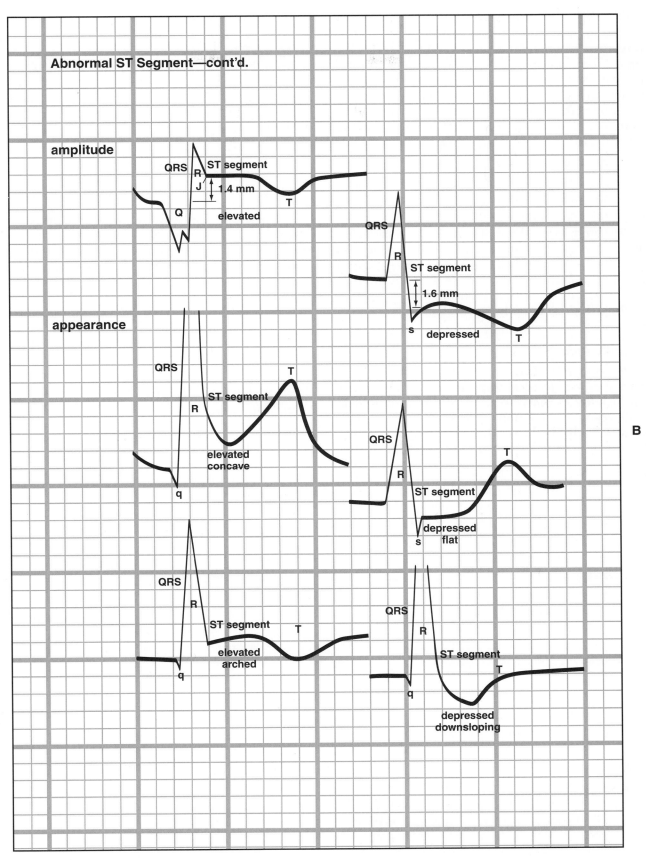

Figure 3-14, cont'd   Abnormal ST segment.

Characteristics

Relationship to cardiac anatomy and physiology. The PR segment (Figure 3-15) represents the time from the end of atrial depolarization to the onset of ventricular depolarization during which the electrical impulse progresses from the AV node through the bundle of His, bundle branches, and Purkinje network to the ventricular myocardium.

Description

Onset and end. The onset of the PR segment begins with the end of the P wave and ends with the onset of the QRS complex.

Duration. The duration normally varies from about 0.02 to 0.10 second. It may be greater than 0.10 second if there is a delay in the progression of the electrical impulse through the AV node, bundle of His, or, rarely, the bundle branches.

Amplitude. Normally, the PR segment is flat (isoelectric).

Significance

A PR segment of 0.10-second duration or less indicates that the electrical impulse has been conducted through the AV junction normally and without delay. A PR segment exceeding 0.10 second in duration indicates a delay in the conduction of the electrical impulse through the AV junction or, rarely, the bundle branches.

Notes

_____

_____

_____

_____

_____

_____

TP Segment

> **KEY DEFINITION**
>
> *A TP segment is the interval between two successive P-QRST complexes, during which electrical activity of the heart is absent.*

Characteristics

Relationship to cardiac anatomy and physiology. A TP segment (Figure 3-16) represents the time from the end of ventricular repolarization to the onset of the following atrial depolarization, during which electrical activity of the heart is absent. A TP segment includes a U wave when one is present, after the T wave.

Description

Onset and end. The TP segment begins with the end of the T wave and ends with the onset of the following P wave.

Duration. The duration is 0.0 to 0.40 second or greater and is dependent on the heart rate and the configuration of the P waves and the QRS-T complexes. When the heart rate is fast, the TP segment is shorter than when the heart rate is slow. For example, when the heart rate is about 120 or greater, the TP segment is absent, with the P wave immediately following the T wave or buried in it. With a heart rate of 60 or less, the TP segment is about 0.4 second or greater.

Amplitude. Usually, the TP segment is flat (isoelectric) unless a U wave is present.

Significance

A TP segment indicates the absence of any electrical activity of the heart. The TP segment is used as the baseline reference for the determination of ST segment elevation or depression.

Notes

_____

_____

_____

_____

_____

_____

_____

_____

_____

_____

_____

_____

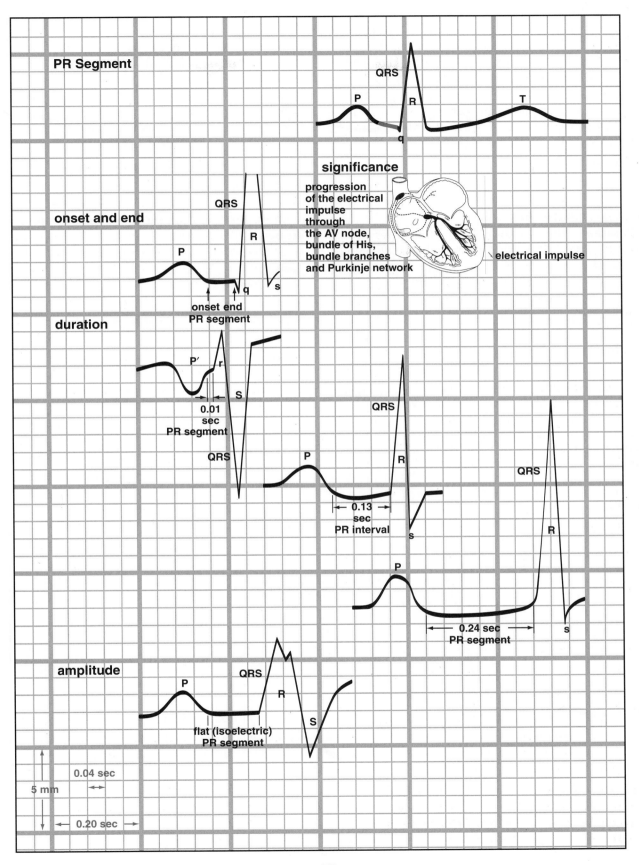

Figure 3-15 PR segment.

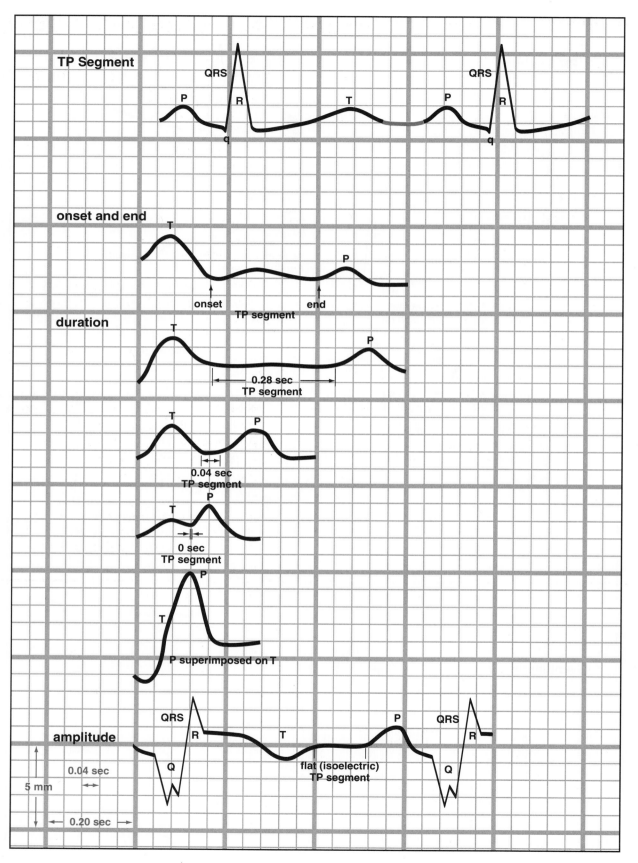

Figure 3-16 TP segment.

CHAPTER REVIEW QUESTIONS

1. Wide, notched P waves may be caused by:
   A. systemic hypertension
   B. mitral and aortic valvular disease
   C. acute MI
   D. all of the above

2. The normal PR interval is between:
   A. 0.8 and 0.24 second
   B. 0.8 and 0.16 second
   C. 0.12 and 0.20 second
   D. 0.10 and 0.24 second

3. An ectopic P wave represents atrial depolarization occurring in:
   A. an abnormal sequence
   B. an abnormal direction
   C. all of the above
   D. none of the above

4. A normal QRS complex represents normal:
   A. repolarization of the atria
   B. depolarization of the ventricles
   C. repolarization of the ventricles
   D. depolarization of the atria

5. The time taken for the depolarization of the interventricular septum plus depolarization of the ventricle from the endocardium to the epicardium under the facing lead is called the:
   A. ventricular activation time
   B. septal excitation time
   C. atrial repolarization phase
   D. none of the above

6. Aberrant ventricular conduction may occur in:
   A. sinus bradycardia with PVCs
   B. atrial tachycardia and PACs
   C. PVCs
   D. all of the above

7. Which one of the following accessory conduction pathways is not involved in causing ventricular preexcitation with associated delta waves?
   A. accessory AV pathways
   B. bundles of Kent
   C. atrio-His fibers
   D. nodoventricular/fasciculoventricular fibers

8. Myocardial ischemia, acute MI, excess serum potassium, and administration of procainamide can cause an abnormal _____ on the ECG.
   A. P wave
   B. QRS complex
   C. T wave
   D. U wave

9. A U wave indicates that repolarization of the ventricles has occurred. An abnormally tall U wave may be present in:
   A. hypothermia, vertigo
   B. hypokalemia, cardiomyopathy
   C. cardiac tamponade, diabetes
   D. CVA, syncope

10. A delay of progression of the electrical impulse through the AV node or bundle of His would show on an ECG as a(n):
    A. prolonged QRS complex
    B. peaked T wave
    C. elevated ST segment
    D. prolonged PR interval

11. An abnormal ST segment indicates:
    A. abnormal ventricular repolarization
    B. abnormal atrial repolarization
    C. abnormal ventricular depolarization
    D. none of the above

4 ECG Interpretation: Arrhythmia Determination

CHAPTER OBJECTIVES

Upon completion of all or part of this chapter, you should be able to complete the following objectives:

1. List the seven steps in determining an arrhythmia.
2. Define heart rate and describe the following methods of determining it:
   6-second count method
   Heart rate calculator ruler method
   Triplicate method
   R-R interval method
     Seconds method
     Small square method
     Large square method
     Conversion table method
3. List and describe two methods of determining the ventricular rhythm.
4. Define the following terms as they apply to ventricular rhythm:
   Essentially regular
   Irregular
5. List and describe the three steps in identifying and analyzing the P, P', F, and f waves.
6. Define the basic differences between the following components of the ECG, including shape, width, height, relationship to the QRS complexes, and rate and rhythm:

Normal P wave	Atrial fibrillation waves
Abnormal P wave	"Coarse"
Atrial flutter waves	"Fine"

7. List and describe the steps in determining the PR intervals and the AV conduction ratio.
8. Define the following normal and abnormal PR intervals:
   Normal and abnormal PR intervals
   RP' intervals
9. Give the causes of a PR interval less than 0.12 second in duration and one greater than 0.20 second.
10. Define the following terms:

Atrioventricular (AV) block	Third-degree AV block
Variable AV block	Dropped beat
Isoelectric line	Wenckebach AV block
Incomplete AV block	AV dissociation
Complete AV block	AV conduction ratio
First-degree AV block	Accessory conduction
Second-degree AV block	pathway

11. List and describe the three steps in identifying and analyzing the QRS complexes.

12. List the most likely site or sites of origin (or pace-maker sites) of arrhythmias under the following circumstances:
    Upright P waves preceding each QRS complex in lead II
    Negative P waves preceding each QRS complex in lead II
    Negative P waves following each QRS complex in lead II
    QRS complexes occurring without any P waves

Atrial flutter waves
Atrial fibrillation waves
Normal QRS complexes with no set relationship to the P waves
Slightly widened QRS complexes (0.10 to 0.12 seconds in duration) with no set relationship to the P waves
Widened QRS complexes (greater than 0.12 second in duration and bizarre) with no set relationship to the P waves

---

Box 4-1 contains an outline of the steps used in interpreting an electrocardiogram (ECG) to determine the presence of an arrhythmia and its identity. The ECG interpretation may be performed in the order shown or in accordance with local prehospital or hospital protocols.

STEP ONE: DETERMINE THE HEART RATE

◆ Calculate the heart rate by determining the number of ventricular depolarizations (QRS complexes), or beats, that occur in the ECG in 1 minute.

The heart rate can be determined by using the 6-second count method, a heart rate calculator ruler, the R-R interval method, or the triplicate method.

The 6-Second Count Method

The 6-second count method is the simplest way of determining the heart rate and is generally considered the fastest, with the exception of the heart rate calculator ruler method. The 6-second count method, however, is the least accurate. This method can be used when the rhythm is either regular or irregular.

The short, vertical lines (or some other similar marking) at the top of most ECG papers divide the ECG paper strip into 3-second intervals (Figure 4-1) when the paper is run at a standard speed of 25 mm per second. Two of these intervals are equal to a 6-second interval. When the ECG strip is run at 50 mm per second, four of these "3-second" intervals are equal to a 6-second interval.

Calculate the heart rate by determining the number of R-R intervals (or cardiac cycles) in a 6-second interval and multiplying this number by 10 (Figure 4-2). The result is the heart rate in beats per minute. If premature beats are present in the 6-second interval, they should be included in the R-R interval count.

The heart rate calculated by this method is almost always an approximation of the actual heart rate.

Example. If there are exactly eight R-R intervals in a 6-second interval, the heart rate is:

$$8 \times 10 = 80 \text{ beats per minute}$$

Example. If there are ten and a half R-R intervals in a 6-second interval, the heart rate is:

$$10.5 \times 10 = 105 \text{ beats per minute}$$

To obtain a more accurate heart rate when the rate is extremely slow and/or the rhythm is grossly irregular, determine the number of R-R intervals in a longer interval, such as a 12-second interval, and adjust the multiplier accordingly.

Example. If there are six and a half R-R intervals in a 12-second interval, the heart rate is:

$$6.5 \times 5 = 32.5 \text{ or, rounded off, 33 beats per minute}$$

BOX

4-1   Arrhythmia Determination

Step One: Determine the heart rate
Step Two: Determine the ventricular rhythm
Step Three: Identify and analyze the P, P', F, or f waves
  1. Identify the P, P', F, or f waves
  2. Determine the atrial rate and rhythm
  3. Note the association of the P, P', F, or f waves to the QRS complexes
Step Four: Determine the PR or RP' intervals and AV conduction ratio
  1. Determine the PR intervals
  2. Assess the equality of the PR intervals
  3. Determine the AV conduction ratio
Step Five: Identify and analyze the QRS complexes
  1. Identify the QRS complexes
  2. Note the duration and shape of the QRS complexes
  3. Assess the equality of the QRS complexes
Step Six: Determine the site of origin of the arrhythmia
Step Seven: Identify the arrhythmia
Step Eight: Evaluate the significance of the arrhythmia

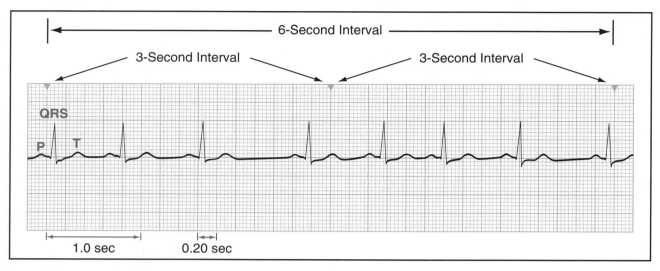

Figure 4-1 Intervals of 3 and 6 seconds at an ECG recording speed of 25 mm per second.

In adults, a heart rate less than 60 beats per minute indicates bradycardia; a heart rate above 100 per minute indicates tachycardia.

The Heart Rate Calculator Ruler Method

A heart rate calculator ruler, such as the one shown in Figure 4-3, is a device that can be used to determine the heart rate rapidly and accurately. This method is most accurate if the rhythm is regular. The directions printed on the ruler should be followed (e.g., "Third complex from arrow is rate/min."). Premature beats should not be included in the QRS complexes used in determining the heart rate by this method, if possible.

The R-R Interval Method

The R-R interval may be used four different ways to determine the heart rate. The rhythm must be regular if the calculation of the heart rate is to be accurate. The two R waves used for measuring the R-R interval should be those of the underlying rhythm and not those of premature beats, if possible. The four methods are as follows:

◆ METHOD 1

Measure the distance in seconds between the peaks of two consecutive R waves and divide this number into 60 to obtain the heart rate (Figure 4-4).

Example. If the distance between the peaks of two consecutive R waves is 0.56 second, the heart rate is:
60/0.56 = 107 beats per minute

◆ METHOD 2

Count the large squares (0.20-second spaces) between the peaks of two consecutive R waves and divide this number into 300 to obtain the heart rate (Figure 4-5).

Example. If there are 2.5 large squares between the peaks of two consecutive R waves, the heart rate is:
300/2.5 = 120 beats per minute

◆ METHOD 3

Count the small squares (0.04-second spaces) between the peaks of two consecutive R waves and divide this number into 1500 to obtain the heart rate (Figure 4-6).

Example. If there are 19 small squares between the peaks of two consecutive R waves, the heart rate is:
1500/19 = 78.9 or, rounded off, 80 beats per minute

◆ METHOD 4

Count the small squares (0.04-second spaces) between the peaks of two consecutive R waves and, using a rate conversion table (Table 4-1), convert the number of small squares into the heart rate (Figure 4-7).

Example. If there are 17 small squares between the peaks of two consecutive R waves, the heart rate is 88 beats per minute.

The Triplicate Method

The triplicate method of determining the heart rate will be accurate only if the rhythm is regular

Text continued on page 79

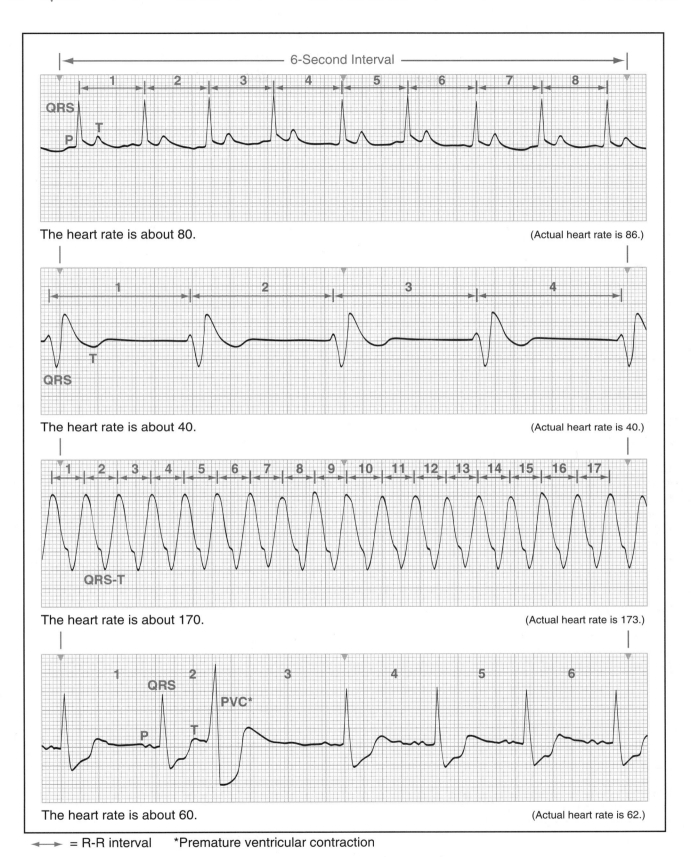

Figure 4-2 6-second count method.

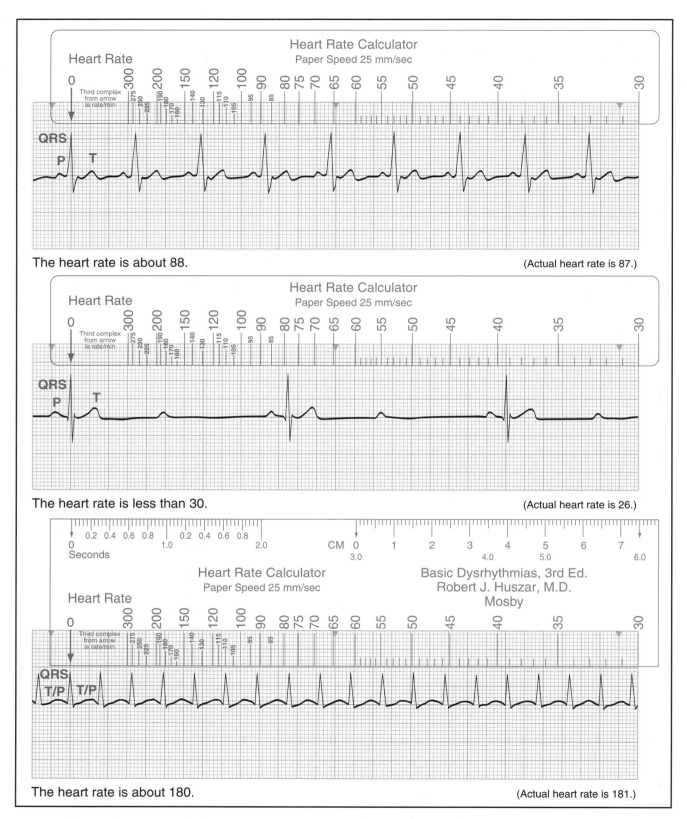

The heart rate is about 88.   (Actual heart rate is 87.)

The heart rate is less than 30.   (Actual heart rate is 26.)

The heart rate is about 180.   (Actual heart rate is 181.)

Figure 4-3   Heart rate calculator ruler method.

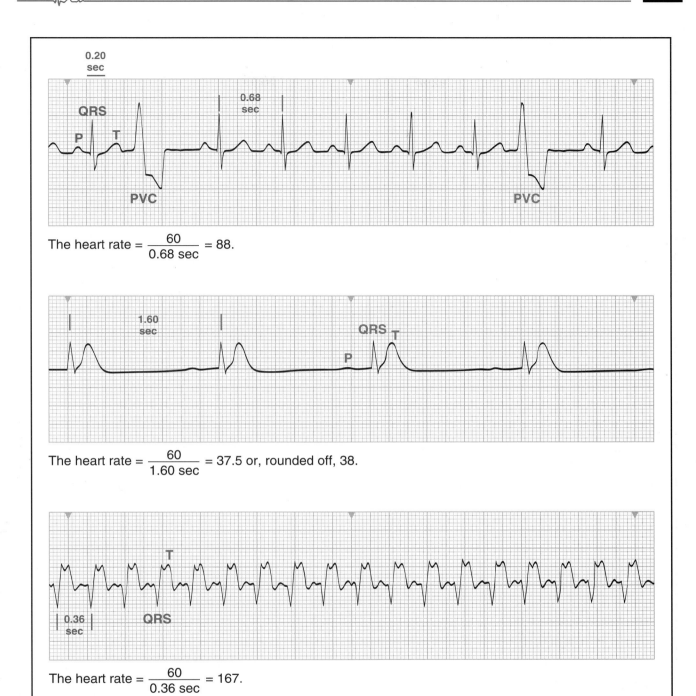

The heart rate = $\dfrac{60}{0.68 \text{ sec}}$ = 88.

The heart rate = $\dfrac{60}{1.60 \text{ sec}}$ = 37.5 or, rounded off, 38.

The heart rate = $\dfrac{60}{0.36 \text{ sec}}$ = 167.

Figure 4-4   R-R interval method 1.

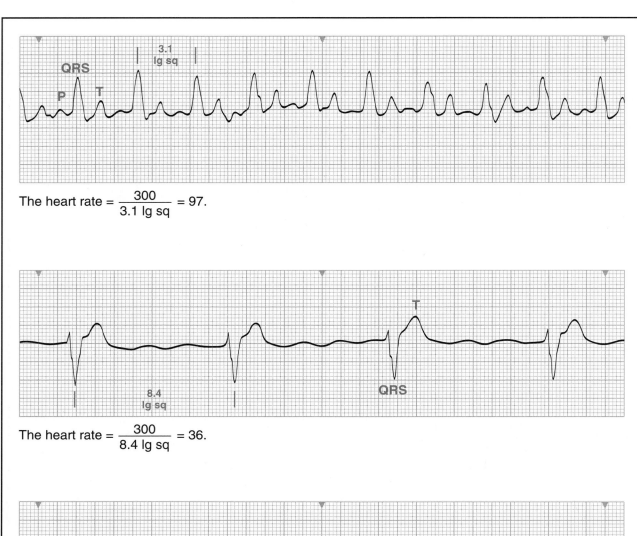

The heart rate = $\dfrac{300}{3.1 \text{ lg sq}}$ = 97.

The heart rate = $\dfrac{300}{8.4 \text{ lg sq}}$ = 36.

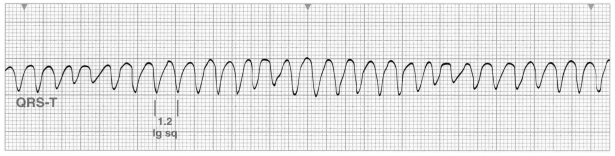

The heart rate = $\dfrac{300}{1.2 \text{ lg sq}}$ = 250.

Figure 4-5 R-R interval method 2.

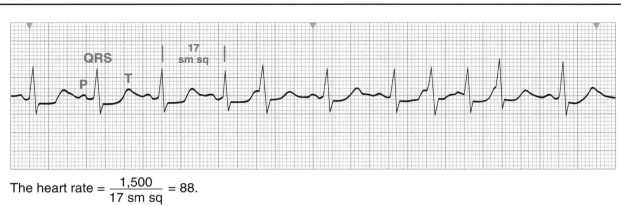

The heart rate = $\dfrac{1,500}{17 \text{ sm sq}}$ = 88.

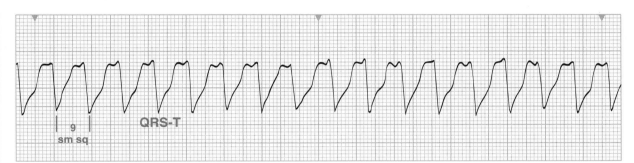

The heart rate = $\dfrac{1,500}{9 \text{ sm sq}}$ = 167.

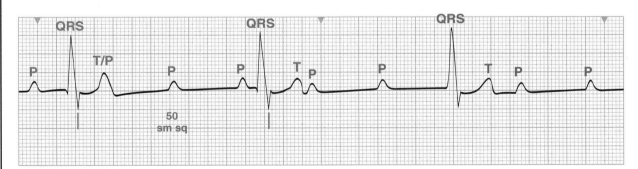

The heart rate = $\dfrac{1,500}{50 \text{ sm sq}}$ = 30.

Figure 4-6 R-R interval method 3.

TABLE

4-1 Conversion of the Number of Small Squares (0.04-Second Spaces) Between the Peaks of Two Consecutive R Waves Into the Heart Rate

0.04-sec Spaces	Heart Rate/min	0.04-sec Spaces	Heart Rate/min
5	300	27	56
6	250	28	54
7	214	29	52
8	188	30	50
9	167	31	48
10	150	32	47
11	136	33	45
12	125	34	44
13	115	35	43
14	107	36	42
15	100	37	41
16	94	38	40
17	88	39	39
18	84	40	38
19	79	41	37
20	75	42	36
21	72	43	35
22	68	44	34
23	65	45	33
24	63	47	32
25	60	48	31
26	58	50	30

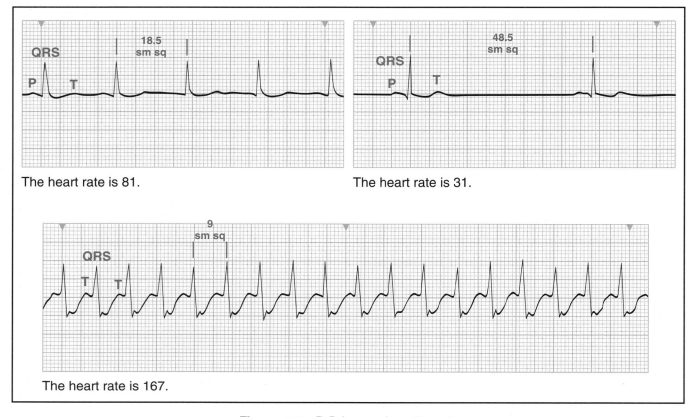

The heart rate is 81.

The heart rate is 31.

The heart rate is 167.

Figure 4-7   R-R interval method 4.

(Figure 4-8). The heart rate per minute is determined as follows:

1. Select an R wave that lines up with a dark vertical line, and label it "A."
2. Number the next six dark vertical lines consecutively from left to right: "300," "150," "100," "75," "60," and "50." These numbers represent heart rate in beats per minute.
3. Identify the first R wave to the right of the R wave labeled "A," and label this R wave "B."
4. Identify the numbered dark vertical lines on either side of the wave labeled "B."
5. Estimate the distance of the R wave labeled "B" from the nearest of the two adjacent numbered dark vertical lines with respect to the total distance between them (e.g., one quarter, one third, or one half of the total distance).
6. Estimate the heart rate by equating the estimated distance of the R wave labeled "B" from the nearest adjacent numbered, dark vertical line to beats per minute.

Example. If the R wave labeled "B" is half way between the "150" dark vertical line and the "100" dark vertical line, the heart rate is about 125 beats per minute.

Example. If the R wave labeled "B" is a third of the way between the "75" dark vertical line and the "60" dark vertical line, the heart rate is about 70 beats per minute.

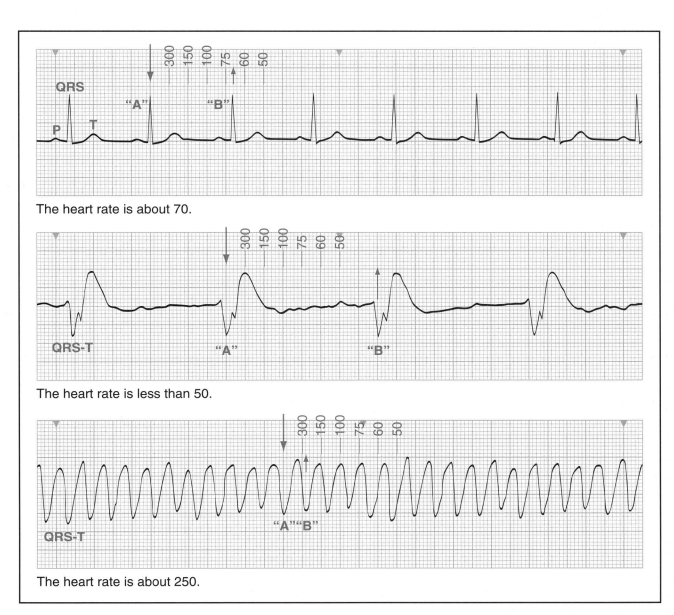

Figure 4-8 Triplicate method.

Notes

_____

_____

_____

_____

_____

_____

_____

_____

STEP TWO: DETERMINE THE VENTRICULAR RHYTHM

◆ Determine the ventricular rhythm by:
1. (a) Estimating the R-R intervals; (b) measuring them using ECG calipers or, if calipers are not available, a pencil and paper; or (c) counting the small squares between the R waves and then
2. Comparing the R-R intervals to each other

The simplest way to determine the ventricular rhythm is to first estimate the width of one of the R-R intervals, preferably one located on the left side of the ECG strip (Figure 4-9). Then visually compare the R-R intervals in the rest of the strip to the one first determined, in a systematic way from left to right.

If ECG calipers are used, first place one tip of the calipers on the peak of one R wave; then adjust the ECG calipers so that the other tip rests on the peak of the adjacent R wave on the right. Then, without changing the distance between the tips of the calipers, compare the other R-R intervals to the R-R interval first measured.

If a pencil and paper are used, place the straight edge of the paper horizontally, close to the peaks of the R waves, and mark off the distance between two consecutive R waves (the R-R interval) with the pencil. Then compare this R-R interval to the other R-R intervals in the ECG strip.

The last method of determining the ventricular rhythm is to count the number of small squares (0.04 second/small square) between the R waves and then to compare the width of the R-R intervals with each other.

The ventricular rhythm as determined using one of the methods above may be regular or irregular.

◆ If the shortest and longest R-R intervals vary by less than 0.16 second (four small squares) in a given ECG strip, the rhythm is considered to be "essentially regular" (Figure 4-10). (Thus the R-R intervals of an "essentially regular" rhythm may be precisely equal or slightly unequal.)

◆ If the shortest and longest R-R intervals vary by more than 0.16 second, the rhythm is considered to be irregular. The rhythm may be _slightly irregular, occasionally irregular, regularly irregular,_ or _irregularly irregular_ (Figure 4-11). Other terms used interchangeably to describe an irregularly irregular rhythm are _grossly_ and _totally_ irregular. These terms apply to atrial as well as ventricular rhythms.

Notes

_____

_____

_____

_____

_____

_____

_____

_____

_____

STEP THREE: IDENTIFY AND ANALYZE THE P, P', F, OR f WAVES

◆ Identify the P, P', F, or f waves
◆ Determine the atrial rate and rhythm
◆ Note the association of the P, P', F, or f waves to the QRS complexes

A normal P wave is a positive, smoothly rounded wave in lead II (Figure 4-12). It is 0.5 to 2.5 mm high and 0.10 second or less wide. It typically appears before each QRS complex, but it may occur singly without a QRS complex after it, as in atrioventricular (AV) block. An AV block is a condition in which there is a complete or incomplete (partial) block in the conduction of electrical impulses from the atria to the ventricles through the AV junction or the bundle branches (see Chapter 9).

An abnormal P wave may be positive, negative, or flat (isoelectric) in lead II (Figure 4-13). It may be smoothly rounded, peaked, or deformed (i.e., wide and notched). Its height may be normal (0.5 to 2.5 mm) or abnormal (less than 0.5 mm or greater than 2.5 mm). Its duration may be normal (0.10 second or less) or abnormal (greater than 0.10 second). Like a normal P wave, it may appear before the QRS complex or occur alone without a QRS complex following it. Unlike a normal P wave, however, an abnormal P wave may regularly appear after each QRS complex or be buried (or "hidden") in the QRS complex.

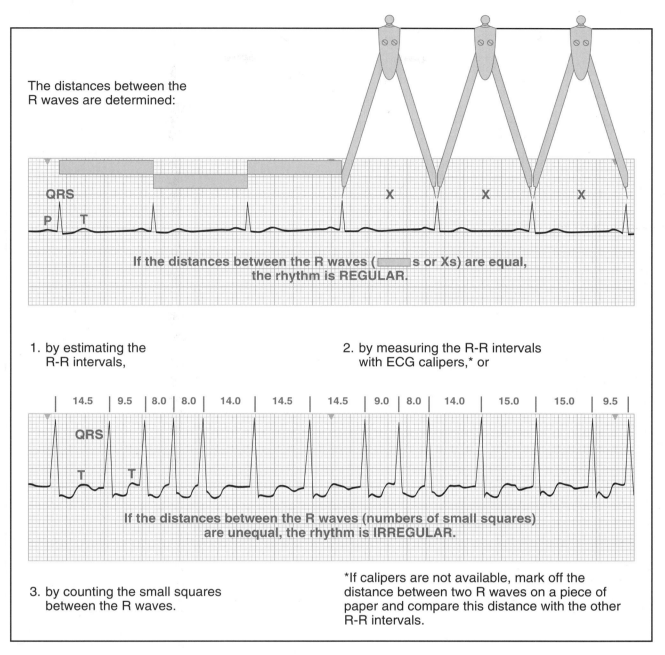

The distances between the R waves are determined:

If the distances between the R waves (▭s or Xs) are equal, the rhythm is REGULAR.

1. by estimating the R-R intervals,

2. by measuring the R-R intervals with ECG calipers,* or

| 14.5 | 9.5 | 8.0 | 8.0 | 14.0 | 14.5 | 14.5 | 9.0 | 8.0 | 14.0 | 15.0 | 15.0 | 9.5 |

If the distances between the R waves (numbers of small squares) are unequal, the rhythm is IRREGULAR.

3. by counting the small squares between the R waves.

*If calipers are not available, mark off the distance between two R waves on a piece of paper and compare this distance with the other R-R intervals.

Figure 4-9   Determining the rhythm.

The origin of the P waves is determined by observing the positivity or negativity of the P waves in lead II as follows (Table 4-2):

◆ If the P waves are positive (upright) in lead II, they usually originate in the sinoatrial (SA) node or upper or middle right atrium. They may appear normal or abnormal (peaked or wide and notched). When such P waves have a set relationship to the QRS complexes, they always precede the QRS complexes.

◆ If the P waves are negative (inverted) in lead II, they usually originate in the lower right atrium,

left atrium, AV junction, or ventricles. They may precede, follow, or be buried in the QRS complexes associated with them.

A P wave that originates in the SA node, whether it appears normal or abnormal, is designated as a "P wave" or a "P" in the figures. A P wave that originates in the atria, AV junction, or ventricles, on the other hand, is designated as a "P' wave" or a "P'" in the figures, regardless of its appearance.

If P waves are present, determine the atrial rate and rhythm and whether each QRS complex is regularly

Regular Rhythms

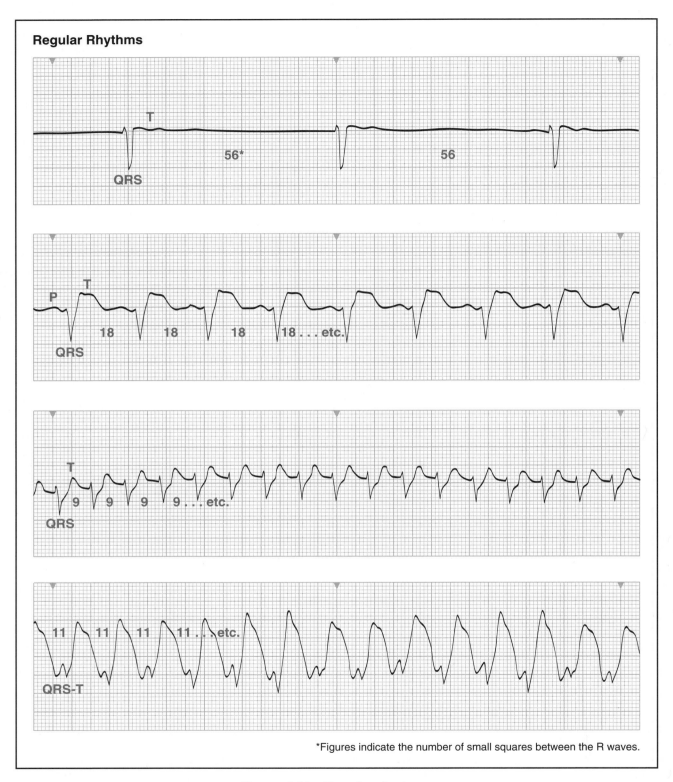

*Figures indicate the number of small squares between the R waves.

Figure 4-10 Regular rhythms.

Irregular Rhythms

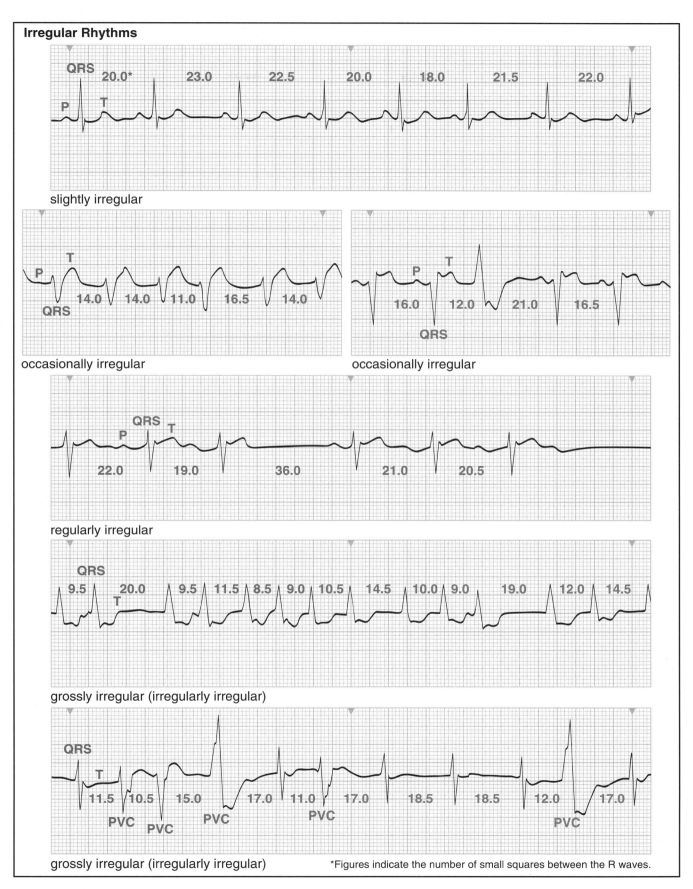

slightly irregular

occasionally irregular

occasionally irregular

regularly irregular

grossly irregular (irregularly irregular)

grossly irregular (irregularly irregular)

*Figures indicate the number of small squares between the R waves.

Figure 4-11 Irregular rhythms.

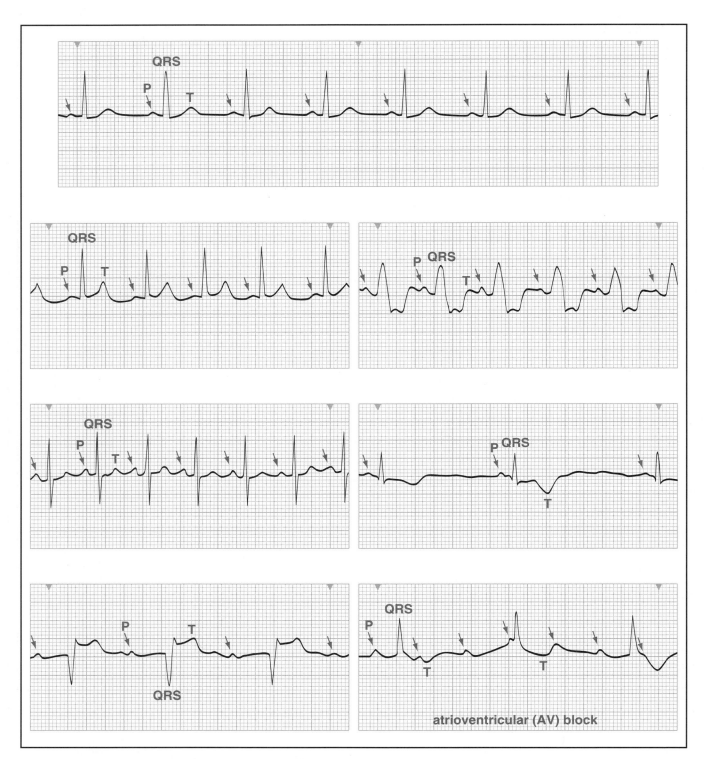

Figure 4-12 Normal P waves.

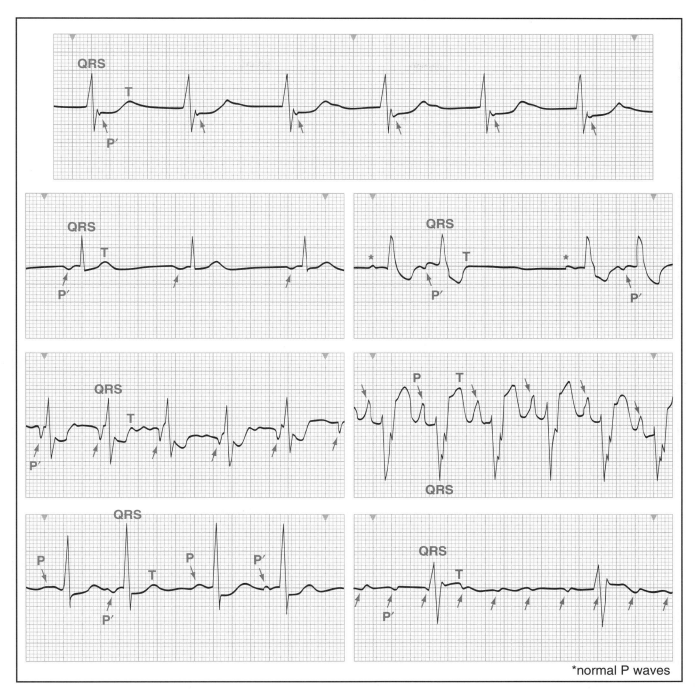

Figure 4-13 Abnormal P waves.

accompanied by a P wave. The rate of the P waves is usually that of the QRS complexes, but it may be less; if an AV block is present, it may be greater.

If P waves are absent, determine if atrial flutter (F) or fibrillation (f) waves are present (Figure 4-14). Atrial flutter waves are typically negative, V-shaped waves followed by positive, sharply pointed atrial T waves in lead II. The rate of the F waves is usually between 240 and 350 per minute. Their rhythm is

typically regular. QRS complexes commonly occur regularly after every other or every fourth F wave, but they may occur irregularly at varying F wave-to-QRS complex ratios if a variable AV block is present.

Atrial fibrillation waves are irregularly shaped, rounded waves, each dissimilar in configuration and amplitude to the other. If the f waves are less than 1 mm high, they are called *fine* fibrillatory waves; if they are greater than 1 mm high, they are called

4-2   Appearance of the P Waves Relative to Their Site of Origin

Site of Origin of the P Wave	Appearance in Lead II	P wave Location
SA node (P wave)	Positive (upright)	Precedes the QRS complex
Upper or middle right atrium (P′ wave)	Normal, peaked, or wide and notched	
Lower right atrium or left atrium (P′ wave)	Negative (inverted)	Precedes the QRS complex
AV junction (P′ wave)		
Upper part	Negative (inverted)	Precedes the QRS complex
Middle or distal part	Absent	Is buried in the QRS complex
Distal part	Negative (inverted)	Follows the QRS complex
Ventricles (P′ wave)	Negative (inverted)	Follows the QRS complex

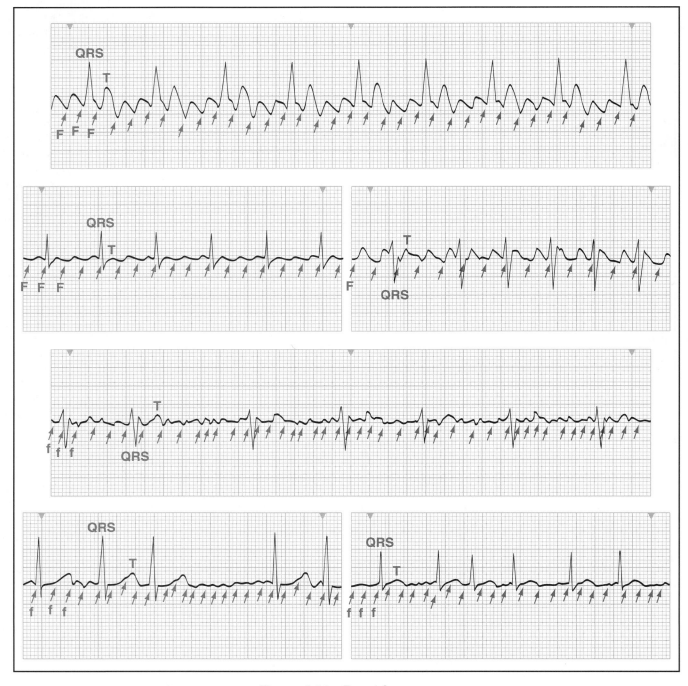

Figure 4-14   F and f waves.

coarse fibrillatory waves. If the f waves are extremely fine, they may not be identified as such, and the sections of the ECG between the T waves and QRS complexes may appear only slightly wavy or even flat (isoelectric).

The rate of the f waves is usually between 350 and 600 (average 400) per minute, and their rhythm is extremely irregular. Typically, in atrial fibrillation, the QRS complexes occur irregularly with no set pattern, reflecting the extremely irregular atrial rhythm. See Chapter 6 for a full description of F and f waves.

Notes

_____

_____

_____

_____

_____

_____

_____

STEP FOUR: DETERMINE THE PR OR RP' INTERVALS AND ATRIOVENTRICULAR CONDUCTION RATIO

◆ Determine the PR intervals by measuring the distance in seconds between the onset of the P wave and the onset of the first wave of the QRS complex, be it a Q, R, or QS wave
◆ Determine if all of the P waves are followed by QRS complexes
◆ Compare the PR intervals to determine if all PR intervals are equal in duration
◆ Determine the AV conduction ratio by noting the number of P (or F) waves followed by QRS complexes in a given set of P (or F) waves

A normal PR interval is 0.12 to 0.20 second in duration (Figure 4-15). It indicates that the electrical impulse causing the P wave originated in the SA node or upper or middle part of the atria. It also indicates that the conduction of the electrical impulse through the AV node and the bundle of His is normal. When the heart rate is fast, the PR interval is shorter than when it is slow.

A PR interval less than 0.12 second or one greater than 0.20 second is abnormal (Figure 4-16).
◆ If the PR interval is less than 0.12 second, it indicates (1) that the electrical impulse originated in the lower part of the atria or in the AV junction or (2) that the electrical impulse progressed from the atria to the ventricles through an abnormal accessory conduction pathway and not through the AV node and bundle of His or the AV node alone.
◆ If the PR interval is greater than 0.20 second, it indicates a delay in the conduction of the electrical impulse through the AV node, bundle of His, or, rarely, the bundle branches. When this occurs and the PR intervals are equal, a first-degree AV block is present (Table 4-3).

If a P wave follows the QRS complex, the P prime or P' wave, an RP' interval is present, indicating that the electrical impulse responsible for the P' wave and QRS complex has originated in the lower part of the AV junction or in the ventricles. An RP' interval is usually 0.20 second or less.

If a QRS complex does not follow a P wave, a PR interval is absent. This indicates a blockage of the conduction of the electrical impulse through the AV node, bundle of His, or bundle branches into the ventricles. If QRS complexes follow some P waves and not others, an incomplete AV block (second-degree AV block) is present. There are several kinds of second-degree AV blocks—type I AV block (Wenckebach AV block) and type II AV block (the two classic forms) and 2:1 and advanced AV block. Often type I and type II AV blocks are referred to as *Mobitz type I* and *Mobitz type II* AV blocks, respectively (see Chapter 9).
◆ If the PR intervals are unequal, determine if there is an increase in their duration until a P wave is not followed by a QRS complex (nonconducted P wave or dropped beat). This indicates that there is, typically, a progressive delay in the conduction of the electrical impulse through the AV node (or, less commonly, the bundle of His or bundle branches) into the ventricles until conduction is completely blocked. This kind of second-degree AV block, which occurs cyclically, is called a type I AV block (Wenckebach AV block).
◆ If the PR intervals are equal, the second-degree AV block is either a type II AV block, a 2:1 AV block, or an advanced AV block. To determine which one is present, the AV conduction ratio is determined. This is the number of P waves followed by QRS complexes in a given set of P waves. The following are examples of AV conduction ratios (Figure 4-17).
  ◇ If all P waves are followed by QRS complexes, the AV conduction ratio is 1:1.
  ◇ If, for every two P waves one is followed by a QRS complex, the AV conduction ratio is 2:1.
  ◇ If, for every three P waves two are followed by QRS complexes, the AV conduction ratio is 3:2.

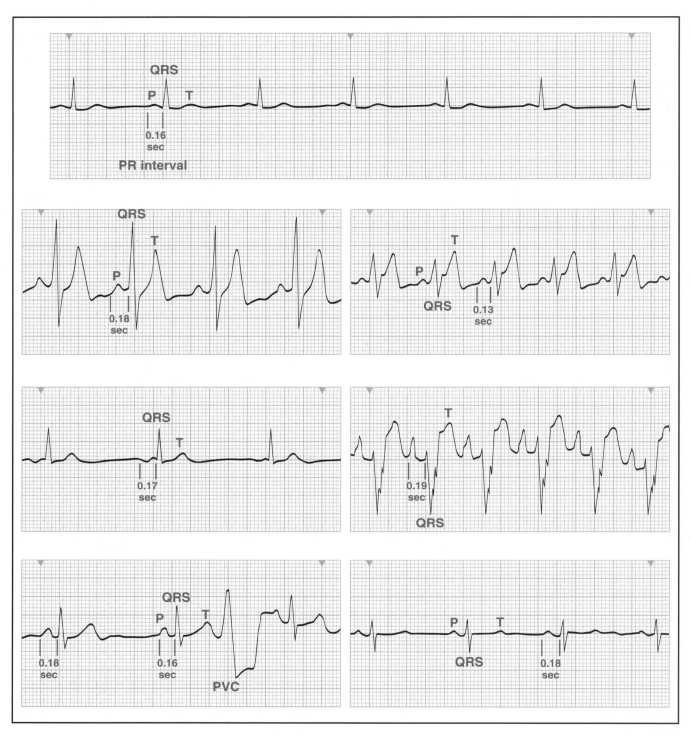

Figure 4-15   Normal PR intervals.

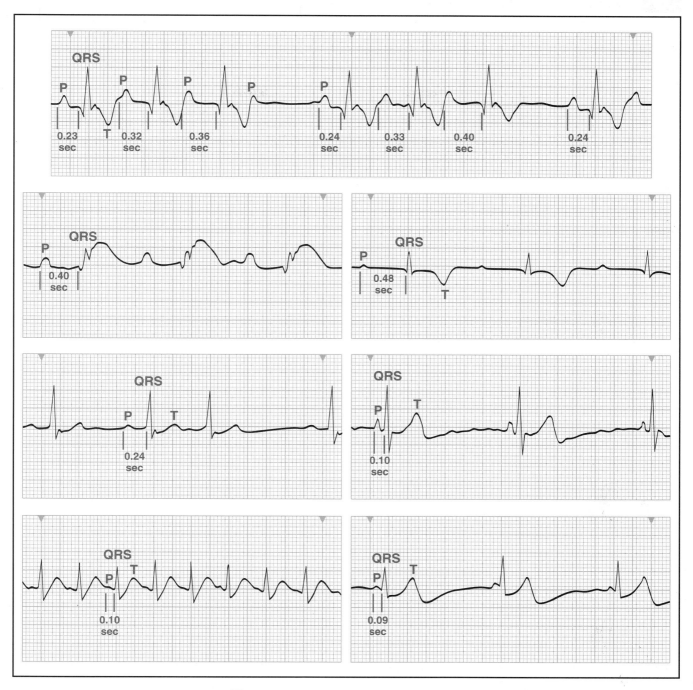

Figure 4-16 Abnormal PR intervals.

4-3 PR Intervals and AV Conduction Ratios in Relation to AV Blocks

AV Block	PR Intervals	AV Conduction Ratio
First-degree AV block	Prolonged, equal	1:1
Second-degree AV block		
Type I AV block (Wenckebach)	Gradually lengthening	5:4, 4:3, 3:2 *or* 6:5, 7:6, etc.
Type II AV block	Equal	3:2, 4:3, 5:4, etc.
2:1 AV block	Equal	2:1
Advanced AV block	Equal	3:1, 4:1, 5:1, etc.
Third-degree AV block	No relationship of P to R waves	None

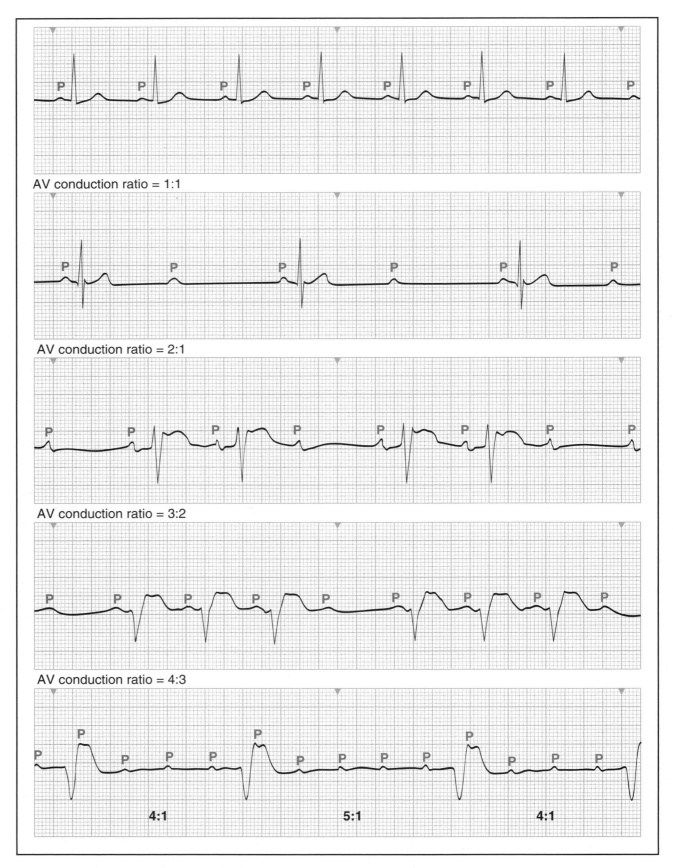

AV conduction ratio = 1:1

AV conduction ratio = 2:1

AV conduction ratio = 3:2

AV conduction ratio = 4:3

4:1   5:1   4:1

Figure 4-17   Examples of AV conduction ratios.

◇ If, for every four P waves three are followed by QRS complexes and one is not, the AV conduction ratio is 4:3.

◇ If, for every five P waves, one is followed by a QRS complex, the AV conduction ratio is 5:1.

If the AV conduction ratio is 3:2, 4:3, 5:4, etc., a type II AV block is present. If the AV conduction ratio is 2:1, a 2:1 AV block is present. If the AV conduction ratio is 3:1, 4:1, 5:1, etc., an advanced AV block is present.

If QRS complexes are present but do not regularly precede or follow the P waves, a complete AV block (third-degree AV block) is present. Another term used to describe the condition when QRS complexes occur totally unrelated to the P, P′, or F waves is *AV dissociation.*

Notes

_____

_____

_____

_____

_____

_____

_____

_____

STEP FIVE: IDENTIFY AND ANALYZE THE QRS COMPLEXES

◆ Identify the QRS complexes.

◆ Note the duration and shape of the QRS complexes. The QRS complexes may be normal (0.10 second or less wide) or abnormal (greater than 0.10 second wide and bizarre appearing).

◆ Compare the QRS complexes to determine if all QRS complexes are equal in duration and shape or if one or more of the QRS complexes differ from the others.

A normal QRS complex, one that is 0.10 second or less in width (Figure 4-18), indicates that the electrical impulse responsible for it originated in the SA node, atria, or AV junction (i.e., supraventricular in origin) and that the electrical impulse progressed normally through the ventricles.

An abnormal QRS complex, one that is 0.12 second or greater in width and bizarre in appearance, indicates that the electrical impulse responsible for it progressed through the ventricles abnor-

mally. The cause may be any one of the following arrhythmias:

KEY DEFINITION

◆ **Ventricular arrhythmias.** *Ectopic or escape beats and rhythms originating in the ventricles.*

◆ **Supraventricular arrhythmias.** *Arrhythmias originating in the SA node, atria, or AV junction with one of the following:*

◇ **Bundle branch block.** *A block in the conduction of electrical impulses through the right or left bundle branch caused by heart disease.*

◇ **Intraventricular conduction defect (IVCD).** *A delay or blockage of conduction of electrical impulses through the myocardium caused by heart disease (myocardial infarction, fibrosis, and hypertrophy), electrolyte imbalance, and excessive administration of certain drugs.*

◇ **Aberrant ventricular conduction (aberrancy).** *A transient bundle branch block caused by the arrival of electrical impulses at a bundle branch while it is still in the refractory stage.*

◇ **Ventricular preexcitation.** *Disfigurement (slurring and sometimes notching) of the initial upstroke (or downstroke) of the QRS complex by a delta wave caused by premature depolarization of the ventricles. This results when an electrical impulse in the atria bypasses the AV junction or bundle of His, entering the ventricles via an abnormal accessory conduction pathway.*

If all of the QRS complexes are equal and normal in duration and shape, they are most likely supraventricular in origin (i.e., in the SA node, atria, or AV junction). If all of the QRS complexes are equal and abnormal in duration and shape, their origin may be either (1) ventricular or (2) supraventricular with bundle branch block, intraventricular conduction defect, aberrancy, or ventricular preexcitation.

If, amongst QRS complexes that are equal and normal in duration and shape, QRS complexes occur that are abnormal in duration and shape, the origin of the abnormal QRS complexes may be either (1) ventricular (e.g., premature ventricular contractions) or (2) supraventricular with aber-

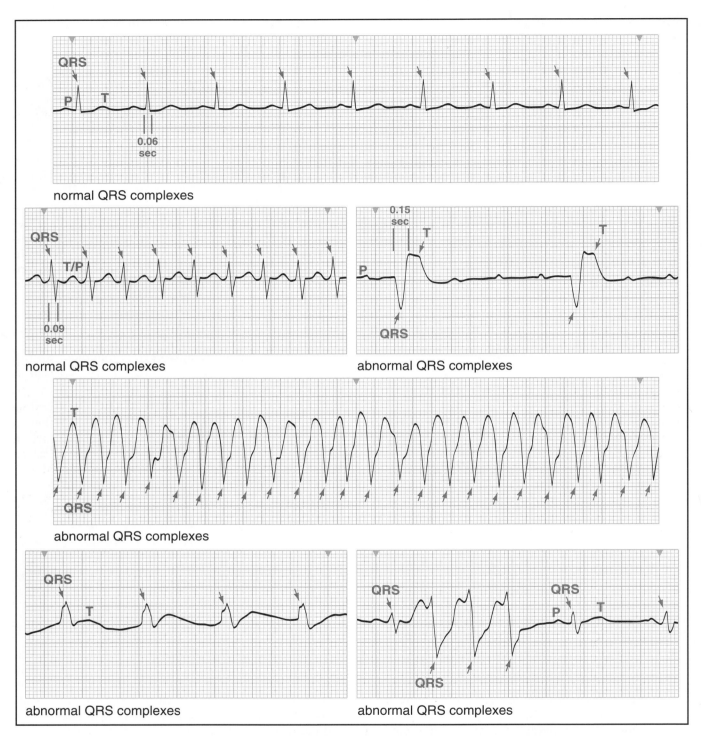

Figure 4-18   Identifying the QRS complexes.

rancy (e.g., atrial and junctional premature contractions with aberrancy).

One of the clues as to whether the abnormal complexes are supraventricular or ventricular in origin is the presence of P waves. If P waves precede or immediately follow the abnormal QRS complexes, the origin of the electrical impulses responsible for the QRS complexes are most likely supraventricular. On the other hand, if no P waves are associated with the abnormal QRS complexes, these QRS complexes are most likely ventricular in origin.

Notes

_____

_____

_____

_____

_____

_____

_____

_____

STEP SIX: DETERMINE THE SITE OF ORIGIN OF THE ARRHYTHMIA

◆ Determine the site of origin of the arrhythmia by analyzing the P waves, the QRS complexes, and their association to each other.

If P waves are associated with the QRS complexes (i.e., the P waves regularly precede or follow the QRS complexes), the site of origin (or pacemaker site) of the arrhythmia is that of the P waves (Figure 4-19). Conversely, if the P waves are not associated with the QRS complexes (i.e., the P waves and the QRS complexes occur independently of each other [AV dissociation]), or if the P waves are absent, the site of origin of the arrhythmia is that of the QRS complexes (Figure 4-20).

The electrical impulses causing the P waves may have originated in the SA node or an ectopic or escape pacemaker in the atria, AV junction, or ventricles. The site of origin of the electrical impulses responsible for the P waves can usually be deduced by noting the direction of the P waves in lead II and their relationship to the QRS complexes. Table 4-4 summarizes the determination of the pacemaker site of arrhythmias with P waves associated with the QRS complexes.

◆ If the P waves are upright (positive) in lead II, the electrical impulses responsible for them may have originated either in the SA node or upper or middle right atrium. When upright P waves have a set relationship to the QRS complexes, they always precede the QRS complexes. The PR interval may be normal (0.12 to 0.20 second), prolonged (greater than 0.20 second, indicating first-degree AV block), or short (less than 0.12 second, indicating an accessory conduction pathway).

◆ If the P waves are negative (inverted) in lead II (P'), the electrical impulses responsible for them may have originated in the lower part of the atria near the AV junction, in the AV junction itself, or in the ventricles. The exact location of the site of origin of negative P' waves can be deduced by analyzing their relationship to the QRS complexes in lead II as follows:

◇ If the negative P' waves regularly precede the QRS complexes, the electrical impulses responsible for the P' waves (and the QRS complexes as well) may have originated either in the lower part of the atria near the AV junction or in the proximal part of the AV junction itself. Typically, the P'R interval is less than 0.12 second, but it may be greater if first-degree AV block is present.

◇ If the negative P' waves regularly follow the QRS complexes, the electrical impulses responsible for the P' waves (and the QRS complexes as well) may have originated either in the distal part of the AV junction or in the ventricles. If the QRS complexes are greater than 0.12 second in duration and appear bizarre, it is more likely that the P' waves originated in the ventricles. The RP' intervals are usually less than 0.20 second.

◇ If the negative P' waves have no set relationship to the QRS complexes, occurring at a rate different from that of the QRS complexes (i.e., AV dissociation), the electrical impulses responsible for the P' waves may have originated either in the lower part of the atria near the AV junction or in the AV junction. The electrical impulses responsible for the QRS complexes may have originated in the AV junction or the ventricles.

◆ If atrial flutter or fibrillation waves are present, the electrical impulses responsible for them have originated in the atria.

If the QRS complexes have no set relationship to the P waves, occurring at a rate different from that of the P waves, or if P waves are absent, the electrical impulses causing the QRS complexes may have originated in an ectopic or escape pacemaker in the AV junction or ventricles (i.e., bundle branch, Purkinje network, or ventricular myocardium).

The site of origin of the electrical impulses responsible for such QRS complexes can be deduced by noting the duration and shape of the QRS complex and whether or not a preexisting bundle branch block, an intraventricular conduction defect, or aberrant ventricular conduction is present. Often, the pacemaker site of wide and bizarre QRS complexes, occurring independently of the P waves or in their absence, cannot be determined with accuracy based on an ECG obtained from a single monitoring lead II. In such instances, a 12-lead ECG or lead MCL1 is extremely helpful. Table 4-5 summarizes the determination of the pacemaker site of arrhythmias with QRS complexes not associated with P waves.

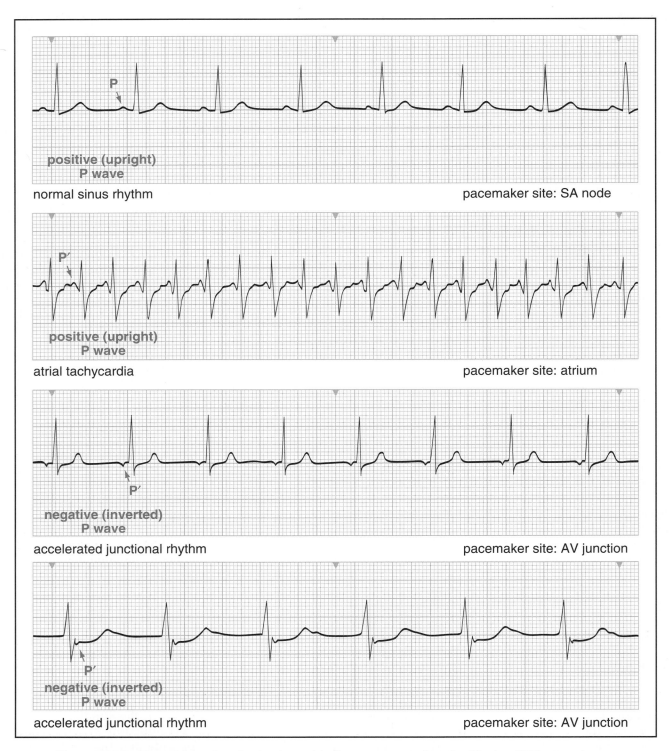

normal sinus rhythm   pacemaker site: SA node

atrial tachycardia   pacemaker site: atrium

accelerated junctional rhythm   pacemaker site: AV junction

accelerated junctional rhythm   pacemaker site: AV junction

Figure 4-19 Examples of arrhythmias with P waves associated with the QRS complexes.

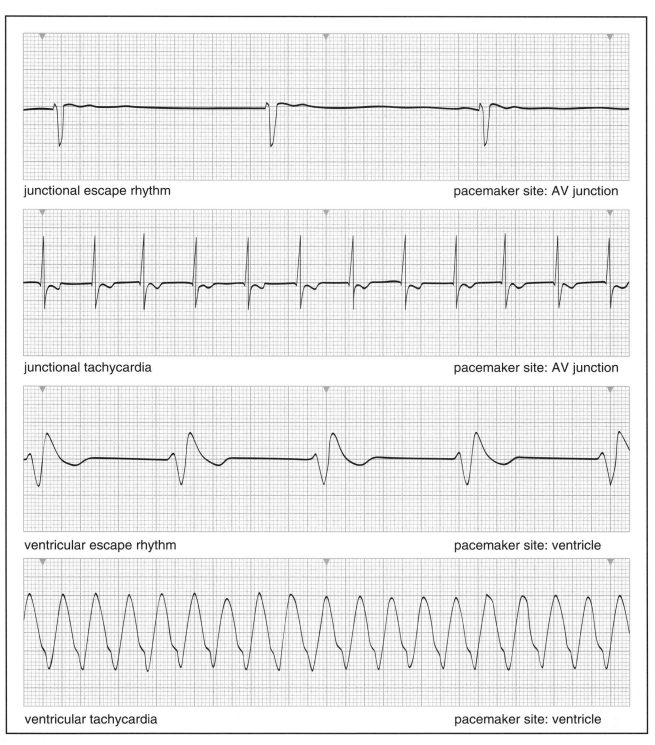

junctional escape rhythm   pacemaker site: AV junction

junctional tachycardia   pacemaker site: AV junction

ventricular escape rhythm   pacemaker site: ventricle

ventricular tachycardia   pacemaker site: ventricle

Figure 4-20 Examples of arrhythmias with QRS complexes not associated with P waves.

TABLE

4-4 Determination of the Pacemaker Site of Arrhythmias With P Waves Associated With the QRS Complexes

Pacemaker Site	Direction of P Waves in Lead II	P/QRS Relationship	PR Interval
SA node or Upper or middle right atrium	Positive (upright)	P precedes QRS complex	0.12-0.20 sec or greater or less than 0.12 sec*
Lower atria or Proximal AV junction	Negative (inverted)	P precedes QRS complex	Less than 0.12 sec
Distal AV junction or Ventricles	Negative (inverted)	P follows QRS complex	None (RP' interval, <0.20 sec)

*In association with an accessory conduction pathway.

TABLE

4-5 Determination of the Pacemaker Site of Arrhythmias With QRS Complexes Not Associated With P Waves

Pacemaker Site	QRS Complex	
	Duration	Appearance
AV junction	0.10 sec or less	Normal
AV junction* or Proximal bundle branch	0.10-0.12 sec	Normal
AV junction† or Distal bundle branch, Purkinje network, or ventricular myocardium	Greater than 0.12 sec	Bizarre

*In association with a preexisting incomplete bundle branch block, an intraventricular conduction defect, or aberrant ventricular conduction.
†In association with a preexisting complete bundle branch block, an intraventricular conduction defect, or aberrant ventricular conduction.

◆ If the QRS complexes are 0.10 second or less in duration, the electrical impulses responsible for the QRS complexes most likely have originated in the AV junction.

◆ If the QRS complexes are between 0.10 and 0.12 second in duration, the electrical impulses responsible for the QRS complexes may have originated in the AV junction (in which case, a preexisting incomplete bundle branch block, an intraventricular conduction defect, or aberrant ventricular conduction has to be present) or in the proximal part of a bundle branch in the ventricles near the bundle of His.

◆ If the QRS complexes are greater than 0.12 second in duration and appear bizarre, the electrical impulses responsible for the QRS complexes may have originated in the AV junction (in which case, a preexisting complete bundle branch block, an intraventricular conduction defect, or aberrant ventricular conduction has to be present) or in the distal part of a bundle branch, the Purkinje network, or ventricular myocardium.

Notes

_____

_____

_____

_____

STEP SEVEN: IDENTIFY THE ARRHYTHMIA

The identification of arrhythmias is presented in detail in Chapters 5 through 9.

STEP EIGHT: EVALUATE THE SIGNIFICANCE OF THE ARRHYTHMIA

The evaluation of the significance of arrhythmias is presented in detail in Chapter 5 through 9.

CHAPTER REVIEW QUESTIONS

1. The heart rate can be determined by:
   A. the 6-second count method
   B. a heart rate calculator ruler
   C. the R-R interval method
   D. all of the above

2. In adults, a heart rate less than _____ beats per minute indicates _____, and a heart rate greater than _____ per minute indicates _____.
   A. 60, bradycardia; 120, tachycardia
   B. 50, tachycardia; 120, bradycardia
   C. 60, bradycardia; 100, tachycardia
   D. 50, bradycardia; 100, bradycardia

3. The rhythm must be regular if the calculation of the heart rate is to be accurate using the _____ method.
   A. triplicate
   B. R-R interval
   C. both of the above
   D. none of the above

4. If there are four large squares between the peaks of two consecutive R waves, the heart rate is _____ beats per minute.
   A. 50
   B. 75
   C. 100
   D. 150

5. The rate of the P waves is:
   A. the same as that of the QRS complexes
   B. sometimes less than the rate of QRS complexes
   C. greater than the QRS rate in AV block
   D. all of the above

6. If QRS complexes are present but do not regularly precede or follow the P waves:
   A. a complete AV block is present
   B. the AV conduction ratio should be calculated
   C. an incomplete AV block is present
   D. none of the above

7. If atrial flutter or fibrillation waves are present, the electrical impulses responsible for them have originated in the:
   A. ventricle
   B. atria
   C. septum
   D. bundle of His

8. The pacemaker site of inverted P waves in lead II is in the:
   A. ventricles
   B. lower atria
   C. AV junction
   D. all of the above

9. A PR interval of less than 0.12 second indicates that the pacemaker site of the P wave is in the:
   A. AV junction
   B. lower right atrium near the AV node
   C. upper right atrium with an accessory AV pathway present
   D. all of the above

10. If the QRS complexes are 0.10 second or less in duration, the electrical impulses responsible for the QRS complexes most likely have originated in the:
    A. SA node
    B. Purkinje network
    C. AV junction in the presence of a right bundle branch block
    D. interventricular septum

11. A QRS that has a bizarre appearance and a duration greater than 0.12 second most likely has a pacemaker site in (the):
    A. AV junction in the presence of aberrant ventricular conduction
    B. Purkinje network
    C. ventricular myocardium
    D. all of the above

12. If, for every three P waves two are followed by QRS complexes, the AV conduction ratio is:
    A. 2:1
    B. 3:1
    C. 3:2
    D. 2:3

Sinus Node Arrhythmias

CHAPTER OBJECTIVES

Upon completion of all or part of this chapter, you should be able to complete the following objective:
1. Define and give the diagnostic characteristics, cause, and clinical significance of the following arrhythmias:
   Normal sinus rhythm (NSR)
   Sinus arrhythmia
   Sinus bradycardia
   Sinus arrest
   Sinoatrial (SA) exit block
   Sinus tachycardia

NORMAL SINUS RHYTHM

KEY DEFINITION

Normal sinus rhythm (NSR) *(Figure 5-1)* is the normal rhythm of the heart, originating in the sinoatrial (SA) node, and characterized by a heart rate of 60 to 100 beats per minute.

Diagnostic Characteristics

Heart rate. The heart rate is 60 to 100 beats per minute.

Rhythm. The atrial and ventricular rhythms are essentially regular.

Pacemaker site. The pacemaker site is the SA node.

P waves. The sinus P waves are identical and precede each QRS complex. They are positive (upright) in lead II.

PR intervals. The PR intervals are normal (0.12 to 0.20 second) and generally constant but may vary slightly with the heart rate.

R-R and P-P intervals. The R-R intervals may be equal or vary slightly. The difference between the longest and shortest R-R (or P-P) interval is less than 0.16 second in normal sinus rhythm.

QRS complexes. A QRS complex typically follows each P wave. The QRS complexes are normal (0.10 second or less) unless a preexisting intraventricular conduction disturbance (such as a bundle branch block) is present, in which case the QRS complexes are abnormal (greater than 0.10 second).

Clinical Significance

Normal sinus rhythm with a palpable pulse is of no clinical significance and requires no specific treatment per se. If a pulse is not palpable in the presence of a normal sinus rhythm as shown on the electrocardiogram (ECG), the treatment is that of pulseless electrical activity (PEA), which is described later.

Normal Sinus Rhythm

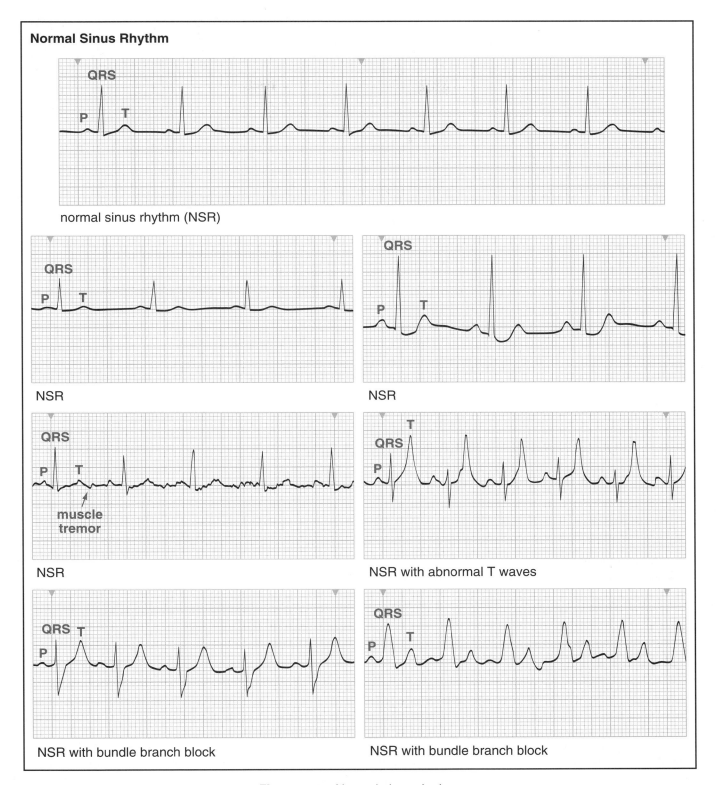

normal sinus rhythm (NSR)

NSR

NSR

NSR

NSR with abnormal T waves

NSR with bundle branch block

NSR with bundle branch block

Figure 5-1 Normal sinus rhythm.

Notes

_____

_____

_____

_____

_____

_____

_____

_____

SINUS ARRHYTHMIA

> **KEY DEFINITION**
>
> **Sinus arrhythmia** *(Figure 5-2) is an irregularity of the heart beat caused by a cyclic increase and decrease in the rate of a sinus rhythm.*

Diagnostic Characteristics

Heart rate. The heart rate is 60 to 100 beats per minute. Occasionally, the heart rate may slow to less than 60 and increase to over 100 beats per minute. Typically, the heart rate increases during inspiration and decreases during expiration.

Rhythm. The atrial and ventricular rhythms are regularly irregular as the heart rate gradually increases and slows; the changes in rate occur in cycles.

Pacemaker site. The pacemaker site is the SA node.

P waves. The sinus P waves are identical and precede each QRS complex. They are positive (upright) in lead II. Sinus arrhythmia is considered to be present when the difference between the longest and shortest P-P (or R-R) interval is greater than 0.16 second.

PR intervals. The PR intervals are normal and constant.

R-R intervals. The R-R intervals are unequal. The most common type of sinus arrhythmia is related to respiration in which the R-R intervals become shorter during inspiration as the heart rate increases and longer during expiration as the heart rate decreases. In another, less common type of sinus arrhythmia, the R-R intervals become shorter and longer without any relation to respiration. The difference between the longest and shortest R-R interval is greater than 0.16 second in sinus arrhythmia.

QRS complexes. A QRS complex normally follows each P wave. The QRS complexes are normal unless a preexisting intraventricular conduction disturbance (such as a bundle branch block) is present.

Cause of Arrhythmia

The most common type of sinus arrhythmia, the one related to respiration, is a normal phenomenon commonly seen in children, young adults, and elderly individuals. It is caused by the changes in vagal tone that occur during respiration. The vagal tone decreases during inspiration, causing the heart rate to increase, and increases during expiration, causing the heart rate to decrease.

The other, less common type of sinus arrhythmia is not related to respiration. It may occur in healthy individuals, but it is more commonly found in adult patients with heart disease, especially after acute inferior myocardial infarction (MI), or in patients receiving certain drugs, such as digitalis and morphine.

Clinical Significance

Usually, sinus arrhythmia is of no clinical significance per se and generally does not require treatment. Marked sinus arrhythmia may cause palpitations, dizziness, and even syncope.

Notes

_____

_____

_____

_____

_____

SINUS BRADYCARDIA

> **KEY DEFINITION**
>
> **Sinus bradycardia** *(Figure 5-3) is an arrhythmia originating in the SA node, characterized by a rate of less than 60 beats per minute.*

Diagnostic Characteristics

Heart rate. The heart rate is less than 60 beats per minute.

Rhythm. The rhythm is essentially regular, but it may be irregular if sinus arrhythmia is also present.

Pacemaker site. The pacemaker site is the SA node.

P waves. The sinus P waves are identical and precede each QRS complex. They are positive (upright) in lead II.

PR intervals. The PR intervals are normal and constant. However, they tend to be at the upper limits of normal.

Sinus Arrhythmia

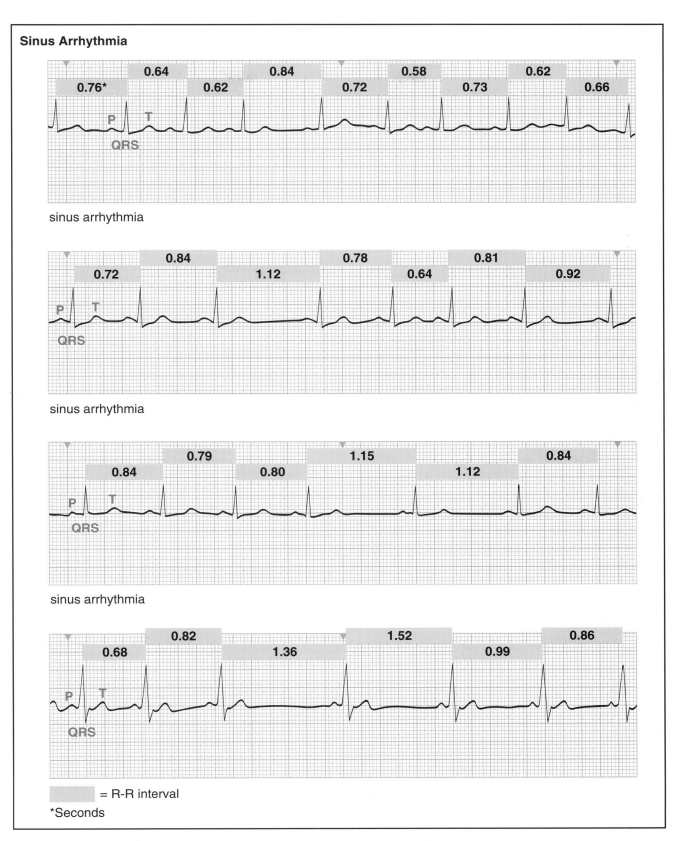

sinus arrhythmia

sinus arrhythmia

sinus arrhythmia

= R-R interval

*Seconds

Figure 5-2 Sinus arrhythmia.

Sinus Bradycardia

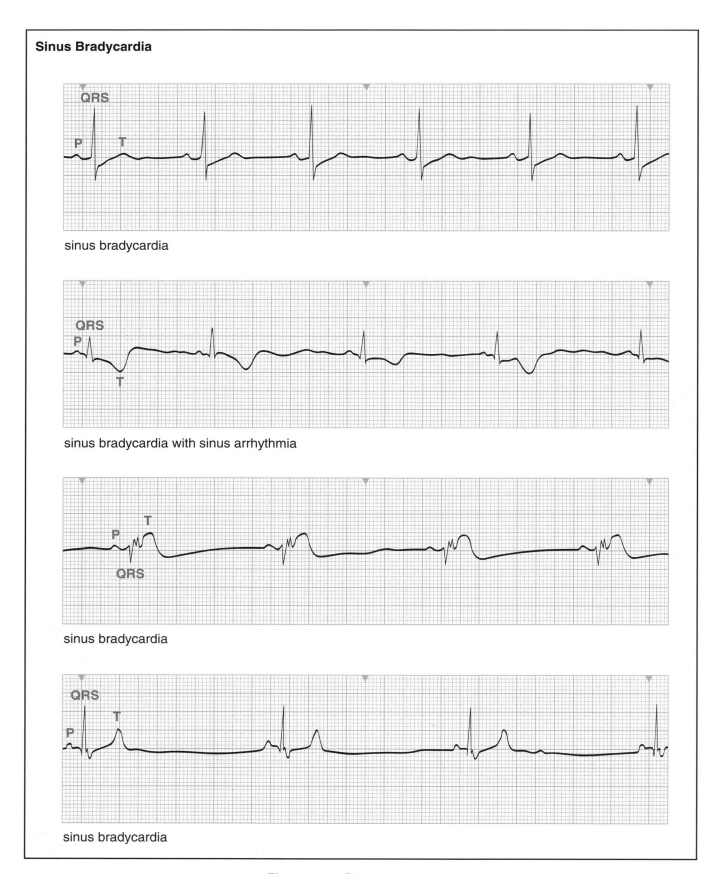

sinus bradycardia

sinus bradycardia with sinus arrhythmia

sinus bradycardia

sinus bradycardia

Figure 5-3 Sinus bradycardia.

R-R intervals. The R-R intervals are usually equal but may vary.

QRS complexes. A QRS complex normally follows each P wave. The QRS complexes are normal unless a preexisting intraventricular conduction disturbance (such as a bundle branch block) is present.

Cause of Arrhythmia

Sinus bradycardia may be caused by any of the following:

◆ Excessive inhibitory vagal (parasympathetic) tone on the SA node as may be caused by carotid sinus stimulation, vomiting, Valsalva maneuvers, or neurocardiogenic (vasovagal) syncope (sudden loss of consciousness after extreme emotional stress or prolonged standing)
◆ Decrease in sympathetic tone on the SA node as may be caused by β-blockers (e.g., atenolol, metoprolol, propranolol)
◆ Administration of calcium channel blockers (e.g., diltiazem, verapamil, nefedipine)
◆ Digitalis toxicity
◆ Disease in the SA node, such as sick sinus syndrome
◆ Acute inferior and right ventricular MI
◆ Hypothyroidism (myxedema)
◆ Hypothermia
◆ Hypoxia
◆ During sleep and in trained athletes

Clinical Significance

Sinus bradycardia with a heart rate between 50 to 59 beats per minute (mild sinus bradycardia) usually does not produce symptoms by itself. Such a bradycardia without symptoms is an *asymptomatic* bradycardia. In the presence of acute MI, mild sinus bradycardia may actually be beneficial in some patients because of the decrease in the workload of the heart, which reduces the oxygen requirements of the myocardium, minimizes the extension of the infarction, and lessens the predisposition to certain arrhythmias.

If the heart rate is 30 to 45 beats per minute or less (marked sinus bradycardia), hypotension with a marked reduction in cardiac output and decreased perfusion of the brain and other vital organs may occur. This may result in the following signs, symptoms, and conditions:

◆ Dizziness, lightheadedness, decreased level of consciousness, or syncope
◆ Shortness of breath
◆ Chest pain
◆ Hypotension
◆ Shock
◆ Pulmonary congestion
◆ Congestive heart failure
◆ Acute MI

◆ Predisposition to more serious arrhythmias (i.e., premature ventricular contractions, ventricular tachycardia or fibrillation, or ventricular asystole)

When symptoms occur, the bradycardia is called a *symptomatic* bradycardia regardless of the heart rate. Symptomatic sinus bradycardia, whatever the heart rate, must be treated promptly with atropine or a transcutaneous pacemaker to reverse the consequences of reduced cardiac output and to prevent the occurrence of serious ventricular arrhythmias.

Notes

_____

_____

_____

_____

_____

_____

_____

_____

SINUS ARREST AND SINOATRIAL EXIT BLOCK

> ### KEY DEFINITION
>
> **Sinus arrest** *(Figure 5-4)* is an arrhythmia caused by episodes of failure in the automaticity of the SA node, resulting in bradycardia, asystole, or both.
>
> **Sinoatrial (SA) exit block** *(Figure 5-4)* is an arrhythmia caused by a block in the conduction of the electrical impulse from the SA node to the atria, resulting (like sinus arrest) in bradycardia, asystole, or both.

Diagnostic Characteristics

Heart rate. The heart rate is usually 60 to 100 beats per minute but may be less.

Rhythm. The rhythm is irregular when sinus arrest or SA exit block is present.

Pacemaker site. The pacemaker site is the SA node.

P waves. The sinus P waves of the underlying rhythm are identical and precede each QRS complex. If an electrical impulse is not generated by the SA node (sinus arrest), or if it is generated by the SA

**Sinus Arrest and
Sinoatrial Exit Block**

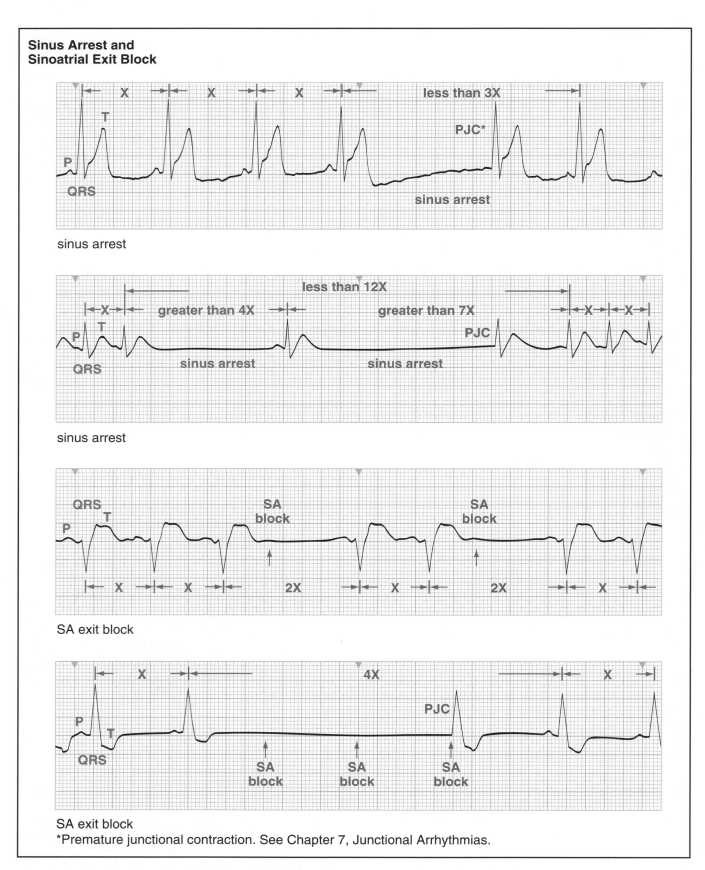

Figure 5-4 Sinus arrest and SA exit block.

node but blocked from entering the atria (SA exit block), atrial depolarization does not occur and, consequently, neither does a P wave (dropped P wave). Often, it is difficult to distinguish sinus arrest from SA exit block when a P wave does not occur. Typically, an SA exit block is indicated by the absence of the normally expected sinus P wave(s) on the ECG.

In addition, the long P-P interval caused by SA exit block is twice (or a multiple of) the P-P interval of the underlying rhythm because the underlying rhythm remains undisturbed. The long P-P interval caused by sinus arrest is, typically, not a multiple of the P-P interval of the underlying rhythm because the timing of the SA node is reset by the arrest.

PR intervals. The PR intervals are those of the underlying rhythm and may be normal or abnormal.

R-R intervals. The R-R intervals are unequal when sinus arrest or SA exit block is present.

QRS complexes. A QRS complex normally follows each P wave. The QRS complexes are normal unless a preexisting intraventricular conduction disturbance (such as a bundle branch block) is present. A QRS complex is absent when a P wave does not occur.

Cause of Arrhythmia

Sinus arrest results from a marked depression in the automaticity of the SA node. SA exit block results from a block in the conduction of the electrical impulse from the SA node into the atria.

Sinus arrest or SA exit block may be precipitated by any of the following:

◆ Increase in vagal (parasympathetic) tone on the SA node
◆ Hypoxia
◆ Hyperkalemia
◆ Excessive dose of digitalis, β-blockers (e.g., atenolol, metoprolol, propranolol), or quinidine
◆ Damage to the SA node or adjacent atrium from acute inferior and right ventricular MI, acute myocarditis, or degenerative forms of fibrosis

Clinical Significance

Transient sinus arrest and SA exit block may have no clinical significance per se if an AV junctional escape pacemaker takes over promptly. If a ventricular escape pacemaker takes over with a slow heart rate or if an escape pacemaker does not take over at all, resulting in transient ventricular asystole, lightheadedness may occur, followed by syncope. The signs and symptoms, clinical significance, and management of sinus arrest and SA exit block with excessively slow heart rates are the same as those in symptomatic sinus bradycardia (i.e., atropine or a transcutaneous pacemaker).

Intermittent sinus arrest or SA exit block can, however, progress to prolonged sinus arrest accompanied by lack of electrical activity of the atria (atrial standstill). If a junctional or ventricular escape pacemaker does not take over, ventricular asystole occurs, requiring immediate treatment.

Notes

_____

_____

_____

_____

_____

_____

_____

_____

_____

_____

SINUS TACHYCARDIA

> **KEY DEFINITION**
>
> **Sinus tachycardia *(Figure 5-5)* is an arrhythmia originating in the SA node, characterized by a rate of over 100 beats per minute.**

Diagnostic Characteristics

Heart rate. The heart rate is over 100 beats per minute and may be as high as 180 beats per minute or greater with extreme exertion. The onset and termination of sinus tachycardia are typically gradual. Vagal maneuvers, such as carotid sinus massage, may cause transient slowing of the heart rate, with a gradual return to the prestimulation rate after the carotid massage.

Rhythm. The rhythm is essentially regular.

Pacemaker site. The pacemaker site is the SA node.

P waves. The sinus P waves are usually normal but may be slightly taller and more peaked than usual. The sinus P waves are identical and precede each QRS complex. They are positive (upright) in lead II. When the heart rate is very rapid, the sinus P waves may be buried in the preceding T waves (buried P waves) and not be easily identified. Such combined T and P waves are identified as "T/P" waves.

Sinus Tachycardia

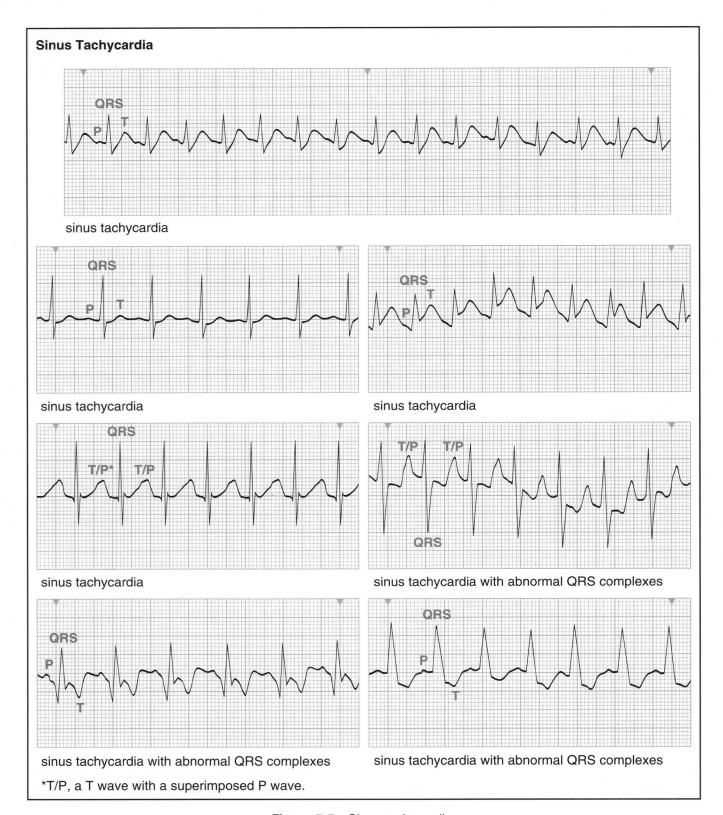

sinus tachycardia

sinus tachycardia

sinus tachycardia

sinus tachycardia

sinus tachycardia with abnormal QRS complexes

sinus tachycardia with abnormal QRS complexes

sinus tachycardia with abnormal QRS complexes

*T/P, a T wave with a superimposed P wave.

Figure 5-5   Sinus tachycardia.

PR intervals. The PR intervals are normal and constant. They are shorter when the heart rate is fast than when the rate is slow.

R-R intervals. The R-R intervals may be equal but may vary slightly.

QRS complexes. The QRS complexes are normal unless a preexisting intraventricular conduction disturbance (such as a bundle branch block) or aberrant ventricular conduction is present. A QRS complex normally follows each P wave. Sinus tachycardia with abnormal QRS complexes may resemble ventricular tachycardia.

Cause of Arrhythmia

Sinus tachycardia in adults is a normal response of the heart to the demand for increased blood flow, as in exercise and exertion. It may also be caused by any of the following:

◆ Ingestion of stimulants (e.g., coffee, tea, and alcohol) or smoking
◆ Increase in catecholamines and sympathetic tone resulting from excitement, anxiety, pain, or stress
◆ Excessive dose of an anticholinergic drug (e.g., atropine) or a sympathomimetic drug (e.g., dopamine, epinephrine, isoproterenol, norepinephrine, or cocaine)
◆ Congestive heart failure
◆ Pulmonary embolism
◆ Myocardial ischemia or acute MI
◆ Fever
◆ Thyrotoxicosis
◆ Anemia
◆ Hypovolemia
◆ Hypoxia
◆ Hypotension or shock

Clinical Significance

Sinus tachycardia per se in healthy individuals is a benign arrhythmia and does not require treatment.

When its cause is removed or treated, sinus tachycardia resolves gradually and spontaneously. Because a rapid heart rate increases the workload of the heart, the oxygen requirements of the heart are increased. For this reason, sinus tachycardia in acute MI may increase myocardial ischemia and the frequency and severity of chest pain, cause an extension of the infarct or even pump failure (e.g., congestive heart failure, hypotension, and cardiogenic shock), or predispose the patient to more serious arrhythmias.

Treatment of sinus tachycardia should be directed to correcting the underlying cause of the arrhythmia.

Notes

_____

_____

_____

_____

_____

_____

_____

_____

_____

_____

_____

_____

SUMMARY

For a brief summary of the various sinus node arrhythmias discussed in this chapter, see Table 5-1.

TABLE

5-1 Typical Diagnostic ECG Features of Sinus Node Arrhythmias

Arrhythmia	Heart Rate (bpm)	Rhythm	P waves	PR Intervals	QRS Complexes
Normal sinus rhythm	60-100	Regular	Normal	Normal	Normal
Sinus arrhythmia	60-100	Irregular	Normal	Normal	Normal
Sinus bradycardia	<60	Regular	Normal	Normal	Normal
Sinus arrest, SA exit block	60-100	Irregular	Normal	Normal	Normal
Sinus tachycardia	100-180	Regular	Normal; may be peaked	Normal	Normal

*SA, Sinoatrial.

TREATMENT ALGORITHMS

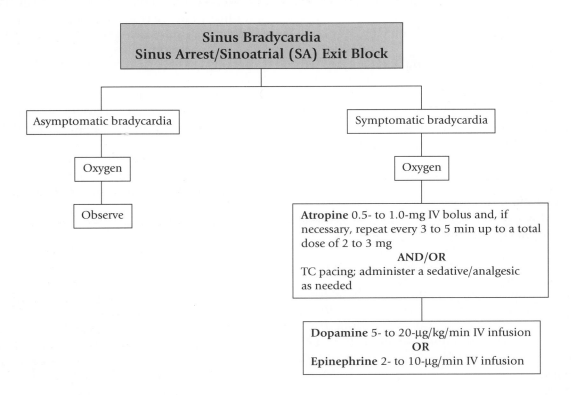

**Sinus Bradycardia
Sinus Arrest/Sinoatrial (SA) Exit Block**

Asymptomatic bradycardia

Oxygen

Observe

Symptomatic bradycardia

Oxygen

Atropine 0.5- to 1.0-mg IV bolus and, if necessary, repeat every 3 to 5 min up to a total dose of 2 to 3 mg
AND/OR
TC pacing; administer a sedative/analgesic as needed

Dopamine 5- to 20-µg/kg/min IV infusion
OR
Epinephrine 2- to 10-µg/min IV infusion

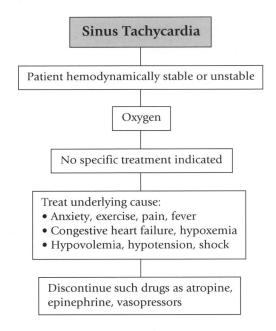

Sinus Tachycardia

Patient hemodynamically stable or unstable

Oxygen

No specific treatment indicated

Treat underlying cause:
• Anxiety, exercise, pain, fever
• Congestive heart failure, hypoxemia
• Hypovolemia, hypotension, shock

Discontinue such drugs as atropine, epinephrine, vasopressors

CHAPTER REVIEW QUESTIONS

1. Typically, the heart rate _____ during inspiration and _____ during expiration.
   A. increases; increases
   B. increases; decreases
   C. decreases; increases
   D. decreases; decreases

2. The most common type of sinus arrhythmia, the one related to respiration, is:
   A. caused by the sympathetic effect on the SA node
   B. extremely rare in children
   C. a normal phenomenon commonly seen in young adults
   D. all of the above

3. Another less common type of sinus arrhythmia is not related to respiration. It may occur in healthy individuals but is more commonly found in adult patients:
   A. with heart disease
   B. with an acute MI
   C. on digitalis
   D. all of the above

4. An arrhythmia originating in the SA node with a regular rate of less than 60 beats per minutes is called:
   A. sinus bradycardia
   B. sinus arrest
   C. first-degree AV block
   D. junctional escape rhythm

5. Sinus bradycardia may be caused by:
   A. excessive inhibitory vagal tone on the SA node
   B. decrease in sympathetic tone on the SA node
   C. hypothermia
   D. all of the above

6. The heart rate in a mild sinus bradycardia is _____ to _____ beats per minute.
   A. 30; 39
   B. 40; 49
   C. 50; 59
   D. 60; 69

7. A patient with marked sinus bradycardia who is symptomatic will likely have:
   A. hypothermia and chest pain
   B. hypotension and decreased cerebral perfusion
   C. hypoxia and increased central venous pressure (CVP)
   D. hypertension and decreased cerebral perfusion

8. Symptomatic sinus bradycardia must be promptly treated with:
   A. isoproterenol and epinephrine
   B. atropine and transcutaneous pacing
   C. lidocaine and oxygen
   D. dopamine and diltiazem (or verapamil)

9. An arrhythmia caused by episodes of failure in the automaticity of the SA node resulting in bradycardia or asystole is called:
   A. marked sinus arrhythmia
   B. Wenckebach phenomenon
   C. sinus arrest
   D. none of the above

10. Sinoatrial (SA) exit block may result from toxicity of the medication(s):
    A. quinidine
    B. digitalis
    C. atenolol
    D. all of the above

6 Atrial Arrhythmias

CHAPTER OUTLINE

Wandering Atrial Pacemaker
Premature Atrial Contractions
Atrial Tachycardia (Ectopic and Multifocal)
Atrial Flutter

Atrial Fibrillation
Summary
Treatment Algorithms

CHAPTER OBJECTIVES

Upon completion of all or part of this chapter, you should be able to complete the following objective:
1. Define and give the diagnostic characteristics, cause, and clinical significance of the following arrhythmias:
   Wandering atrial pacemaker (WAP)
   Premature atrial contractions (PACs)
   Atrial tachycardia
      Ectopic atrial tachycardia
      Multifocal atrial tachycardia (MAT)
   Atrial flutter
   Atrial fibrillation

WANDERING ATRIAL PACEMAKER

KEY DEFINITION

A wandering atrial pacemaker (WAP) (Figure 6-1) is an arrhythmia originating in pacemakers that shift back and forth between the sinoatrial (SA) node and an ectopic pacemaker in the atria or atrioventricular (AV) junction. It is characterized by P waves of varying size, shape, and direction in any one lead.

Diagnostic Characteristics

Heart rate. The heart rate is usually 60 to 100 beats per minute but may be slower. Usually, the heart rate gradually slows slightly when the pacemaker site shifts from the SA node to the atria or AV junction and increases as the pacemaker site shifts back to the SA node.

Rhythm. The rhythm is usually irregular, but, rarely, it may be regular.

Pacemaker site. The pacemaker site shifts back and forth between the SA node and an ectopic pacemaker in the atria or AV junction.

P waves. The P waves gradually change in size, shape, and direction over the duration of several beats. They vary in lead II from normal, positive (upright) P waves to abnormal, negative (inverted) P waves, or even become buried in the QRS complexes as the pacemaker site shifts from the SA node to the atria or AV junction. These changes occur in reverse as the pacemaker site shifts back to the SA node.

The P waves other than those arising in the SA node are ectopic P waves (P' waves). The changing configuration of the P waves distinguishes a WAP from a normal sinus rhythm in which the P waves remain constant in size, shape, and direction throughout a lead.

PR intervals. The duration of the PR intervals usually decreases gradually from about 0.20 second to about 0.12 second or less as the pacemaker site shifts

Wandering Atrial Pacemaker

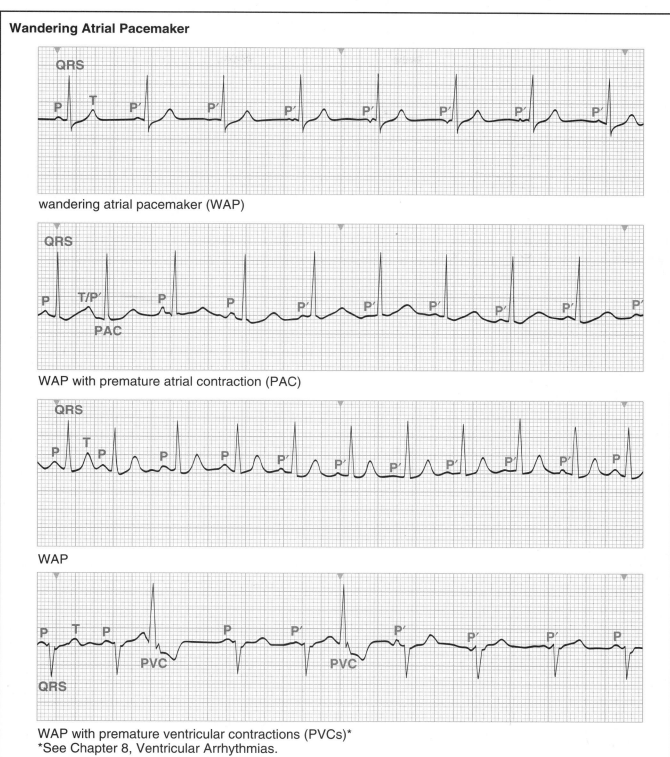

wandering atrial pacemaker (WAP)

WAP with premature atrial contraction (PAC)

WAP

WAP with premature ventricular contractions (PVCs)*
*See Chapter 8, Ventricular Arrhythmias.

Figure 6-1 Wandering atrial pacemaker.

from the SA node to the lower part of the atria or AV junction. The duration of the intervals then gradually increases as the pacemaker site shifts back to the SA node.

R-R intervals. The R-R intervals (and P-P intervals as well) are usually unequal, but they may be equal. They usually increase in duration as the pacemaker site shifts from the SA node to the atria or AV junction and decrease as the pacemaker shifts back to the SA node.

QRS complexes. The QRS complexes are normal unless a preexisting intraventricular conduction disturbance (such as a bundle branch block) is present. A QRS complex normally follows each P wave.

Cause of Arrhythmia

A WAP may be a normal phenomenon seen in the very young or the elderly and in athletes. It is caused in the majority of cases by the inhibitory vagal (parasympathetic) effect of respiration on the SA node and AV junction. It may also be caused by the administration of digitalis.

Clinical Significance

A WAP is usually not clinically significant, and treatment is not indicated. When the heart rate slows excessively, the signs and symptoms, clinical significance, and management are the same as those in symptomatic sinus bradycardia.

Notes

_____
_____
_____
_____
_____
_____
_____
_____
_____
_____
_____
_____
_____
_____
_____
_____
_____

PREMATURE ATRIAL CONTRACTIONS

KEY DEFINITION

A premature atrial contraction (PAC) (Figure 6-2) is an extra P-QRS complex consisting of an abnormal (sometimes normal) P wave followed by a normal or abnormal QRS complex, occurring earlier than the next expected beat of the underlying rhythm, usually a sinus rhythm. A PAC is generally followed by a noncompensatory pause. PACs, which can originate in a single or multiple ectopic pacemakers in the atria, are also called premature atrial beats (PABs) or complexes.

Diagnostic Characteristics

Heart rate. The heart rate is that of the underlying rhythm.

Rhythm. The rhythm is irregular when PACs are present.

Pacemaker site. The pacemaker site of the PAC is an ectopic pacemaker in any part of the atria outside the SA node. PACs may originate from a single ectopic pacemaker site or from multiple sites in the atria.

P waves. A PAC is diagnosed when a P wave accompanied by a QRS complex occurs earlier than the next expected sinus P wave. The premature P wave is called an *ectopic P wave (P')*. Although the P' waves of the PACs may resemble the normal sinus P waves, they are generally different. The size, shape, and direction of the P' waves depend on the location of the pacemaker site. For example, they may appear positive (upright) and quite normal in lead II if the pacemaker site is near the SA node but negative (inverted) if the pacemaker site is near the AV junction, the result of retrograde atrial depolarization. P' waves originating in the same atrial ectopic pacemaker are usually identical. The P' waves precede the QRS complexes and are frequently buried in the preceding T waves, distorting them and often making these T waves more peaked and pointed than the other nonaffected ones. A P' wave followed by a QRS complex is said to be a *conducted* PAC.

If the atrial ectopic pacemaker discharges too soon after the preceding QRS complex—early in diastole, for example—the AV junction or bundle branches may not be repolarized sufficiently to conduct the premature electrical impulse into the ventricles normally. Thus, being still refractory from conducting the previous electrical impulse, the AV junction or

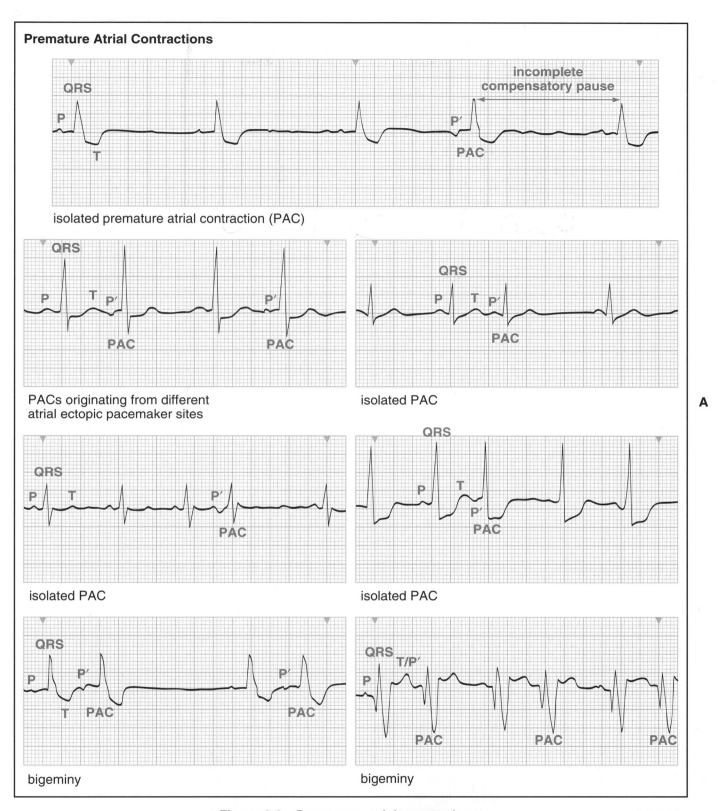

Figure 6-2 Premature atrial contractions.

Continued

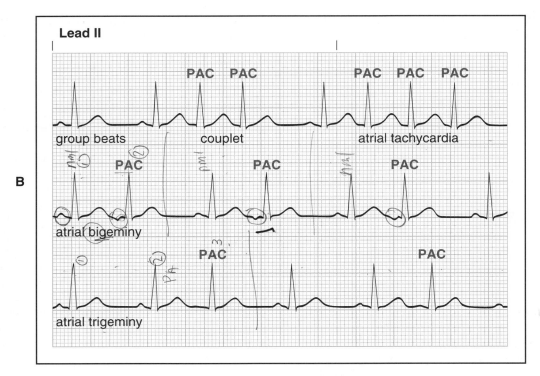

Figure 6-2, cont'd Premature atrial contractions.

bundle branches may either slow the conduction of the premature electrical impulse, prolonging the PR interval (first-degree AV block), or block it completely (complete AV block).

When complete AV block occurs, the P' wave is not followed by a QRS complex. Such a PAC is called a *nonconducted* or *blocked* PAC. Nonconducted PACs are commonly the cause of unexpected pauses in the electrocardiogram (ECG), suggesting sinus arrest or SA exit block.

The interval between the P wave of the QRS complex preceding the PAC and the P' wave of the PAC—the P-P' interval—is typically shorter than the P-P interval of the underlying rhythm. Because the PAC usually depolarizes the SA node prematurely, the timing of the SA node is reset, causing the next cycle of the SA node to begin anew at this point. When this occurs, the next expected P wave of the underlying rhythm appears earlier than it would have if the SA node had not been disturbed. The resulting P'-P interval is called an *incomplete compensatory pause* or a *noncompensatory pause*. This interval may be equal to the P-P interval of the underlying rhythm, or it may be slightly longer because of the depressing effect on the automaticity of the SA node brought on by its being depolarized prematurely. Because of the incomplete compensatory pause, the interval between the P waves of the underlying rhythm preceding and following the PAC is less than twice the P-P interval of the underlying rhythm.

Less commonly, the SA node is not depolarized by the PAC so that its timing is not reset, allowing the next P wave of the underlying rhythm to appear at the time expected. Such a P'-P interval is said to be *fully compensatory*, or a *full compensatory pause*. In this case, the interval between the P waves of the underlying rhythm occurring before and after the PAC is twice the P-P interval of the underlying rhythm. A full compensatory pause may also occur, even if the SA node is prematurely depolarized, if the automaticity of the SA node is excessively depressed after its premature depolarization.

PR intervals. The PR intervals of the PACs may be normal but they usually differ from those of the underlying rhythm. The PR interval of a PAC varies from about 0.20 second when the pacemaker site is near the SA node to about 0.12 second when the pacemaker is near the AV junction. The PAC's PR interval may be greater than 0.20 second if there is a delay in AV conduction (first-degree AV block).

R-R and P-P intervals. The R-R intervals are unequal when PACs are present. The interval between the P wave of the underlying rhythm preceding a PAC and the P' wave of the PAC—the P-P' interval (coupling interval)—varies depending on the ectopic pacemaker's rate of spontaneous depolarization and its location in the atria. Generally, the coupling intervals of PACs originating in the same ectopic pacemaker site are equal.

QRS complexes. The QRS complex of the PAC usually resembles that of the underlying rhythm because the conduction of the electrical impulse through the bundle branches is usually unchanged. If the atrial ectopic pacemaker discharges very soon after the preceding QRS complex, the bundle branches may not be repolarized sufficiently to conduct the electrical impulse of the PAC normally. If this occurs, the electrical impulse may only be conducted down one bundle branch, usually the left one, and blocked in the other. The result is a wide and bizarre-appearing QRS complex that resembles a right bundle branch block. Such a PAC, called a *premature atrial contraction with aberrancy* (or with *aberrant ventricular conduction*), can mimic a premature ventricular contraction (PVC) (see Premature Ventricular Contractions, p. 147).

Usually, a QRS complex follows each P' wave (conducted PACs), but a QRS complex may be absent because of a temporary complete AV block (nonconducted PACs). A nonconducted PAC is also called a *blocked* or *dropped* PAC.

Frequency and pattern of occurrence of PACs. The following are the various forms in which PACs may appear:

◆ **Isolated:** PACs may occur singly (isolated beats).
◆ **Group beats:** The PACs may occur in groups of two or more consecutive beats. Two PACs in a row are called a *couplet*. When three or more PACs occur in succession, atrial tachycardia is considered to be present.
◆ **Repetitive beats:** PACs may alternate with the QRS complexes of the underlying rhythm (atrial bigeminy) or occur after every two QRS complexes (atrial trigeminy) or after every three QRS complexes of the underlying rhythm (atrial quadrigeminy).

Cause of Arrhythmia

Common causes of PACs include the following. Often, however, they appear without apparent cause.

◆ Increase in catecholamines and sympathetic tone
◆ Infections
◆ Emotion
◆ Stimulants (e.g., alcohol, caffeine, and tobacco)
◆ Sympathomimetic drugs (e.g., epinephrine, isoproterenol, and norepinephrine)
◆ Electrolyte imbalance
◆ Hypoxia
◆ Digitalis toxicity
◆ Cardiovascular disease (such as myocardial ischemia, acute myocardial infarction (MI), or early congestive heart failure)
◆ Dilated or hypertrophied atria resulting from increased atrial pressure commonly caused by mitral stenosis or an atrial septal defect

The electrophysiological mechanism responsible for PACs is either enhanced automaticity or reentry.

Clinical Significance

Isolated PACs may occur in persons with apparently healthy hearts and are not significant. In persons with heart disease, however, frequent PACs may indicate enhanced automaticity of the atria, or a reentry mechanism resulting from a variety of causes, such as congestive heart failure or acute MI. In addition, such PACs may warn of or initiate more serious supraventricular arrhythmias, such as atrial tachycardia, atrial flutter, atrial fibrillation, or paroxysmal supraventricular tachycardia (PSVT).

If nonconducted PACs are frequent and the heart rate is less than 50 beats per minute, the signs and symptoms, clinical significance, and management are the same as those of symptomatic sinus bradycardia.

Because PACs with wide and bizarre-appearing QRS complexes (i.e., aberrancy) often resemble PVCs (see p. 147), care must be taken to identify such PACs correctly so as not to treat them inappropriately as PVCs.

Notes

_____

_____

_____

_____

ATRIAL TACHYCARDIA (ECTOPIC AND MULTIFOCAL)

> **KEY DEFINITION**
>
> **Atrial tachycardia *(Figure 6-3)* is an arrhythmia originating in an ectopic pacemaker in the atria with a rate between 160 to 240 beats per minute. It includes ectopic atrial tachycardia and multifocal atrial tachycardia (MAT).**

Diagnostic Characteristics

Heart rate. The atrial rate is usually 160 to 240 beats per minute but may be slower, especially in MAT. The ventricular rate is usually the same as that of the atria, but it may be slower, often half the atrial rate because of a 2:1 AV block. Because atrial tachycardia commonly starts and ends gradually, it is

Atrial Tachycardia
(Ectopic Atrial Tachycardia, Multifocal Atrial Tachycardia)

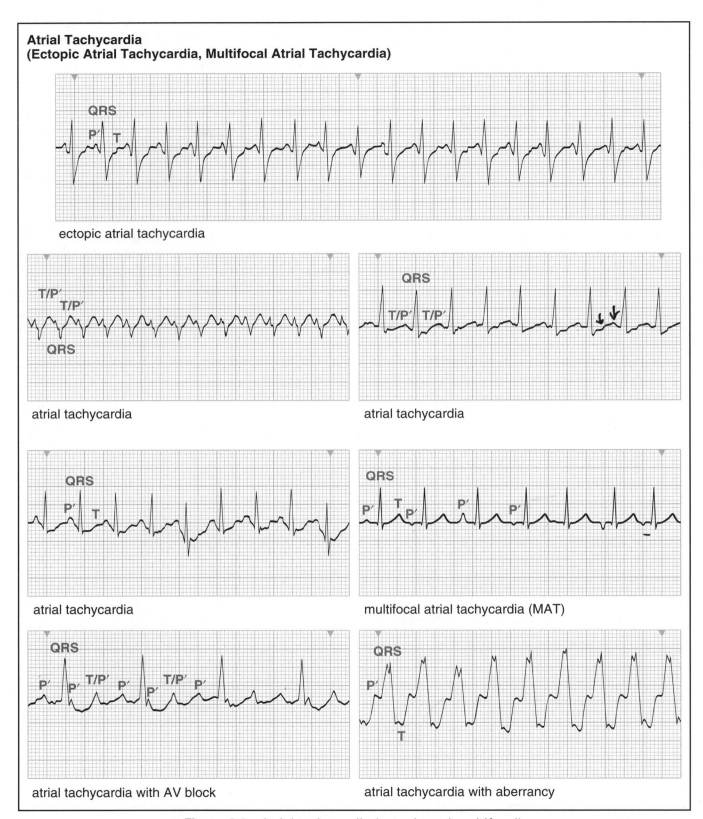

ectopic atrial tachycardia

atrial tachycardia

atrial tachycardia

atrial tachycardia

multifocal atrial tachycardia (MAT)

atrial tachycardia with AV block

atrial tachycardia with aberrancy

Figure 6-3   Atrial tachycardia (ectopic and multifocal).

called a *nonparoxysmal atrial tachycardia*. By definition, three or more consecutive PACs are considered to be atrial tachycardia.

Vagal maneuvers, such as carotid sinus massage, by increasing the parasympathetic (vagal) tone, do not terminate atrial tachycardia abruptly nor slow the atrial rate, but they do impede AV conduction and result in an AV block.

Rhythm. The atrial rhythm is essentially regular. The ventricular rhythm is usually regular if the AV conduction ratio is constant, but it may be irregular if a variable AV block or MAT is present.

Pacemaker site. The pacemaker site is an ectopic pacemaker in any part of the atria outside the SA node. Atrial tachycardia may occasionally originate in more than one atrial ectopic pacemaker site. One that originates in a single ectopic pacemaker site is called an *ectopic atrial tachycardia;* one originating in three or more different ectopic pacemaker sites is called a *multifocal atrial tachycardia (MAT)*. The activity of the SA node is completely suppressed by atrial tachycardia.

P waves. The ectopic P waves in atrial tachycardia usually differ from normal sinus P waves. The size, shape, and direction of the P' waves vary, depending on the location of the pacemaker site. They may appear positive (upright) and quite normal in lead II if the pacemaker site is near the SA node, but negative (inverted) if they originate near the AV junction.

The P' waves are usually identical in ectopic atrial tachycardia and precede each QRS complex. In MAT, on the other hand, the P' waves usually vary in size, shape, and direction in each given lead. The P' waves are often not easily identified because they are buried in the preceding T or U waves or QRS complexes. Normal sinus P waves are absent.

P wave–QRS complex relationship. In most untreated atrial tachycardias not caused by digitalis intoxication, and in which the atrial rate is less than 200 per minute, the AV conduction ratio is 1:1. When the atrial rate is greater than 200 per minute, a 2:1 AV conduction ratio is common. (A 2:1 AV conduction ratio indicates that for every two P' waves, one is followed by a QRS complex.) When the AV block occurs only during the tachycardia, the arrhythmia is called *atrial tachycardia with block.*

The cause of the AV block is the relatively long refractory period of the AV junction, which prevents the conduction of all of the rapidly occurring atrial electrical impulses into the ventricles *(physiological AV block).*

If there is a preexisting AV block because of cardiac disease, if digitalis excess is the cause of the atrial tachycardia (i.e., ectopic atrial tachycardia), or if certain drugs (e.g., digitalis, β-blockers, or calcium channel blockers) have been administered, 2:1 AV block may occur at atrial rates less than 200 per minute.

Higher-degree AV block (e.g., 3:1, 4:1, and so forth) or variable AV block may also occur, particularly in atrial tachycardia caused by digitalis toxicity.

PR intervals. The PR intervals are usually normal and constant in ectopic atrial tachycardia. In MAT, the PR intervals usually vary slightly in each given lead. They may vary from 0.20 second to less than 0.12 second, depending on the pacemaker site. Occasionally, the PR intervals are prolonged (greater than 0.20 second), particularly when the atrial rate is extremely rapid. This occurs when the atrial impulses reach the AV junction while it is in the relative refractory period, thereby increasing the AV conduction time. In addition, a preexisting first-degree AV block may be present. A shorter than normal PR interval may be present when atrial tachycardia is relatively slow, when it occurs in healthy young individuals, or when ventricular preexcitation is present.

R-R intervals. The R-R intervals are usually equal in ectopic atrial tachycardia if the AV conduction ratio is constant (i.e., 2:1, 2:1, 2:1, and so forth). But if the AV conduction ratio varies (as in atrial tachycardia with varying AV block [i.e., 3:1, 2:1, 4:1, 3:1, and so forth]), the R-R intervals will be unequal. The R-R intervals will also vary in each given lead if MAT is present.

QRS complexes. The QRS complexes are normal unless a preexisting intraventricular conduction disturbance (such as a bundle branch block), aberrant ventricular conduction, or ventricular preexcitation is present. If the QRS complexes are abnormal only during the tachycardia, the arrhythmia is called *atrial tachycardia with aberrancy* (or *with aberrant ventricular conduction*). Atrial tachycardia with abnormal QRS complexes may resemble ventricular tachycardia (see p. 151).

Cause of Arrhythmia

In general, the causes of atrial tachycardia are essentially the same as those of PACs. Like PACs, atrial tachycardia may occur in persons with apparently healthy hearts, as well as in those with diseased hearts.

Most often, atrial tachycardia occurs in patients with the following conditions:

◆ Digitalis toxicity
◆ Metabolic abnormalities (including acute alcohol abuse)
◆ Electrolyte disturbances
◆ Hypoxemia
◆ Chronic lung disease
◆ Coronary artery disease (especially after an acute MI)
◆ Rheumatic heart disease

Atrial tachycardia caused by digitalis toxicity is often associated with a 2:1 or higher-degree AV block or a varying AV block. Atrial tachycardia with AV block may also occur in patients with significant heart disease, such as coronary artery disease or cor pulmonale. MAT is most often associated with respiratory failure, as in decompensated chronic obstructive pulmonary disease (COPD); it is rarely caused by digitalis excess. The electrophysiological mechanism responsible for atrial tachycardia is either enhanced automaticity or reentry.

Clinical Significance

The signs and symptoms in atrial tachycardia depend on the presence or absence of heart disease, the nature of the heart disease, the ventricular rate, and the duration of the arrhythmia. Frequently, atrial tachycardia is accompanied by feelings of palpitations, nervousness, or anxiety.

When the ventricular rate is very rapid, the ventricles are unable to fill completely during diastole, resulting in a significant reduction of the cardiac output and a decrease in perfusion of the brain and other vital organs. This decrease in body perfusion may cause confusion, dizziness, lightheadedness, shortness of breath, near-syncope or syncope, and, in patients with coronary artery disease, it may cause angina, congestive heart failure, or MI.

In addition, because a rapid heart rate increases the workload of the heart, the oxygen requirements of the myocardium are usually increased in atrial tachycardia. Because of this, in addition to the consequences of decreased cardiac output, atrial tachycardia in acute MI may increase myocardial ischemia and the frequency and severity of chest pain; bring about the extension of the infarct; cause congestive heart failure, hypotension, or cardiogenic shock; or predispose the patient to serious ventricular arrhythmias.

Symptomatic atrial tachycardia must be treated promptly to reverse the consequences of the reduced cardiac output and increased workload of the heart and to prevent the occurrence of serious ventricular arrhythmias. As noted earlier, atrial tachycardia with wide QRS complexes may resemble ventricular tachycardia. A 12-lead ECG or lead MCL$_1$ may be useful in making a differentiation in this situation by helping to identify the presence or absence of P waves in lead V$_1$ in particular.

Notes

_____

_____

_____

_____

_____

ATRIAL FLUTTER

> ### KEY DEFINITION
>
> **Atrial flutter _(Figures 6-4 and 6-5) is an arrhythmia arising in an ectopic pacemaker or the site of a rapid reentry circuit in the atria, characterized by rapid abnormal flutter (F) waves with a sawtooth appearance and, usually, a slower, regular ventricular response._**

Diagnostic Characteristics

Heart rate. Usually, the atrial rate is between 240 and 360 (average, 300) F waves per minute, but it may be slower or faster. The ventricular rate is commonly about 150 beats per minute (half the atrial rate because of a 2:1 AV block) in an uncontrolled (untreated) atrial flutter and about 60 to 75 in a controlled (treated) one or one with a preexisting AV block. Rarely, the ventricular rate may be over 240 beats per minute, the same as the atrial rate, if the atrial rate is relatively slow and a 1:1 AV conduction ratio is present. Vagal maneuvers, such as carotid sinus massage, often produce a slowing of the ventricular rate in stepwise increments.

Rhythm. The atrial rhythm is typically regular, but it may be irregular. The ventricular rhythm is usually regular if the AV conduction ratio is constant, but it may be grossly irregular if a variable AV block is present.

Pacemaker site. The pacemaker site is an ectopic pacemaker in part of the atria outside of the SA node. Commonly, it is located low in the atria near the AV node. The activity of the SA node is completely suppressed by atrial flutter.

Characteristics of atrial F waves. The characteristics of atrial F waves include the following:

◆ **Relationship to cardiac anatomy and physiology:** An atrial F wave represents depolarization of the atria in an abnormal direction followed by atrial repolarization. Depolarization of the atria commonly begins near the AV node and progresses across the atria in a retrograde direction. Normal P waves are absent.

◆ **Onset and end:** The onset and end of the F waves cannot be determined with certainty.

◆ **Components:** The F wave consists of an abnormal atrial depolarization wave corresponding to an ectopic P wave followed by an atrial T wave (Ta) of atrial repolarization.

◆ **Direction:** The first part of the F wave, corresponding to an ectopic P wave, is commonly neg-

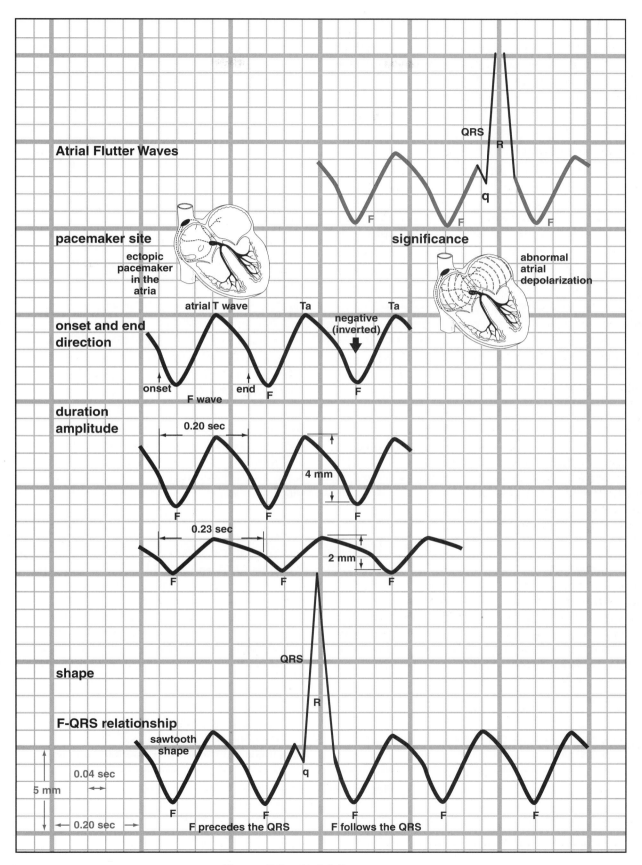

Figure 6-4 Atrial flutter waves.

Atrial Flutter

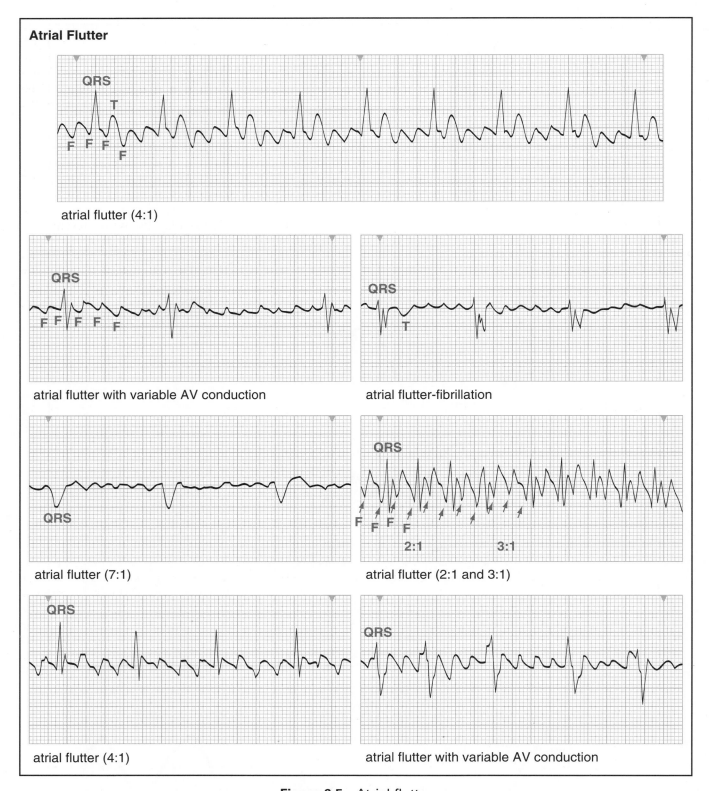

atrial flutter (4:1)

atrial flutter with variable AV conduction

atrial flutter-fibrillation

atrial flutter (7:1)

atrial flutter (2:1 and 3:1)

atrial flutter (4:1)

atrial flutter with variable AV conduction

Figure 6-5   Atrial flutter.

ative (inverted) in lead II and followed by a positive (upright) wave, the atrial T wave.
- **Duration:** The duration varies according to the rate of the F waves.
- **Amplitude:** The amplitude, measured from peak to peak of the F wave, varies greatly from less than 1 mm to over 5 mm.
- **Shape:** The atrial F waves have a sawtooth appearance. The typical F wave consists of a negative (inverted), V-shaped ectopic atrial wave immediately followed by an upright, peaked atrial T wave in lead II. An isoelectric line is seldom present between the waves. Typically, the first, downward part of the F wave is shorter and more abrupt than the second, upward part. F waves are generally identical in shape and size in any given lead but may occasionally vary slightly. Atrial fibrillation may occur during atrial flutter and vice versa. Such a mixture of atrial flutter and fibrillation is called *atrial flutter-fibrillation.*
- **F wave–QRS complex relationship:** The F waves precede, are buried in, and follow the QRS complexes and may be superimposed on the T waves or ST segments. The AV conduction ratio in most instances of atrial flutter is commonly 2:1, which indicates that for every two F waves, one is followed by a QRS complex.

The discrepancy in the rate of F waves and the QRS complexes is the result of the long refractory period of the AV junction, which prevents the conduction of all the rapidly occurring atrial electrical impulses into the ventricles (physiological AV block).

Rarely, the AV conduction ratio in untreated atrial flutter is 1:1. The AV block may be greater (i.e., 3:1, 4:1, and so forth) or even variable because of disease of the AV node, increased vagal (parasympathetic) tone, and certain drugs (e.g., digitalis, β-blockers, or calcium channel blockers).

The AV conduction ratio is usually constant in any given lead, producing a regular ventricular rhythm. If the AV conduction ratio varies, the ventricular rhythm will be irregular. When there is a 2:1 or 1:1 AV conduction ratio, the sawtooth pattern of the F waves may be distorted by the QRS complexes and T waves, making the F waves difficult to recognize. On rare occasions when a complete AV block is present and the atria and ventricles beat independently, there is no set relation between the F waves and the QRS complexes. When this occurs, AV dissociation is present.

FR intervals. FR intervals are usually equal but may vary.

R-R intervals. The R-R intervals are equal if the AV conduction ratio is constant, but if the AV conduction ratio varies, the R-R intervals are unequal.

QRS complexes. The QRS complexes are normal unless a preexisting intraventricular conduction disturbance (such as a bundle branch block), aberrant ventricular conduction, or ventricular preexcitation is present. Atrial flutter with a rapid ventricular response and abnormal QRS complexes may resemble ventricular tachycardia.

Cause of Arrhythmia

Chronic (persistent) atrial flutter is most commonly seen in middle-aged and elderly persons with the following conditions:
- Advanced rheumatic heart disease, particularly if mitral or tricuspid valvular disease is present
- Coronary or hypertensive heart disease

Transient (paroxysmal) atrial flutter usually indicates the presence of cardiac disease; however, it may occasionally occur in apparently healthy persons. The arrhythmia may also be associated with the following:
- Cardiomyopathy
- Atrial dilatation from any cause
- Thyrotoxicosis
- Digitalis toxicity (rarely)
- Hypoxia
- Acute or chronic cor pulmonale
- Congestive heart failure
- Damage to the SA node or atria because of pericarditis or myocarditis
- Alcoholism

Atrial flutter may be initiated by a PAC. The electrophysiological mechanism responsible for atrial flutter is either enhanced automaticity or reentry.

Clinical Significance

The signs and symptoms and clinical significance of atrial flutter with a rapid ventricular response are the same as those of atrial tachycardia. In addition, in 2:1 atrial flutter, in particular, the atria do not regularly contract and empty, as they normally do, during the last part of ventricular diastole, completely filling the ventricles just before they contract. The loss of this "atrial kick" may result in incomplete filling of the ventricles before they contract, causing a reduction of the cardiac output by as much as 25%.

Notes

_____

_____

_____

_____

_____

_____

ATRIAL FIBRILLATION

> **KEY DEFINITION**
>
> Atrial fibrillation *(Figures 6-6 and 6-7) is
> an arrhythmia arising in multiple ectopic
> pacemakers or sites of rapid reentry cir-
> cuits in the atria, characterized by very
> rapid abnormal atrial fibrillation (f) waves
> and an irregular, often rapid ventricular re-
> sponse.*

Diagnostic Characteristics

Heart rate. Typically, the atrial rate is 350 to 600 (average, 400) f waves per minute, but it can be as high as 700. The ventricular rate is commonly about 160 to 180 (or as high as 200) beats per minute in an uncontrolled (untreated) atrial fibrillation and about 60 to 70 in a controlled (treated) one, or one with a preexisting AV block. If the ventricular rate is greater than 100 per minute, atrial fibrillation is considered to be "fast"; if it is less than 60, it is considered to be "slow." Carotid sinus massage often slows the ventricular rate.

Rhythm. The atrial rhythm is irregularly (or grossly) irregular. The ventricular rhythm is almost always irregularly irregular in untreated atrial fibrillation.

Pacemaker site. The pacemaker sites, multiple ectopic pacemakers in the atria outside of the SA node, generate electrical impulses chaotically. The activity of the SA node is completely suppressed by atrial fibrillation.

Characteristics of atrial f waves. Characteristics of atrial f waves include the following:

◆ **Relationship to cardiac anatomy and physiology:** Atrial f waves represent abnormal, chaotic, and incomplete depolarizations of small individual groups (or islets) of atrial muscle fibers. Because organized depolarizations of the atria are absent, P waves and organized atrial contractions are absent.

◆ **Onset and end:** The onset and end of the f waves cannot be determined with certainty.

◆ **Direction:** The direction of the f waves varies from positive (upright) to negative (inverted) at random.

◆ **Duration:** The duration of the f waves varies greatly and cannot be determined with accuracy.

◆ **Amplitude:** The amplitude varies from less than 1 millimeter to several millimeters. If the f waves are small (less than 1 mm), they are called *fine* fibrillatory waves; if they are large (1 mm or greater), they are called *coarse* fibrillatory waves. If

the f waves are so small or "fine" that they are not recorded, the sections of the ECG between the QRS complexes may appear as a wavy or flat (iso-electric) line.

◆ **Shape:** The f waves are irregularly shaped, rounded (or pointed), and dissimilar.

◆ **f wave–QRS complex relationship:** The f waves precede, are buried in, and follow the QRS complexes and are superimposed on the ST segments and T waves. Typically, in atrial fibrillation, fewer than one half or one third of the atrial electrical impulses are conducted through the AV junction into the ventricles, and these, at random. This results in a grossly irregular ventricular rhythm. The main reason for this is the long refractory period of the AV junction, which prevents the conduction of all the rapidly occurring atrial electrical impulses into the ventricles (physiological AV block).

R-R intervals. The R-R intervals are typically unequal. When atrial fibrillation is complicated by a second-degree, type I AV block, the R-R intervals progressively decrease in duration over a cycle of three or more R-R intervals, each cycle following an exceptionally wide R-R interval. When only two R-R intervals occur in a cycle, the ventricular rhythm assumes a roughly bigeminal appearance.

QRS complexes. The QRS complexes are normal unless a preexisting intraventricular conduction disturbance (such as a bundle branch block), aberrant ventricular conduction, or ventricular preexcitation is present. Atrial fibrillation with a rapid ventricular response and abnormal QRS complexes may resemble ventricular tachycardia, except for the irregular rhythm.

Cause of Arrhythmia

Atrial fibrillation is commonly associated with the following:

◆ Advanced rheumatic heart disease (particularly with mitral stenosis)
◆ Hypertensive or coronary heart disease (with or without acute MI)
◆ Thyrotoxicosis

Less commonly, atrial fibrillation may occur in the following:

◆ Cardiomyopathy
◆ Acute myocarditis and pericarditis
◆ Chest trauma
◆ Pulmonary disease
◆ Digitalis toxicity (rarely)

Whatever the underlying form of heart disease, atrial fibrillation is commonly associated with congestive heart failure. In a small percentage of cases, atrial fibrillation may occur in apparently normal individuals after excessive ingestion of alcohol and caffeine, during emotional stress, and sometimes without any apparent cause.

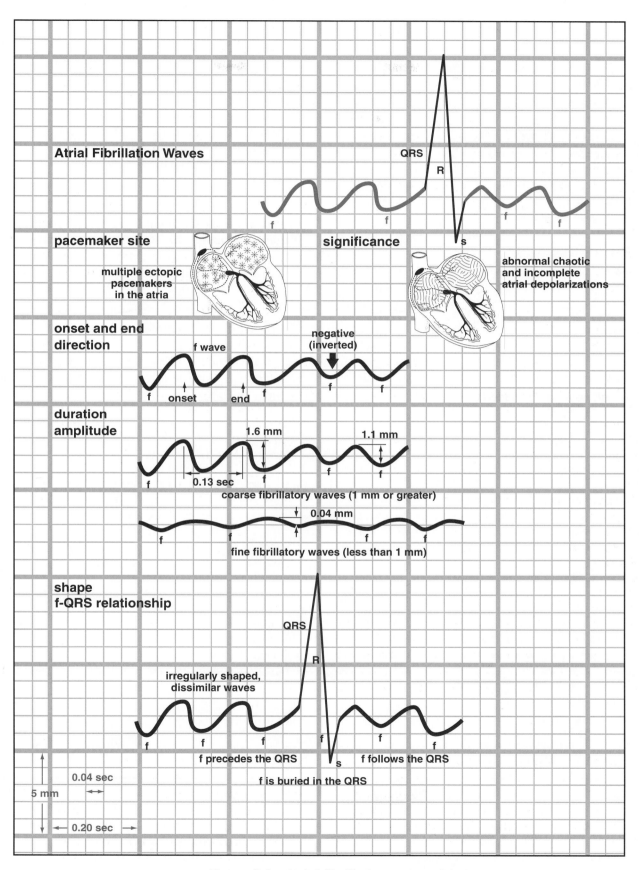

Figure 6-6 Atrial fibrillation waves.

Atrial Fibrillation

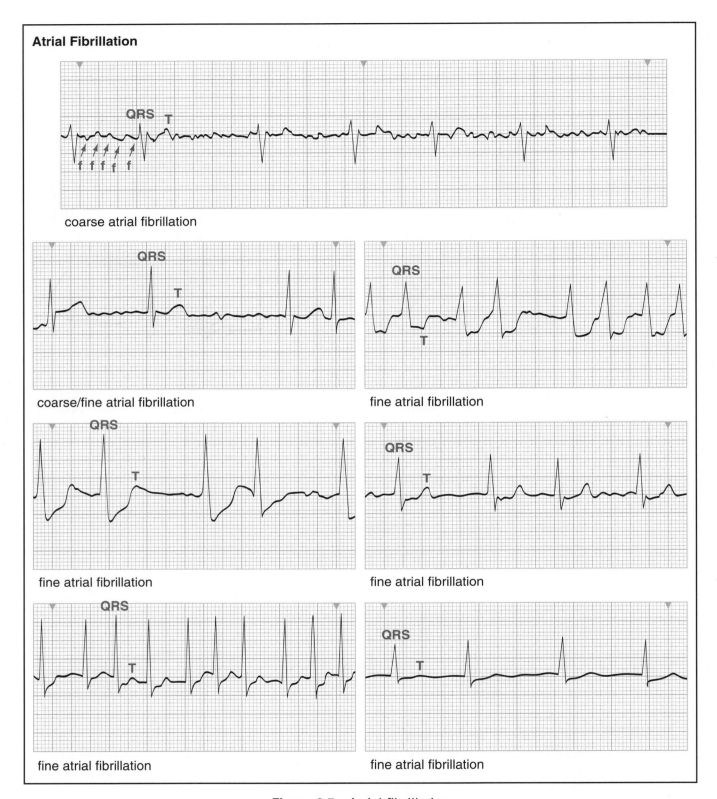

coarse atrial fibrillation

coarse/fine atrial fibrillation

fine atrial fibrillation

fine atrial fibrillation

fine atrial fibrillation

fine atrial fibrillation

fine atrial fibrillation

Figure 6-7   Atrial fibrillation.

Atrial fibrillation may be intermittent, even occurring in short bursts or paroxysms, as does paroxysmal supraventricular tachycardia (PSVT), or it may be chronic (persistent). The electrophysiological mechanism responsible for atrial fibrillation is either enhanced automaticity or reentry.

Clinical Significance

The signs and symptoms and clinical significance of atrial fibrillation with a rapid ventricular response are the same as those of atrial tachycardia. In addition, in atrial fibrillation, the atria do not regularly contract and empty, as they normally do, during the last part of ventricular diastole, completely filling the ventricles just before they contract. The loss of this "atrial kick" may result in incomplete filling of the ventricles before they contract, causing a reduction of the cardiac output by as much as 25%. A small percentage of patients with persistent atrial fibrillation may develop atrial thrombi with peripheral arterial embolization.

SUMMARY

Table 6-1 summarizes the diagnostic characteristics of the various atrial arrhythmias discussed in his chapter.

Notes

_____

_____

_____

_____

_____

_____

TABLE

6-1   Typical Diagnostic ECG Features of Atrial Arrhythmias

Arrhythmia	Heart Rate (bpm)	Rhythm	P Waves	P'R Intervals	QRS Complexes
Wandering atrial pacemaker	60-100	Irregular	Varying from normal to inverted	Varying from 0.20 to 0.12 sec	Normal
Atrial tachycardia	160-240	Regular (irregular in MAT)	Normal or abnormal (varying from normal to inverted in MAT)	Normal, constant (varying from 0.20 to ≤ 0.12 sec in MAT)	Normal
Atrial flutter	60-150	Usually regular; may be irregular	Atrial flutter waves	FR intervals: usually equal	Normal
Atrial fibrillation	60-180	Irregular	Atrial fibrillation waves	None	Normal

MAT, Multifocal atrial tachycardia.

TREATMENT ALGORITHMS

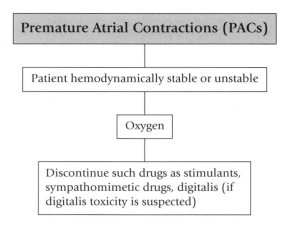

Atrial Tachycardia Without Block

Patient hemodynamically stable
Heart rate over 150 beats/min

Patient hemodynamically unstable
Heart rate over 150 beats/min or less

Oxygen

Oxygen

Diltiazem 20-mg (0.25-mg/kg) IV bolus over 2 min and, if necessary, administer in 15 min a 25-mg (0.35-mg/kg) IV bolus over 2 min, followed by an IV infusion at a rate of 5 to 15 mg/h
OR
One of the following **β-blockers:**
• **Esmolol** 0.5-mg/kg IV bolus over 1 min, followed by an IV infusion at a rate of 0.05 mg/kg/min; repeat the bolus twice, 5 min between each bolus, while increasing the rate of the IV infusion 0.05 mg/kg/min after each bolus; then, if necessary, increase the IV infusion by 0.05 mg/kg/min every 5 min to a maximum of 0.30 mg/kg/min
• **Atenolol** 5 mg IV over 5 min and repeat in 10 min for a total dose of 10 mg
• **Metoprolol** 5 mg IV over 2 to 5 min and repeat every 5 min up to a total dose of 15 mg
OR
Amiodarone 150-mg IV infusion over 10 min, followed by a 1-mg/min IV infusion

Amiodarone 150-mg IV infusion over 10 min, followed by a 1-mg/min IV infusion
OR
Diltiazem 20-mg (0.25-mg/kg) IV bolus over 2 min and, if necessary, administer in 15 min a 25-mg (0.35-mg/kg) IV bolus over 2 min, followed by an IV infusion at a rate of 5 to 15 mg/h

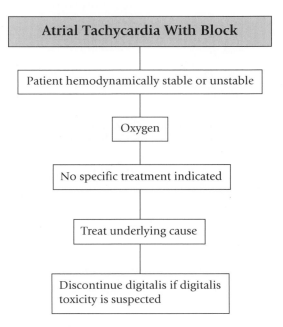

Atrial Tachycardia With Block

Patient hemodynamically stable or unstable

Oxygen

No specific treatment indicated

Treat underlying cause

Discontinue digitalis if digitalis toxicity is suspected

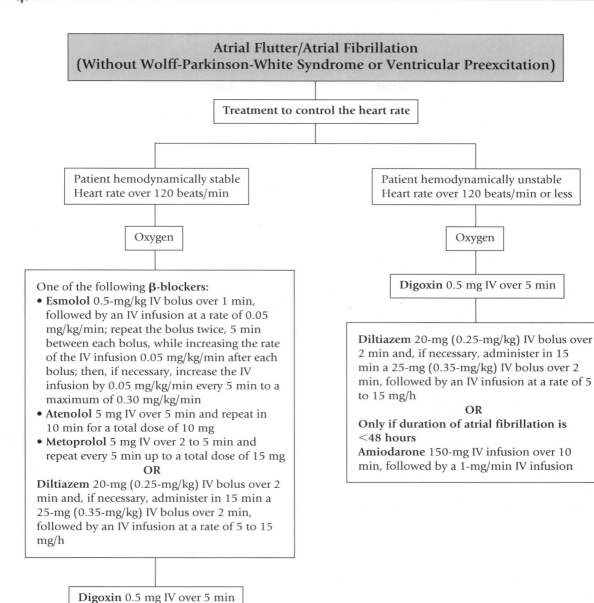

Atrial Flutter/Atrial Fibrillation
(Without Wolff-Parkinson-White Syndrome or Ventricular Preexcitation)

Treatment to control the heart rate

Patient hemodynamically stable
Heart rate over 120 beats/min

Oxygen

One of the following β-blockers:
- **Esmolol** 0.5-mg/kg IV bolus over 1 min, followed by an IV infusion at a rate of 0.05 mg/kg/min; repeat the bolus twice, 5 min between each bolus, while increasing the rate of the IV infusion 0.05 mg/kg/min after each bolus; then, if necessary, increase the IV infusion by 0.05 mg/kg/min every 5 min to a maximum of 0.30 mg/kg/min
- **Atenolol** 5 mg IV over 5 min and repeat in 10 min for a total dose of 10 mg
- **Metoprolol** 5 mg IV over 2 to 5 min and repeat every 5 min up to a total dose of 15 mg
OR
Diltiazem 20-mg (0.25-mg/kg) IV bolus over 2 min and, if necessary, administer in 15 min a 25-mg (0.35-mg/kg) IV bolus over 2 min, followed by an IV infusion at a rate of 5 to 15 mg/h

Digoxin 0.5 mg IV over 5 min

Patient hemodynamically unstable
Heart rate over 120 beats/min or less

Oxygen

Digoxin 0.5 mg IV over 5 min

Diltiazem 20-mg (0.25-mg/kg) IV bolus over 2 min and, if necessary, administer in 15 min a 25-mg (0.35-mg/kg) IV bolus over 2 min, followed by an IV infusion at a rate of 5 to 15 mg/h
OR
Only if duration of atrial fibrillation is <48 hours
Amiodarone 150-mg IV infusion over 10 min, followed by a 1-mg/min IV infusion

Atrial Flutter/Atrial Fibrillation
(Without Wolff-Parkinson-White Syndrome or Ventricular Preexcitation)

Treatment to convert the rhythm: atrial fibrillation <48 hours and atrial flutter of any duration

---

Patient hemodynamically stable
Heart rate over 120 beats/min

Oxygen

Ibutilide
- If patient's weight ≥60 kg (≥132 lb), **ibutilide** 1.0 mg IV over 10 min and repeat 10 min after first infusion, if necessary
- If patient's weight <60 kg (<132 lb), ibutilide 0.1 mg/kg IV over 10 min and repeat 10 min after first infusion, if necessary

OR

Amiodarone 150-mg IV infusion over 10 min, followed by a 1-mg/min IV infusion

OR

Procainamide 20- to 30-mg/min IV infusion up to a total dose of 17 mg/kg

---

Synchronized shock 50-100 J for atrial flutter and 100-200 J for atrial fibrillation; repeat as necessary at 100 J, 200 J, 300 J, etc.; administer a sedative/ analgesic before cardioversion

---

Patient hemodynamically unstable
Heart rate over 120 beats/min or less

Oxygen

Synchronized shock 50-100 J for atrial flutter and 100-200 J for atrial fibrillation; repeat as necessary at 100 J, 200 J, 300 J, etc.; administer a sedative/ analgesic before cardioversion

OR

Amiodarone 150-mg IV infusion over 10 min, followed by a 1-mg/min IV infusion

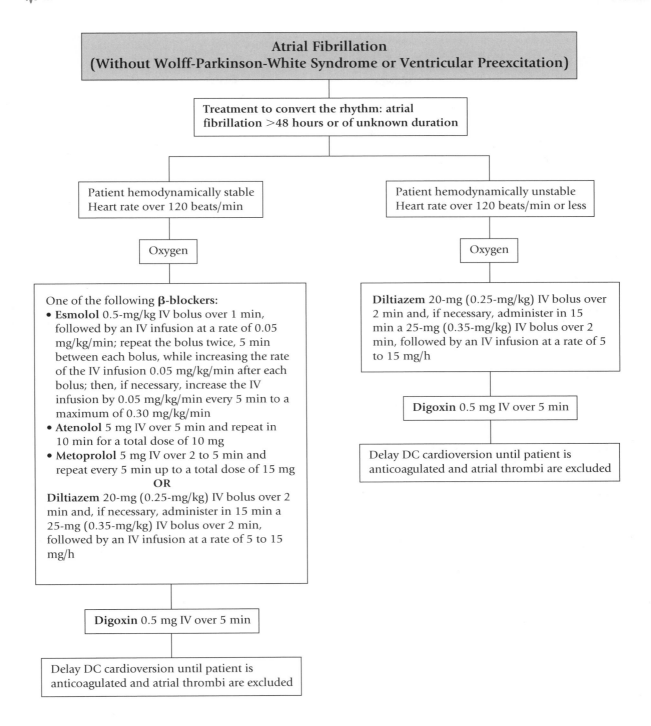

Atrial Fibrillation
(Without Wolff-Parkinson-White Syndrome or Ventricular Preexcitation)

Treatment to convert the rhythm: atrial
fibrillation >48 hours or of unknown duration

Patient hemodynamically stable
Heart rate over 120 beats/min

Oxygen

One of the following β-blockers:
• **Esmolol** 0.5-mg/kg IV bolus over 1 min,
followed by an IV infusion at a rate of 0.05
mg/kg/min; repeat the bolus twice, 5 min
between each bolus, while increasing the rate
of the IV infusion 0.05 mg/kg/min after each
bolus; then, if necessary, increase the IV
infusion by 0.05 mg/kg/min every 5 min to a
maximum of 0.30 mg/kg/min
• **Atenolol** 5 mg IV over 5 min and repeat in
10 min for a total dose of 10 mg
• **Metoprolol** 5 mg IV over 2 to 5 min and
repeat every 5 min up to a total dose of 15 mg
OR
Diltiazem 20-mg (0.25-mg/kg) IV bolus over 2
min and, if necessary, administer in 15 min a
25-mg (0.35-mg/kg) IV bolus over 2 min,
followed by an IV infusion at a rate of 5 to 15
mg/h

Digoxin 0.5 mg IV over 5 min

Delay DC cardioversion until patient is
anticoagulated and atrial thrombi are excluded

Patient hemodynamically unstable
Heart rate over 120 beats/min or less

Oxygen

Diltiazem 20-mg (0.25-mg/kg) IV bolus over
2 min and, if necessary, administer in 15
min a 25-mg (0.35-mg/kg) IV bolus over 2
min, followed by an IV infusion at a rate of 5
to 15 mg/h

Digoxin 0.5 mg IV over 5 min

Delay DC cardioversion until patient is
anticoagulated and atrial thrombi are excluded

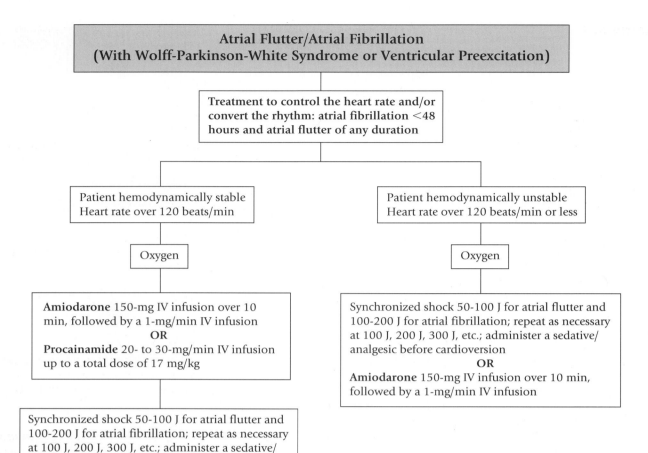

**Atrial Flutter/Atrial Fibrillation
(With Wolff-Parkinson-White Syndrome or Ventricular Preexcitation)**

Treatment to control the heart rate and/or convert the rhythm: atrial fibrillation <48 hours and atrial flutter of any duration

Patient hemodynamically stable
Heart rate over 120 beats/min

Oxygen

Amiodarone 150-mg IV infusion over 10 min, followed by a 1-mg/min IV infusion
OR
Procainamide 20- to 30-mg/min IV infusion up to a total dose of 17 mg/kg

Synchronized shock 50-100 J for atrial flutter and 100-200 J for atrial fibrillation; repeat as necessary at 100 J, 200 J, 300 J, etc.; administer a sedative/analgesic before cardioversion

Patient hemodynamically unstable
Heart rate over 120 beats/min or less

Oxygen

Synchronized shock 50-100 J for atrial flutter and 100-200 J for atrial fibrillation; repeat as necessary at 100 J, 200 J, 300 J, etc.; administer a sedative/analgesic before cardioversion
OR
Amiodarone 150-mg IV infusion over 10 min, followed by a 1-mg/min IV infusion

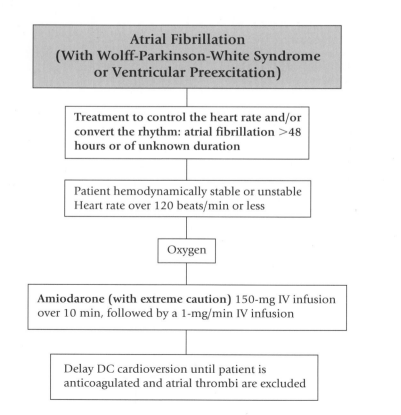

**Atrial Fibrillation
(With Wolff-Parkinson-White Syndrome
or Ventricular Preexcitation)**

Treatment to control the heart rate and/or convert the rhythm: atrial fibrillation >48 hours or of unknown duration

Patient hemodynamically stable or unstable
Heart rate over 120 beats/min or less

Oxygen

Amiodarone (with extreme caution) 150-mg IV infusion over 10 min, followed by a 1-mg/min IV infusion

Delay DC cardioversion until patient is anticoagulated and atrial thrombi are excluded

CHAPTER REVIEW QUESTIONS

1. An arrhythmia originating in pacemakers that shift back and forth between the SA node and an ectopic pacemaker in the atria or AV junction is called a(n):
   A. supraventricular tachycardia
   B. wandering atrial pacemaker
   C. alternating atrial flutter
   D. all of the above

2. The arrhythmia described in question number 1 may be a normal phenomenon seen in:
   A. the very young
   B. the elderly
   C. athletes
   D. all of the above

3. An extra atrial contraction consisting of a positive P wave in lead II followed by a normal or abnormal QRS complex, occurring earlier than the next beat of the underlying rhythm, is called:
   A. a premature junctional contraction
   B. a premature ventricular contraction
   C. a premature atrial contraction
   D. none of the above

4. A nonconducted or blocked PAC is:
   A. found in bradycardiac arrhythmias
   B. a P' wave that is not followed by a QRS complex
   C. always symptomatic in patients
   D. none of the above

5. The QRS complex of a PAC usually resembles that of:
   A. the underlying rhythm
   B. a premature ventricular complex
   C. a right bundle branch block
   D. a left bundle branch block

6. Two PACs in a row are called:
   A. a reentry rhythm
   B. a couplet
   C. bigeminy
   D. atrial tachycardia

7. An arrhythmia originating in an ectopic pacemaker in the atria with an atrial rate between 160 and 240 beats per minute is called:
   A. atrial flutter
   B. junctional tachycardia
   C. sinus tachycardia
   D. atrial tachycardia

8. The reduction in cardiac output accompanying atrial tachycardia can cause:
   A. syncope
   B. lightheadedness
   C. dizziness
   D. all of the above

9. Atrial flutter is characterized by:
   A. an atrial rate slower than the ventricular rate
   B. waves with a sawtooth appearance
   C. an atrial rate between 160 and 240 beats per minute
   D. all of the above

10. An arrhythmia characterized by multiple dissimilar, small atrial waves occuring at 350 or more beats per minute is:
    A. multifocal atrial tachycardia
    B. atrial flutter
    C. atrial fibrillation
    D. ectopic atrial tachycardia

CHAPTER OBJECTIVES

Upon completion of all or part of this chapter, you should be able to complete the following objective:
1. Define and give the diagnostic characteristics, cause, and clinical significance of the following arrhythmias:
   Premature junctional contractions (PJCs)
   Junctional escape rhythm
   Nonparoxysmal junctional tachycardia
     Accelerated junctional rhythm
     Junctional tachycardia
   Paroxysmal supraventricular tachycardia (PSVT)

PREMATURE JUNCTIONAL CONTRACTIONS

KEY DEFINITION

A premature junctional contraction (PJC) (Figure 7-1) is an extra ventricular contraction that originates in an ectopic pacemaker in the atrioventricular (AV) junction and occurs before the next expected beat of the underlying rhythm. It consists of a normal or abnormal QRS complex with or without an abnormal P wave. If a P wave is present, it may precede or follow the QRS complex. PJCs are also called premature junctional beats or complexes.

Diagnostic Characteristics

Heart rate. The heart rate is that of the underlying rhythm.

Rhythm. The rhythm is irregular when PJCs are present.

Pacemaker site. The pacemaker site of the PJC is an ectopic pacemaker in the AV junction.

P waves. P waves may or may not be associated with the PJCs. If they are present, they are abnormal P' waves, varying in size, shape, and direction from normal P waves. The P' waves may precede, be buried in, or, less commonly, follow the QRS complexes of the PJCs (Table 7-1).

A P' wave that occurs before the QRS complex has most likely originated in the proximal, upper part of the AV junction. A P' wave that occurs during or after the QRS complex has most likely originated in the middle or distal part of the AV junction, respectively. If the P' waves precede the QRS complexes, they may be buried in the preceding T waves, distorting them. If the P' waves follow the QRS complexes, they are usually found in the ST segments. Because atrial depolarization occurs in a retrograde fashion, the P' waves that precede or follow the QRS complexes are negative (inverted) in lead II. Absent P' waves indicate that either (1) retrograde atrial depolarizations occurred during the QRS complexes or (2) atrial depolarizations have not occurred because of a retrograde AV block between the ectopic pacemaker site in the AV junction and the atria.

Premature Junctional Contractions

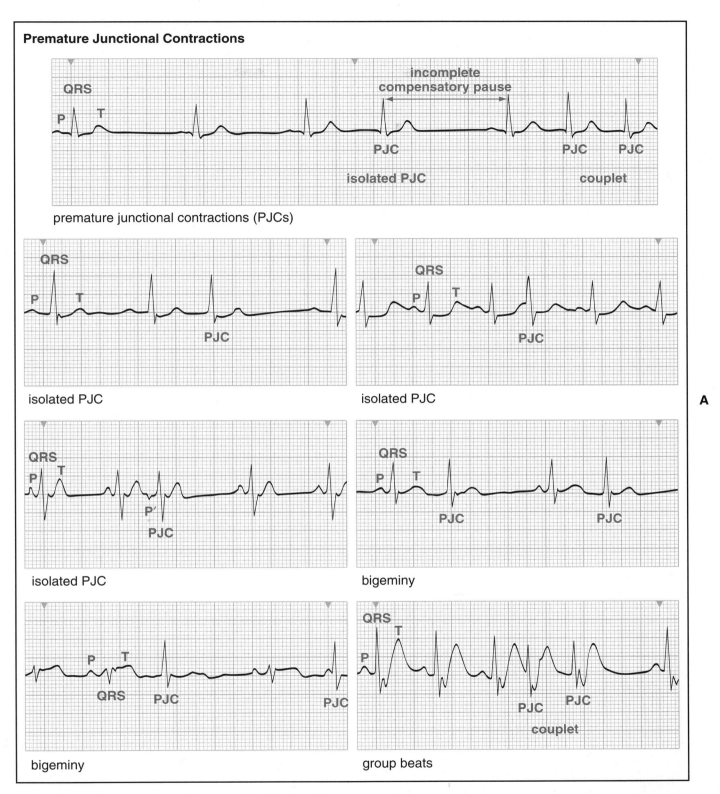

Figure 7-1   Premature junctional contractions.

Continued

A

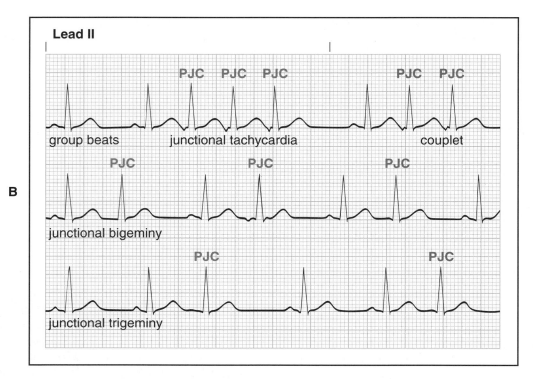

Figure 7-1, cont'd Premature junctional contractions.

7-1   Relationship of P' Waves to the QRS Complexes Depending on Their Site of Origin

Site of Origin of the P' Wave in the AV Junction	P' Wave Location
Upper part	Precedes the QRS complex
Middle or distal part	Is buried in the QRS complex
Distal part	Follows the QRS complex

If the ectopic pacemaker in the AV junction discharges too soon after the preceding QRS complex, the premature P' wave may not be followed by a QRS complex because the bundle of His or bundle branches may not be repolarized sufficiently to conduct an electrical impulse into the ventricles (nonconducted PJC).

PR intervals. If the P' waves of the PJCs precede the QRS complexes, the P'R intervals are usually abnormal (less than 0.12 second). Rarely, the P'R interval may be normal (0.12 to 0.20 second) or even prolonged (greater than 0.20 second). A prolonged PR interval is usually present if there is a delay in the AV conduction (first-degree AV block) below the ectopic pacemaker site. If the P' waves follow the QRS complexes, the RP' intervals are usually less than 0.20 second.

R-R intervals. The R-R intervals are unequal when PJCs are present. The interval between the PJC and the preceding QRS complex (the pre-PJC interval) is shorter than the R-R interval of the underlying rhythm. A full compensatory pause commonly follows a PJC because the sinoatrial (SA) node is usually not depolarized by the PJC. Less commonly, the SA node is depolarized by the PJC, resulting in an incomplete compensatory pause. (See the discussion of full and incomplete compensatory pauses under Premature Atrial Contractions, p. 147.)

QRS complexes. The QRS complex of the PJC usually resembles that of the underlying rhythm. If the ectopic pacemaker in the AV junction discharges too soon after the preceding QRS complex, the bundle branches may not be repolarized sufficiently to conduct the electrical impulse of the PJC normally. If this occurs, the electrical impulse may only be conducted down one bundle branch, usually the left one, and blocked in the other, producing a wide and bizarre-appearing QRS complex that resembles a right bundle branch block.

Such a bizarre-appearing PJC, called a *premature junctional contraction with aberrancy* (or *with aberrant ventricular conduction*), can mimic a premature ventricular contraction (PVC) (see Premature Ventricular Contractions, p. 147). Usually, a QRS complex follows each premature P' wave (conducted PJC), but a QRS complex may be absent because of a transient complete AV block below the ectopic pacemaker site in the AV junction (nonconducted PJC).

Frequency and pattern of occurrence of PJCs. The following are the various forms in which PJCs may appear:

◆ **Isolated:** PJCs may occur singly (isolated beats).
◆ **Group beats:** PJCs may occur in groups of two or more beats in succession. Two PJCs in a row are called a *couplet*. When three or more PJCs occur consecutively, *junctional tachycardia* is considered to be present.
◆ **Repetitive beats:** PJCs may alternate with the QRS complexes of the underlying rhythm *(bigeminy)* or occur after every two QRS complexes *(trigeminy)* or after every three QRS complexes of the underlying rhythm *(quadrigeminy)*.

Cause of Arrhythmia

Occasional PJCs may occur in a healthy person without apparent cause. Common causes of PJCs include the following:

◆ Digitalis toxicity (most common cause)
◆ Enhanced automaticity of the AV junction
◆ Increase in vagal (parasympathetic) tone on the SA node
◆ Excessive dose of certain cardiac drugs (e.g., quinidine and procainamide)
◆ Excessive dose of sympathomimetic drugs (e.g., epinephrine, isoproterenol, and norepinephrine)
◆ Hypoxia
◆ Congestive heart failure
◆ Coronary artery disease (especially following an acute myocardial infarction [MI])

The electrophysiological mechanism responsible for premature junctional contractions is either enhanced automaticity or reentry.

Clinical Significance

Isolated PJCs are not significant. However, if digitalis is being administered, PJCs may indicate digitalis toxicity and enhanced automaticity of the AV junction. Frequent PJCs, more than four to six per minute, may indicate an enhanced automaticity or a reentry mechanism in the AV junction and warn of the appearance of more serious junctional arrhythmias.

Because PJCs with aberrancy resemble PVCs, such PJCs must be correctly identified so that the patient is not treated inappropriately.

Notes

_____

_____

_____

_____

JUNCTIONAL ESCAPE RHYTHM

KEY DEFINITION

Junctional escape rhythm *(Figure 7-2)* is an arrhythmia originating in an escape pacemaker in the AV junction with a rate of 40 to 60 beats per minute. When less than three consecutive QRS complexes arising from the escape pacemaker are present, they are called junctional escape beats *or* complexes.

Diagnostic Characteristics

Heart rate. The heart rate is typically 40 to 60 beats per minute, but it may be less.

Rhythm. The ventricular rhythm is essentially regular.

Pacemaker site. The pacemaker site is an escape pacemaker in the AV junction.

P waves. P waves may be present or absent. If P waves are present but have no relation to the QRS complexes of the junctional escape rhythm, appearing independently at a rate different (typically slower) from that of the junctional rhythm, the pacemaker site of such P waves is the SA node or an ectopic pacemaker in the atria. These P waves are usually positive (upright) in lead II. When the P waves occur independently of the QRS complexes, AV dissociation is present.

AV dissociation indicating independent beating of the atria and ventricles can occur in several situations, including the following:

◆ When the rate of the sinus rhythm drops below the normal inherent rate of the AV junctional pacemaker of 40 to 60 beats per minute. The atrial rate is usually less than the ventricular rate.
◆ When the rate of the sinus rhythm is less than that of an AV junctional pacemaker whose rate has been abnormally increased beyond its inherent

Junctional Escape Rhythm

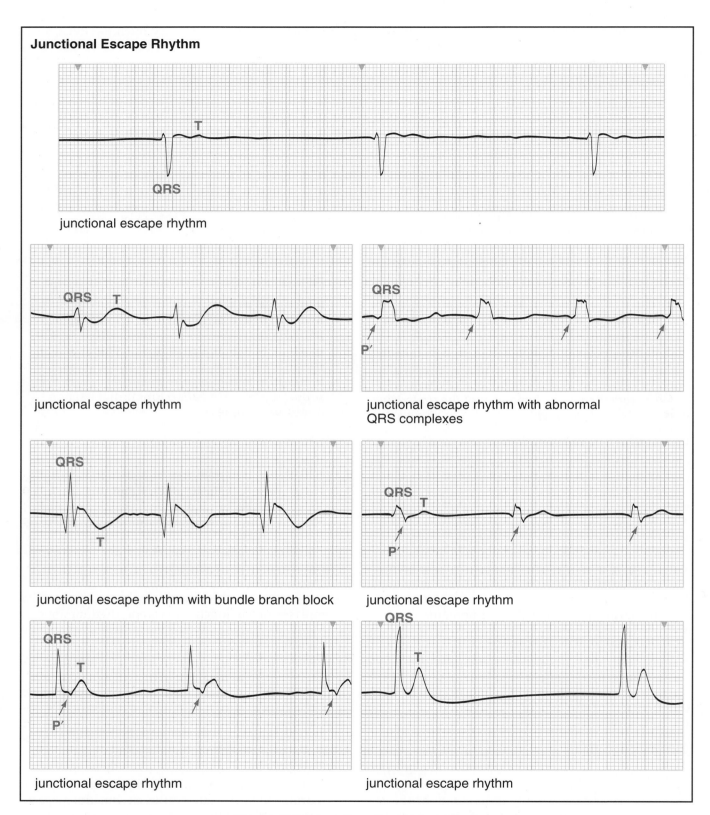

junctional escape rhythm

junctional escape rhythm

junctional escape rhythm with abnormal QRS complexes

junctional escape rhythm with bundle branch block

junctional escape rhythm

junctional escape rhythm

junctional escape rhythm

Figure 7-2 Junctional escape rhythm.

rate. The atrial rate is usually less than the ventricular rate which may range from 60 to 240 beats per minute.

◆ When an AV block is present. The atrial rate may be less or greater than the ventricular rate.

If the P waves regularly precede or follow the QRS complexes and are identical, the electrical impulses responsible for them have originated in the pacemaker site of the junctional escape rhythm. Such P' waves differ from normal P waves in size, shape, and direction. Because the atria depolarize retrogradely when the electrical impulses arise in the AV junction, the P' waves are negative (inverted) in lead II.

P' waves are absent in junctional escape rhythm if the P' waves occur during the QRS complexes, if a complete block in retrograde conduction is present, or if atrial flutter or fibrillation is the underlying atrial rhythm.

PR intervals. If the P' waves regularly precede the QRS complexes, the P'R intervals are abnormal (less than 0.12 second). If the P' waves regularly follow the QRS complexes, the RP' intervals are usually less than 0.20 second.

R-R intervals. The R-R intervals are usually equal.

QRS complexes. The QRS complexes are normal unless a preexisting intraventricular conduction disturbance (such as a bundle branch block) is present. Junctional escape rhythm with abnormal QRS complexes may resemble ventricular escape rhythm.

Cause of Arrhythmia

Junctional escape rhythm is a normal response of the AV junction under the following circumstances:

◆ When the rate of impulse formation of the dominant pacemaker (usually the SA node) drops below that of the escape pacemaker in the AV junction

OR

◆ When the electrical impulses from the SA node or atria fail to reach the AV junction because of sinus arrest, SA exit block, or third-degree (complete) AV block

Generally, when an electrical impulse fails to arrive at the AV junction within approximately 1.0 to 1.5 seconds, the escape pacemaker in the AV junction begins to generate electrical impulses at its inherent firing rate of 40 to 60 beats per minute. The result is one or more junctional escape beats or a junctional escape rhythm.

Clinical Significance

The signs and symptoms and clinical significance of junctional escape rhythm are the same as those in symptomatic sinus bradycardia. Symptomatic junctional escape rhythm must be treated promptly, preferably by transcutaneous or transvenous pacing, to reverse the consequences of the reduced cardiac output.

Notes

_____

_____

_____

_____

NONPAROXYSMAL JUNCTIONAL TACHYCARDIA (ACCELERATED JUNCTIONAL RHYTHM, JUNCTIONAL TACHYCARDIA)

KEY DEFINITION

Nonparoxysmal junctional tachycardia (Figure 7-3) is an arrhythmia originating in an ectopic pacemaker in the AV junction with a regular rhythm and a rate of 60 to 150 beats per minute. It includes accelerated junctional rhythm and junctional tachycardia.

Diagnostic Characteristics

Heart rate. The heart rate is usually 60 to 130 beats per minute, but it may be greater than 130 beats per minute and as high as 150. Nonparoxysmal junctional tachycardia with a heart rate between 60 and 100 beats per minute is commonly called *accelerated junctional rhythm;* one with a rate greater than 100 beats per minute is called *junctional tachycardia.* The onset and termination of nonparoxysmal junctional tachycardia are usually gradual.

Rhythm. The rhythm is essentially regular.

Pacemaker site. The pacemaker site is an ectopic pacemaker in the AV junction.

P waves. P waves may be present or absent. If present, they may have no relation to the QRS complexes of the nonparoxysmal junctional tachycardia, appearing independently at a rate different from that of the junctional rhythm. The pacemaker site of such P waves is the SA node or an ectopic pacemaker in the atria. These P waves are usually positive (upright) in lead II. When the P waves occur independently of the QRS complexes, AV dissociation is present.

If the P waves are identical and regularly precede or follow the QRS complexes, the electrical impulses responsible for them have originated in the pacemaker site of the nonparoxysmal junctional tachycardia. Such P' waves differ from normal P waves in size, shape, and direction. Because the atria depolarize ret-

Nonparoxysmal Junctional Tachycardia
(Accelerated Junctional Rhythm, Junctional Tachycardia)

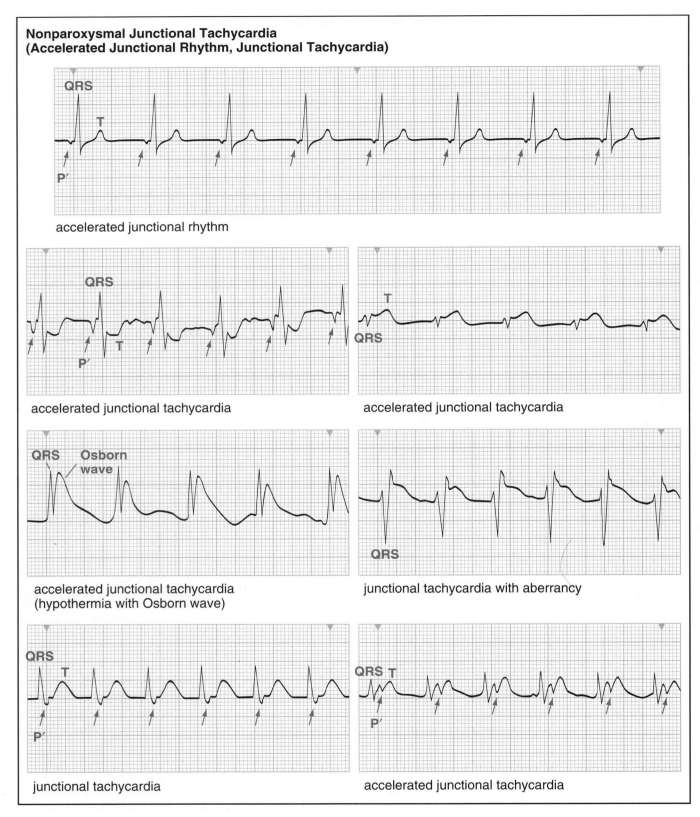

accelerated junctional rhythm

accelerated junctional tachycardia

accelerated junctional tachycardia

accelerated junctional tachycardia
(hypothermia with Osborn wave)

junctional tachycardia with aberrancy

junctional tachycardia

accelerated junctional tachycardia

Figure 7-3 Nonparoxysmal junctional tachycardia (accelerated junctional rhythm, junctional tachycardia).

rogradely when the electrical impulses arise in the AV junction, the P' waves are negative (inverted) in lead II.

P' waves are absent in nonparoxysmal junctional tachycardia if the P' waves occur during the QRS complexes, if a complete block in retrograde conduction is present, or if atrial flutter or atrial fibrillation is the underlying atrial rhythm.

PR intervals. If the P' waves regularly precede the QRS complexes, the P'R intervals are abnormal (less than 0.12 second). If the P' waves regularly follow the QRS complexes, the RP' intervals are usually less than 0.20 second.

R-R intervals. The R-R intervals are usually equal.

QRS complexes. The QRS complexes are normal unless a preexisting intraventricular conduction disturbance (such as a bundle branch block) or aberrant ventricular conduction is present. If abnormal QRS complexes occur only when junctional tachycardia is present, the arrhythmia is called *junctional tachycardia with aberrancy* (or *aberrant ventricular conduction*).

Nonparoxysmal junctional tachycardia with abnormal QRS complexes may resemble accelerated idioventricular rhythm if the heart rate is 60 to 100 beats per minute (accelerated junctional rhythm), or it may resemble ventricular tachycardia if the heart rate is over 100 beats per minute (junctional tachycardia).

Cause of Arrhythmia

Common causes of nonparoxysmal junctional tachycardia include the following:

◆ Digitalis toxicity (most common cause)
◆ Excessive administration of catecholamines
◆ Damage to the AV junction from an inferior MI or rheumatic fever
◆ Electrolyte imbalance (especially hypokalemia)
◆ Hypoxemia

The arrhythmia may begin with one or more PJCs and becomes manifest when the rate of the sinus rhythm becomes slower than that of the ectopic pacemaker. The electrophysiological mechanism responsible for nonparoxysmal junctional tachycardia is most likely enhanced automaticity.

Clinical Significance

Nonparoxysmal junctional tachycardia is clinically significant because it commonly indicates digitalis toxicity. The signs and symptoms and clinical significance of rapid nonparoxysmal junctional tachycardia are the same as those of atrial tachycardia.

In addition, in nonparoxysmal junctional tachycardia, the atria do not regularly contract and empty, as they normally do, during the last part of ventricular diastole, completely filling the ventricles just before they contract. The loss of this "atrial kick" may result in incomplete filling of the ventricles before they contract, causing a reduction of the cardiac output by as much as 25%.

Notes

_____

_____

_____

_____

PAROXYSMAL SUPRAVENTRICULAR TACHYCARDIA

KEY DEFINITION

Paroxysmal supraventricular tachycardia (PSVT) *(Figure 7-4) is an arrhythmia originating at the site of a rapid reentry circuit in the AV junction with a rate between 160 and 240 beats per minute. The PSVT may present as an AV nodal reentry tachycardia (AVNRT) or an AV reentry tachycardia (AVRT) as described below.*

Diagnostic Characteristics

Heart rate. The heart rate is usually 160 to 240 beats per minute and constant. The heart rate, however, may be as low as 110 beats per minute or exceed 240 per minute. The onset and termination of PSVT are typically abrupt, with the onset often being initiated by a premature atrial impulse. A brief period of asystole may follow the termination of the arrhythmia. The rate may be slower during the few beats after onset and before termination. PSVT is characterized by repeated episodes (paroxysms) of tachycardia that last from a few seconds to many hours or days and recur for many years. Vagal maneuvers, such as carotid sinus massage, usually terminate PSVT.

Rhythm. The rhythm is essentially regular.

Pacemaker site. The pacemaker site is a reentry mechanism in the AV junction that may involve the AV node alone or the AV node and an accessory conduction pathway located between the atria and ventricles, as described in Chapter 1. When the reentry mechanism involves only the AV node, the arrhythmia is called *AV nodal reentry tachycardia (AVNRT).* When both the AV node and an accessory conduction pathway are involved in the reentry mechanism, the arrhythmia is called *AV reentry tachycardia (AVRT).*

P waves. P' waves are often absent, being buried in the QRS complex. If present, they are identical and typically follow the QRS complexes. Rarely, the P' waves precede the QRS complexes. The P' waves are generally abnormal, differing from normal P waves

Paroxysmal Supraventricular Tachycardia

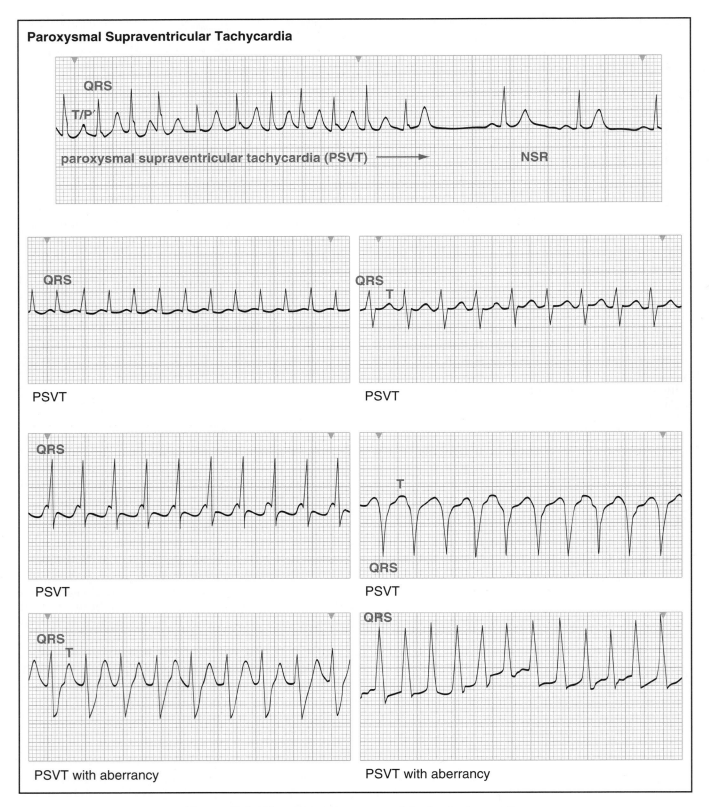

Figure 7-4 Paroxysmal supraventricular tachycardia.

in size, shape, and direction. Because atrial depolarization occurs in a retrograde fashion, the P' waves are negative (inverted) in lead II.

PR intervals. If the P' waves precede the QRS complexes, the P'R intervals are abnormal (less than 0.12 second). If the P' waves follow the QRS complexes, the RP' intervals are usually less than 0.20 second.

R-R intervals. The R-R intervals are usually equal.

QRS complexes. The QRS complexes are normal unless a preexisting intraventricular conduction disturbance (such as a bundle branch block) or aberrant ventricular conduction is present. If abnormal QRS complexes occur only with the tachycardia, the arrhythmia is called *paroxysmal supraventricular tachycardia with aberrancy* (or *aberrant ventricular conduction*). PSVT with abnormal QRS complexes may resemble ventricular tachycardia.

Cause of Arrhythmia

PSVT may occur without apparent cause in healthy persons of any age with no apparent underlying heart disease. In susceptible persons, it may be precipitated by the following:

◆ Increase in catecholamines and sympathetic tone
◆ Overexertion
◆ Stimulants (e.g., alcohol, coffee, and tobacco)
◆ Electrolyte or acid-base abnormalities
◆ Hyperventilation
◆ Emotional stress

The electrophysiological mechanism responsible for PSVT is a reentry mechanism involving the AV node alone, or the AV node in conjunction with an accessory conduction pathway as described above.

Clinical Significance

The signs and symptoms and clinical significance of PSVT are the same as those of atrial tachycardia. In addition, syncope may occur after the termination of PSVT because of the asystole that may follow its termination.

When episodes of PSVT with normal QRS complexes occur where the ECG ordinarily shows ventricular preexcitation (i.e., a short PR interval and a wide QRS complex with a slurred initial component—the delta wave) during sinus or atrial rhythms, the Wolff-Parkinson-White (WPW) syndrome is present.

SUMMARY

Table 7-2 summarizes the diagnostic characteristics of the various junctional arrhythmias in this chapter.

Notes

_____

_____

_____

_____

TABLE

7-2 Typical Diagnostic ECG Features of Junctional Arrhythmias

Arrhythmia	Heart Rate (bpm)	Rhythm	P Waves	P'R/RP' Intervals	QRS Complexes
Junctional escape rhythm	40-60	Regular	Present or absent; if they precede or follow QRS complexes, negative; if no relation to QRS complexes usually normal	If P'R, <0.12 sec If RP', <0.20 sec	Normal
Nonparoxysmal junctional tachycardia	60-150	Regular	Present or absent; if they precede or follow QRS complexes, negative; if no relation to QRS complexes, usually normal	If P'R, <0.12 sec If RP', <0.20 sec	Normal
Paroxysmal supraventricular tachycardia	160-240	Regular	Present or absent; if they precede or follow QRS complexes, negative; if no relation to QRS complexes, usually normal	If P'R, <0.12 sec If RP', <0.20 sec	Normal

TREATMENT ALGORITHMS

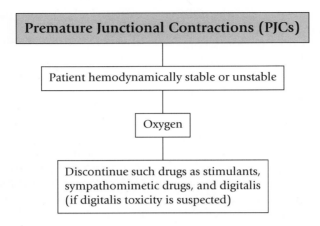

Premature Junctional Contractions (PJCs)

Patient hemodynamically stable or unstable

Oxygen

Discontinue such drugs as stimulants, sympathomimetic drugs, and digitalis (if digitalis toxicity is suspected)

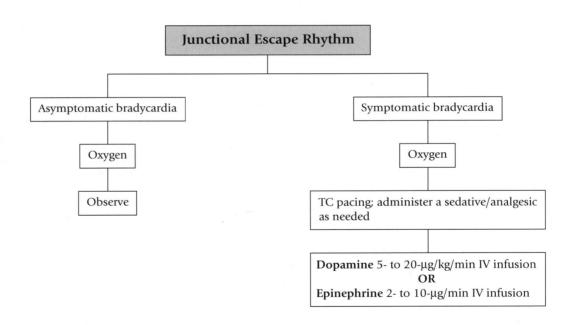

Junctional Escape Rhythm

Asymptomatic bradycardia

Oxygen

Observe

Symptomatic bradycardia

Oxygen

TC pacing; administer a sedative/analgesic as needed

Dopamine 5- to 20-μg/kg/min IV infusion
OR
Epinephrine 2- to 10-μg/min IV infusion

Junctional Tachycardia

Patient hemodynamically stable
Heart rate over 150 beats/min

Oxygen

Amiodarone 150-mg IV infusion over 10 min,
followed by a 1-mg/min IV infusion
OR
One of the following **β-blockers:**
• **Esmolol** 0.5-mg/kg IV bolus over 1 min,
followed by an IV infusion at a rate of 0.05
mg/kg/min; repeat the bolus twice, 5 min
between each bolus, while increasing the rate
of the IV infusion 0.05 mg/kg/min after each
bolus; then, if necessary, increase the IV
infusion by 0.05 mg/kg/min every 5 min to a
maximum of 0.30 mg/kg/min
• **Atenolol** 5 mg IV over 5 min and repeat in
10 min for a total dose of 10 mg
• **Metoprolol** 5 mg IV over 2 to 5 min and
repeat every 5 min up to a total dose of 15 mg

Patient hemodynamically unstable
Heart rate over 150 beats/min or less

Oxygen

Amiodarone 150-mg IV infusion over 10 min,
followed by a 1-mg/min IV infusion

Paroxysmal Supraventricular Tachycardia (PSVT) With Narrow QRS Complexes (Without Wolff-Parkinson-White Syndrome or Ventricular Preexcitation)

Patient hemodynamically stable
Heart rate over 150 beats/min

Oxygen

Vagal maneuvers

Adenosine 6-mg IV bolus over 1 to 3 sec and, if necessary, administer in 1 to 2 min a 12-mg IV bolus over 1 to 3 sec; if necessary, repeat once in 1 to 2 min

Diltiazem 20-mg (0.25-mg/kg) IV bolus over 2 min and, if necessary, administer in 15 min a 25-mg (0.35-mg/kg) IV bolus over 2 min, followed by an IV infusion at a rate of 5 to 15 mg/h

OR

One of the following β-blockers:
- **Esmolol** 0.5-mg/kg IV bolus over 1 min, followed by an IV infusion at a rate of 0.05 mg/kg/min; repeat the bolus twice, 5 min between each bolus, while increasing the rate of the IV infusion 0.05 mg/kg/min after each bolus; then, if necessary, increase the IV infusion by 0.05 mg/kg/min every 5 min to a maximum of 0.30 mg/kg/min
- **Atenolol** 5 mg IV over 5 min and repeat in 10 min for a total dose of 10 mg
- **Metoprolol** 5 mg IV over 2 to 5 min and repeat every 5 min up to a total dose of 15 mg

Digoxin 0.5-mg IV over 5 min

Synchronized shock 50-100 J and repeat as necessary at 100 J, 200 J, 300 J, etc.; administer a sedative/analgesic before cardioversion

Patient hemodynamically unstable
Heart rate over 150 beats/min or less

Oxygen

Vagal maneuvers

Digoxin 0.5-mg IV over 5 min

Amiodarone 150-mg IV infusion over 10 min, followed by a 1-mg/min IV infusion

OR

Diltiazem 20-mg (0.25-mg/kg) IV bolus over 2 min and, if necessary, administer in 15 min a 25-mg (0.35-mg/kg) IV bolus over 2 min, followed by an IV infusion at a rate of 5 to 15 mg/h

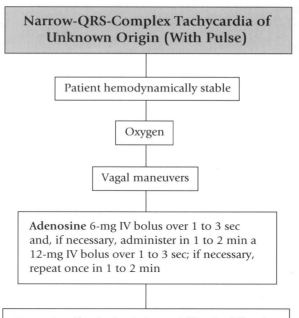

Narrow-QRS-Complex Tachycardia of Unknown Origin (With Pulse)

Patient hemodynamically stable

Oxygen

Vagal maneuvers

Adenosine 6-mg IV bolus over 1 to 3 sec and, if necessary, administer in 1 to 2 min a 12-mg IV bolus over 1 to 3 sec; if necessary, repeat once in 1 to 2 min

Determine if arrhythmia is caused by the following:
- Atrial tachycardia without block
- Paroxysmal supraventricular tachycardia (PSVT)
- Junctional tachycardia

CHAPTER REVIEW QUESTIONS

1. Absent P' waves in a junctional arrhythmia indicate:
   A. retrograde atrial depolarizations occurred during the QRS complexes
   B. atrial depolarizations have not occurred because of a retrograde AV block
   C. either of the above
   D. none of the above

2. If the ectopic pacemaker in the AV junction discharges too soon after the preceding QRS complex:
   A. a premature ventricular contraction will occur
   B. a premature atrial contraction with aberrancy occurs
   C. the premature P' wave may not be followed by a QRS complex
   D. none of the above

3. An extra contraction that originates in an ectopic pacemaker in the AV junction, occurring before the next expected beat of the underlying rhythm, is called:
   A. a premature atrial contraction
   B. a premature junctional contraction
   C. a premature ventricular contraction
   D. none of the above

4. The QRS complex of a PJC:
   A. resembles a premature ventricular contraction if aberrant ventricular conduction is present
   B. precedes or follows the P' wave associated with it
   C. usually resembles that of the underlying rhythm
   D. all of the above

5. PJCs are caused by:
   A. digitalis toxicity
   B. increased parasympathetic tone on the SA node
   C. sympathomimetic drugs
   D. all of the above

6. More than four to six PJCs per minute may indicate:
   A. enhanced automaticity in the AV junction
   B. a reentry mechanism in the AV junction
   C. that more serious junctional arrhythmias may occur
   D. all of the above

7. An arrhythmia originating in an escape pacemaker in the AV junction with a rate of 40 to 60 beats per minute is called a(n):
   A. agonal rhythm
   B. junctional bradycardia
   C. junctional escape rhythm
   D. complete AV block

8. An arrhythmia consisting of narrow QRS complexes occurring at a rate of 55 beats per minute and P waves occurring independently at a slower rate is called:
   A. a junctional escape rhythm
   B. a supraventricular arrhythmia
   C. atrioventricular (AV) dissociation
   D. all of the above

9. A common cause of nonparoxysmal junctional tachycardia is:
   A. acute anterior MI
   B. digitalis toxicity
   C. damage to the SA node
   D. all of the above

10. Paroxysmal supraventricular tachycardia (PSVT) is characterized by:
    A. a heart rate between 60 and 130 beats per minute
    B. a reentry mechanism in the bundle of His
    C. an abrupt onset and termination
    D. all of the above

CHAPTER OBJECTIVES

Upon completion of all or part of this chapter, you should be able to complete the following objective:
1. Define and give the diagnostic characteristics, cause, and clinical significance of the following arrhythmias:
   Premature ventricular contractions (PVCs)
   Ventricular tachycardia (VT)
   Ventricular fibrillation (VF)
   Accelerated idioventricular rhythm (AIVR)
   Ventricular escape rhythm
   Ventricular asystole

PREMATURE VENTRICULAR CONTRACTIONS

KEY DEFINITION

A premature ventricular contraction (PVC) (Figure 8-1) is an extra ventricular contraction consisting of an abnormally wide and bizarre QRS complex that originates in an ectopic pacemaker in the ventricles. It occurs earlier than the next expected beat of the underlying rhythm and is usually followed by a compensatory pause.

Diagnostic Characteristics

Heart rate. The heart rate is that of the underlying rhythm.

Rhythm. The rhythm is typically irregular when PVCs are present.

Pacemaker site. The pacemaker site of the PVC is an ectopic pacemaker in the ventricles, specifically in the bundle branches, Purkinje network, or ventricular myocardium. PVCs may originate from a single ectopic pacemaker site or from multiple sites in the ventricles.

P waves. P waves may be present or absent. If present, they are usually of the underlying rhythm and have no relation to the PVCs. Typically, the PVCs do not disturb the P-P cycle of the underlying rhythm, so the P waves continue without disruption during and after the PVCs and occur at their expected time.

Uncommonly, the electrical impulse responsible for the PVC enters the atria, depolarizing them retrogradely. This results in a P wave that follows the QRS complex of the PVC at an RP' interval of about 0.20 second, but often the P' wave is buried in the QRS complex. Because atrial depolarization occurs in a retrograde fashion, these P' waves are negative (inverted) in lead II. The electrical impulse of the PVC may also depolarize the sinoatrial (SA) node,

Premature Ventricular Contractions

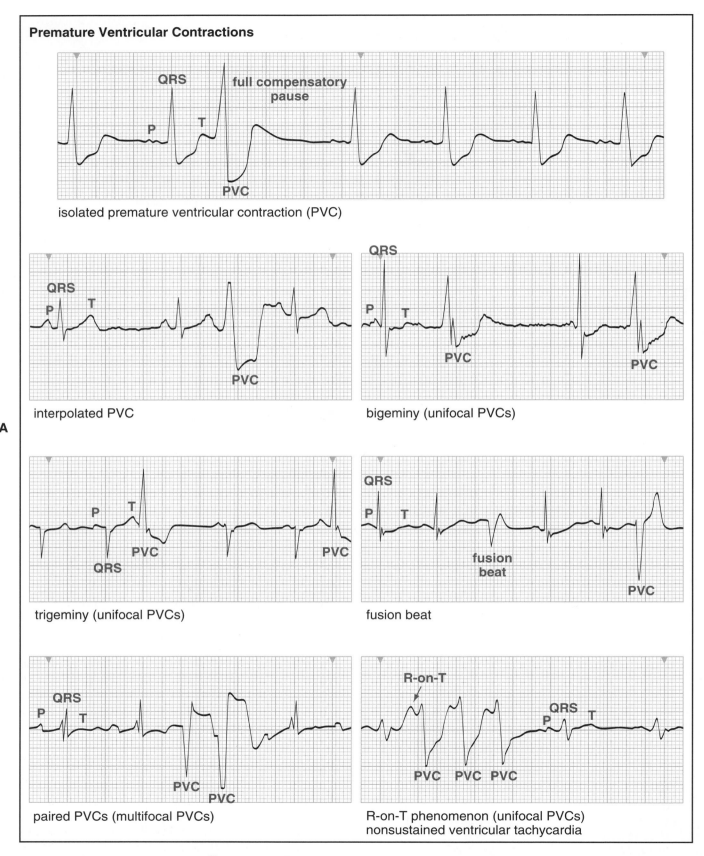

isolated premature ventricular contraction (PVC)

interpolated PVC

bigeminy (unifocal PVCs)

trigeminy (unifocal PVCs)

fusion beat

paired PVCs (multifocal PVCs)

R-on-T phenomenon (unifocal PVCs)
nonsustained ventricular tachycardia

A

Figure 8-1 Premature ventricular contractions.

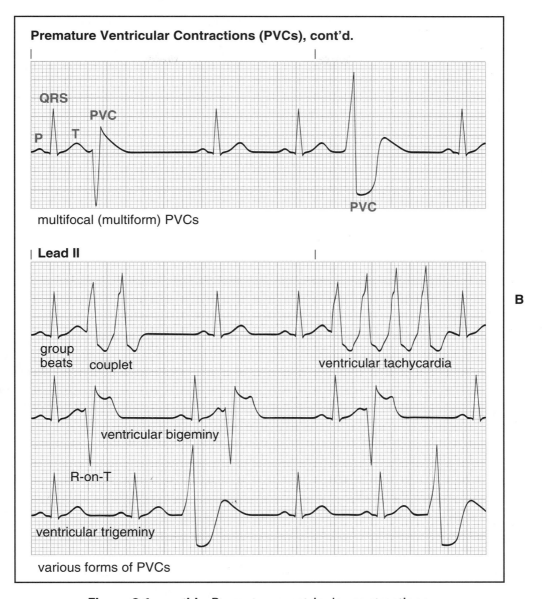

Figure 8-1, cont'd Premature ventricular contractions.

momentarily suppressing it, so that the next P wave of the underlying rhythm appears later than expected.

Often the P waves of the underlying rhythm are obscured by the PVCs, but sometimes they appear as notches on the ST segment or T wave of the PVCs. This provides a clue that the premature ectopic complex is a PVC and not a premature atrial contraction with aberrant ventricular conduction. In a premature atrial contraction, a P wave typically precedes the QRS complex.

PR intervals. No PR intervals are associated with the PVCs.

R-R intervals. The R-R intervals are unequal when PVCs are present. The R-R interval between the PVC and the preceding QRS complex of the underlying rhythm is usually shorter than that of the underlying rhythm. This R-R interval is called the *coupling interval.* PVCs with the same coupling interval in a given ECG lead usually originate from the same ectopic pacemaker site.

A full compensatory pause commonly follows a PVC because the SA node is often not depolarized prematurely by the PVC (i.e., the P wave of the underlying rhythm that follows the PVC appears at the expected time). Consequently, the interval between the P waves of the underlying rhythm occurring before and after the PVC is twice the P-P interval of the underlying rhythm. Rarely, when the SA node is depolarized by the PVC, an incomplete compensatory pause occurs.

A combination of a full compensatory pause and a P wave of the underlying rhythm superimposed on a premature ectopic beat with a wide and bizarre QRS complex helps to make a positive diagnosis of a PVC.

QRS complexes. The QRS complex of the PVC typically appears prematurely (and without a preceding ectopic P wave) before the next expected QRS complex of the underlying rhythm. The QRS complex is nearly always 0.12 second or greater in duration. Because of the abnormal direction and sequence of ventricular depolarization, the QRS complex is also distorted and bizarre, often with notching, appearing different from the QRS complex of the underlying rhythm.

An abnormal QRS complex is usually followed by an abnormal ST segment and a large T wave, opposite in direction to the major deflection of the QRS complex.

The shape of a PVC often resembles that of a right or left bundle branch block. For example, the QRS complex of a PVC originating from the left ventricle resembles that of a right bundle branch block. Likewise, a PVC originating in the right ventricle has a QRS complex resembling that of a left bundle branch block. However, the QRS complex of a PVC arising from a bundle branch appears only slightly bizarre (fascicular PVC). A PVC arising from the ventricles near the bifurcation of the bundle of His may appear relatively normal.

PVCs that originate from the same ectopic pacemaker site *(unifocal)* usually have QRS complexes that are identical and preceded by equal (constant) coupling intervals in any given lead. These PVCs are called *uniform PVCs.* Occasionally, PVCs arising from the same ectopic pacemaker site may differ from each other because of changing depolarization pathways within the ventricles—a common abnormality present in severe myocardial disease. Such PVCs with constant coupling intervals but differing QRS complexes are called *multiform PVCs.* When PVCs originate in two or more ectopic pacemaker sites *(multifocal),* they characteristically have different QRS complexes with varying coupling intervals in the same lead. Such PVCs, also commonly seen in severe myocardial disease, are also called *multiform PVCs.*

When a PVC occurs at about the same time that an electrical impulse of the underlying rhythm is activating the ventricles, depolarization of the ventricles occurs simultaneously in two directions. This results in a QRS complex that has the characteristics of both the PVC and the QRS complex of the underlying rhythm. Such a QRS complex is called a *ventricular fusion beat.* The presence of ventricular fusion beats provides evidence in favor of a premature ectopic contraction be-

ing ventricular in origin and not supraventricular with aberrant ventricular conduction.

Frequency and pattern of occurrence of PVCs. The following are the various forms in which PVCs may appear:

- ◆ **Infrequent:** The PVCs may be infrequent (less than five beats per minute).
- ◆ **Frequent:** The PVCs may be frequent (five or more beats per minute).
- ◆ **Isolated:** The PVCs may occur singly (isolated).
- ◆ **Group beats:** The PVCs may occur in groups of two or more in succession. Groups of two or more PVCs are called *ventricular group beats* or *bursts* or *salvos of PVCs.* Two PVCs in a row are called *paired PVCs* or a *couplet.* A group of three or more consecutive PVCs is considered to be *ventricular tachycardia (VT).*
- ◆ **Repetitive beats:** If PVCs alternate with the QRS complexes of the underlying rhythm, *ventricular bigeminy* is present. If, in ventricular bigeminy, the PVCs follow the QRS complexes of the underlying rhythm at precisely the same intervals, *coupling* is said to be present. *Ventricular trigeminy* occurs when there is one PVC for every two QRS complexes of the underlying rhythm, or one QRS complex of the underlying rhythm for every two PVCs. When there is one PVC for every three QRS complexes of the underlying rhythm, *quadrigeminy* is present.
- ◆ **R-on-T phenomenon:** The term *R-on-T phenomenon* is used to indicate that a PVC has occurred during the vulnerable period of ventricular repolarization—the relative refractory period of the ventricles that coincides with the downslope of the T wave. During this period, the myocardium is at its greatest electrical nonuniformity, a condition in which some of the ventricular muscle fibers may be completely repolarized, others may be only partially repolarized, and still others may be completely refractory. Stimulation of the ventricles at this point by an intrinsic electrical impulse such as that generated by a PVC or by an extrinsic impulse from a cardiac pacemaker or an electrical countershock may result in nonuniform conduction of the electrical impulse through the muscle fibers.

In such nonuniform conduction of the electrical impulse through the muscle fibers, some of the fibers will be able to conduct the electrical impulse normally, whereas others will only be able to conduct them slowly or not at all. Thus a reentry mechanism will be established that may precipitate repetitive ventricular contractions and result in ventricular tachycardia or fibrillation.

- ◆ **End-diastolic PVCs:** A PVC that occurs at about the same time that ventricular depolarization of the underlying rhythm is expected to occur is called an *end-diastolic PVC*. This usually results in a ventricular fusion beat. End-diastolic PVCs tend to occur when the underlying rhythm is relatively rapid.

◆ **Interpolated PVCs:** A PVC occurring between two normally conducted QRS complexes without greatly disturbing the underlying rhythm is called an *interpolated PVC*. This tends to occur when the underlying rhythm is relatively slow. The R-R interval that includes the PVC is often slightly greater than that of the underlying rhythm, but a full compensatory pause usually does not occur.

Cause of Arrhythmia

PVCs may occur in healthy persons with apparently healthy hearts and without apparent cause. PVCs, especially if they are frequent, may be caused by the following:

◆ Increase in catecholamines and sympathetic tone (as in emotional stress)
◆ Stimulants (alcohol, caffeine, and tobacco)
◆ Myocardial ischemia or acute myocardial infarction (MI)
◆ Congestive heart failure
◆ Excessive administration of digitalis or sympathomimetic drugs (epinephrine, isoproterenol, and norepinephrine)
◆ Increase in vagal (parasympathetic) tone
◆ Hypoxia
◆ Acidosis
◆ Hypokalemia
◆ Hypomagnesemia

The electrophysiological mechanism responsible for PVCs in the above conditions is either enhanced automaticity or reentry.

Clinical Significance

Isolated PVCs in patients with no underlying heart disease usually have no significance and usually require no treatment. However, in the presence of heart disease, such as an acute MI or ischemic episode, and drug intoxication (e.g., digitalis), PVCs may indicate the presence of enhanced ventricular automaticity, a reentry mechanism, or both, and may herald the appearance of such life-threatening arrhythmias as ventricular tachycardia or fibrillation.

At times, premature atrial and junctional contractions with aberrant ventricular conduction may mimic PVCs because of the abnormally wide and bizarre-appearing QRS complexes that resemble right or left bundle branch block. The presence of P waves or a notch in the preceding T wave and an incomplete compensatory pause helps to differentiate PACs and PJCs with abnormal QRS complexes from PVCs.

Notes

_____

_____

_____

_____

_____

_____

VENTRICULAR TACHYCARDIA

> ### KEY DEFINITION
>
> **Ventricular tachycardia (VT or V TACH) (Figure 8-2) is an arrhythmia originating in an ectopic pacemaker in the ventricles with a rate between 110 and 250 beats per minute. The QRS complexes are abnormally wide and bizarre.**

Diagnostic Characteristics

Heart rate. The heart rate in VT is over 100 beats per minute, usually between 110 and 250 beats per minute. VT exists if three or more consecutive PVCs are present, occurring at a rate greater than 100 beats per minute. The onset and termination of VT may or may not be abrupt. VT may occur in paroxysms of three or more consecutive PVCs separated by the underlying rhythm, or it they may persist for a long period. VT lasting for three consecutive beats or less than 30 seconds is called *nonsustained* or *paroxysmal VT*. When VT lasts for more than 30 seconds, it is called a *sustained VT*.

Rhythm. The rhythm is usually regular, but it may be slightly irregular.

Pacemaker site. The pacemaker site of VT is an ectopic pacemaker in the bundle branches, Purkinje network, or ventricular myocardium.

P waves. P waves may be present or absent. If present, they usually have no set relation to the QRS complexes of the VT, appearing between the QRS complexes at a rate different from that of the VT. The pacemaker site of such P waves is the SA node or an ectopic or escape pacemaker in the atria or atrioventricular (AV) junction. These P waves may be positive (upright) or negative (inverted) in lead II. P waves are often difficult to detect in VT, especially if it is rapid. When the P waves occur independently of the QRS complexes, AV dissociation is present. Rarely, identical P waves regularly follow

Ventricular Tachycardia

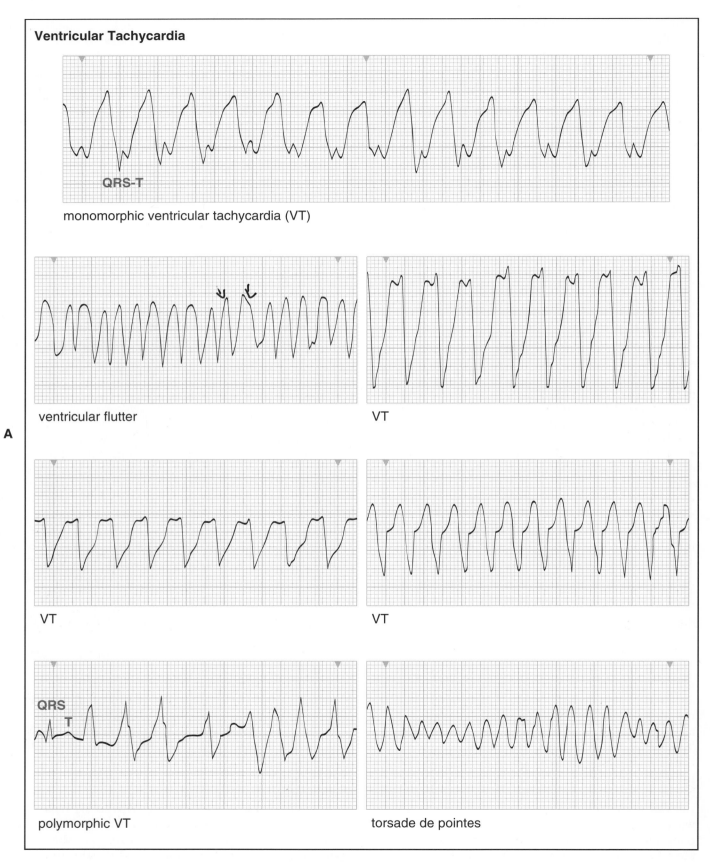

monomorphic ventricular tachycardia (VT)

ventricular flutter

VT

VT

VT

polymorphic VT

torsade de pointes

A

Figure 8-2   Ventricular tachycardia.

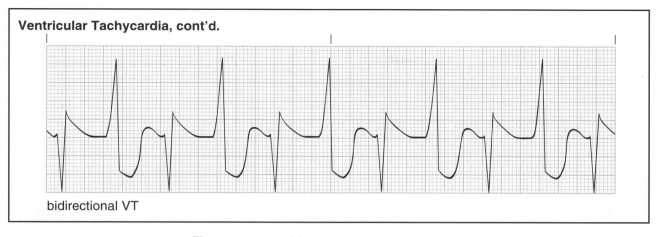

Ventricular Tachycardia, cont'd.

bidirectional VT

B

Figure 8-2, cont'd Ventricular tachycardia.

the QRS complexes. The electrical impulses responsible for them have most likely originated in the ectopic pacemaker site of the VT. Such P waves differ from normal P waves in size, shape, and direction. Because the atria are depolarized in a retrograde manner by the electrical impulse entering the atria from the ventricles through the AV junction (retrograde AV conduction), the P waves are negative (inverted) in lead II.

PR intervals. If P waves are present and occur independently of the QRS complexes, no PR intervals are present. If P waves regularly follow the QRS complexes, the RP intervals are usually less than 0.20 second.

R-R intervals. The R-R intervals may be equal or vary slightly.

QRS complexes. The QRS complexes exceed 0.12 second and are usually distorted and bizarre, often with notching. They are followed by large T waves, opposite in direction to the major deflection of the QRS complexes. Usually, the QRS complexes are identical, but, occasionally, one or more QRS complexes differ in size, shape, and direction, especially at the onset or end of VT. These are most likely fusion beats.

Occasionally, an electrical impulse of the underlying rhythm is conducted from the atria to the ventricles through the AV junction, producing a normal-appearing QRS complex (0.10 second or less) among the abnormal QRS complexes of the VT. Such a QRS complex is called a *capture beat.* The R-R interval between the QRS complex of the VT preceding the capture beat and the QRS complex of the capture beat is usually less than that of the VT. The presence of capture or ventricular fusion beats provides evidence that the tachycardia is most likely ventricular in origin and not a supraventricular tachycardia with aberrant ventricular conduction.

KEY DEFINITION

Several forms of VT exist, depending on the configuration of the QRS complexes. They include the following:

- **Monomorphic VT:** VT with QRS complexes that are of the same or almost the same shape, size, and direction.
- **Bidirectional VT:** VT with two distinctly different forms of QRS complexes alternating with each other, indicating that they originated in two different ventricular ectopic pacemakers.
- **Polymorphic VT:** VT in which the QRS complexes differ markedly in shape, size, and direction from beat to beat.
- **Torsade de pointes:** A form of polymorphic VT characterized by QRS complexes that gradually change back and forth from one shape, size, and direction to another over a series of beats. *Torsade de pointes*, literally translated from the French, means "twisting around a point." It typically occurs when the QT interval of the underlying rhythm is abnormally prolonged, usually 0.5 second, the result of severe slowing of myocardial repolarization.
- **Ventricular flutter:** A very rapid VT with sawtooth–like QRS complexes of similar shape, size, and direction.

Cause of Arrhythmia

VT usually occurs in the presence of the following:
- Significant cardiac disease, such as the following:
  - ◇ Coronary artery disease, particularly in the setting of acute MI and especially if hypoxia or acidosis is present

◇ Cardiomyopathy, mitral valve prolapse, and congenital heart disease

◇ Left ventricular hypertrophy, valvular heart disease, and congestive heart failure

◆ Digitalis toxicity

◆ QT interval prolongation from various causes, including the following:

◇ Excessive administration of quinidine, procainamide, disopyramide, phenothiazines, and tricyclic antidepressants

◇ Bradyarrhythmias (marked sinus bradycardia and third-degree AV block with slow ventricular escape rhythm)

◇ Electrolyte disturbances (hypokalemia)

◇ Liquid protein diets

◇ Central nervous system disorders (subarachnoid hemorrhage and intracranial trauma)

The torsade de pointes form of VT is particularly prone to occur following administration of such antiarrhythmic agents as disopyramide, quinidine, procainamide, and sotalol, or other agents that prolong the QT interval.

The electrophysiological mechanism responsible for VT is either enhanced automaticity, reentry, or triggered activity.

A PVC can initiate VT when the PVC occurs during the vulnerable period of ventricular repolarization coincident with the peak of the T wave (i.e., the R-on-T phenomenon, described in the section on PVCs). Often, VT may occur without preexisting or precipitating PVCs.

Clinical Significance

The signs and symptoms in VT vary, depending on the nature and severity of the underlying cardiac disease, such as acute MI or congestive heart failure. VT may cause or aggravate existing angina pectoris, acute MI, or congestive heart failure; produce hypotension or shock; or terminate in VF or asystole. The patient with VT may often experience feelings of impending death. The torsade de pointes form of VT tends to terminate and recur spontaneously.

In VT, the atria do not regularly contract and empty, as they normally do, during the last part of ventricular diastole, completely filling the ventricles just before they contract. The loss of this "atrial kick" results in incomplete filling of the ventricles before they contract, causing a reduction of the cardiac output by as much as 25%. This reduction in cardiac output often compounds the already low cardiac output frequently seen in the diseased hearts in which VT tends to occur. When the cardiac output is so low in VT that it is unable to produce a blood pressure or palpable pulse, it is termed *pulseless VT*.

Because VT is considered a life-threatening arrhythmia, often initiating or degenerating into ventricular fibrillation (VF) or asystole, VT and its underlying causes must be treated immediately. Pulseless VT should be treated the same as VF (i.e., cardiac arrest).

At times, a supraventricular tachycardia (e.g., sinus, atrial, and junctional tachycardias, atrial flutter, and paroxysmal supraventricular tachycardia) with wide QRS complexes caused by a preexisting intraventricular conduction disturbance (such as a bundle branch block), aberrant ventricular conduction, or ventricular preexcitation may mimic VT. Atrial fibrillation with wide QRS complexes and a rapid ventricular rate may also mimic VT, but usually the grossly irregular rhythm of atrial fibrillation provides a clue to its true identity.

The presence of certain features common to VT, namely AV dissociation, a QRS-complex duration greater than 0.12 second (and especially if it is greater than 0.14 second), and capture or ventricular fusion beats, helps to differentiate VT from a supraventricular tachycardia with wide QRS complexes. A 12-lead ECG or lead MCL_1 is also useful in making a differentiation in this situation by helping to determine the presence or absence of P waves and, if present, their relationship to the QRS complexes.

Notes

_____

_____

_____

_____

_____

_____

_____

_____

_____

_____

_____

_____

_____

_____

_____

_____

_____

VENTRICULAR FIBRILLATION

KEY DEFINITION

Ventricular fibrillation (VF or V-FIB) *(Figures 8-3 and 8-4) is an arrhythmia arising in numerous ectopic pacemakers in the ventricles, characterized by very rapid abnormal VF (f) waves and no QRS complexes.*

Diagnostic Characteristics

Heart rate. No coordinated ventricular beats are present. The ventricles contract from about 300 to 500 times a minute in an unsynchronized, uncoordinated, and haphazard manner. The fibrillating ventricles are often described as resembling a "bag of worms."

Rhythm. The rhythm is grossly (totally) irregular.

Pacemaker site. The pacemaker sites of VF are multiple ectopic pacemakers in the Purkinje network and ventricular myocardium.

PR intervals. PR intervals are absent.

R-R intervals. R-R intervals are absent.

QRS complexes. QRS complexes are absent.

Characteristics of VF waves include the following:

◆ **Relationship to cardiac anatomy and physiology:** VF waves represent abnormal, chaotic, and incomplete ventricular depolarizations caused by haphazard depolarization of small individual groups (or islets) of muscle fibers. Because organized depolarizations of the atria and ventricles are absent, distinct P waves, QRS complexes, ST segments, and T waves and organized atrial and ventricular contractions are absent.

◆ **Onset and end:** The onset and end of the VF waves often cannot be determined with certainty.

◆ **Direction:** The direction of the VF waves varies at random from positive (upright) to negative (inverted).

◆ **Duration:** The duration of VF waves cannot be measured with certainty.

◆ **Amplitude:** The amplitude varies from less than 1 mm to about 10 mm. Generally, if the VF waves are small (less than 3 mm), the arrhythmia is called *fine VF.* If the VF waves are large (greater than 3 mm), it is called *coarse VF.* Such coarse VF, whose fibrillatory waves appear as large, narrow, rounded waves measuring 10 mm or more in amplitude, is sometimes referred to as *ventricular flutter,* and occurs when VT degenerates into VF. If the VF waves are so small or "fine" that they are not recorded, the ECG appears as a wavy or flat (isoelectric) line resembling ventricular asystole.

◆ **Shape:** The VF waves are of varying shape, appearing bizarre, rounded or pointed, and markedly dissimilar.

Cause of Arrhythmia

VF, one of the most common causes of cardiac arrest, usually occurs in the following:

◆ Significant cardiac disease, such as the following:
  ◇ Coronary artery disease (i.e., myocardial ischemia and acute MI—the most common cause of VF)
  ◇ Third-degree AV block with a slow ventricular escape rhythm
  ◇ Cardiomyopathy, mitral valve prolapse, and cardiac trauma (penetrating or blunt)
◆ Cardiac, medical, and traumatic conditions as a terminal event
◆ Excessive dose of digitalis, quinidine, or procainamide
◆ Hypoxia
◆ Acidosis
◆ Electrolyte imbalance (hypokalemia and hyperkalemia)
◆ During anesthesia, cardiac and noncardiac operations, cardiac catheterization, and cardiac pacing
◆ Following cardioversion or accidental electrocution

The electrophysiological mechanism responsible for VF is either enhanced automaticity or reentry.

A PVC can initiate VF when the PVC occurs during the vulnerable period of ventricular repolarization coincident with the peak of the T wave (i.e., the R-on-T phenomenon), particularly when electrical instability of the heart has been altered by ischemia or acute MI. Sustained VT may also precipitate VF. Often, VF may begin without preexisting or precipitating PVCs or VT.

Clinical Significance

Organized ventricular depolarization and contraction and, consequently, cardiac output cease at the moment VF occurs, resulting in the sudden disappearance of the pulse and blood pressure. VF results in faintness, followed within seconds by loss of consciousness, seizures, apnea, and, if the arrhythmia remains untreated, death. *Ventricular fibrillation must be treated immediately!*

The significance of coarse versus fine VF is that coarse VF, indicating a recent onset of the arrhythmia, is more apt to be reversed by defibrillation shock than is fine VF, which indicates that the arrhythmia has been present for some time. Sometimes the distinction between coarse and fine VF cannot be made because of the limitations of the monitoring equipment.

Because fine VF may resemble ventricular asystole, VF must be correctly identified using at least two ECG

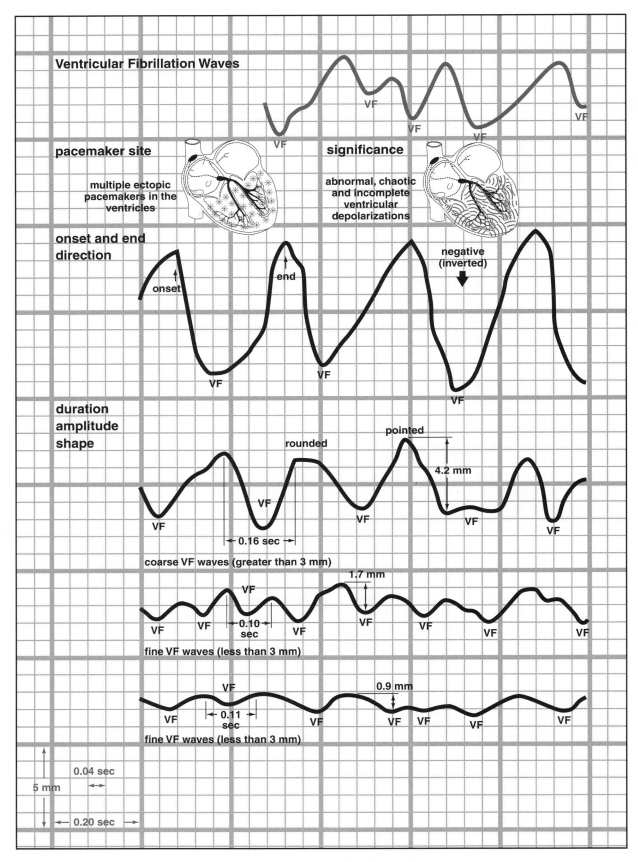

Ventricular Fibrillation Waves

pacemaker site

multiple ectopic pacemakers in the ventricles

significance

abnormal, chaotic and incomplete ventricular depolarizations

onset and end direction

onset

end

negative (inverted)

VF

VF

VF

duration amplitude shape

rounded

pointed

4.2 mm

0.16 sec

coarse VF waves (greater than 3 mm)

VF

1.7 mm

0.10 sec

fine VF waves (less than 3 mm)

VF

0.9 mm

0.11 sec

fine VF waves (less than 3 mm)

0.04 sec

5 mm

0.20 sec

Figure 8-3   Ventricular fibrillation waves.

Ventricular Fibrillation

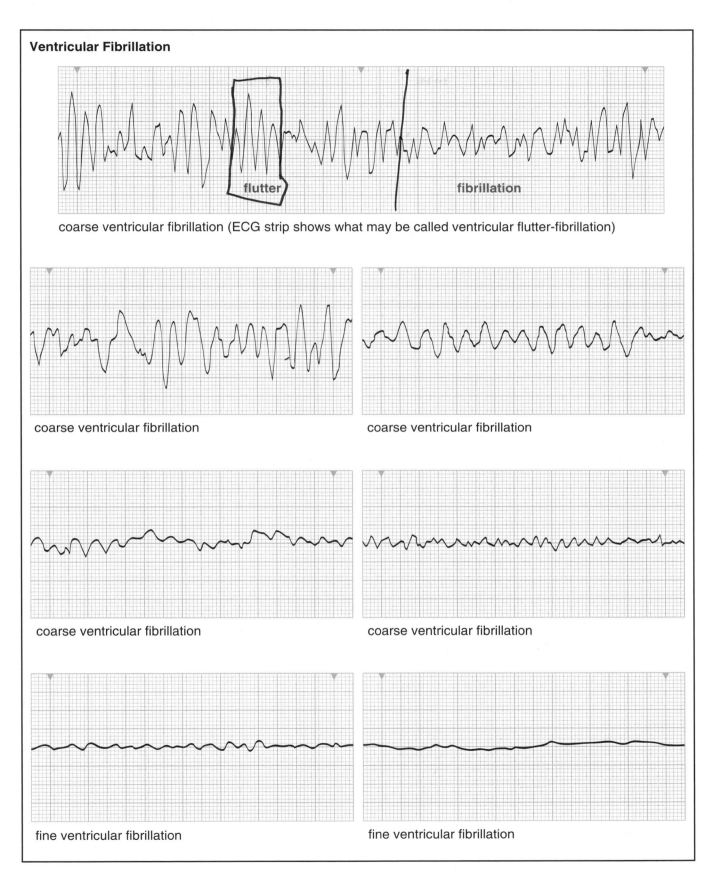

coarse ventricular fibrillation (ECG strip shows what may be called ventricular flutter-fibrillation)

coarse ventricular fibrillation

coarse ventricular fibrillation

coarse ventricular fibrillation

coarse ventricular fibrillation

fine ventricular fibrillation

fine ventricular fibrillation

Figure 8-4 Ventricular fibrillation.

leads (i.e., lead II and leads I or III) so that the patient is not inappropriately treated for ventricular asystole.

In addition, ECG artifacts produced by loose or dry electrodes, broken ECG leads, or patient movement or muscle tremor may also resemble VF. A rapid assessment of the patient, including a check of the patient's pulse, must be performed immediately after the ECG-indicated onset of VF to confirm the arrhythmia before treating the patient for cardiac arrest.

Notes

_____

_____

_____

_____

_____

_____

_____

_____

_____

_____

_____

ACCELERATED IDIOVENTRICULAR RHYTHM (ACCELERATED VENTRICULAR RHYTHM, IDIOVENTRICULAR TACHYCARDIA, SLOW VENTRICULAR TACHYCARDIA)

KEY DEFINITION

Accelerated idioventricular rhythm (Figure 8-5) is an arrhythmia originating in an ectopic pacemaker in the ventricles with a rate between 40 and 100 beats per minute.

Diagnostic Characteristics

Heart rate. The heart rate in accelerated idioventricular rhythm is between 40 and 100 beats per minute. The onset and termination of accelerated idioventricular rhythm are usually gradual, but the arrhythmia may begin abruptly after a PVC.

Rhythm. The rhythm is essentially regular, but it may be irregular.

Pacemaker site. The pacemaker site is an ectopic pacemaker in the bundle branches, Purkinje network, or ventricular myocardium.

P waves. P waves may be present or absent. If present, they have no relation to the QRS complexes of the accelerated idioventricular rhythm, appearing independently at a rate different from that of the QRS complexes (AV dissociation).

The pacemaker site of such P waves is the SA node or an ectopic or escape pacemaker in the atria or AV junction. These P waves may be positive (upright) or negative (inverted) in lead II.

PR intervals. If P waves are present and occur independently of the QRS complexes, no PR intervals are present.

R-R intervals. The R-R intervals may be equal or may vary.

QRS complexes. The QRS complexes typically exceed 0.12 second and are bizarre, but they may be only slightly wider than normal (greater than 0.10 second but less than 0.12 second) if the pacemaker site is in the bundle branches below the bundle of His. Fusion beats may be present if a supraventricular rhythm is present, and particularly if its rate is about the same as that of the accelerated idioventricular rhythm. When this occurs, the cardiac rhythm alternates between the supraventricular rhythm and the accelerated idioventricular rhythm. Fusion beats most commonly occur at the onset and end of the arrhythmia.

Cause of Arrhythmia

Accelerated idioventricular rhythm can occur under the following conditions:
◆ Acute MI (relatively common)
◆ When the firing rate of the dominant pacemaker (usually the SA node) or escape pacemaker in the AV junction becomes less than that of the ventricular ectopic pacemaker
◆ When a sinus arrest, SA exit block, or third-degree (complete) AV block develops
◆ Digitalis toxicity

The electrophysiological mechanism responsible for accelerated idioventricular rhythm is probably enhanced automaticity.

Clinical Significance

Accelerated idioventricular rhythm occurring in acute MI usually requires no treatment because it is self-limited in most cases. Because it does not affect the course or prognosis of the MI, it is considered rela-

Accelerated Idioventricular Rhythm (Accelerated Ventricular Rhythm, Idioventricular Tachycardia, Slow Ventricular Tachycardia)

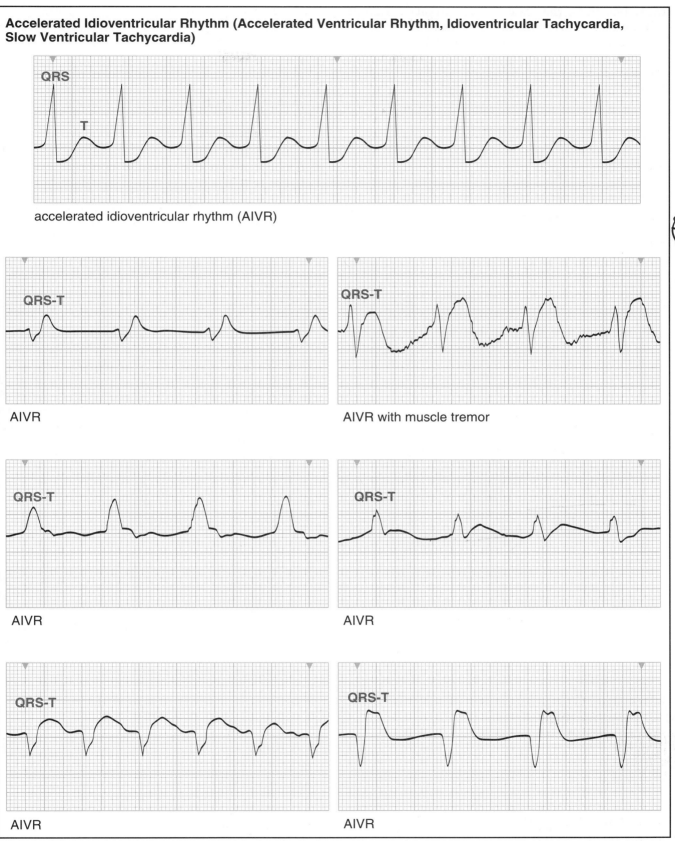

Figure 8-5 Accelerated idioventricular rhythm (accelerated ventricular rhythm, idioventricular tachycardia, slow ventricular tachycardia).

tively benign. If the patient does, however, become symptomatic, accelerated idioventricular rhythm should be treated as one would treat VT.

Notes

_____

_____

_____

_____

_____

_____

_____

_____

_____

VENTRICULAR ESCAPE RHYTHM (IDIOVENTRICULAR RHYTHM)

KEY DEFINITION

Ventricular escape rhythm _(Figure 8-6)_ is an arrhythmia originating in an escape pacemaker in the ventricles with a rate of less than 40 beats per minute. When less than three consecutive QRS complexes arising from the escape pacemaker are present, they are called ventricular escape beats _or_ complexes.

Diagnostic Characteristics

Heart rate. The heart rate is less than 40 beats per minute, usually between 30 and 40 beats per minute, but it may be less.

Rhythm. The rhythm is usually regular, but it may be irregular.

Pacemaker site. The pacemaker site of ventricular escape rhythm is an escape pacemaker in the bundle branches, Purkinje network, or ventricular myocardium.

P waves. P waves may be present or absent. If present, they have no set relation to the QRS complexes of the ventricular escape rhythm, appearing independently at a rate different from that of the QRS complexes. The pacemaker site of such P waves is the SA node or an ectopic or escape pacemaker in the atria

or AV junction. These P waves may be positive (upright) or negative (inverted) in lead II. They precede, are buried in, or follow the QRS complexes haphazardly. When the atria and ventricles thus beat independently, AV dissociation is present.

PR intervals. PR intervals are absent.

R-R intervals. The R-R intervals may be equal or may vary.

QRS complexes. The QRS complexes exceed 0.12 second and are bizarre. Sometimes the shape of the QRS complexes varies in any given lead.

Cause of Arrhythmia

Ventricular escape rhythm can occur under either of the following conditions:

◆ When the rate of impulse formation of the dominant pacemaker (usually the SA node) and escape pacemaker in the AV junction becomes less than that of the escape pacemaker in the ventricles

◆ When the electrical impulses from the SA node, atria, and AV junction fail to reach the ventricles because of a sinus arrest, SA exit block, or third-degree (complete) AV block

Generally, when an electrical impulse fails to arrive in the ventricles within approximately 1.5 to 2.0 seconds, an escape pacemaker in the ventricles takes over at its inherent firing rate of 30 to 40 beats per minute. The result is one or more ventricular escape beats or a ventricular escape rhythm.

Ventricular escape rhythm also occurs in advanced heart disease and is often the cardiac arrhythmia that is present in a dying heart, the so-called _agonal rhythm_, just before the appearance of the final arrhythmia—ventricular asystole.

Clinical Significance

Ventricular escape rhythm is generally symptomatic. Hypotension with marked reduction in cardiac output and decreased perfusion of the brain and other vital organs may occur, resulting in syncope, shock, or congestive heart failure. Ventricular escape rhythm must be treated promptly, preferably with a transcutaneous pacemaker, to reverse the consequences of the reduced cardiac output.

Notes

_____

_____

_____

_____

_____

_____

Ventricular Escape Rhythm (Idioventricular Rhythm)

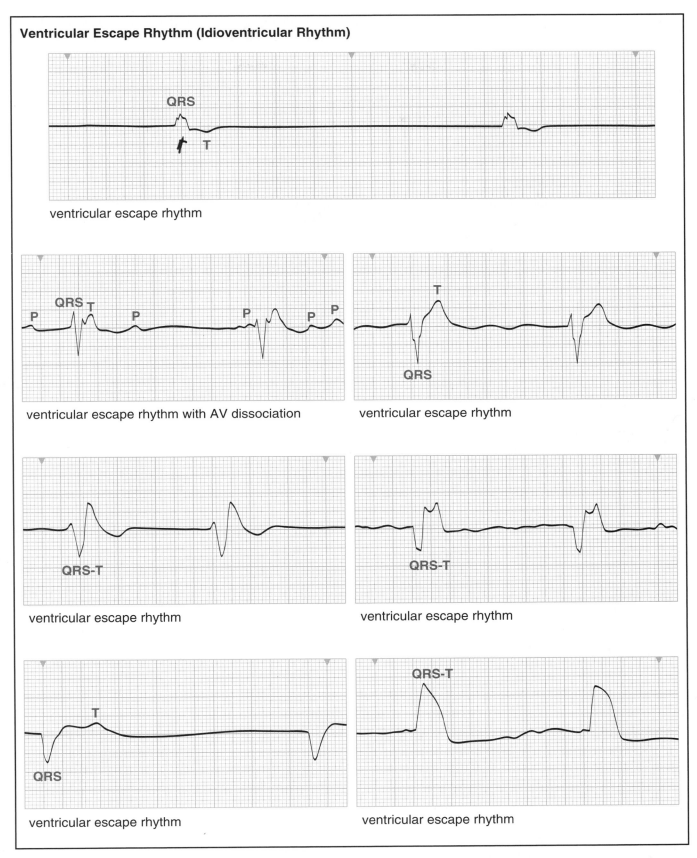

ventricular escape rhythm

ventricular escape rhythm with AV dissociation

ventricular escape rhythm

ventricular escape rhythm

ventricular escape rhythm

ventricular escape rhythm

ventricular escape rhythm

Figure 8-6   Ventricular escape rhythm.

VENTRICULAR ASYSTOLE (CARDIAC STANDSTILL)

> ### KEY DEFINITION
>
> **Ventricular asystole (Figure 8-7) is the absence of all electrical activity within the ventricles.**

Diagnostic Characteristics

Heart rate. Heart rate is absent.

Rhythm. Rhythm is absent.

Pacemaker site. A pacemaker site in the ventricles is absent. If P waves are present, their pacemaker site is the SA node or an ectopic or escape pacemaker in the atria or AV junction.

P waves. P waves may be present or absent.

PR intervals. PR intervals are absent.

R-R intervals. R-R intervals are absent.

QRS complexes. QRS complexes are absent.

Cause of Arrhythmia

Ventricular asystole, one of the common causes of cardiac arrest, may occur in advanced cardiac disease as a primary event in the following situations:

◆ When the dominant pacemaker (usually the SA node) and/or the escape pacemaker in the AV junction fail to generate electrical impulses

◆ When the electrical impulses are blocked from entering the ventricles because of a third-degree (complete) AV block and an escape pacemaker in the ventricles fails to take over

In the dying heart, ventricular asystole is usually the final event that occurs after such arrythmias as:

◆ VT

◆ VF

◆ Pulseless electrical activity*

◆ Ventricular escape rhythm

Ventricular asystole may also follow the termination of tachyarrhythmias by whatever means—drugs, defibrillation shock, or synchronized countershock.

Clinical Significance

Organized ventricular depolarization and contraction and, consequently, cardiac output and a palpable pulse are absent in ventricular asystole. The occurrence of sudden ventricular asystole in a conscious person results in faintness, followed within seconds by loss of consciousness, seizures, apnea (Adams-Stokes syndrome), and, if the arrhythmia remains untreated, death. *Ventricular asystole must be treated immediately.*

Notes

_____

_____

_____

SUMMARY

Table 8-1 summarizes the diagnostic characteristics of the various ventricular arrhythmias discussed in this chapter.

---

*Pulseless electrical activity, a life-threatening condition, is the absence of effective ventricular contraction, cardiac output, and pulse in the presence of some form of electrical activity of the heart as shown on the ECG. See the discussion of Pulseless Electrical Activity in Chapter 10.

TABLE

8-1 Typical Diagnostic ECG Features of Ventricular Arrhythmias

Arrhythmia	Heart Rate (bpm)	Rhythm	P Waves	PR Intervals	QRS Complexes
Ventricular tachycardia	110-250	Regular	Present or absent; no relation to QRS complexes	None	Abnormal, >0.12 sec
Ventricular fibrillation	None	None	Present or absent	None	Ventricular fibrillation waves
Accelerated idioventricular rhythm	40-100	Regular	Present or absent; no relation to QRS complexes	None	Abnormal, >0.12 sec
Ventricular escape rhythm	<40	Regular	Present or absent; no relation to QRS complexes	None	Abnormal, >0.12 sec
Ventricular asystole	None	None	Present or absent	None	None

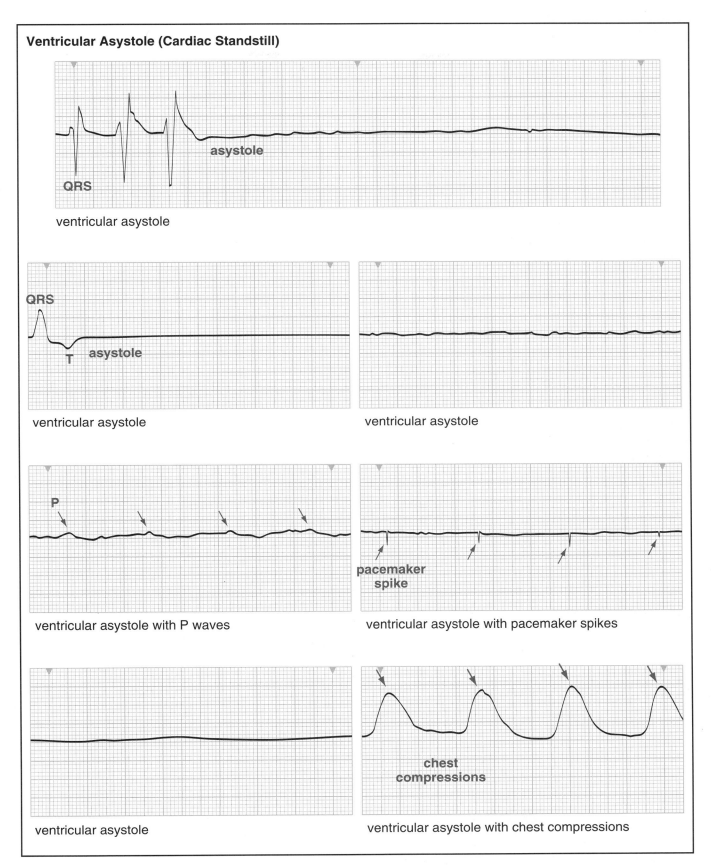

Figure 8-7 Ventricular asystole (cardiac standstill).

TREATMENT ALGORITHMS

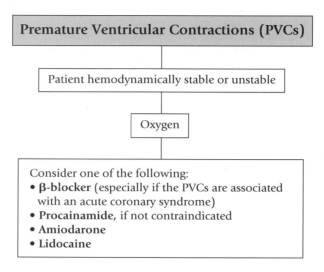

Premature Ventricular Contractions (PVCs)

Patient hemodynamically stable or unstable

Oxygen

Consider one of the following:
- **β-blocker** (especially if the PVCs are associated with an acute coronary syndrome)
- **Procainamide,** if not contraindicated
- **Amiodarone**
- **Lidocaine**

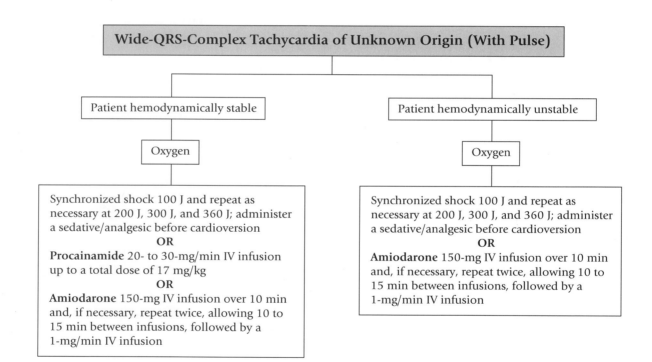

Wide-QRS-Complex Tachycardia of Unknown Origin (With Pulse)

Patient hemodynamically stable

Oxygen

Synchronized shock 100 J and repeat as necessary at 200 J, 300 J, and 360 J; administer a sedative/analgesic before cardioversion
OR
Procainamide 20- to 30-mg/min IV infusion up to a total dose of 17 mg/kg
OR
Amiodarone 150-mg IV infusion over 10 min and, if necessary, repeat twice, allowing 10 to 15 min between infusions, followed by a 1-mg/min IV infusion

Patient hemodynamically unstable

Oxygen

Synchronized shock 100 J and repeat as necessary at 200 J, 300 J, and 360 J; administer a sedative/analgesic before cardioversion
OR
Amiodarone 150-mg IV infusion over 10 min and, if necessary, repeat twice, allowing 10 to 15 min between infusions, followed by a 1-mg/min IV infusion

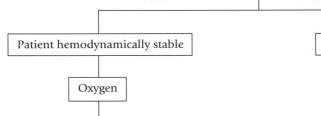

Ventricular Tachycardia (VT), Monomorphic (With Pulse)

Patient hemodynamically stable	Patient hemodynamically unstable
Oxygen	Oxygen

Patient hemodynamically stable:

Synchronized shock 100 J and repeat as necessary at 200 J, 300 J, and 360 J; administer a sedative/analgesic before cardioversion

OR

Procainamide 20- to 30-mg/min IV infusion up to a total dose of 17 mg/kg

OR

Amiodarone 150-mg IV infusion over 10 min and, if necessary, repeat twice, allowing 10 to 15 min between infusions, followed by a 1-mg/min IV infusion

OR

Lidocaine 75- to 100-mg (1.0- to 1.5-mg/kg) IV bolus slowly and, if necessary, repeat a 25- to 50-mg (0.5- to 0.75-mg/kg) IV bolus slowly every 5 to 10 min up to a total dose of 3 mg/kg

Patient hemodynamically unstable:

Synchronized shock 100 J and repeat as necessary at 200 J, 300 J, and 360 J; administer a sedative/analgesic before cardioversion

OR

Amiodarone 150-mg IV infusion over 10 min and, if necessary, repeat twice, allowing 10 to 15 min between infusions, followed by a 1-mg/min IV infusion

OR

Lidocaine 75- to 100-mg (1.0- to 1.5-mg/kg) IV bolus slowly and, if necessary, repeat a 25- to 50-mg (0.5- to 0.75-mg/kg) IV bolus slowly every 5 to 10 min up to a total dose of 3 mg/kg

Ventricular Tachycardia (VT), Polymorphic (With Pulse)
Normal Baseline QT Interval

Patient hemodynamically stable

Oxygen

Synchronized shock 100 J and repeat as necessary at 200 J, 300 J, and 360 J; administer a sedative/analgesic before cardioversion

OR

One of the following **β-blockers** (especially if polymorphic VT is associated with an acute coronary syndrome):

- **Esmolol** 0.5-mg/kg IV bolus over 1 min, followed by an IV infusion at a rate of 0.05 mg/kg/min; repeat the bolus twice, 5 min between each bolus, while increasing the rate of the IV infusion 0.05 mg/kg/min after each bolus; then, if necessary, increase the IV infusion by 0.05 mg/kg/min every 5 min to a maximum of 0.30 mg/kg/min
- **Atenolol** 5 mg IV over 5 min and repeat in 10 min for a total dose of 10 mg
- **Metoprolol** 5 mg IV over 2 to 5 min and repeat every 5 min up to a total dose of 15 mg

OR

Procainamide 20- to 30-mg/min IV infusion up to a total dose of 17 mg/kg

OR

Amiodarone 150-mg IV infusion over 10 min and, if necessary, repeat twice, allowing 10 to 15 min between infusions, followed by a 1-mg/min IV infusion

OR

Lidocaine 75- to 100-mg (1.0- to 1.5-mg/kg) IV bolus slowly and, if necessary, repeat a 25- to 50-mg (0.5- to 0.75-mg/kg) IV bolus slowly every 5 to 10 min up to a total dose of 3 mg/kg

Patient hemodynamically unstable

Oxygen

Synchronized shock 100 J and repeat as necessary at 200 J, 300 J, and 360 J; administer a sedative/analgesic before cardioversion

OR

Amiodarone 150-mg IV infusion over 10 min and, if necessary, repeat twice, allowing 10 to 15 min between infusions, followed by a 1-mg/min IV infusion

OR

Lidocaine 75- to 100-mg (1.0- to 1.5-mg/kg) IV bolus slowly and, if necessary, repeat a 25- to 50-mg (0.5- to 0.75-mg/kg) IV bolus slowly every 5 to 10 min up to a total dose of 3 mg/kg

Ventricular Tachycardia (VT), Polymorphic (With Pulse)
Prolonged Baseline QT Interval
Torsade de Pointes (TdP) (With Pulse)

Patient hemodynamically stable or unstable

Oxygen

Magnesium sulfate 1- to 2-g IV infusion over 5 to 60 min, if indicated, followed by a 0.5- to 1.0-g IV infusion over 1 hr

TC overdrive pacing; administer a sedative/ analgesic before cardioversion
AND
Consider administration of one of the following **β-blockers:**
- **Esmolol** 0.5-mg/kg IV bolus over 1 min, followed by an IV infusion at a rate of 0.05 mg/kg/min; repeat the bolus twice, 5 min between each bolus, while increasing the rate of the IV infusion 0.05 mg/kg/min after each bolus; then, if necessary, increase the IV infusion by 0.05 mg/kg/min every 5 min to a maximum of 0.30 mg/kg/min
- **Atenolol** 5 mg IV over 5 min and repeat in 10 min for a total dose of 10 mg
- **Metoprolol** 5 mg IV over 2 to 5 min and repeat every 5 min up to a total dose of 15 mg

Discontinue such antiarrhythmic agents as the following:
- Amiodarone, disopyramide
- Procainamide, quinidine, sotalol
- Any other agent that prolongs the QT interval (e.g., phenothiazines, tricyclic antidepressants, etc.)
AND
Correct any electrolyte imbalance

Unsynchronized shock 200 J and repeat as necessary at 200-300 J and 360 J; administer a sedative/analgesic before cardioversion

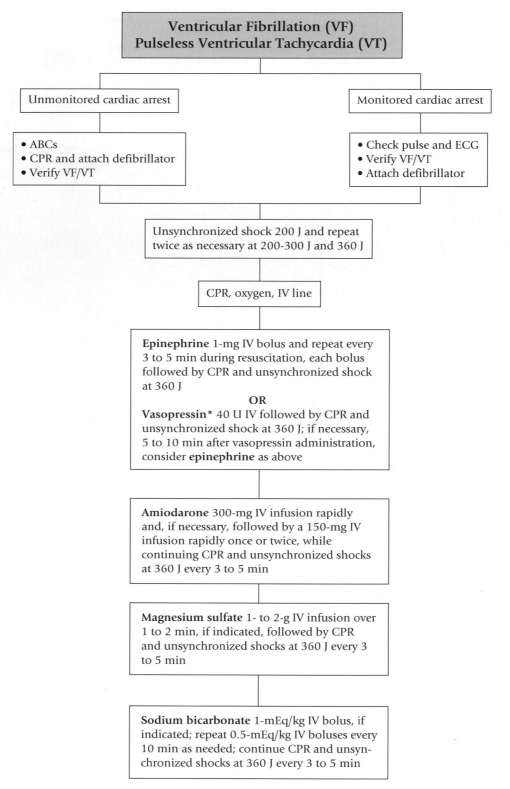

Ventricular Fibrillation (VF)
Pulseless Ventricular Tachycardia (VT)

Unmonitored cardiac arrest

- ABCs
- CPR and attach defibrillator
- Verify VF/VT

Monitored cardiac arrest

- Check pulse and ECG
- Verify VF/VT
- Attach defibrillator

Unsynchronized shock 200 J and repeat
twice as necessary at 200-300 J and 360 J

CPR, oxygen, IV line

Epinephrine 1-mg IV bolus and repeat every
3 to 5 min during resuscitation, each bolus
followed by CPR and unsynchronized shock
at 360 J
OR
Vasopressin* 40 U IV followed by CPR and
unsynchronized shock at 360 J; if necessary,
5 to 10 min after vasopressin administration,
consider **epinephrine** as above

Amiodarone 300-mg IV infusion rapidly
and, if necessary, followed by a 150-mg IV
infusion rapidly once or twice, while
continuing CPR and unsynchronized shocks
at 360 J every 3 to 5 min

Magnesium sulfate 1- to 2-g IV infusion over
1 to 2 min, if indicated, followed by CPR
and unsynchronized shocks at 360 J every 3
to 5 min

Sodium bicarbonate 1-mEq/kg IV bolus, if
indicated; repeat 0.5-mEq/kg IV boluses every
10 min as needed; continue CPR and unsynchronized shocks at 360 J every 3 to 5 min

*At the time of publication of this book, vasopressin has not
been approved for use in the treatment of cardiac arrest in
the United States.

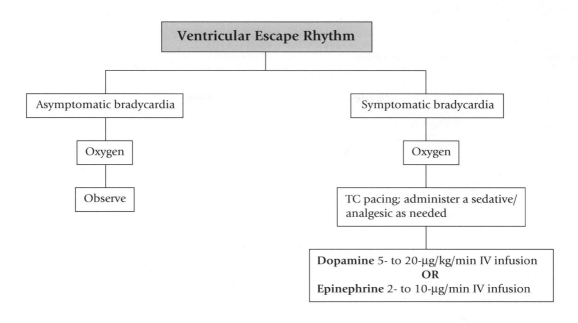

Ventricular Escape Rhythm

Asymptomatic bradycardia

Oxygen

Observe

Symptomatic bradycardia

Oxygen

TC pacing; administer a sedative/ analgesic as needed

Dopamine 5- to 20-μg/kg/min IV infusion
OR
Epinephrine 2- to 10-μg/min IV infusion

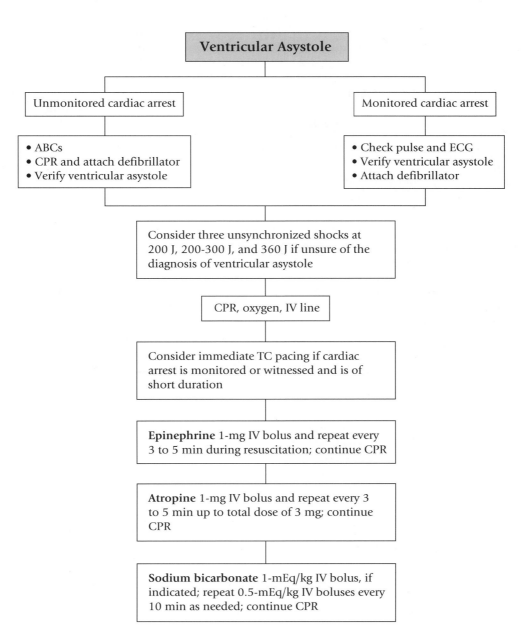

Ventricular Asystole

Unmonitored cardiac arrest

- ABCs
- CPR and attach defibrillator
- Verify ventricular asystole

Monitored cardiac arrest

- Check pulse and ECG
- Verify ventricular asystole
- Attach defibrillator

Consider three unsynchronized shocks at 200 J, 200-300 J, and 360 J if unsure of the diagnosis of ventricular asystole

CPR, oxygen, IV line

Consider immediate TC pacing if cardiac arrest is monitored or witnessed and is of short duration

Epinephrine 1-mg IV bolus and repeat every 3 to 5 min during resuscitation; continue CPR

Atropine 1-mg IV bolus and repeat every 3 to 5 min up to total dose of 3 mg; continue CPR

Sodium bicarbonate 1-mEq/kg IV bolus, if indicated; repeat 0.5-mEq/kg IV boluses every 10 min as needed; continue CPR

CHAPTER REVIEW QUESTIONS

1. An extra contraction consisting of an abnormally wide and bizarre QRS complex originating in an ectopic pacemaker in the ventricles is called a:
   A. PAC
   B. PJC
   C. PVC
   D. none of the above
2. Identical PVCs that originate from a single ectopic pacemaker site are called:
   A. multifocal
   B. unifocal
   C. multiform
   D. isolated
3. A PVC may:
   A. trigger ventricular fibrillation if it occurs on the T wave
   B. depolarize the SA node, momentarily suppressing it, so that the next P wave of the underlying rhythm appears later than expected
   C. all of the above
   D. none of the above
4. A PVC that appears relatively normal usually originates:
   A. near the bifurcation of the bundle of His
   B. in the Purkinje network
   C. in the AV junction
   D. in the SA node
5. A QRS that has characteristics of both the PVC and a QRS complex of the underlying rhythm is called a(n):
   A. fascicular PVC
   B. multifocal PVC
   C. ventricular fusion beat
   D. isolated PVC
6. Groups of two or more PVCs are called:
   A. ventricular group beats
   B. bursts
   C. salvos
   D. all of the above
7. A reentry mechanism in the ventricles may be responsible for:
   A. repetitive ventricular contractions
   B. ventricular tachycardia
   C. ventricular fibrillation
   D. all of the above
8. A form of ventricular tachycardia characterized by QRS complexes that gradually change back and forth from one shape and direction to another over a series of beats is called:
   A. multiform ventricular tachycardia
   B. torsade de pointes
   C. bigeminy
   D. none of the above
9. When the ventricles contract between 300 and 500 times a minute in an unsynchronized, uncoordinated manner:
   A. a life-threatening arrhythmia is present
   B. ventricular fibrillation is present
   C. defibrillation is indicated immediately
   D. all of the above
10. The following is true of an asymptomatic accelerated idioventricular rhythm:
    A. defibrillation should be attempted immediately
    B. it is often benign
    C. the heart rate is usually over 100 beats per minute
    D. it usually develops during second-degree type II AV block
11. A symptomatic ventricular arrhythmia with a heart rate and pulse of less than 40 beats per minute is called:
    A. accelerated idioventricular rhythm
    B. ventricular escape rhythm
    C. pulseless electrical activity of the heart
    D. ventricular asystole

CHAPTER OBJECTIVES

Upon completion of all or part of this chapter, you should be able to complete the following objective:
1. Define and give the diagnostic characteristics, cause, and clinical significance of the following arrhythmias:
   First-degree AV block
   Second-degree, type I AV block (Wenckebach)
   Second-degree, type II AV block
   Second-degree, 2:1 and advanced AV block
   Third-degree (complete AV block)
   Pacemaker rhythm

FIRST-DEGREE AV BLOCK

> ### KEY DEFINITION
>
> **First-degree atrioventricular (AV) *block* (Figure 9-1) is an arrhythmia in which there is a constant delay in the conduction of electrical impulses, usually through the AV node. It is characterized by abnormally prolonged PR intervals that are greater than 0.20 second and constant.**

Diagnostic Characteristics

Heart rate. The heart rate is that of the underlying sinus or atrial rhythm. The atrial and ventricular rates are typically the same.

Rhythm. The rhythm is that of the underlying rhythm.

Pacemaker site. The pacemaker site is that of the underlying rhythm.

P waves. The P waves are identical and precede each QRS complex.

PR intervals. The PR intervals are prolonged (greater than 0.20 second) and usually do not vary from beat to beat.

R-R intervals. The R-R intervals are those of the underlying rhythm.

QRS complexes. The QRS complexes are usually normal, but they may be abnormal (rarely) because of a preexisting intraventricular conduction disturbance (such as a bundle branch block). Typically, the AV conduction ratio is 1:1 (i.e., a QRS complex follows each P wave).

Cause of Arrhythmia

First-degree AV block usually represents a delay in the conduction of the electrical impulses through the AV node (nodal AV block), and thus the QRS complexes

First-Degree AV Block

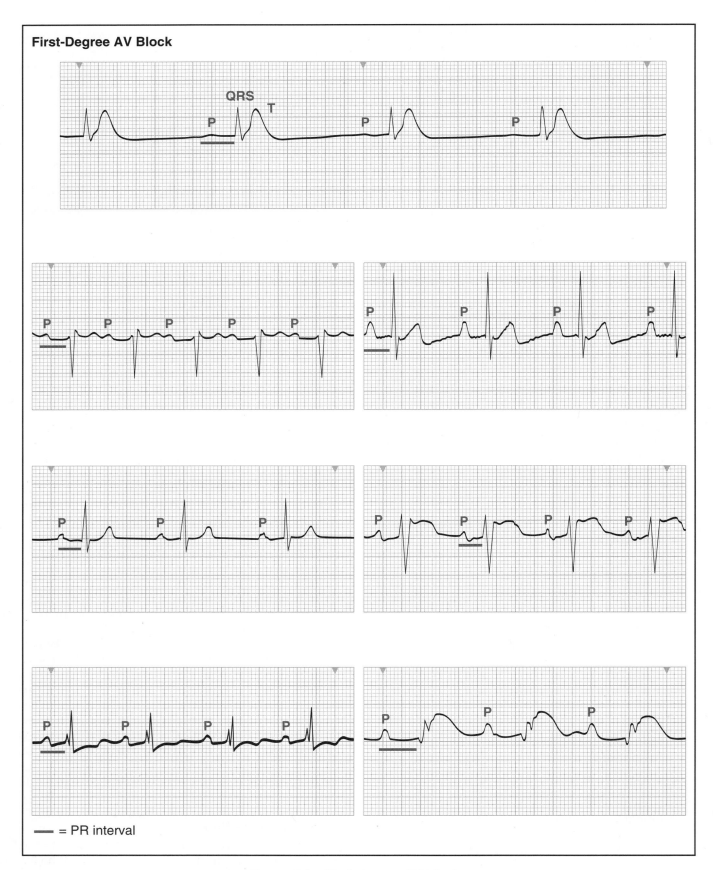

—— = PR interval

Figure 9-1   First-degree AV block.

are typically normal—unless a preexisting intraventricular conduction disturbance (such as a bundle branch block) is present. Infrequently, the AV block may occur below the AV node (infranodal AV block) in the His-Purkinje system of the ventricles (i.e., bundle of His or bundle branches).

Although first-degree AV block may appear without any apparent cause, it can occur in the following:

- Acute inferior or right ventricular myocardial infarction (MI) because of the effect of an increase in vagal (parasympathetic) tone and ischemia on the AV node
- Ischemic heart disease in general
- Excessive inhibitory vagal (parasympathetic) tone from whatever cause
- Digitalis toxicity
- Administration of certain drugs, such as amiodarone, β-blockers (e.g., atenolol, metoprolol, propranolol), or calcium channel blockers (e.g., diltiazem, verapamil, nifedipine)
- Electrolyte imbalance (hyperkalemia)
- Acute rheumatic fever or myocarditis

Clinical Significance

First-degree AV block produces no signs or symptoms per se and usually requires no specific treatment. However, any underlying cause should be corrected, if possible. Because it can progress to a higher-degree AV block under certain conditions (e.g., excessive administration of β-blockers or calcium channel blockers and acute inferior or right ventricular MI), the patient may require observation and ECG monitoring.

Notes

_____

_____

_____

_____

_____

_____

_____

_____

_____

_____

_____

_____

SECOND-DEGREE, TYPE I AV BLOCK (WENCKEBACH)

> ### KEY DEFINITION
>
> **Second-degree, type I AV block *(Wenckebach)* (Figure 9-2) is an arrhythmia in which there is a progressive delay following each P wave in the conduction of electrical impulses through the AV node until conduction is completely blocked. This arrhythmia is characterized by progressive lengthening of the PR intervals until a QRS complex fails to appear after a P wave. The sequence of increasing PR intervals and absent QRS complex is repetitive. Second-degree, type I AV block is also referred to as Mobitz type I *second-degree AV block.***

Diagnostic Characteristics

Heart rate. The atrial rate is that of the underlying sinus or atrial rhythm. The ventricular rate is typically less than that of the atria.

Rhythm. The atrial rhythm is essentially regular. The ventricular rhythm is usually irregular.

Pacemaker site. The pacemaker site is that of the underlying rhythm.

P waves. The P waves are identical and precede the QRS complexes when they occur.

PR intervals. The PR intervals gradually lengthen until a QRS complex fails to appear following a P wave (nonconducted P wave or dropped beat) (Table 9-1). Following the pause produced by the nonconducted P wave, the sequence begins anew.

R-R intervals. The R-R intervals are unequal. As the PR intervals gradually lengthen, the R-R intervals typically decrease gradually until the P wave is not conducted. The cycle then repeats itself. The reason for the progressive decrease in the R-R intervals is that the PR intervals do not increase in such increments as to maintain the R-R intervals at the same duration as that of the first one immediately following the nonconducted P wave. This characteristic cyclic decrease in the R-R intervals may also be seen in atrial fibrillation complicated by a Wenckebach block.

Rarely, the R-R interval may remain constant until the nonconduction of the P wave. The R-R interval that includes the nonconducted P wave is usually less than the sum of two of the R-R intervals of the underlying rhythm.

**Second-Degree AV Block
(Type I AV Block [Wenckebach])**

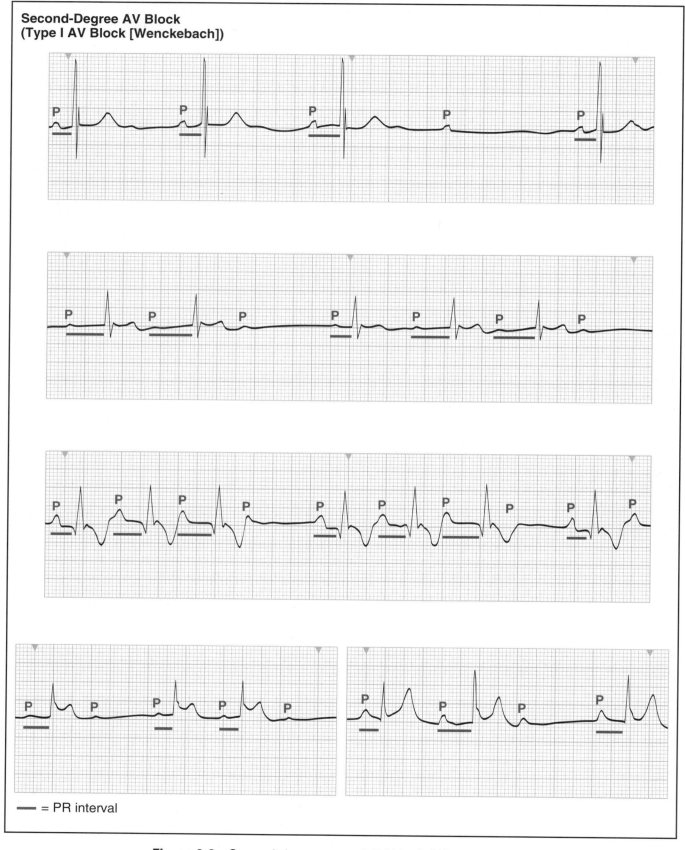

— = PR interval

Figure 9-2 Second-degree, type I AV block (Wenckebach).

QRS complexes. The QRS complexes are typically normal, but they may be abnormal (rarely) because of a preexisting intraventricular conduction disturbance (such as a bundle branch block). Commonly, the AV conduction ratio is 5:4, 4:3, or 3:2, but it may be 6:5, 7:6, etc. An AV conduction ratio of 5:4, for example, indicates that for every five P waves, four are followed by QRS complexes. The repetitive sequence of two or more beats in a row followed by a dropped beat is called *group beating*. The AV conduction ratio may be fixed or may vary in any given lead.

Cause of Arrhythmia

Type I second-degree AV block most commonly represents defective conduction of the electrical impulses through the AV node (nodal AV block), and thus the QRS complexes are typically normal unless a preexisting intraventricular conduction disturbance (such as a bundle branch block) is present. The AV block may infrequently occur below the AV node (infranodal AV block) in the His-Purkinje system of the ventricles (i.e., bundle of His or bundle branches).

Type I second-degree AV block often occurs, as does first-degree AV block, in the following:

◆ Acute inferior or right ventricular MI because of the effect of an increase in vagal (parasympathetic) tone and ischemia on the AV node
◆ Ischemic heart disease in general
◆ Excessive inhibitory vagal (parasympathetic) tone from whatever cause
◆ Digitalis toxicity
◆ Administration of certain drugs, such as amiodarone, β-blockers (e.g., atenolol, metoprolol, propranolol), or calcium channel blockers (e.g., diltiazem, verapamil, nifedipine)
◆ Electrolyte imbalance (hyperkalemia)
◆ Acute rheumatic fever or myocarditis

Clinical Significance

Type I second-degree AV block is usually transient and reversible. Although it produces few if any symptoms per se, it can progress to a higher-degree AV block. For this reason, the patient requires observation and ECG monitoring. Type I AV block does respond to atropine if it is necessary to increase the heart rate.

Notes

_____

_____

_____

_____

_____

_____

SECOND-DEGREE, TYPE II AV BLOCK

KEY DEFINITION

Second-degree, type II AV block *(Figure 9-3)* is an arrhythmia in which a complete block of conduction of the electrical impulses occurs in one bundle branch and an intermittent block in the other. This produces (1) an AV block characterized by regularly or irregularly absent QRS complexes, commonly producing an AV conduction ratio of 4:3 or 3:2, and (2) a bundle branch block. Second-degree, type II AV block is also referred to as Mobitz type II second-degree AV block.

Diagnostic Characteristics

Heart rate. The atrial rate is that of the underlying sinus, atrial, or junctional rhythm. The ventricular rate is typically less than the atrial rate.

Rhythm. The atrial rhythm is essentially regular. The ventricular rhythm is usually irregular.

Pacemaker site. The pacemaker site is that of the underlying rhythm.

P waves. The P waves are identical and precede the QRS complexes when they occur.

PR intervals. The PR intervals may be normal or prolonged (greater than 0.20 second). They are usually constant (Table 9-1).

R-R intervals. The R-R intervals are equal except for those that include the nonconducted P waves (dropped beats); these are equal to or slightly less than twice the R-R interval of the underlying rhythm.

QRS complexes. The QRS complexes are typically abnormal (greater than 0.12 second) because of a bundle branch block. Rarely, the QRS complex may be normal (0.10 second or less) if the AV block is at the level of the bundle of His and a preexisting intraventricular conduction disturbance (such as a bundle branch block) is not present. Commonly, the AV conduction ratio is 4:3 or 3:2, but it may be 5:4, 6:5, 7:6, and so forth. An AV conduction ratio of 4:3, for example, indicates that for every four P waves, three are followed by QRS complexes. The repetitive sequence of two or more beats in a row followed by a dropped beat is called *group beating*. The AV conduction ratio may be fixed, or it may vary within any given lead.

Second-Degree AV Block
(Type II AV Block)

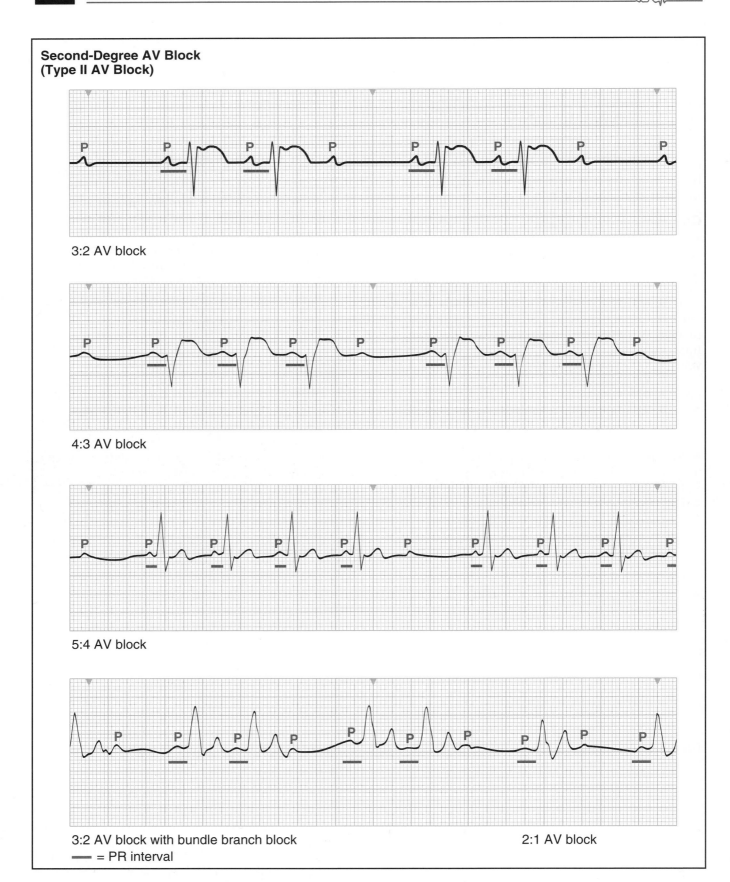

3:2 AV block

4:3 AV block

5:4 AV block

3:2 AV block with bundle branch block

2:1 AV block

▬ = PR interval

Figure 9-3   Second-degree, type II AV block.

Cause of Arrhythmia

Type II second-degree AV block usually occurs below the bundle of His in the bundle branches (infranodal AV block). It represents an intermittent block of conduction of the electrical impulses through one bundle branch and a complete block in the other. This produces an intermittent AV block with abnormally wide and bizarre QRS complexes.

Commonly, type II second-degree AV block is the result of extensive damage to the bundle branches following an acute anterior MI, and, unlike type I second-degree AV block, is not the result of an acute inferior or right ventricular MI or increased vagal (parasympathetic) tone or drug toxicity on the AV node. Rarely, the AV block occurs at the level of the bundle of His. When this occurs, the QRS complexes are normal (0.10 second or less) unless a preexisting intraventricular conduction disturbance (such as a bundle branch block) is present.

Clinical Significance

The signs and symptoms of type II second-degree AV block with excessively slow heart rates are the same as those in symptomatic sinus bradycardia. Because type II second-degree AV block is more serious than type I AV block, often progressing to a third-degree AV block and even ventricular asystole, a standby cardiac pacemaker is indicated for asymptomatic patients, and temporary cardiac pacing is required immediately for symptomatic patients, especially in the setting of an acute anterior MI. Atropine is usually not effective in reversing a type II AV block.

Notes

_____

_____

_____

_____

_____

_____

_____

_____

_____

_____

_____

_____

_____

_____

SECOND-DEGREE 2:1 AND ADVANCED AV BLOCK

KEY DEFINITION

Second-degree 2:1 *and* advanced AV block (Figure 9-4) are arrhythmias caused by the defective conduction of electrical impulses through the AV node or the bundle branches or both. This produces an AV block characterized by regularly or irregularly absent QRS complexes, commonly producing an AV conduction ratio of 2:1, 3:1, or greater, with or without a bundle branch block. 2:1 and advanced AV blocks are not considered to be of the classic type I or type II AV block.

Diagnostic Characteristics

Heart rate. The atrial rate is that of the underlying sinus, atrial, or junctional rhythm. The ventricular rate is typically less than the atrial rate.

Rhythm. The atrial rhythm is essentially regular. The ventricular rhythm may be regular or irregular. The ventricular rhythm is irregular when the AV block is intermittent, causing a varying AV conduction ratio.

Pacemaker site. The pacemaker site is that of the underlying rhythm.

P waves. The P waves are identical and precede the QRS complexes when they occur.

PR intervals. The PR intervals may be normal or prolonged (greater than 0.20 second); they are constant (Table 9-1).

R-R intervals. The R-R intervals may be equal or may vary.

QRS complexes. The QRS complexes may be normal or abnormal because of a bundle branch block. Commonly, the AV conduction ratios are even numbers, such as 2:1, 4:1, 6:1, 8:1, and so forth, but may be uneven numbers, such as 3:1 or 5:1. An AV conduction ratio of 3:1, for example, indicates that for every three P waves, one is followed by a QRS complex. The AV conduction ratio may be fixed, or it may vary in any given lead. The AV block is identified by the AV conduction ratio present (e.g., 2:1, 3:1, 4:1, or 6:1 AV block). An AV block with a 2:1 AV conduction ratio is termed a *2:1 AV block.* A 3:1 or higher AV block is called an *advanced AV block.*

Cause of Arrhythmia

2:1 and advanced AV blocks with normal QRS complexes usually represent defective conduction of the electrical impulses through the AV node (nodal

Second-Degree AV Block
(2:1 and High-Degree [Advanced] AV Block)

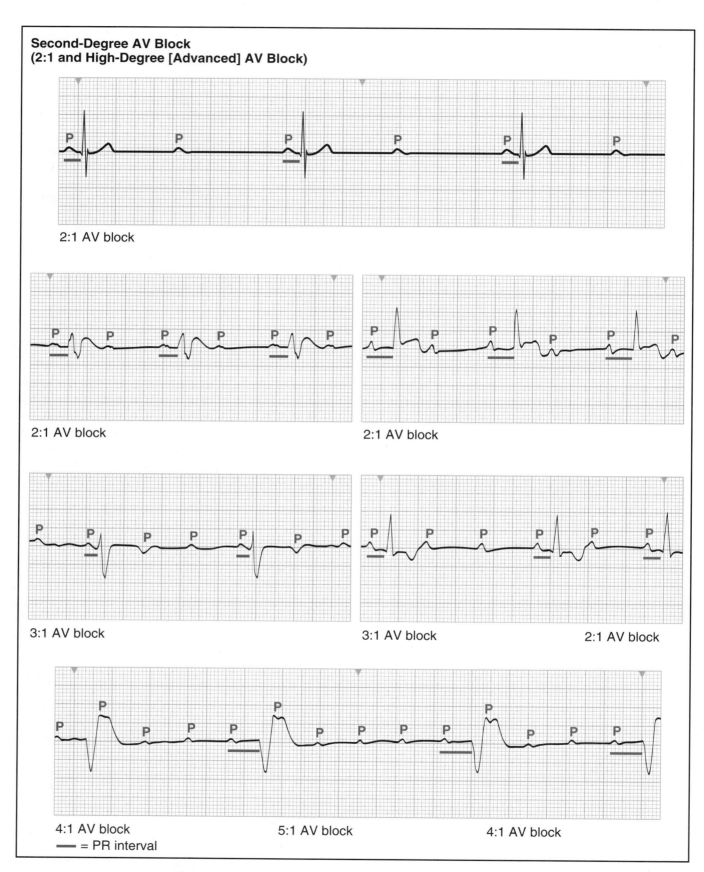

2:1 AV block

2:1 AV block

2:1 AV block

3:1 AV block

3:1 AV block

2:1 AV block

4:1 AV block

5:1 AV block

4:1 AV block

▬ = PR interval

Figure 9-4 Second-degree, 2:1 and advanced AV block.

AV block) and are often associated with a second-degree, type I AV block. They are commonly caused by the following:

◆ Acute inferior or right ventricular MI because of the effect of an increase in vagal (parasympathetic) tone and ischemia on the AV node
◆ Ischemic heart disease in general
◆ Excessive inhibitory vagal (parasympathetic) tone from whatever cause
◆ Digitalis toxicity
◆ Administration of certain drugs, such as amiodarone, β-blockers (e.g., atenolol, metoprolol, propranolol), or calcium channel blockers (e.g., diltiazem, verapamil, nifedipine)
◆ Electrolyte imbalance (hyperkalemia)
◆ Acute rheumatic fever or myocarditis

2:1 and advanced AV blocks with wide QRS complexes usually represent defective conduction of the electrical impulses through the bundle branches (infranodal AV block) and are often associated with a second-degree, type II AV block. Acute anterior MI is commonly the cause of such AV blocks. 2:1 and advanced AV blocks with wide QRS complexes may also be the result of AV node dysfunction, as in type I AV block (nodal AV block), accompanied by a preexisting intraventricular conduction disturbance (such as a bundle branch block).

Clinical Significance

When the heart rate is excessively slow in 2:1 and advanced second-degree AV blocks, the signs and symptoms are the same as those in symptomatic sinus bradycardia. 2:1 and advanced AV blocks with normal QRS complexes may often be transient. Atropine is usually effective in reversing the arrhythmia.

Because 2:1 and advanced AV blocks with wide QRS complexes frequently progress to a third-degree AV block and even ventricular asystole, a standby cardiac pacemaker is indicated for asymptomatic patients, and temporary cardiac pacing is required immediately for symptomatic patients, especially in the setting of an acute anterior MI. Atropine is usually not effective in reversing 2:1 and advanced AV blocks with wide QRS complexes.

Notes

_____

_____

_____

_____

_____

THIRD-DEGREE AV BLOCK (COMPLETE AV BLOCK)

> **KEY DEFINITION**
>
> **Third-degree AV block *(Figure 9-5)* is the complete absence of conduction of the electrical impulses through the AV node, bundle of His, or bundle branches, characterized by independent beating of the atria and ventricles.**

Diagnostic Characteristics

Heart rate. The atrial rate is that of the underlying sinus, atrial, or junctional rhythm. The ventricular rate is typically 40 to 60 beats per minute, but it may be as slow as 30 to 40 or less. The ventricular rate is usually less than that of the atrial rate.

Rhythm. The atrial rhythm may be regular or irregular, depending on the underlying sinus, atrial, or junctional rhythm. The ventricular rhythm is essentially regular. The atrial and ventricular rhythms are independent of each other (AV dissociation).

Pacemaker site. If P waves are present, they may have originated in the SA node or an ectopic or escape pacemaker in the atria or AV junction. The pacemaker site of the QRS complexes is an escape pacemaker in the AV junction, bundle branches, Purkinje network, or ventricular myocardium, below the AV block.

Generally, if the third-degree AV block is at the level of the AV node, the escape pacemaker is usually infranodal, in the bundle of His. If the third-degree AV block is at the level of the bundle of His or bundle branches, the escape pacemaker is in the ventricles distal to the site of the AV block. If the escape pacemaker is in the AV junction (i.e., junctional escape rhythm), the heart rate is 40 to 60 beats per minute. If the escape pacemaker is in the ventricles (i.e., bundle branches, Purkinje network, or ventricular myocardium [ventricular escape rhythm]), the heart rate is 30 to 40 beats per minute or less.

P waves. P waves or atrial flutter or fibrillation waves may be present. When present, they have no relation to the QRS complexes, appearing independently at a rate different from that of the QRS complexes (AV dissociation).

PR intervals. The PR intervals vary widely because the P waves and QRS complexes occur independently (Table 9-1).

R-R and P-P intervals. The R-R intervals are usually equal and independent of the P-P intervals.

**Third-Degree AV Block
(Complete AV Block)**

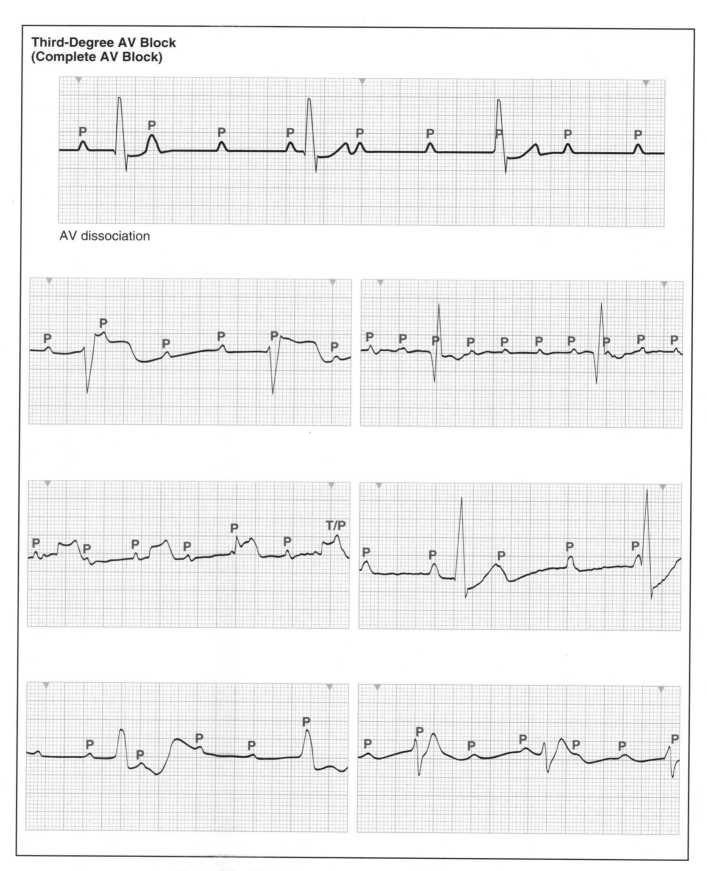

AV dissociation

Figure 9-5 Third-degree AV block (complete AV block).

QRS complexes. The QRS complexes typically exceed 0.12 second and are bizarre if the escape pacemaker site is in the ventricles or if the escape pacemaker site is in the AV junction and a preexisting intraventricular conduction disturbance (such as a bundle branch block) is present. But the QRS complexes may be normal (0.10 second or less) if the pacemaker site is above the bundle branches in the AV junction and no bundle branch block is present.

Cause of Arrhythmia

Third-degree AV block represents a complete block of the conduction of the electrical impulses from the atria to the ventricles at the level of the AV node (nodal AV block) or bundle of His or bundle branches (infranodal AV block). It may be transient and reversible or permanent.

Transient and reversible third-degree AV block is usually associated with normal QRS complexes and a heart rate of 45 to 60 beats per minute (i.e., junctional escape rhythm). It is commonly caused by a complete block of conduction of the electrical impulses through the AV node. This can result from the following:

◆ Acute inferior or right ventricular MI because of the effect of an increase in vagal (parasympathetic) tone and ischemia on the AV node
◆ Ischemic heart disease in general
◆ Excessive inhibitory vagal (parasympathetic) tone from whatever cause
◆ Digitalis toxicity
◆ Administration of certain drugs, such as amiodarone, β-blockers (e.g., atenolol, metoprolol, propranolol), or calcium channel blockers (e.g., diltiazem, verapamil, nifedipine)
◆ Electrolyte imbalance (hyperkalemia)
◆ Acute rheumatic fever or myocarditis

Permanent or chronic third-degree AV block is usually associated with wide QRS complexes and a heart rate of 30 to 40 beats per minute or less (i.e., ventricular escape rhythm). It is commonly caused by a complete block of conduction of electrical impulses through both bundle branches. The most likely causes include the following:

◆ Acute anterior MI
◆ Chronic degenerative changes in the bundle branches present in the elderly (Lenègre's disease and Lev's disease)

Permanent third-degree AV block usually does not result from increased vagal (parasympathetic) tone or drug toxicity.

Clinical Significance

The signs and symptoms of third-degree AV block are the same as those in symptomatic sinus bradycardia, except that third-degree AV block can be more omi-nous, especially when it is associated with wide and bizarre QRS complexes. If an AV junctional or ventricular escape pacemaker does not take over following a sudden onset of third-degree AV block, ventricular asystole will occur. This results in faintness, followed within seconds by loss of consciousness, seizures, apnea (*Adams-Stokes syndrome*), and death if an escape pacemaker does not respond or ventricular asystole is not immediately treated

Temporary cardiac pacing is required immediately for treatment of symptomatic third-degree AV block with wide QRS complexes (regardless of cause) and for asymptomatic third-degree AV block with wide QRS complexes in a setting of an acute anterior MI. Otherwise, a standby cardiac pacemaker is indicated. Third-degree AV block with narrow QRS complexes does respond to atropine occasionally if it is caused by an acute inferior or right ventricular MI.

Notes

_____

_____

_____

_____

_____

PACEMAKER RHYTHM

KEY DEFINITION

A pacemaker rhythm *(Figure 9-6)* consists of the beats and rhythm produced by a cardiac pacemaker.

◆ TYPES OF PACEMAKERS

There are two basic kinds of pacemakers: *fixed rate* and *demand*. Fixed rate pacemakers are designed to fire constantly at a preset rate without regard to the patient's own electrical activity of the heart. Demand pacemakers have a sensing device that senses the heart's electrical activity and fires at a preset rate only when the heart's electrical activity drops below a predetermined rate level.

Pacemakers can be either *single-chamber* pacemakers that pace either the ventricles or atria or *dual-chambered* pacemakers that pace both the atria and ventricles. Examples of commonly used pacemakers from each category are described below, with the In-

Pacemaker Rhythm

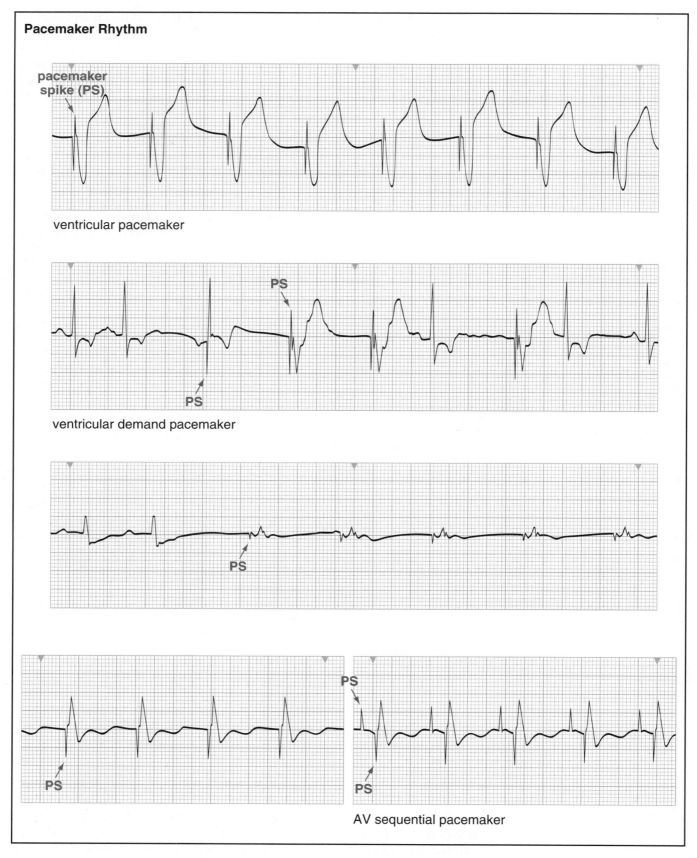

pacemaker
spike (PS)

ventricular pacemaker

ventricular demand pacemaker

AV sequential pacemaker

Figure 9-6 Pacemaker rhythm.

tersociety Commission for Heart Disease Resources (ICHD) code noted. The codes can be deciphered as follows:

◆ The first of the three letters of the code indicates which chamber is paced (A = atria, V = ventricles, D = both atria and ventricles)

◆ The second letter indicates which chamber is sensed (A = atria, V = ventricles, D = both atria and ventricles)

◆ The third letter indicates the response of the pacemaker to a P wave or QRS complex (I = pacemaker output is inhibited by the P wave or QRS complex, D = pacemaker output is inhibited by a QRS complex and triggered by a P wave)

Single-Chamber Pacemakers

Atrial demand pacemaker (AAI). A pacemaker that senses spontaneously occurring P waves and paces the atria when they do not appear.

Ventricular demand pacemaker (VVI). A pacemaker that senses spontaneously occurring QRS complexes and paces the ventricles when they do not appear.

Dual-Chambered Pacemakers

Atrial synchronous ventricular pacemaker (VDD). A pacemaker that senses spontaneously occurring P waves and QRS complexes and paces the ventricles when QRS complexes fail to appear following spontaneously occurring P waves, as in complete AV block. In this type of pacemaker, the pacing of the ventricles is synchronized with the P waves so the ventricular contractions follow the atrial contractions in a normal sequence.

AV sequential pacemaker (DVI). A pacemaker that senses spontaneously occurring QRS complexes and paces both the atria and ventricles (the atria first, followed by the ventricles following a short delay) when QRS complexes do not appear.

Optimal sequential pacemaker (DDD). A pacemaker that senses spontaneously occurring P waves and QRS complexes and (1) paces the atria when P waves fail to appear, as in sinus node dysfunction, and (2) paces the ventricles when QRS complexes fail to appear following spontaneously occurring or paced P waves. In this type of pacemaker, like the VDD pacemaker, the pacing of the ventricles is synchronized with the atrial activity so the ventricular contractions follow the atrial contractions in a normal sequence.

Diagnostic Features

Heart rate. The heart rate produced by a permanently implanted cardiac pacemaker is usually between 60 and 70 beats per minute, depending on its preset rate of firing. If the pacemaker rate is greater

than 90 beats per minute, it is probably malfunctioning.

Rhythm. The ventricular rhythm produced by a pacemaker that is pacing constantly is regular. The ventricular rate may be irregular when the pacemaker is pacing on demand (i.e., pacing only when P waves and/or QRS complexes fail to appear).

Pacemaker site. The pacemaker site of a cardiac pacemaker is an electrode usually located in the tip of the pacemaker lead, commonly positioned in the apex of the right ventricular cavity (ventricular pacemaker), in the right atrium (atrial pacemaker), or in both (dual chamber pacemaker).

Pacemaker spikes. The electrical discharge from a cardiac pacemaker produces a narrow, often biphasic spike. A pacemaker lead positioned in the atria produces a pacemaker spike followed by a small, often flattened P wave; a pacemaker lead positioned in the ventricles produces a pacemaker spike followed by a wide (0.12 second or greater) and bizarre QRS complex. A P wave or QRS complex following a pacemaker spike indicates "capturing" by the cardiac pacemaker. A pacemaker spike not followed by a P wave or QRS complex indicates the pacemaker is discharging but not capturing. In a fixed-rate pacemaker, the pacemaker spikes occur at regular intervals.

> **KEY POINT**
>
> *It has been noted that in certain cardiac monitors and cardiographs, the pacemaker spikes are not discernable as such. The manual supplied with such a device should be consulted for further information.*

In a demand pacemaker, the pacemaker spikes in the atria and/or ventricles occur at regular intervals or occur intermittently interspersed with the patient's own electrical activity of the heart.

P waves. P waves may be present or absent. If present, they may be spontaneously occurring or induced by a pacemaker lead positioned in the atria. When not followed by inherent QRS complexes, spontaneously occurring P waves are usually followed by pacemaker-induced QRS complexes. This indicates that a dual-chamber VDD or DDD pacemaker is present. A narrow, often biphasic spike—the pacemaker spike—precedes pacemaker-induced P waves. These P waves may be followed by the inherent QRS complexes or pacemaker-induced QRS complexes, as seen in dual-chamber DVI or DDD pacemakers. A ventricular pacemaker usually does not produce a retrograde, inverted P wave.

PR intervals. The PR intervals of the underlying rhythm may be normal (0.12 to 0.20 second) or abnormal, depending on the arrhythmia. The PR intervals in atrial synchronous and dual-paced, AV sequential pacemakers are within normal limits.

R-R intervals. The R-R intervals of the pacemaker rhythm are equal. When the pacemaker-induced QRS complexes are interspersed among the patient's normally occurring QRS complexes, the R-R intervals are unequal.

QRS complexes. The QRS complexes of the underlying rhythm may be normal (0.10 second or less in width) or abnormal. Pacemaker-induced QRS complexes are typically greater than 0.12 second in width and bizarre. Preceding each pacemaker-induced QRS complex is a narrow deflection, often biphasic—the pacemaker spike—representing the electrical discharge of the pacemaker. If only the atria are being paced, the QRS complexes are those of the underlying rhythm. These are normal unless a preexisting intraventricular conduction disturbance (such as a bundle branch block) is present.

Clinical Significance

A pacemaker rhythm indicates that the patient's heart is being electronically paced. Cardiac pacemakers are usually permanently implanted in patients to correct an underlying third-degree AV block or episodes of symptomatic bradycardia.

Typically, a 2½- to 3-inch diameter bulge is present, usually in the upper, right anterior chest wall, indicating an implanted cardiac pacemaker.

The presence of pacemaker spikes followed by a QRS complex indicates that the patient's heart rate is being regulated by a cardiac pacemaker. When a normal or wide and bizarre QRS complex follows every pacemaker spike or every paced P wave (as seen in single-chamber pacing) or every pair of pacemaker spikes (as seen in dual-chamber pacing), the pacemaker is apparently functioning normally even if the patient's own P waves and QRS complexes are interspersed between the pacemaker spikes and associated QRS complexes.

Some of the problems that can occur with cardiac pacemakers include the following:

◆ The presence of pacemaker spikes that are not followed by P waves or QRS complexes indicates a malfunctioning pacemaker, one whose electric impulses are unable to stimulate the heart to depolarize; the failure to capture most likely results from the current output from the pacemaker being adjusted too low

◆ Complete absence of pacemaker spikes in the presence of bradycardia or ventricular asystole indicates battery failure

◆ A pacemaker spike rate of over 300 per minute, causing a ventricular tachyarrhythmia, can occur in older models of pacemakers. This indicates a malfunction in the electrical impulse generating circuit, usually the result of low battery power. Such a malfunctioning pacemaker is known as a *runaway pacemaker.*

◆ Failure of a demand pacemaker to shut off when the patient has adequate electrical activity of the heart indicates a failure in the pacemaker's sensing circuit. The danger here is that the pacemaker spikes may fall on the vulnerable period of the cardiac cycle, triggering a life-threatening arrhythmia.

No treatment is necessary if the cardiac pacemaker is functioning properly. Appropriate treatment may be necessary if the pacemaker is malfunctioning and an underlying bradyarrhythmia, ventricular asystole, or ventricular fibrillation is present. Antiarrhythmic drugs may be administered without inhibiting the heart's response to the pacemaker. When delivering a defibrillatory shock or countershock, the defibrillator paddles should be placed about 2 inches away from the cardiac pacemaker and not directly over it.

SUMMARY

Table 9-1 summarizes the diagnostic characteristics of the various atrial arrhythmias discussed in this chapter.

Figure 9-7 is an algorithm on how to determine the degree and type of AV block that is present by analyzing the P waves, QRS complexes, and PR intervals.

Notes:

_____

_____

_____

_____

_____

_____

_____

_____

_____

_____

_____

_____

_____

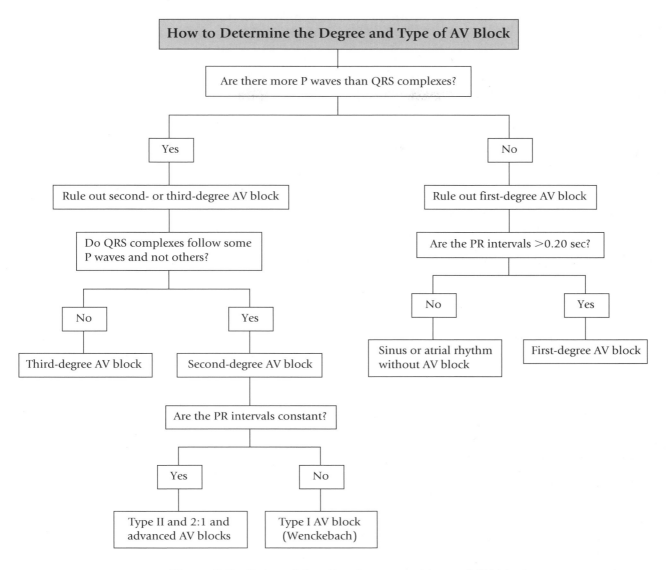

Figure 9-7 Determining the degree and type of AV block.

9-1 Typical Diagnostic ECG Features of First-, Second-, and Third-Degree AV Blocks

AV Block	PR Intervals	AV Conduction Ratio	QRS Complex
First-degree AV block	Prolonged, constant	1:1	Usually normal
Second-degree AV block			
Type I AV block (Wenckebach)	Gradually lengthening	5:4, 4:3, 3:2 or 6:5, 7:6, etc.	Usually normal
Type II AV block	Constant	3:2, 4:3, 5:4, etc.	Typically abnormal
2:1 AV block	Constant	2:1	Normal or abnormal
Advanced AV block	Constant	3:1, 4:1, 5:1, etc.	Normal or abnormal
Third-degree AV block	No relationship of P to R waves	None	Normal or abnormal

TREATMENT ALGORITHMS

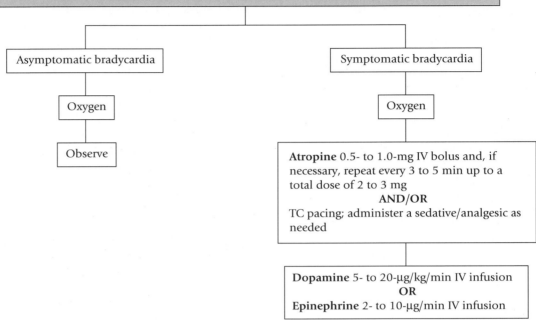

Second-Degree, Type I AV Block (Wenckebach) / Second-Degree, 2:1 and Advanced AV Block With Narrow QRS Complexes / Third-Degree AV Block With Narrow QRS Complexes

Asymptomatic bradycardia
- Oxygen
- Observe

Symptomatic bradycardia
- Oxygen
- **Atropine** 0.5- to 1.0-mg IV bolus and, if necessary, repeat every 3 to 5 min up to a total dose of 2 to 3 mg
  AND/OR
  TC pacing; administer a sedative/analgesic as needed
- **Dopamine** 5- to 20-µg/kg/min IV infusion
  OR
  Epinephrine 2- to 10-µg/min IV infusion

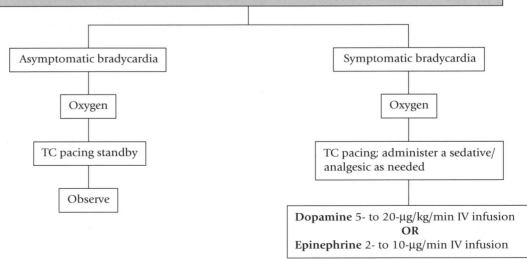

Second-Degree, Type II AV Block / Second-Degree, 2:1 and Advanced AV Block With Wide QRS Complexes / Third-Degree AV Block With Wide QRS Complexes

Asymptomatic bradycardia
- Oxygen
- TC pacing standby
- Observe

Symptomatic bradycardia
- Oxygen
- TC pacing; administer a sedative/analgesic as needed
- **Dopamine** 5- to 20-µg/kg/min IV infusion
  OR
  Epinephrine 2- to 10-µg/min IV infusion

CHAPTER REVIEW QUESTIONS

1. An arrhythmia that occurs commonly in acute inferior MI because of the effect of an increase in vagal (parasympathetic) tone and ischemia on the AV node is called:
   A. chronic third-degree AV block
   B. second-degree, type II AV block
   C. first-degree AV block
   D. ventricular tachycardia

2. An arrhythmia in which there is a progressive delay following each P wave in the conduction of electrical impulses through the AV node until the conduction of electrical impulses is completely blocked is called a:
   A. first-degree AV block
   B. second-degree, type I AV block
   C. second-degree, type II AV block
   D. third-degree AV block

3. Second-degree, type I AV block is usually transient and reversible, yet the patient should be monitored and observed because:
   A. it can progress to a higher-degree AV block
   B. it can progress to ventricular tachycardia
   C. it is symptomatic
   D. none of the above

4. An arrhythmia in which a complete block of conduction of electrical impulses occurs in one bundle branch and an intermittent block occurs in the other is called:
   A. first-degree AV block
   B. second-degree, type I AV block
   C. second-degree, type II AV block
   D. third-degree AV block

5. If a second-degree, type II AV block presents in the setting of an acute anteroseptal MI, the immediate treatment in a symptomatic patient is:
   A. temporary cardiac pacing
   B. atropine
   C. an isoproterenol drip
   D. all of the above

6. A second-degree, advanced AV block has an AV conduction ratio of:
   A. 8:1 or greater
   B. 4:1 or 6:1
   C. 3:1 or 4:1
   D. all of the above

7. The absence of conduction of electrical impulses through the AV node, bundle of His, or bundle branches, characterized by independent beating of the atria and ventricles, is called a:
   A. second-degree, type I AV block
   B. second-degree, type II AV block
   C. third-degree AV block
   D. first-degree AV block

8. An escape pacemaker in the AV junction has a firing rate of _____ beats per minute.
   A. 100 to 120
   B. 80 to 100
   C. 60 to 80
   D. 40 to 60

9. If an AV junctional or ventricular escape pacemaker does not take over following a sudden onset of third-degree AV block, ventricular asystole will occur, resulting in:
   A. ventricular escape rhythm
   B. Adams-Stokes syndrome
   C. bundle branch block
   D. atrial arrest

10. A pacemaker that senses spontaneous occurring P waves and QRS complexes and (1) paces the atria when P waves fail to appear and (2) paces the ventricles when QRS complexes fail to appear following spontaneously occurring or paced P waves is called a(n):
    A. optimal sequential pacemaker (DDD)
    B. AV sequential pacemaker (DVI)
    C. atrial synchronous ventricular pacemaker (VDD)
    D. ventricular demand pacemaker (VVI)

Clinical Significance and Treatment of Arrhythmias

CHAPTER OBJECTIVES

Upon completion of all or part of this chapter, you should be able to complete the following objectives:

1. Discuss the clinical significance of the following bradycardias, the indications for their treatment, and their treatment:
Sinus bradycardia
Sinus arrest/sinoatrial (SA) exit block
Second-degree, type I atrioventricular (AV) block (Wenckebach)
Second-degree, type II AV block
Second-degree, 2:1 and advanced AV block
  With narrow QRS complexes
  With wide QRS complexes
Third-degree AV block
  With narrow QRS complexes
  With wide QRS complexes
Junctional escape rhythm
Ventricular escape rhythm

2. Discuss the clinical significance of the following tachycardias, the indications for their treatment, and their treatment:
Sinus tachycardia
Atrial tachycardia with block
Narrow-QRS-complex tachycardia of unknown origin (with pulse)

3. Discuss the clinical significance of the following tachycardias, the indications for their treatment, and their treatment based on whether the patient is hemodynamically stable or unstable:
Atrial tachycardia without block
Atrial flutter with or without Wolff-Parkinson-White (WPW) syndrome or ventricular preexcitation
Atrial fibrillation with or without WPW syndrome or ventricular preexcitation
  Less than 48 hours in duration
  Greater than 48 hours in duration

CHAPTER OBJECTIVES—cont'd

Paroxysmal supraventricular tachycardia (PSVT) with narrow QRS complexes

Junctional tachycardia

4. Discuss the clinical significance of the following tachycardias, the indications for their treatment, and their treatment based on whether the patient is hemodynamically stable or unstable:

Wide-QRS-complex tachycardia of unknown origin (with pulse)

Ventricular tachycardia (VT), monomorphic (with pulse)

VT, polymorphic (with pulse)

Normal QT interval

Prolonged QT interval

Torsade de Pointes (TdP) (with pulse)

5. Discuss the clinical significance of the following tachycardias, the indications for their treatment, and their treatment:

Premature atrial contractions (PACs)

Premature junctional contractions (PJCs)

Premature ventricular contractions (PVCs)

6. Discuss the clinical significance of the following arrhythmias, the indications for their treatment, and their treatment based on whether the patient has suffered a monitored versus an unmonitored cardiac arrest:

Ventricular fibrillation/pulseless ventricular tachycardia (VF/VT)

Ventricular asystole

Pulseless electrical activity

The arrhythmia treatment protocols presented in this section are based on the recommendations of the following:

◆ The 2000 National Conference on Standards and Guidelines for Cardiopulmonary Resuscitation (CPR) and Emergency Cardiac Care (ECC).

◆ Ryan TJ, et al: ACC/AHA guidelines for the management of patients with acute myocardial infarction: a report of the American College of Cardiology/American Heart Association Task Force on Practice Guidelines (Committee on Management of Acute Myocardial Infarction), *J Am Coll Cardiol* 28:1328-1428, 1996 (1999 update available at *www.acc.org*).

◆ Guidelines 2000 for Cardiopulmonary Resuscitation and Emergency Cardiovascular Care, International Consensus on Science.

These treatment protocols may be used as guidelines for the development of local or regional protocols for the management of arrhythmias during the prehospital and in-hospital phase of emergency cardiac care. Management may deviate from these treatment protocols or include additional treatment modalities when the physician in charge of the patient determines if such a deviation or addition is in the best interests of the patient.

The treatment sections in this chapter differentiate between prehospital and in-hospital emergency cardiac care. The drugs and techniques authorized for in-hospital care only are indicated by the icon shown here. However, the scheme of authorization may be changed at the discretion of the medical control of the prehospital advanced life support system.

Part I of this chapter includes the arrhythmias present in situations that do not involve cardiac arrest: hemodynamically stable and unstable bradycardias and tachycardias and premature ectopic beats.

Part II includes arrhythmias present in cardiac arrest: ventricular fibrillation/pulseless ventricular tachycardia, ventricular asystole, and pulseless electrical activity.

Following Part II are the arrhythmia treatment protocols presented in Parts I and II in summary and algorithm formats.

PART I

BRADYCARDIAS

Clinical Significance of Bradycardias

A bradycardia with a heart rate between 50 to 59 beats per minute (*mild bradycardia*) usually does not produce symptoms by itself. If the heart rate slows to 30 to 45 beats per minute or less (*marked bradycardia*), the cardiac output may drop significantly, causing the systolic blood pressure to fall to 80 to 90 mm Hg or less and signs and symptoms of decreased perfusion of the body, especially of the vital organs, to appear. The skin may become pale, cold, and clammy; the pulse may be weak or absent; and the patient may be agitated, lightheaded, confused, or unconscious. The patient may experience chest pain and also become dyspneic.

In the presence of an acute myocardial infarction (MI), mild bradycardia may actually be beneficial in some patients because of the decrease in the workload of the heart, which reduces the oxygen requirements of the myocardium, minimizes the extension of the infarction, and lessens the predisposition to certain arrhythmias. Marked bradycardia, however, may result in hypotension, with a marked reduction of cardiac output leading to congestive heart failure, loss of consciousness, and shock, and predispose the patient to more serious arrhythmias (i.e., premature ventricular contractions (PVCs), ventricular tachycardia or fibrillation, or ventricular asystole).

If sinus arrest or sinoatrial (SA) exit block is prolonged or second-degree atrioventricular (AV) block suddenly progresses to a third-degree AV block, and if an escape pacemaker in the AV junction (junctional escape rhythm) or ventricles (ventricular escape rhythm) does not take over, ventricular asystole will follow.

Indications for Treatment of Bradycardias

Treatment is usually not indicated for a bradycardia if the heart rate is 60 beats per minute or less and none of the signs and symptoms listed below is present. However, treatment of bradycardia, regardless of cause, is indicated immediately if the heart rate is less than 60 beats per minute and one or more of the following signs or symptoms are present (such a bradycardia is considered a *symptomatic bradycardia*):

◆ Hypotension (systolic blood pressure less than 90 mm Hg)
◆ Congestive heart failure
◆ Chest pain or dyspnea
◆ Signs and symptoms of decreased cardiac output (e.g., decreased level of consciousness)
◆ PVCs, particularly in the setting of an acute MI

Treatment to increase the heart rate may also be indicated if the heart rate is somewhat above 60 beats per minute and one or more of the above signs and symptoms are present. This may result if the heart rate is too slow relative to the existing metabolic needs. Such a slow heart rate is called a *symptomatic "relative" bradycardia* and requires immediate treatment.

Treatment may not be indicated even if the heart rate falls below 50 beats per minute if the systolic blood pressure remains greater than 100 mm Hg and stable; if congestive heart failure, chest pain, and dyspnea are not present; if agitation, lightheadedness, confusion, and loss of consciousness are absent; and if frequent PVCs do not occur. Such a bradycardia is considered to be an *asymptomatic bradycardia*.

Transcutaneous Pacing

Transcutaneous pacing (TCP) is usually effective in the treatment of all symptomatic bradycardias, regardless of cause. The indications for TCP are as follows:

◆ TCP is indicated in the treatment of all symptomatic bradycardias
◆ TCP is indicated in the initial treatment of the following symptomatic bradycardias with wide QRS complexes, commonly the result of disruption of the electrical conduction system below the AV node, secondary to an acute anterior MI involving the interventricular septum:
  ◇ Second-degree, type II AV block
  ◇ Second-degree, 2:1 and advanced AV block with wide QRS complexes
  ◇ Third-degree AV block with wide QRS complexes
◆ TCP should be considered in the initial treatment of symptomatic bradycardias associated with acute MI and in situations in which intravenous (IV) access is difficult or delayed, or when it should be avoided in the setting of an acute MI in anticipation of thrombolytic therapy
◆ TCP is the treatment of choice in symptomatic bradycardias in patients with heart transplants because atropine sulfate is ineffective in such patients
◆ TCP is not indicated in bradycardia caused by hypothermia

Atropine Sulfate

Atropine sulfate may or may not be effective or indicated in the treatment of symptomatic bradycardias depending on the cause of the bradycardia and the site of the AV block. The effectiveness of and indications for atropine sulfate are as follows:

◆ Atropine sulfate is usually effective in the treatment of the following symptomatic bradycardias and is indicated in their initial treatment:
  ◇ Sinus bradycardia and sinus arrest/SA exit block resulting from an increase in vagal (parasympathetic) tone on the SA node secondary to an inferior or right ventricular MI and/or SA node dysfunction usually caused by an acute right ventricular MI
  ◇ Second-degree, type I AV block (Wenckebach); second-degree, 2:1 and advanced AV block with narrow QRS complexes; and third-degree AV block with narrow QRS complexes. The cause of these AV blocks is commonly an increase in vagal (parasympathetic) tone on the AV node and/or an AV node dysfunction secondary to an acute inferior or right ventricular MI.
◆ Atropine sulfate is usually not effective (nor indicated) in the treatment of the following bradycardias that result from disruption of the electrical conduction system below the AV node, secondary to an acute anterior MI involving the interventric-

ular septum:

◇ Second-degree, type II AV block
◇ Second-degree, 2:1 and advanced AV block with wide QRS complexes
◇ Third-degree AV block with wide QRS complexes

In such second-degree AV blocks (which have a propensity to progress rapidly to complete third-degree AV block without warning) and third-degree AV blocks, particularly in the setting of an acute anterior MI involving the interventricular septum, the attachment of a transcutaneous pacemaker is indicated immediately, whether or not the bradycardia is symptomatic.

◆ Atropine sulfate should be used with caution in patients with acute MI because of the possibility of an excessive increase in the heart rate, with the potential of increasing myocardial ischemia and precipitating ventricular tachycardia or ventricular fibrillation. TCP is preferred in such patients and in those in which IV access is difficult or delayed, or in situations when it should be avoided in the setting of an acute MI in anticipation of thrombolytic therapy (see *Transcutaneous Pacing*, p. 190).

◆ Atropine sulfate is ineffective in the treatment of bradycardia in patients with heart transplants because parasympathetic activity has no role in the production of bradycardia in such patients whose transplanted hearts have been denervated and are not connected to their own parasympathetic nervous system. TCP is the treatment of choice in symptomatic bradycardias in such patients. Catecholamines such as dopamine hydrochloride and epinephrine are also effective in treating symptomatic bradycardias in patients with transplanted hearts.

◆ In addition to use in treatment of symptomatic bradycardias, atropine sulfate is also indicated for treatment of the nausea and vomiting associated with administration of morphine sulfate. If atropine sulfate is contraindicated for any reason, such as a preexisting tachycardia or an acute coronary syndrome without bradycardia, hydroxyzine hydrochloride or thiethylperazine may be substituted.

Sinus Bradycardia
Sinus Arrest/SA Exit Block
Second-Degree, Type I AV Block (Wenckebach)
Second-Degree, 2:1 and Advanced AV Block With Narrow QRS Complexes
Third-Degree AV Block With Narrow QRS Complexes

◆ **TREATMENT**

If the bradycardia is symptomatic:
1. Administer high-concentration oxygen.
2. Administer a 0.5- to 1.0-mg IV bolus of **atropine sulfate** IV rapidly. Repeat every 3 to 5 minutes until the heart rate increases to 60 to 100 beats per minute or the maximum dose of 2 to 3 mg (0.03 to 0.04 mg/kg) of atropine has been administered.

AND/OR

Initiate TCP. If the patient is unable to tolerate TCP and is conscious and not hypotensive, administer a sedative such as **midazolam** or **diazepam** as follows:

◆ Administer 1 to 2 mg of midazolam IV slowly over at least 2 minutes and repeat every 3 to 5 minutes, titrated to produce sedation/amnesia.

OR

Administer 5 to 15 mg of diazepam with or without 2 to 5 mg **morphine** IV slowly to produce amnesia/analgesia.

NOTE: If the bradycardia is the result of an inferior or right ventricular infarction and is symptomatic but does not seem to respond to atropine or transcutaneous pacing:

◆ Administer 250 to 500 mL of **normal saline** IV rapidly and repeat up to a total of 1 to 2 L or until the heart rate increases to 60 to 100 beats per minute and the systolic blood pressure is within normal limits.

If the bradycardia, hypotension, or both persist:
3. Start an IV infusion of **dopamine hydrochloride** at an initial rate of 2 to 5μg/kg/min, and adjust the rate of infusion up to 20 μg/kg/min to increase the heart rate to 60 to 100 beats per minute and the systolic blood pressure to within normal limits.

OR

Start an IV infusion of **epinephrine** at an initial rate of 1 to 2 μg per minute, and adjust the rate of infusion up to 10 μg per minute to increase the heart rate to 60 to 100 beats per minute and the systolic blood pressure to within normal limits.

4. Insert a temporary transvenous pacemaker immediately.

Notes

Second-Degree, Type II AV Block
Second-Degree, 2:1 and Advanced AV Block With Wide QRS Complexes
Third-Degree AV Block With Wide QRS Complexes

◆ TREATMENT

If the bradycardia is asymptomatic and the cause of the second- or third-degree AV block with wide QRS complexes is an acute anterior MI involving the interventricular septum:

1. Administer high-concentration oxygen.

AND

Attach a transcutaneous pacemaker, test for ventricular capture and patient tolerance, and put on standby.

If the bradycardia is or becomes symptomatic:

2. Initiate TCP. If the patient is unable to tolerate TCP and is conscious and not hypotensive, administer a sedative such as **midazolam** or **diazepam** as follows:

    ◆ Administer 1 to 2 mg of midazolam IV slowly over at least 2 minutes and repeat every 3 to 5 minutes, titrated to produce sedation/amnesia.

    OR

    Administer 5 to 15 mg of diazepam with or without 2 to 5 mg **morphine** IV slowly to produce amnesia/analgesia.

    NOTE: If TCP is not available, consider the administration of atropine; however, it is usually not effective in second- and third-degree AV blocks with wide QRS complexes.

If the bradycardia, hypotension, or both persist:

3. Start an IV infusion of **dopamine** at an initial rate of 2 to 5 μg/kg/min and adjust the rate of infusion up to 20 μg/kg/min to increase the heart rate to 60 to 100 beats per minute and the systolic blood pressure to within normal limits.

    OR

    Start an IV infusion of **epinephrine** at an initial rate of 1 to 2 μg/min and adjust the rate of infusion up to 10 μg/min to increase the heart rate to 60 to 100 beats per minute and the systolic blood pressure to within normal limits.

4. Insert a temporary transvenous pacemaker immediately.

Notes

_____

_____

_____

_____

Junctional Escape Rhythm
Ventricular Escape Rhythm

◆ TREATMENT

If the bradycardia is symptomatic:

1. Administer high-concentration oxygen.

2. Initiate TCP. If the patient is unable to tolerate TCP and is conscious and not hypotensive, administer a sedative such as **midazolam** or **diazepam** as follows:

    ◆ Administer 1 to 2 mg of midazolam IV slowly over at least 2 minutes and repeat every 3 to 5 minutes, titrated to produce sedation/amnesia.

    OR

    Administer 5 to 15 mg of diazepam with or without 2 to 5 mg **morphine** IV slowly to produce amnesia/analgesia.

If the bradycardia, hypotension, or both persist:

3. Start an IV infusion of **dopamine** at an initial rate of 2 to 5 μg/kg/min and adjust the rate of infusion up to 20 μg/kg/min to increase the heart rate to 60 to 100 beats per minute and the systolic blood pressure to within normal limits.

    OR

    Start an IV infusion of **epinephrine** at an initial rate of 1 to 2 μg/min and adjust the rate of infusion up to 10 μg/min to increase the heart rate to 60 to 100 beats per minute and the systolic blood pressure to within normal limits.

4. Insert a temporary transvenous pacemaker immediately.

Notes

_____

_____

_____

TACHYCARDIAS

Clinical Significance of Tachycardias

The signs and symptoms in a tachycardia depend on the presence or absence of heart disease, the nature of the heart disease, the ventricular rate, and the duration of the tachycardia. Frequently, a tachycardia is accompanied by feelings of palpitations, nervousness, or anxiety.

A tachycardia with a heart rate over 150 beats per minute may cause the cardiac output to drop significantly because of the inability of the ventricles to fill completely during the extremely short diastole that results from the very rapid beating of the heart. Consequently, the systolic blood pressure may fall to 80 to 90 mm Hg or less, and signs and symptoms of decreased perfusion of the body, especially of the brain and other vital organs, may occur. The skin may become pale, cold, and clammy; the pulse may become weak or disappear; and the patient may become agitated, confused, lightheaded, or unconscious, or may experience chest pain and become dyspneic.

In addition, because a rapid heart rate increases the workload of the heart, the oxygen requirements of the myocardium are usually increased in a tachycardia. Thus in addition to the consequences of decreased cardiac output, a tachycardia in an acute MI may increase myocardial ischemia and the frequency and severity of chest pain; bring about the extension of the infarct; cause congestive heart failure, hypotension, or cardiogenic shock; or predispose the patient to serious ventricular arrhythmias.

Another reason for low cardiac output in certain tachycardias (atrial flutter, atrial fibrillation, paroxysmal supraventricular tachycardia [PSVT], and junctional and ventricular tachycardias) is that because an atrial contraction does not precede each ventricular contraction as it normally does (the so-called "atrial kick"), the ventricles do not fill completely during diastole. Consequently, the cardiac output may drop by as much as 25%.

Indications for Treatment of Tachycardias

Specific treatment of atrial tachycardia without block, atrial flutter, atrial fibrillation, PSVT, and junctional tachycardia is indicated if the heart rate is greater than 150 beats per minute or even as low as 100 to 120 beats per minute and, particularly, if signs and symptoms of decreased cardiac output or increased workload of the heart are associated with the tachycardia.

Treatment of ventricular tachycardia, however, is indicated immediately, regardless of whether signs and symptoms of decreased cardiac output are present, because of its potential of initiating or degenerating into ventricular fibrillation.

No specific treatment of sinus tachycardia and atrial tachycardia with block is indicated.

Precautions and Contraindications in Drug Therapy

Certain drugs, such as β-blockers, calcium channel blockers, and procainamide, may be contraindicated and/or require caution in their administration under certain conditions. The contraindications and/or precautions for these drugs are listed in boxes 10-1 to 10-3.

BOX

10-1 Administration of Calcium Channel Blockers

Calcium channel blockers are contraindicated:
- If hypotension or cardiogenic shock is present
- If second- or third-degree AV block, sinus node dysfunction, atrial flutter or fibrillation associated with ventricular or atrio-His preexcitation or a wide-QRS-complex tachycardia is present
- If β-blockers are being administered intravenously, or
- If there is a history of bradycardia

Calcium channel blockers should be used cautiously, if at all, in patients with congestive heart failure and those receiving oral β-blockers.

The patient's blood pressure and pulse must be monitored frequently during and after the administration of a calcium channel blocker.

If hypotension occurs with a calcium channel blocker, place the patient in a Trendelenburg position and administer 1 g of calcium chloride IV slowly, IV fluids, and a vasopressor.

If bradycardia, AV block, or asystole occurs, refer to the appropriate treatment protocol.

BOX

10-2 Administration of β-Blockers

β-blockers are contraindicated:
- If bradycardia (heart rate <60 beats/min) is present
- If hypotension (systolic blood pressure <100 mm Hg is present
- If PR interval >0.24 second or second- or third-degree AV block is present
- If severe congestive heart failure (left and/or right heart failure) is present
- If bronchospasm or a history of asthma is present
- If severe chronic obstructive pulmonary disease (COPD) is present
- If intravenous calcium channel blockers have been administered within a few hours

The patient's blood pressure and pulse must be monitored frequently during and after the administration of a β-blocker.

If hypotension occurs with a β-blocker, place the patient in a Trendelenburg position and administer a vasopressor.

If bradycardia, AV block, or asystole occurs, refer to the appropriate treatment protocol.

10-3   Administration of Procainamide

Do not administer procainamide if any of the following are present:
- Hypotension
- Pulmonary edema
- Unconsciousness
- Prolonged QT interval
- Torsade de pointes

Sinus Tachycardia

◆ TREATMENT

No specific treatment of sinus tachycardia is indicated.
1. Treat the underlying cause of the tachycardia (anxiety, exercise, pain, fever, congestive heart failure, hypoxemia, hypovolemia, hypotension, or shock).
If excessive amounts of drugs, such as atropine, epinephrine, or a vasopressor, have been administered:
2. Discontinue such drugs.

Notes

_____

_____

_____

_____

_____

Atrial Tachycardia With Block

◆ TREATMENT

No specific treatment of atrial tachycardia with block is indicated.
1. Treat the underlying cause of the tachycardia.
If digitalis toxicity is suspected:
2. Discontinue digitalis.

Notes

_____

_____

_____

_____

_____

Narrow-QRS-Complex Tachycardia of Unknown Origin (With Pulse)

◆ TREATMENT

Patient hemodynamically stable:

If the patient's condition is hemodynamically stable—that is, the patient is conscious and has a pulse, the systolic blood pressure is greater than 100 mm Hg, and pulmonary edema and signs and symptoms of decreased cardiac output or an acute coronary syndrome are absent:
1. Administer high-concentration oxygen.
2. Attempt vagal maneuvers, such as unilateral carotid sinus massage (preferably of the right carotid sinus), or have the patient perform the Valsalva maneuver, cough, or take a deep breath while in a head-down tilt position. ECG monitoring and an IV line must be in place, and atropine and antiarrhythmic drugs must be immediately available before vagal maneuvers are performed. The technique of immersing the patient's face in ice water ("diving reflex") may also be tried, but only if ischemic heart disease is not present or suspected.

CAUTION!

Verify the absence of known carotid artery disease or carotid bruits before attempting carotid sinus massage!

AUTHOR'S NOTE

Because of the possibility of dislodging an atheromatous plaque or an embolus to the brain while massaging a carotid sinus, it is preferable to massage the right carotid sinus to spare the dominant left side of the brain should there be an undetected plaque or thrombus in the left carotid artery.

If the vagal maneuvers are unsuccessful and the patient remains stable:
3. Administer an AV node depressant such as **adenosine.**
   - Administer a 6-mg bolus of adenosine IV rapidly over 1 to 3 seconds.

        AND

     If the initial dose is not immediately effective, administer in 1 to 2 minutes a 12-mg bolus of adenosine IV rapidly over 1 to 3 seconds. Repeat the 12-mg bolus of adenosine a second time in 1 to 2 minutes if needed.

If the arrhythmia converts to a sinus rhythm at any time, indicating that PSVT is present, continue with the appropriate step in the section on *Paroxysmal Supraventricular Tachycardia With Narrow QRS Complexes,* p. 196.

If the heart rate slows because of an AV nodal block at any time, indicating that an atrial or junctional tachycardia is present, continue with the treatment plans outlined in either the section on *Atrial Tachycardia Without Block* (below) or *Junctional Tachycardia* (p. 198) as appropriate.

Notes

_____

_____

_____

_____

_____

_____

_____

_____

_____

_____

Atrial Tachycardia Without Block

◆ TREATMENT

Patient hemodynamically stable:

If the heart rate is over 150 beats per minute

AND

The patient's condition is hemodynamically stable—that is, the patient is conscious and has a pulse, the systolic blood pressure is greater than 100 mm Hg, and pulmonary edema and signs and symptoms of decreased cardiac output or an acute coronary syndrome are absent:

1. Administer high-concentration oxygen.
2. Administer a calcium channel blocker such as **diltiazem** if not contraindicated.
   ◆ Administer a 20-mg (0.25-mg/kg) bolus of diltiazem IV slowly over 2 minutes. If the initial dose is not effective in 15 minutes and no adverse effects have occurred, repeat a second 25-mg (0.35-mg/kg) bolus of diltiazem IV slowly over 2 minutes.

NOTE: In elderly patients (>60 years of age) the boluses of diltiazem should be administered slowly over 3 to 4 minutes.

AND

Start a maintenance IV infusion of diltiazem at a rate of 5 to 15 mg per hour to maintain the heart rate within normal limits.

OR

Administer a β-**blocker** if not contraindicated.
◆ Administer a 0.5-mg/kg bolus of **esmolol** IV over 1 minute, followed by an IV infusion of esmolol at 0.05 mg/kg/min and repeat the 0.5-mg/kg bolus of esmolol IV twice at 5-minute intervals while increasing the IV infusion of esmolol 0.05 mg/kg/min after each bolus of esmolol. After the third bolus of esmolol, increase the IV infusion of esmolol 0.05 mg/kg/min every 5 minutes to a maximum infusion of 0.30 mg/kg/min, if necessary, and then titrate the esmolol infusion to maintain the heart rate within normal limits.

OR

Administer 5 mg **atenolol** IV over 5 minutes and repeat in 10 minutes to a total dose of 10 mg, if needed.

OR

Administer 5 mg **metoprolol** IV over 2 to 5 minutes and repeat twice every 5 minutes to a total dose of 15 mg, if needed.

AND

Monitor the pulse, blood pressure, and ECG while administering the drug. Stop the administration of the β-blocker if the systolic blood pressure falls below 100 mm Hg.

OR

Administer an antiarrhythmic drug such as **amiodarone.**
◆ Administer a loading dose of 150 mg of amiodarone IV over 10 minutes.

AND

Start an IV infusion of amiodarone at a rate of 1 mg per minute.

Patient hemodynamically unstable:

If the heart rate is over 150 beats per minute or less

AND

The patient is hemodynamically unstable—that is, the patient is hypotensive (systolic blood pressure of less than 90 mm Hg) with evidence of poor peripheral perfusion or has signs and symptoms of congestive heart failure or an acute coronary syndrome:

1. Administer high-concentration oxygen.
2. Administer an antiarrhythmic drug such as **amiodarone.**
   ◆ Administer a loading dose of 150 mg of amiodarone IV over 10 minutes.

AND

Start an IV infusion of amiodarone at a rate of 1 mg per minute.

OR

Administer a calcium channel blocker such as **diltiazem** if not contraindicated.

◆ Administer a 20-mg (0.25-mg/kg) bolus of diltiazem IV slowly over 2 minutes. If the initial dose is not effective in 15 minutes and no adverse effects have occurred, repeat a second 25-mg (0.35-mg/kg) bolus of diltiazem IV over 2 minutes.

NOTE: In elderly patients (>60 years of age) the boluses of diltiazem should be administered slowly over 3 to 4 minutes.

AND

Start a maintenance IV infusion of diltiazem at a rate of 5 to 15 mg per hour to maintain the heart rate within normal limits.

Notes

_____

_____

_____

_____

Paroxysmal Supraventricular Tachycardia With Narrow QRS Complexes
(Without Wolff-Parkinson-White Syndrome or Ventricular Preexcitation)

◆ **TREATMENT**

Patient hemodynamically stable:

If the heart rate is over 150 beats per minute

AND

The patient's condition is hemodynamically stable—that is, the patient is conscious and has a pulse, the systolic blood pressure is greater than 100 mm Hg, and pulmonary edema and signs and symptoms of decreased cardiac output or an acute coronary syndrome are absent:

1. Administer high-concentration oxygen.
2. Attempt vagal maneuvers, such as unilateral carotid sinus massage (preferably of the right carotid sinus), or have the patient perform the Valsalva maneuver, cough, or take a deep breath while in a head-down tilt position. ECG monitoring and an IV line must be in place, and atropine and antiarrhythmic drugs must be immediately available before vagal maneuvers are performed. The technique of immersing the patient's face in ice water ("diving reflex") may also be tried but only if ischemic heart disease is not present or suspected.

> **CAUTION!**
>
> **Verify the absence of known carotid artery disease or carotid bruits before attempting carotid sinus massage!**

If the vagal maneuvers are unsuccessful and the patient remains stable:

3. Administer an AV node depressant such as **adenosine.**

◆ Administer a 6-mg bolus of adenosine IV rapidly over 1 to 3 seconds.

AND

If the initial dose is not immediately effective, administer in 1 to 2 minutes a 12-mg bolus of adenosine IV rapidly over 1 to 3 seconds. Repeat the 12-mg bolus of adenosine a second time in 1 to 2 minutes, if needed.

If vagal maneuvers and adenosine are not effective and the patient continues to be stable:

4. Administer a calcium channel blocker such as **diltiazem** if not contraindicated.

◆ Administer a 20-mg (0.25-mg/kg) bolus of diltiazem IV slowly over 2 minutes. If the initial dose is not effective in 15 minutes and no adverse effects have occurred, repeat a second 25-mg (0.35-mg/kg) bolus of diltiazem IV over 2 minutes.

NOTE: In elderly patients (>60 years of age) the boluses of diltiazem should be administered slowly over 3 to 4 minutes.

AND

Start a maintenance IV infusion of diltiazem at a rate of 5 to 15 mg per hour to maintain the heart rate within normal limits.

OR

Administer a β-**blocker** if not contraindicated.

◆ Administer a 0.5-mg/kg bolus of **esmolol** IV over 1 minute, followed by an IV infusion of esmolol at 0.05 mg/kg/min and repeat the 0.5-mg/kg bolus of esmolol IV twice at 5-minute intervals while increasing the IV infusion of esmolol 0.05 mg/kg/min after each bolus of esmolol. After the third bolus of esmolol IV, increase the IV infusion of esmolol 0.05 mg/kg/min every 5 minutes to a maximum infusion of 0.30 mg/kg/min, if necessary, and then titrate the esmolol infusion to maintain the heart rate within normal limits.

OR

Administer 5 mg **atenolol** IV over 5 minutes and

repeat in 10 minutes to a total dose of 10 mg, if needed.

OR

Administer 5 mg **metoprolol** IV over 2 to 5 minutes and repeat twice every 5 minutes to a total dose of 15 mg, if needed.

AND

Monitor the pulse, blood pressure, and ECG while administering the drug. Stop the administration of the β-blocker if the systolic blood pressure falls below 100 mm Hg.

AND

5. Administer an initial digitalization dose of 0.5 mg **digoxin** IV over 5 minutes.

If vagal maneuvers, adenosine, diltiazem or a β-blocker, and digoxin are not effective and the patient continues to be stable:

6. Deliver a synchronized shock (50 or 100 joules [J]). In the conscious patient, premedicate the patient before cardioversion, using a sedative such as **midazolam** or **diazepam** as follows:

◆ Administer 1 to 2 mg of midazolam IV slowly over at least 2 minutes and repeat every 3 to 5 minutes, titrated to produce sedation/amnesia before cardioversion.

OR

Administer 5 to 15 mg of diazepam with or without 2 to 5 mg IV **morphine** slowly to produce amnesia/analgesia before cardioversion.

AND

Repeat the synchronized shock as often as necessary at progressively increasing energy levels as appropriate (100 or 200 J, 300 J, and 360 J).

AUTHOR'S NOTE

The energy levels indicated are for monophasic waveform cardioversion. Biphasic shocks should be delivered at equivalent energy levels.

Notes

_____

_____

_____

_____

_____

_____

_____

_____

Patient hemodynamically unstable:

If the heart rate is over 150 beats per minute or less

AND

The patient is hemodynamically unstable—that is, the patient is hypotensive (systolic blood pressure of less than 90 mm Hg) with evidence of poor peripheral perfusion or has signs and symptoms of congestive heart failure or an acute coronary syndrome:

1. Administer high-concentration oxygen.
2. Attempt vagal maneuvers, such as unilateral carotid sinus massage (preferably of the right carotid sinus), or have the patient perform the Valsalva maneuver, cough, or take a deep breath while in a head-down tilt position. ECG monitoring and an IV line must be in place and atropine and antiarrhythmic drugs must be immediately available before vagal maneuvers are performed. The technique of immersing the patient's face in ice water ("diving reflex") may also be tried but only if ischemic heart disease is not present or suspected.

CAUTION!

Verify the absence of known carotid artery disease or carotid bruits before attempting carotid sinus massage!

---

3. Administer an initial digitalization dose of 0.5 mg IV **digoxin** over 5 minutes.
4. Administer an antiarrhythmic drug such as **amiodarone.**

◆ Administer an IV loading dose of 150 mg of amiodarone over 10 minutes with caution.

AND

Start an IV infusion of amiodarone at a rate of 1 mg per minute.

OR

Administer a calcium channel blocker such as **diltiazem** with caution, if not contraindicated.

◆ Administer a 20-mg (0.25-mg/kg) bolus of diltiazem IV slowly over 2 minutes. If the initial dose is not effective in 15 minutes and no adverse effects have occurred, repeat a second 25-mg (0.35-mg/kg) bolus of IV diltiazem over 2 minutes.

NOTE: In elderly patients (>60 years of age) the boluses of diltiazem should be administered over 3 to 4 minutes.

AND

Start a maintenance IV infusion of diltiazem at a rate of 5 to 15 mg per hour to maintain the heart rate within normal limits.

Notes

_____

_____

_____

_____

_____

_____

_____

_____

_____

_____

Junctional Tachycardia

◆ TREATMENT

Patient hemodynamically stable:

If the heart rate is over 150 beats per minute

AND

The patient's condition is hemodynamically stable—that is, the patient is conscious and has a pulse, the systolic blood pressure is greater than 100 mm Hg, and pulmonary edema and signs and symptoms of decreased cardiac output or an acute coronary syndrome are absent:

1. Administer high-concentration oxygen.
2. Administer an antiarrhythmic drug such as **amiodarone.**
   ◆ Administer a loading dose of 150 mg of amiodarone IV over 10 minutes.

   AND

   Start an IV infusion of amiodarone at a rate of 1 mg per minute.

   OR

Administer a β-**blocker** if not contraindicated.
   ◆ Administer a 0.5-mg/kg bolus of **esmolol** IV over 1 minute, followed by an IV infusion of esmolol at 0.05 mg/kg/min and repeat the 0.5-mg/kg bolus of esmolol IV twice at 5-minute intervals while increasing the IV infusion of esmolol 0.05 mg/kg/min after each bolus of esmolol. After the third bolus of esmolol IV, increase the IV infusion of esmolol 0.05 mg/kg/min every 5 minutes to a maximum infusion of 0.30 mg/kg/min, if necessary, and then titrate the esmolol infusion to maintain the heart rate within normal limits.

   OR

Administer 5 mg **atenolol** IV over 5 minutes and repeat in 10 minutes to a total dose of 10 mg, if needed.

OR

Administer 5 mg **metoprolol** IV over 2 to 5 minutes and repeat twice every 5 minutes to a total dose of 15 mg, if needed.

AND

Monitor the pulse, blood pressure, and ECG while administering the drug. Stop the administration of the β-blocker if the systolic blood pressure falls below 100 mm Hg.

Patient hemodynamically unstable:

If the heart rate is over 150 beats per minute or less

AND

The patient is hemodynamically unstable—that is, the patient is hypotensive (systolic blood pressure of less than 90 mm Hg) with evidence of poor peripheral perfusion or has signs and symptoms of congestive heart failure or an acute coronary syndrome:

1. Administer high-concentration oxygen.
2. Administer an antiarrhythmic drug such as **amiodarone.**
   ◆ Administer a loading dose of 150 mg of amiodarone IV over 10 minutes.

   AND

   Start an IV infusion of amiodarone at a rate of 1 mg per minute.

Notes

_____

_____

_____

Atrial Flutter/Atrial Fibrillation
(Without Wolff-Parkinson-White Syndrome or Ventricular Preexcitation)

◆ TREATMENT TO CONTROL THE HEART RATE

Patient hemodynamically stable:

If the heart rate is over 120 beats per minute

AND

The patient's condition is hemodynamically stable—that is, the patient is conscious and has a pulse, the systolic blood pressure is greater than 100 mm Hg, and pulmonary edema and signs and symptoms of decreased cardiac output or an acute coronary syndrome are absent:

1. Administer high-concentration oxygen.
2. Administer a β-**blocker** if not contraindicated.
   ◆ Administer a 0.5-mg/kg bolus of **esmolol** IV over 1 minute, followed by an IV infusion of esmolol at 0.05 mg/kg/min and repeat the

0.5-mg/kg bolus of esmolol IV twice at 5-minute intervals while increasing the IV infusion of esmolol 0.05 mg/kg/min after each bolus of esmolol. After the third bolus of esmolol IV, increase the IV infusion of esmolol 0.05 mg/kg/min every 5 minutes to a maximum infusion of 0.30 mg/kg/min, if necessary, and then titrate the esmolol infusion to maintain the heart rate within normal limits.

OR

Administer 5 mg **atenolol** IV over 5 minutes and repeat in 10 minutes to a total dose of 10 mg, if needed.

OR

Administer 5 mg **metoprolol** IV over 2 to 5 minutes and repeat twice every 5 minutes to a total dose of 15 mg, if needed.

AND

Monitor the pulse, blood pressure, and ECG while administering the drug. Stop the administration of the β-blocker if the systolic blood pressure falls below 100 mm Hg.

OR

Administer a calcium channel blocker such as **diltiazem** if not contraindicated.

◆ Administer a 20-mg (0.25-mg/kg) bolus of diltiazem IV slowly over 2 minutes. If the initial dose is not effective in 15 minutes and no adverse effects have occurred, repeat a second 25-mg (0.35-mg/kg) bolus of diltiazem IV slowly over 2 minutes.

NOTE: In elderly patients (>60 years of age) the boluses of diltiazem should be administered slowly over 3 to 4 minutes.

AND

Start a maintenance IV infusion of diltiazem at a rate of 5 to 15 mg per hour to maintain the heart rate within normal limits.

3. Administer an initial digitalization dose of 0.5 mg **digoxin** IV over 5 minutes.

Patient hemodynamically unstable:

If the heart rate is over 120 beats per minute or less

AND

The patient is hemodynamically unstable—that is, the patient is hypotensive (systolic blood pressure of less than 90 mm Hg) with evidence of poor peripheral perfusion or has signs and symptoms of congestive heart failure or an acute coronary syndrome:

1. Administer high-concentration oxygen.
2. Administer an initial digitalization dose of 0.5 mg **digoxin** IV over 5 minutes.
3. Administer a calcium channel blocker such as **diltiazem** if not contraindicated.

◆ Administer a 20-mg (0.25-mg/kg) bolus of diltiazem IV slowly over 2 minutes. If the initial

dose is not effective in 15 minutes and no adverse effects have occurred, repeat a second 25-mg (0.35-mg/kg) bolus of diltiazem IV slowly over 2 minutes.

NOTE: In elderly patients (>60 years of age) the boluses of diltiazem should be administered slowly over 3 to 4 minutes.

AND

Start a maintenance IV infusion of diltiazem at a rate of 5 to 15 mg per hour to maintain the heart rate within normal limits.

OR

Administer an antiarrhythmic drug such as **amiodarone**, but only if atrial fibrillation has been present for less than 48 hours.

◆ Administer a loading dose of 150 mg of amiodarone IV over 10 minutes.

AND

Start an IV infusion of amiodarone at a rate of 1 mg per minute.

Notes

_____

_____

_____

_____

_____

_____

Atrial Flutter/Atrial Fibrillation
(Without Wolff-Parkinson-White Syndrome or
Ventricular Preexcitation)

◆ TREATMENT TO CONVERT THE RHYTHM

Atrial Fibrillation <48 Hours and Atrial Flutter of Any Duration

Patient hemodynamically stable:

If the heart rate is over 120 beats per minute

AND

The patient's condition is hemodynamically stable—that is, the patient is conscious and has a pulse, the systolic blood pressure is greater than 100 mm Hg, and pulmonary edema and signs and symptoms of decreased cardiac output or an acute coronary syndrome are absent:

1. Administer high-concentration oxygen.
2. Administer a short-acting antiarrhythmic such as **ibutilide.**

If the patient weighs ≥60 kg (≥132 lb), administer 1 mg of ibutilide IV over 10 minutes and repeat in 10 minutes if necessary after completion of the first infusion.

If the patient weighs <60 kg (<132 lb), administer 0.1 mg/kg of ibutilide IV over 10 minutes and repeat in 10 minutes if necessary after completion of the first infusion.

OR

Administer an antiarrhythmic drug such as **amiodarone.**

◆ Administer a loading dose of 150 mg of amiodarone IV over 10 minutes.

AND

Start an IV infusion of amiodarone at a rate of 1 mg per minute.

OR

Administer an antiarrhythmic drug such as **procainamide hydrochloride** if not contraindicated.

◆ Start an IV infusion of procainamide at a rate of 20 to 30 mg/min.

AND

Continue the infusion of procainamide until:
◆ Atrial flutter or atrial fibrillation is converted
◆ A total dose of 17 mg/kg of procainamide has been administered (1.2 g of procainamide for a 70-kg patient)
◆ Side effects from the procainamide appear (such as hypotension)
◆ The QRS complex widens by 50% of its original width, or
◆ The PR or QT interval lengthens by 50% of its original length

AND

Start a maintenance IV infusion of procainamide if indicated, at a rate of 1 to 4 mg per minute to prevent the recurrence of atrial flutter or atrial fibrillation.

If one of the antiarrhythmic drugs is unsuccessful in converting atrial flutter or atrial fibrillation:

3. Deliver a low-energy synchronized shock (50 or 100 J for atrial flutter, 100 or 200 J for atrial fibrillation). In the conscious patient, premedicate the patient before cardioversion, using a sedative such as **midazolam** or **diazepam** as follows:
◆ Administer 1 to 2 mg of midazolam IV slowly over at least 2 minutes and repeat every 3 to 5 minutes, titrated to produce sedation/amnesia before cardioversion.

OR

Administer 5 to 15 mg of diazepam with or without 2 to 5 mg **morphine** IV slowly to produce amnesia/analgesia before cardioversion.

AND

Repeat the synchronized shock as often as necessary at progressively increasing energy levels as appropriate (100 J, 200 J, and so forth, up to 360 J).

Notes

_____

_____

_____

_____

_____

_____

_____

_____

_____

_____

Patient hemodynamically unstable:

If the heart rate is over 120 beats per minute or less

AND

The patient is hemodynamically unstable—that is, the patient is hypotensive (systolic blood pressure of less than 90 mm Hg) with evidence of poor peripheral perfusion or has signs and symptoms of congestive heart failure or an acute coronary syndrome:

1. Administer high-concentration oxygen.

AND

Consider immediate DC cardioversion or administration of an antiarrhythmic drug.

2. Deliver a low-energy synchronized shock (50 or 100 J for atrial flutter, 100 or 200 J for atrial fibrillation). If the patient is conscious, consider premedicating the patient before cardioversion, using a sedative such as **midazolam** or **diazepam** as follows:
◆ Administer 1 to 2 mg of midazolam IV slowly over at least 2 minutes and repeat every 3 to 5 minutes, titrated to produce sedation/amnesia before cardioversion.

OR

Administer 5 to 15 mg of diazepam with or without 2 to 5 mg **morphine** IV slowly to produce amnesia/analgesia before cardioversion.

AND

Repeat the synchronized shock as often as necessary at progressively increasing energy levels as appropriate (100 J, 200 J, and so forth, up to 360 J).

3. Administer an antiarrhythmic drug such as **amiodarone.**

◆ Administer a loading dose of 150 mg of amiodarone IV over 10 minutes.

AND

Start an IV infusion of amiodarone at a rate of 1 mg per minute.

If amiodarone is unsuccessful in converting atrial flutter or atrial fibrillation:

◆ Perform **DC cardioversion** as above in Step 2.

Notes

_____

_____

_____

_____

_____

Atrial Fibrillation >48 Hours or of Unknown Duration

Patient hemodynamically stable:

If the heart rate is over 120 beats per minute

AND

The patient's condition is hemodynamically stable—that is, the patient is conscious and has a pulse, the systolic blood pressure is greater than 100 mm Hg, and pulmonary edema and signs and symptoms of decreased cardiac output or an acute coronary syndrome are absent:

1. Administer high-concentration oxygen.
2. Administer a β-**blocker** if not contraindicated.
   - ◆ Administer a 0.5-mg/kg bolus of **esmolol** IV over 1 minute, followed by an IV infusion of esmolol at 0.05 mg/kg/min and repeat the 0.5-mg/kg bolus of esmolol IV twice at 5-minute intervals while increasing the IV infusion of esmolol 0.05 mg/kg/min after each bolus of esmolol. After the third bolus of esmolol IV, increase the IV infusion of esmolol 0.05 mg/kg/min every 5 minutes to a maximum infusion of 0.30 mg/kg/min, if necessary, and then titrate the esmolol infusion to maintain the heart rate within normal limits.

     OR

     Administer 5 mg **atenolol** IV over 5 minutes and repeat in 10 minutes to a total dose of 10 mg, if needed.

     OR

     Administer 5 mg **metoprolol** IV over 2 to 5 minutes and repeat twice every 5 minutes to a total dose of 15 mg, if needed.

     AND

     Monitor the pulse, blood pressure, and ECG while administering the drug. Stop the administration of the β-blocker if the systolic blood pressure falls below 100 mm Hg.

     OR

   Administer a calcium channel blocker such as **diltiazem** if not contraindicated.

   - ◆ Administer a 20-mg (0.25-mg/kg) bolus of diltiazem IV slowly over 2 minutes. If the initial dose is not effective in 15 minutes and no adverse effects have occurred, repeat a second 25-mg (0.35-mg/kg) bolus of diltiazem IV slowly over 2 minutes.

NOTE: In elderly patients (>60 years of age) the boluses of diltiazem should be administered slowly over 3 to 4 minutes.

AND

Start a maintenance IV infusion of diltiazem at a rate of 5 to 15 mg per hour to maintain the heart rate within normal limits.

3. Administer an initial digitalization dose of 0.5 mg **digoxin** IV over 5 minutes.
4. Delay DC cardioversion until the patient is anticoagulated and atrial thrombi are excluded.

Patient hemodynamically unstable:

If the heart rate is over 120 beats per minute or less

AND

The patient is hemodynamically unstable—that is, the patient is hypotensive (systolic blood pressure of less than 90 mm Hg) with evidence of poor peripheral perfusion or has signs and symptoms of congestive heart failure or an acute coronary syndrome:

1. Administer high-concentration oxygen.
2. Administer a calcium channel blocker such as **diltiazem** if not contraindicated.
   - ◆ Administer a 20-mg (0.25-mg/kg) bolus of diltiazem IV slowly over 2 minutes. If the initial dose is not effective in 15 minutes and no adverse effects have occurred, repeat a second 25-mg (0.35-mg/kg) bolus of diltiazem IV slowly over 2 minutes.

NOTE: In elderly patients (>60 years of age) the boluses of diltiazem should be administered slowly over 3 to 4 minutes.

AND

Start a maintenance IV infusion of diltiazem at a rate of 5 to 15 mg per hour to maintain the heart rate within normal limits.

3. Administer an initial digitalization dose of 0.5 mg **digoxin** IV over 5 minutes.
4. Delay DC cardioversion until the patient is anticoagulated and atrial thrombi are excluded.

Notes

_____

_____

_____

_____

_____

_____

_____

_____

_____

Atrial Flutter/Atrial Fibrillation
(With Wolff-Parkinson-White Syndrome or
Ventricular Preexcitation)

◆ TREATMENT TO CONTROL THE HEART RATE AND/OR CONVERT THE RHYTHM

Atrial Fibrillation <48 Hours and Atrial Flutter of Any Duration

Patient hemodynamically stable:

If the heart rate is over 120 beats per minute

AND

The patient's condition is hemodynamically stable—that is, the patient is conscious and has a pulse, the systolic blood pressure is greater than 100 mm Hg, and pulmonary edema and signs and symptoms of decreased cardiac output or an acute coronary syndrome are absent:

1. Administer high-concentration oxygen.
2. Administer an antiarrhythmic drug such as **amiodarone.**
   - ◆ Administer a loading dose of 150 mg of amiodarone IV over 10 minutes.

AND

   Start an IV infusion of amiodarone at a rate of 1 mg per minute.

OR

Administer an antiarrhythmic drug such as **procainamide** if not contraindicated.
   - ◆ Start an IV infusion of procainamide at a rate of 20 to 30 mg/min.

AND

   Continue the infusion of procainamide until:
   - ◆ Atrial flutter or atrial fibrillation is converted
   - ◆ A total dose of 17 mg/kg of procainamide has been administered (1.2 g of procainamide for a 70-kg patient)
   - ◆ Side effects from the procainamide appear (such as hypotension)
   - ◆ The QRS complex widens by 50% of its original width, or
   - ◆ The PR or QT interval lengthens by 50% of its original length

AND

   Start a maintenance IV infusion of procainamide if indicated, at a rate of 1 to 4 mg per minute to prevent the recurrence of atrial flutter or atrial fibrillation.

If one of the antiarrhythmic drugs is unsuccessful in converting atrial flutter or atrial fibrillation:

3. Deliver a low-energy synchronized shock (50 or 100 J for atrial flutter, 100 or 200 J for atrial fibrillation).

In the conscious patient, premedicate the patient before cardioversion as follows, using a sedative such as **midazolam** or **diazepam:**
   - ◆ Administer 1 to 2 mg of midazolam IV slowly over at least 2 minutes and repeat every 3 to 5 minutes, titrated to produce sedation/amnesia before cardioversion.

OR

Administer 5 to 15 mg of diazepam with or without 2 to 5 mg **morphine** IV slowly to produce amnesia/analgesia before cardioversion.

AND

Repeat the synchronized shock as often as necessary at progressively increasing energy levels as appropriate (100 J, 200 J, and so forth, up to 360 J).

Patient hemodynamically unstable:

If the heart rate is over 120 beats per minute or less

AND

The patient is hemodynamically unstable—that is, the patient is hypotensive (systolic blood pressure of less than 90 mm Hg) with evidence of poor peripheral perfusion or has signs and symptoms of congestive heart failure or an acute coronary syndrome:

1. Administer high-concentration oxygen.

AND

   Consider immediate DC cardioversion or administration of an antiarrhythmic drug.

2. Deliver a low-energy synchronized shock (50 or 100 J for atrial flutter, 100 or 200 J for atrial fibrillation). If the patient is conscious, consider premedicating the patient before cardioversion, using a sedative such as **midazolam** or **diazepam** as follows:
   - ◆ Administer 1 to 2 mg of midazolam IV slowly over at least 2 minutes and repeat every 3 to 5 minutes, titrated to produce sedation/amnesia before cardioversion.

OR

Administer 5 to 15 mg of diazepam with or without 2 to 5 mg **morphine** IV slowly to produce amnesia/analgesia before cardioversion.

AND

Repeat the synchronized shock as often as necessary at progressively increasing energy levels as appropriate (100 J, 200 J, and so forth, up to 360 J).

3. Administer an antiarrhythmic drug such as **amiodarone.**
   - ◆ Administer a loading dose of 150 mg of amiodarone IV over 10 minutes.

AND

   Start an IV infusion of amiodarone at a rate of 1 mg/min.

If amiodarone is unsuccessful in converting atrial flutter or atrial fibrillation:
   - ◆ Perform DC cardioversion as above in Step 2.

Notes

_____

_____

_____

_____

Atrial Fibrillation >48 Hours or of Unknown Duration

Patient hemodynamically stable or unstable:

If the heart rate is over 120 beats per minute or less:

1. Administer high-concentration oxygen.
2. Administer an antiarrhythmic drug such as **amiodarone** with extreme caution.
   - ◆ Administer a loading dose of 150 mg of amiodarone IV over 10 minutes.

      AND

     Start an IV infusion of amiodarone at a rate of 1 mg/min.
3. Delay **DC cardioversion** until the patient is anticoagulated and atrial thrombi are excluded.

Notes

_____

_____

_____

_____

_____

_____

_____

Wide-QRS-Complex Tachycardia of Unknown Origin (With Pulse)

◆ TREATMENT

Patient hemodynamically stable:

If the patient's condition is hemodynamically stable—that is, the patient is conscious and has a pulse, the systolic blood pressure is greater than 100 mm Hg, and pulmonary edema and signs and symptoms of decreased cardiac output or an acute coronary syndrome are absent:

1. Administer high-concentration oxygen.

      AND

   Consider immediate DC cardioversion or administration of an antiarrhythmic drug.
2. Deliver a synchronized shock (100 J). In the conscious patient, premedicate the patient before cardioversion as follows, using a sedative such as **midazolam** or **diazepam**:
   - ◆ Administer 1 to 2 mg of midazolam IV slowly over at least 2 minutes and repeat every 3 to 5 minutes, titrated to produce sedation/amnesia before cardioversion.

      OR

     Administer 5 to 15 mg of diazepam with or without 2 to 5 mg **morphine** IV slowly to produce amnesia/analgesia before cardioversion.

      AND

   Repeat the synchronized shock as often as necessary at progressively increasing energy levels (200 J, 300 J, and 360 J).

If the wide-QRS-complex tachycardia persists and the patient remains hemodynamically stable and has a pulse:
   - ◆ Administer an antiarrhythmic drug such as **procainamide** or **amiodarone** as in Step 3 below while continuing the delivery of synchronized shocks.

If the wide-QRS-complex tachycardia persists and the patient is or becomes hemodynamically unstable and has a pulse:
   - ◆ Continue with an antiarrhythmic drug such as **amiodarone** as in Step 3 below while continuing the delivery of synchronized shocks.

If the wide-QRS-complex tachycardia persists and the patient becomes pulseless at any time:
   - ◆ Continue with section B, _Monitored Cardiac Arrest_ under _Ventricular Fibrillation/Pulseless Tachycardia_, p. 213.

3. Administer an antiarrhythmic drug such as **procainamide** if not contraindicated.
   - ◆ Start an IV infusion of procainamide at a rate of 20 to 30 mg per minute (up to 50 mg per minute, if necessary).

      AND

     Continue the infusion of procainamide until:
     - ◆ The wide-QRS-complex tachycardia is suppressed
     - ◆ A total dose of 17 mg/kg of procainamide has been administered (1.2 g of procainamide for a 70-kg patient)
     - ◆ Side effects from the procainamide appear (such as hypotension)
     - ◆ The QRS complex widens by 50% of its original width, or
     - ◆ The PR or QT interval lengthens by 50% of its original length

If procainamide is successful in suppressing the wide-QRS-complex tachycardia:
   - ◆ Start a maintenance IV infusion of procainamide at a rate of 1 to 4 mg/min.

      OR

Administer an antiarrhythmic drug such as **amiodarone.**

◆ Administer a loading dose of 150 mg of amiodarone IV over 10 minutes and repeat two to three times if necessary, allowing 10 to 15 minutes between infusions.

AND

Start an IV infusion of amiodarone at a rate of 1 mg/min.

If procainamide or amiodarone is unsuccessful in suppressing the wide-QRS-complex tachycardia and the patient remains stable, or if at any time while administrating procainamide or amiodarone the patient's condition becomes hemodynamically unstable and synchronized shocks were not delivered initially:

◆ Immediately deliver a synchronized shock (100 J), premedicating the patient first, if necessary, as above in Step 2.

AND

Repeat the synchronized shock as often as necessary at progressively increasing energy levels (200 J, 300 J, and 360 J).

If one of the shocks or procainamide or amiodarone is successful in terminating the wide-QRS-complex tachycardia:

4. Continue or start a maintenance IV infusion of procainamide or amiodarone as appropriate.

Patient hemodynamically unstable:

If the patient is conscious (or unconscious) and has a pulse, but with a hemodynamically unstable condition—that is, the patient is hypotensive (systolic blood pressure of less than 90 mm Hg) with evidence of poor peripheral perfusion or has signs and symptoms of congestive heart failure or an acute coronary syndrome:

1. Administer high-concentration oxygen.

AND

Consider immediate DC cardioversion or administration of an antiarrhythmic drug.

2. Deliver a synchronized shock (100 J). If the patient is conscious, consider premedicating the patient before cardioversion as follows, using a sedative such as **midazolam** or **diazepam:**

◆ Administer 1 to 2 mg of midazolam IV slowly over at least 2 minutes and repeat every 3 to 5 minutes, titrated to produce sedation/amnesia before cardioversion.

OR

Administer 5 to 15 mg of diazepam with or without 2 to 5 mg **morphine** IV slowly to produce amnesia/analgesia before cardioversion.

Administration of a sedative should not delay cardioversion if it is indicated immediately by the patient's condition!

AND

Repeat the synchronized shock as often as necessary at progressively increasing energy levels (200 J, 300 J, and 360 J).

If the wide-QRS-complex tachycardia persists and the patient remains hemodynamically unstable and has a pulse:

◆ Continue with an antiarrhythmic drug such as **amiodarone** as in Step 3 below while continuing the delivery of synchronized shocks.

If the wide-QRS-complex tachycardia persists and the patient becomes pulseless at any time:

◆ Continue with section B, *Monitored Cardiac Arrest* under *Ventricular Fibrillation/Pulseless Tachycardia,* p. 213.

3. Administer an antiarrhythmic drug such as **amiodarone.**

◆ Administer a loading dose of 150 mg of amiodarone IV over 10 minutes and repeat two to three times if necessary, allowing 10 to 15 minutes between infusions.

AND

Start an IV infusion of amiodarone at a rate of 1 mg/min.

If amiodarone is unsuccessful in suppressing the wide-QRS-complex tachycardia and the patient remains hemodynamically unstable and synchronized shocks were not delivered initially:

◆ Immediately deliver a synchronized shock (100 J), premedicating the patient first, if necessary, as above in Step 2.

AND

Repeat the synchronized shock as often as necessary at progressively increasing energy levels (200 J, 300 J, and 360 J).

If one of the shocks or amiodarone is successful in terminating the wide-QRS-complex tachycardia:

4. Continue or start a maintenance IV infusion of amiodarone.

Notes

Ventricular Tachycardia, Monomorphic (With Pulse)

◆ **TREATMENT**

Patient hemodynamically stable:

If the patient's condition is hemodynamically stable—that is, the patient is conscious and has a pulse, the systolic blood pressure is greater than 100 mm Hg, and pulmonary edema and signs and symptoms of decreased cardiac output or an acute coronary syndrome are absent:

1. Administer high-concentration oxygen.

   AND

   Consider immediate DC cardioversion or administration of an antiarrhythmic drug.

2. Deliver a synchronized shock (100 J). In the conscious patient, premedicate the patient before cardioversion as follows, using a sedative such as **midazolam** or **diazepam:**

   ◆ Administer 1 to 2 mg of midazolam IV slowly over at least 2 minutes and repeat every 3 to 5 minutes, titrated to produce sedation/amnesia before cardioversion.

   OR

   Administer 5 to 15 mg of diazepam with or without 2 to 5 mg **morphine** IV slowly to produce amnesia/analgesia before cardioversion.

   AND

   Repeat the synchronized shock as often as necessary at progressively increasing energy levels (200 J, 300 J, and 360 J).

If ventricular tachycardia persists and the patient remains hemodynamically stable and has a pulse:

   ◆ Administer an antiarrhythmic drug such as **procainamide, amiodarone,** or **lidocaine** as in Step 3 below while continuing the delivery of synchronized shocks.

If ventricular tachycardia persists and the patient is or becomes hemodynamically unstable and has a pulse:

   ◆ Administer an antiarrhythmic drug such as **amiodarone** or **lidocaine** as in Step 3 below while continuing the delivery of synchronized shocks.

If ventricular tachycardia persists and the patient becomes pulseless at any time:

   ◆ Continue with section B, *Monitored Cardiac Arrest* under *Ventricular Fibrillation/Pulseless Tachycardia,* p. 213.

3. Administer an antiarrhythmic drug such as **procainamide** if not contraindicated.

   ◆ Start an IV infusion of procainamide at a rate of 20 to 30 mg per minute (up to 50 mg per minute, if necessary).

   AND

   Continue the infusion of procainamide until:

   ◆ Ventricular tachycardia is suppressed
   ◆ A total dose of 17 mg/kg of procainamide has been administered (1.2 g of procainamide for a 70-kg patient)
   ◆ Side effects from the procainamide appear (such as hypotension)
   ◆ The QRS complex widens by 50% of its original width, or

   ◆ The PR or QT interval lengthens by 50% of its original length

If procainamide is successful in suppressing ventricular tachycardia:

   ◆ Start a maintenance IV infusion of procainamide at a rate of 1 to 4 mg/min.

   OR

Administer an antiarrhythmic drug such as **amiodarone.**

   ◆ Administer a loading dose of 150 mg of amiodarone IV over 10 minutes, and repeat two to three times if necessary, allowing 10 to 15 minutes between infusions.

   AND

   Start an IV infusion of amiodarone at a rate of 1 mg/min.

   OR

Administer an antiarrhythmic drug such as **lidocaine.**

   ◆ Administer a 1.0- to 1.5-mg/kg bolus (75 to 100 mg) of lidocaine IV slowly, and repeat a 0.5- to 0.75-mg/kg bolus (25 to 50 mg) of lidocaine IV slowly every 5 to 10 minutes until the ventricular tachycardia is suppressed or a total dose of 3 mg/kg of lidocaine has been administered.

If lidocaine is successful in suppressing the ventricular tachycardia:

   ◆ Start a maintenance infusion of lidocaine (1 g of lidocaine in 500 mL of D_5W [2 mg/mL]) at a rate of 2 mg/min (1 mL/min of the diluted lidocaine solution) to prevent the recurrence of the ventricular tachycardia. If additional boluses of lidocaine were administered initially, increase the rate of the lidocaine infusion by 1-mg increments for each additional 1-mg/kg dose of lidocaine to a maximum rate of 4 mg/min.

If procainamide, amiodarone, or lidocaine is unsuccessful in suppressing ventricular tachycardia and the patient remains stable, or if at any time while administrating procainamide, amiodarone, or lidocaine, the patient's condition becomes hemodynamically unstable and synchronized shocks were not delivered initially:

   ◆ Immediately deliver a synchronized shock (100 J), premedicating the patient first, if necessary, as above in Step 2.

   AND

   Repeat the synchronized shock as often as necessary at progressively increasing energy levels (200 J, 300 J, and 360 J).

If one of the shocks or procainamide, amiodarone, or lidocaine is successful in terminating ventricular tachycardia:

4. Continue or start a maintenance IV infusion of procainamide, amiodarone, or lidocaine as appropriate.

Patient hemodynamically unstable:

If the patient is conscious (or unconscious) and has a pulse, but with a hemodynamically unstable condition—that is, the patient is hypotensive (systolic blood pressure of less than 90 mm Hg) with evidence of poor peripheral perfusion or has signs and symptoms of congestive heart failure or an acute coronary syndrome:

1. Administer high-concentration oxygen.

    AND

    Consider immediate DC cardioversion or administration of an antiarrhythmic drug.

2. Deliver a synchronized shock (100 J). If the patient is conscious, consider premedicating the patient before cardioversion as follows, using a sedative such as **midazolam** or **diazepam:**

    ◆ Administer 1 to 2 mg of midazolam IV slowly over at least 2 minutes and repeat every 3 to 5 minutes, titrated to produce sedation/amnesia before cardioversion.

    OR

    Administer 5 to 15 mg of diazepam with or without 2 to 5 mg **morphine** IV slowly to produce amnesia/analgesia before cardioversion.

Administration of a sedative should not delay cardioversion if it is indicated immediately by the patient's condition!

    AND

    Repeat the synchronized shock as often as necessary at progressively increasing energy levels (200 J, 300 J, and 360 J).

If ventricular tachycardia persists and the patient remains hemodynamically unstable and has a pulse:

    ◆ Administer an antiarrhythmic drug such as **amiodarone** or **lidocaine** as in Step 3 below while continuing the delivery of synchronized shocks.

If ventricular tachycardia persists and the patient becomes pulseless at any time:

    ◆ Continue with section B, *Monitored Cardiac Arrest* under *Ventricular Fibrillation/Pulseless Tachycardia,* p. 213.

3. Administer an antiarrhythmic drug such as **amiodarone.**

    ◆ Administer a loading dose of 150 mg of amiodarone IV over 10 minutes and repeat two to three times if necessary, allowing 10 to 15 minutes between infusions.

    AND

    Start an IV infusion of amiodarone at a rate of 1 mg per minute.

    OR

Administer an antiarrhythmic drug such as **lidocaine.**

    ◆ Administer a 1.0- to 1.5-mg/kg bolus (75 to 100 mg) of lidocaine IV slowly, and repeat a 0.5- to 0.75-mg/kg bolus (25 to 50 mg) of lidocaine IV slowly every 5 to 10 minutes until the ventricular tachycardia is suppressed or a total dose of 3 mg/kg of lidocaine has been administered.

If lidocaine is successful in suppressing the ventricular tachycardia:

    ◆ Start a maintenance infusion of lidocaine (1 g of lidocaine in 500 mL of D_5W [2 mg/mL]) at a rate of 2 mg/min (1 mL/min of the diluted lidocaine solution) to prevent the recurrence of the ventricular tachycardia. If additional boluses of lidocaine were administered initially, increase the rate of the lidocaine infusion by 1-mg increments for each additional 1-mg/kg dose of lidocaine to a maximum rate of 4 mg/min.

If amiodarone or lidocaine is unsuccessful in suppressing ventricular tachycardia and the patient remains hemodynamically unstable and synchronized shocks were not delivered initially:

    ◆ Immediately deliver a synchronized shock (100 J), premedicating the patient first, if necessary, as above in Step 2.

    AND

    Repeat the synchronized shock as often as necessary at progressively increasing energy levels (200 J, 300 J, and 360 J).

If one of the shocks or amiodarone or lidocaine is successful in terminating ventricular tachycardia:

4. Continue or start a maintenance IV infusion of amiodarone or lidocaine as appropriate.

Notes

_____

_____

_____

_____

_____

_____

_____

_____

_____

_____

_____

_____

Ventricular Tachycardia, Polymorphic (With Pulse)
Normal Baseline QT Interval

◆ **TREATMENT**

Patient hemodynamically stable:

If the patient's condition is hemodynamically stable—that is, the patient is conscious and has a pulse, the systolic blood pressure is greater than 100 mm Hg, and pulmonary edema and signs and symptoms of decreased cardiac output or an acute coronary syndrome are absent:

1. Administer high-concentration oxygen.

AND

Consider immediate DC cardioversion or administration of an antiarrhythmic drug while correcting any electrolyte imbalance.

2. Deliver a synchronized shock (200 J). In the conscious patient, premedicate the patient before cardioversion as follows, using a sedative such as **midazolam** or **diazepam**:

◆ Administer 1 to 2 mg of midazolam IV slowly over at least 2 minutes and repeat every 3 to 5 minutes, titrated to produce sedation/amnesia before cardioversion.

OR

◆ Administer 5 to 15 mg of diazepam with or without 2 to 5 mg **morphine** IV slowly to produce amnesia/analgesia before cardioversion.

AND

Repeat the synchronized shock as often as necessary at progressively increasing energy levels (200 to 300 J and 360 J).

If the polymorphic ventricular tachycardia persists and the patient remains hemodynamically stable and has a pulse:

◆ Administer a β-**blocker** or an antiarrhythmic drug such as **procainamide, amiodarone,** or **lidocaine** as in Step 3 below while continuing the delivery of synchronized shocks.

If the polymorphic ventricular tachycardia persists and the patient is or becomes hemodynamically unstable and has a pulse:

◆ Administer an antiarrhythmic drug such as **amiodarone** or **lidocaine** as in Step 3 below while continuing the delivery of synchronized shocks.

If the polymorphic ventricular tachycardia persists and the patient becomes pulseless at any time:

◆ Continue with section B, *Monitored Cardiac Arrest* under *Ventricular Fibrillation/Pulseless Tachycardia,* p. 213.

3. If the polymorphic ventricular tachycardia is associated with an acute coronary syndrome:

◆ Treat the acute coronary syndrome, while correcting the myocardial ischemia, as far as possible.

AND

Administer a β-**blocker** if not contraindicated.

◆ Administer a 0.5-mg/kg bolus of **esmolol** IV over 1 minute, followed by an IV infusion of esmolol at 0.05 mg/kg/min and repeat the 0.5-mg/kg bolus of esmolol IV twice at 5-minute intervals while increasing the IV infusion of esmolol 0.05 mg/kg/min after each bolus of esmolol. After the third bolus of esmolol IV, increase the IV infusion of esmolol 0.05 mg/kg/min every 5 minutes to a maximum infusion of 0.30 mg/kg/min, if necessary, to suppress the polymorphic ventricular tachycardia, and then titrate the esmolol infusion to maintain the heart rate within normal limits.

OR

Administer 5 mg **atenolol** IV over 5 minutes and repeat in 10 minutes to a total dose of 10 mg, if needed.

OR

Administer 5 mg **metoprolol** IV over 2 to 5 minutes and repeat twice every 5 minutes to a total dose of 15 mg, if needed.

AND

Monitor the pulse, blood pressure, and ECG while administering the drug. Stop the administration of the β-blocker if the systolic blood pressure falls below 100 mm Hg.

OR

If the polymorphic ventricular tachycardia is or is not associated with an acute coronary syndrome, administer an antiarrhythmic drug such as **procainamide** if not contraindicated.

◆ Start an IV infusion of procainamide at a rate of 20 to 30 mg/min (up to 50 mg/min, if necessary).

AND

Continue the infusion of procainamide until:

◆ The polymorphic ventricular tachycardia is suppressed
◆ A total dose of 17 mg/kg of procainamide has been administered (1.2 g of procainamide for a 70-kg patient)
◆ Side effects from the procainamide appear (such as hypotension)
◆ The QRS complex widens by 50% of its original width, or
◆ The PR or QT interval lengthens by 50% of its original length

If procainamide is successful in suppressing the polymorphic ventricular tachycardia:

◆ Start a maintenance IV infusion of procainamide at a rate of 1 to 4 mg/min.

OR

Administer an antiarrhythmic drug such as **amiodarone.**

◆ Administer a loading dose of 150 mg of amiodarone IV over 10 minutes and repeat two to three times if necessary, allowing 10 to 15 minutes between infusions.

AND

Start an IV infusion of amiodarone at a rate of 1 mg per minute.

OR

Administer an antiarrhythmic drug such as **lidocaine.**

◆ Administer a 1.0- to 1.5-mg/kg bolus (75 to 100 mg) of lidocaine IV slowly, and repeat a 0.5- to 0.75-mg/kg bolus (25 to 50 mg) of lidocaine IV slowly every 5 to 10 minutes until the ventricular tachycardia is suppressed or a total dose of 3 mg/kg of lidocaine has been administered.

If lidocaine is successful in suppressing the ventricular tachycardia:

◆ Start a maintenance infusion of lidocaine (1 g of lidocaine in 500 mL of D_5W [2 mg/mL]) at a rate of 2 mg/min of lidocaine (1 mL/min of the diluted lidocaine solution) to prevent the recurrence of the ventricular tachycardia. If additional boluses of lidocaine were administered initially, increase the rate of the lidocaine infusion by 1-mg increments for each additional 1-mg/kg dose of lidocaine to a maximum rate of 4 mg/min.

If a β-blocker, procainamide, amiodarone, or lidocaine is unsuccessful in suppressing the polymorphic ventricular tachycardia and the patient remains stable, or if, at any time while administrating the β-blocker, procainamide, amiodarone, or lidocaine, the patient's condition becomes hemodynamically unstable and synchronized shocks were not delivered initially:

◆ Immediately deliver a synchronized shock (200 J), premedicating the patient first, if necessary, as above in Step 2.

AND

Repeat the synchronized shock as often as necessary at progressively increasing energy levels (200 to 300 J and 360 J).

If one of the shocks or a β-blocker, procainamide, amiodarone, or lidocaine is successful in terminating the polymorphic ventricular tachycardia:

4. Continue or start a maintenance IV infusion of the β-blocker, procainamide, amiodarone, or lidocaine as appropriate.

Patient hemodynamically unstable:

If the patient is conscious (or unconscious) and has a pulse, but with a hemodynamically unstable condition—that is, the patient is hypotensive (systolic blood pressure of less than 90 mm Hg) with ev-

idence of poor peripheral perfusion or has signs and symptoms of congestive heart failure or an acute coronary syndrome:

1. Administer high-concentration oxygen.

AND

Consider immediate DC cardioversion or administration of an antiarrhythmic drug while correcting any electrolyte imbalance.

2. Deliver a synchronized shock (200 J). If the patient is conscious, consider premedicating the patient before cardioversion as follows, using a sedative such as **midazolam** or **diazepam:**

◆ Administer 1 to 2 mg of midazolam IV slowly over at least 2 minutes and repeat every 3 to 5 minutes, titrated to produce sedation/amnesia before cardioversion.

OR

Administer 5 to 15 mg of diazepam with or without 2 to 5 mg **morphine** IV slowly to produce amnesia/analgesia before cardioversion.

Administration of a sedative should not delay cardioversion if it is indicated immediately by the patient's condition!

AND

Repeat the synchronized shock as often as necessary at progressively increasing energy levels (200 to 300 J and 360 J).

If ventricular tachycardia persists and the patient remains hemodynamically unstable and has a pulse:

◆ Administer an antiarrhythmic drug such as **amiodarone** or **lidocaine** as in Step 3 below while continuing the delivery of synchronized shocks.

If ventricular tachycardia persists and the patient becomes pulseless at any time:

◆ **Continue with section B,** *Monitored Cardiac Arrest* **under** *Ventricular Fibrillation/Pulseless Tachycardia,* p. 213.

3. Administer an antiarrhythmic drug such as **amiodarone.**

◆ Administer a loading dose of 150 mg of amiodarone IV over 10 minutes and repeat two to three times if necessary, allowing 10 to 15 minutes between infusions.

AND

Start an IV infusion of amiodarone at a rate of 1 mg/min.

OR

Administer an antiarrhythmic drug such as **lidocaine.**

◆ Administer a 1.0- to 1.5-mg/kg bolus (75 to 100 mg) of lidocaine IV slowly, and repeat a 0.5- to 0.75-mg/kg bolus (25 to 50 mg) of lidocaine IV slowly every 5 to 10 minutes until the ventricular tachycardia is suppressed or a total dose of 3 mg/kg of lidocaine has been administered.

If lidocaine is successful in suppressing the ventricular tachycardia:

◆ Start a maintenance infusion of lidocaine (1 g of lidocaine in 500 mL of D$_5$W [2 mg/mL]) at a rate of 2 mg/min (1 mL/min of the diluted lidocaine solution) to prevent the recurrence of the ventricular tachycardia. If additional boluses of lidocaine were administered initially, increase the rate of the lidocaine infusion by 1-mg increments for each additional 1-mg/kg dose of lidocaine to a maximum rate of 4 mg/min.

If amiodarone or lidocaine is unsuccessful in suppressing ventricular tachycardia and the patient remains hemodynamically unstable and synchronized shocks were not delivered initially:

◆ Immediately deliver a synchronized shock (200 J), premedicating the patient first, if necessary, as above in Step 2.

AND

Repeat the synchronized shock as often as necessary at progressively increasing energy levels (200 to 300 J and 360 J).

If one of the shocks or amiodarone or lidocaine is successful in terminating ventricular tachycardia:

4. Continue or start a maintenance IV infusion of amiodarone or lidocaine as appropriate.

Notes

_____

_____

_____

_____

_____

_____

Ventricular Tachycardia, Polymorphic (With Pulse)
Prolonged Baseline QT Interval
Torsade de Pointes (TdP) (With Pulse)

◆ TREATMENT

Patient hemodynamically stable or unstable:

1. Administer high-concentration oxygen.
2. If magnesium deficiency is present or suspected, and the patient is not hypotensive:

◆ Administer a dose of 1 to 2 g (8 to 16 mEq) of **magnesium sulfate,** diluted with 50 to 100 mL of D$_5$W, IV over 5 to 60 minutes.

AND

Follow with a maintenance IV infusion of 0.5 to 1.0 g (4 to 8 mEq) of magnesium sulfate, diluted with 100 mL of D$_5$W, IV to run for 1 hour.

3. Initiate transcutaneous overdrive pacing, if appropriate rate-wise. If the patient is unable to tolerate transcutaneous pacing and is conscious and not hypotensive, administer a sedative such as **midazolam** or **diazepam** as follows:

◆ Administer 1 to 2 mg of midazolam IV slowly over at least 2 minutes and repeat every 3 to 5 minutes, titrated to produce sedation/amnesia.

OR

Administer 5 to 15 mg of diazepam with or without 2 to 5 mg **morphine** IV slowly to produce amnesia/analgesia.

AND

Consider the administration of a β-**blocker** if not contraindicated and hypotension not present.

◆ Administer a 0.5-mg/kg bolus of **esmolol** IV over 1 minute, followed by an IV infusion of esmolol at 0.05 mg/kg/min and repeat the 0.5-mg/kg bolus of esmolol IV twice at 5-minute intervals while increasing the IV infusion of esmolol 0.05 mg/kg/min after each bolus of esmolol. After the third bolus of esmolol IV, increase the IV infusion of esmolol 0.05 mg/kg/min every 5 minutes to a maximum infusion of 0.30 mg/kg/min, if necessary, to suppress the ventricular tachycardia, and then titrate the esmolol infusion to maintain the heart rate within normal limits.

OR

Administer 5 mg **atenolol** IV over 5 minutes and repeat in 10 minutes to a total dose of 10 mg, if needed.

OR

Administer 5 mg **metoprolol** IV over 2 to 5 minutes and repeat twice every 5 minutes to a total dose of 15 mg, if needed.

AND

Monitor the pulse, blood pressure, and ECG while administering the drug. Stop the administration of the β-blocker if the systolic blood pressure falls below 100 mm Hg.

4. Withhold administration of such antiarrhythmic agents as amiodarone, disopyramide, procainamide, quinidine, and sotalol or other agents that prolong the QT interval, such as phenothiazines and tricyclic antidepressants.

AND

Correct any electrolyte imbalance.

If polymorphic ventricular tachycardia or torsade de pointes persists and the patient is or becomes unstable:

5. Deliver an unsynchronized shock (200 J). If the patient is conscious and has not been previously sedated, consider premedicating the patient before

cardioversion as follows, using a sedative such as **midazolam** or **diazepam:**

◆ Administer 1 to 2 mg of midazolam IV slowly over at least 2 minutes and repeat every 3 to 5 minutes, titrated to produce sedation/amnesia before cardioversion.

OR

Administer 5 to 15 mg of diazepam with or without 2 to 5 mg **morphine** IV slowly to produce amnesia/analgesia before cardioversion.

Administration of a sedative should not delay cardioversion if it is indicated immediately by the patient's condition!

AND

Repeat the unsynchronized shock as often as necessary at progressively increasing energy levels (200 to 300 J and 360 J).

If polymorphic ventricular tachycardia or torsade de pointes degenerates into ventricular fibrillation at any time:

6. Continue with section B, *Monitored Cardiac Arrest* under *Ventricular Fibrillation/Pulseless Ventricular Tachycardia*, p. 213.

Notes

_____

_____

_____

_____

_____

_____

_____

PREMATURE ECTOPIC BEATS

Premature Atrial Contractions

Clinical Significance

Single, isolated premature atrial contractions (PACs) are not significant. Frequent PACs may indicate the presence of enhanced atrial automaticity, an atrial reentry mechanism, or both, and herald impending atrial arrhythmias (such as atrial tachycardia, atrial flutter, and atrial fibrillation) and PSVT.

Indications for Treatment

Treatment may be indicated if the premature atrial contractions are frequent (8 to 10 per minute), occur in groups of two or more, or alternate with the QRS complexes of the underlying rhythm (bigeminy).

◆ **TREATMENT**

If stimulants (such as caffeine, tobacco, or alcohol) or excessive amounts of sympathomimetic drugs (such as epinephrine or dopamine) have been administered:

1. Discontinue the stimulants and sympathomimetic drugs.

If digitalis toxicity is suspected:

2. Withhold digitalis.

Notes

_____

_____

_____

_____

_____

_____

Premature Junctional Contractions

Clinical Significance

Single, isolated premature junctional contractions (PJCs) are not significant. Frequent PJCs may indicate the presence of enhanced AV junctional automaticity, an AV junctional reentry mechanism, or both, and herald an impending junctional tachycardia.

Indications for Treatment

Treatment is indicated if the premature junctional contractions are frequent (4 to 6 per minute), occur in groups of two or more, or alternate with the QRS complexes of the underlying rhythm (bigeminy).

◆ **TREATMENT**

If stimulants (such as caffeine, tobacco, or alcohol) or excessive amounts of sympathomimetic drugs (such as epinephrine or dopamine) have been administered:

1. Discontinue the stimulants and sympathomimetic drugs.

If digitalis toxicity is suspected:

2. Withhold digitalis.

Notes

_____

_____

_____

Premature Ventricular Contractions

Clinical Significance

Single PVCs, especially in patients who have no heart disease, are generally not significant. In patients with an acute MI or an ischemic episode, PVCs may indicate the presence of enhanced ventricular automaticity, a ventricular reentry mechanism, or both, and herald the appearance of life-threatening arrhythmias, such as ventricular tachycardia or fibrillation. Although these lethal arrhythmias may occur without warning, they are often initiated by PVCs, especially if the PVCs:

◆ Are frequent (six or more per minute)
◆ Occur in groups of two or more (group beats)
◆ Have different QRS configurations (multiform)
◆ Arise from different ventricular ectopic pacemakers (multifocal)
◆ Are close coupled, or
◆ Fall on the T wave (R-on-T phenomenon)

Indications for Treatment

Treatment should be considered for PVCs in patients in whom an acute MI or ischemic episode is suspected, except for those that occur in conjunction with bradycardias. In such circumstances, first treat the underlying bradycardia. Refer to the appropriate bradycardia treatment. If feasible, identify and correct the following underlying causes of PVCs:

◆ Low serum potassium (hypokalemia)
◆ Low serum magnesium (hypomagnesemia)
◆ Digitalis toxicity
◆ Excessive administration of sympathomimetic drugs (e.g., epinephrine and dopamine)
◆ Hypoxia
◆ Acidosis
◆ Acute coronary syndrome
◆ Congestive heart failure

◆ TREATMENT

If the PVCs are associated with an acute coronary syndrome:

1. Treat the acute coronary syndrome, while correcting the myocardial ischemia, as far as possible.

AND

Consider the administration of a β-**blocker** or **lidocaine**.

If the PVCs are or are not associated with an acute coronary syndrome:

2. Consider the administration of an antiarrhythmic drug such as **procainamide, amiodarone,** or **lidocaine**.

Notes

_____

_____

_____

_____

_____

_____

PART II

CARDIAC ARREST

Ventricular Fibrillation/Pulseless Ventricular Tachycardia

Clinical Significance

Ventricular fibrillation is a life-threatening arrhythmia resulting in chaotic beating of the heart and the immediate end of organized ventricular contractions, cardiac output, and pulse.

Pulseless ventricular tachycardia, like ventricular fibrillation, becomes a life-threatening arrhythmia when the ventricular contractions are unable to maintain an adequate cardiac output and a pulse.

At the moment ventricular fibrillation or pulseless ventricular tachycardia occurs and cardiac output stops, clinical death is present. Biological death occurs within 10 minutes unless cardiopulmonary resuscitation (CPR), unsynchronized shocks, or both are administered within minutes.

Indications for Treatment

Treatment of ventricular fibrillation and pulseless ventricular tachycardia is indicated immediately.

◆ TREATMENT

A. Unmonitored Cardiac Arrest

If the cardiac arrest is witnessed by the resuscitation team, or if cardiac arrest occurred before the arrival of the team and the patient is not being monitored, the following procedures should be performed:

Rescuer One:
1. Assess the patient's responsiveness.
2. Check the patient's ABCs.
3. Perform CPR until the defibrillator paddles or defibrillation pads are applied.

Rescuer Two:
1. Apply the defibrillator paddles or defibrillation pads.
2. Determine the ECG rhythm on the ECG monitor.
3. Verify cardiac arrest by checking the patient's pulse.

If ventricular fibrillation/pulseless ventricular tachycardia is present:
4. Deliver an unsynchronized shock (200 J) immediately, and check the patient's ECG rhythm on the ECG monitor.

AND

If ventricular fibrillation/pulseless ventricular tachycardia persists:
◆ Deliver a second unsynchronized shock (200 to 300 J) immediately, and check the patient's ECG rhythm on the ECG monitor.

AND

If ventricular fibrillation/pulseless ventricular tachycardia persists:
◆ Deliver a third unsynchronized shock (360 J) immediately, and check the patient's ECG rhythm on the ECG monitor and the patient's pulse.

If ventricular fibrillation/pulseless ventricular tachycardia persists:
5. Resume CPR.
6. Intubate the patient.
7. Ventilate with high-concentration oxygen.
8. Establish an IV line and attach ECG electrodes to the patient.
9. Administer 1 mg of **epinephrine** (10 mL of a 1:10,000 solution of epinephrine) IV followed by a 20-mL flush of IV fluid; repeat every 3 to 5 minutes during resuscitation.
   NOTE: If an IV line cannot be established, administer 2.0 to 2.5 mg of epinephrine diluted with 10 mL of normal saline via the tracheal tube, if one is in place, followed by three to four forceful ventilations.
   ◆ Continue CPR for 30 to 60 seconds to circulate the drug.
   ◆ Deliver an unsynchronized shock (360 J), and check the patient's ECG rhythm and pulse; repeat after each administration of epinephrine.

OR

Administer a single dose of 40 U of **vasopressin** IV followed by a 20-mL flush of IV fluid.

◆ Continue CPR for 30 to 60 seconds to circulate the drug.
◆ Deliver an unsynchronized shock (360 J), and check the patient's ECG rhythm and pulse.

If ventricular fibrillation/pulseless ventricular tachycardia persists, resume CPR and:
◆ Deliver an unsynchronized shock (360 J) every 3 to 5 minutes.

If ventricular fibrillation/pulseless ventricular tachycardia persists for 5 to 10 minutes after the dose of vasopressin:
◆ Consider the administration of 1 mg of **epinephrine** (10 mL of a 1:10,000 solution of epinephrine) IV followed by a 20-mL flush of IV fluid; repeat every 3 to 5 minutes during resuscitation.
◆ Continue CPR for 30 to 60 seconds to circulate the drug.
◆ Deliver an unsynchronized shock (360 J), and check the patient's ECG rhythm and pulse; repeat after each administration of epinephrine.

If ventricular fibrillation/pulseless ventricular tachycardia persists:
10. Consider the administration of **amiodarone.**
   ◆ Administer a dose of 300 mg of amiodarone IV rapidly followed by a 20-mL flush of IV fluid and, if necessary, administer one or two supplemental doses of 150 mg of amiodarone, each followed by a 20-mL flush of IV fluid.
   ◆ Continue CPR for 30 to 60 seconds after each administration to circulate the drug.
   ◆ Deliver an unsynchronized shock (360 J) and check the patient's ECG rhythm and pulse; repeat every 3 to 5 minutes after administration of amiodarone.

If pulseless torsade de pointes is present or hypomagnesemia suspected:
11. Consider the administration of **magnesium sulfate.**
   ◆ Administer a dose of 1 to 2 g (8 to 16 mEq) of magnesium sulfate diluted with 100 mL D_5W, IV over 1 to 2 minutes followed by a 20-mL flush of IV fluid.
   ◆ Continue CPR for 30 to 60 seconds to circulate the drug.
   ◆ Deliver an unsynchronized shock (360 J) and check the patient's ECG rhythm and pulse.

If preexisting hyperkalemia or metabolic acidosis is present:

12. Consider the administration of **sodium bicarbonate.**
    ◆ Administer a 1-mEq/kg bolus of sodium bicarbonate IV, and repeat 0.5-mEq/kg boluses of sodium bicarbonate IV every 10 minutes as needed, based on blood gas analyses.
    ◆ Continue CPR for 30 to 60 seconds after each bolus to circulate the drug.
    ◆ Deliver an unsynchronized shock (360 J), and check the patient's ECG rhythm and pulse; repeat after each administration of sodium bicarbonate.

Notes

_____

_____

_____

_____

B. Monitored Cardiac Arrest

If the patient is being monitored and ventricular fibrillation/pulseless ventricular tachycardia occurs:

1. Verify cardiac arrest by checking the patient's pulse while checking the patient's ECG rhythm on the ECG monitor.

If ventricular fibrillation/pulseless ventricular tachycardia is present:

2. Apply the defibrillator paddles or defibrillation pads to the patient.

AND

Deliver an unsynchronized shock (200 J) immediately, and check the patient's ECG rhythm on the ECG monitor.

AND

If ventricular fibrillation/pulseless ventricular tachycardia persists:

Deliver a second unsynchronized shock (200 to 300 J) immediately after the first shock, and check the patient's ECG rhythm on the ECG monitor.

AND

If ventricular fibrillation/pulseless ventricular tachycardia persists:

Deliver a third unsynchronized shock (360 J) immediately after the second shock, and check the patient's ECG rhythm on the ECG monitor and the patient's pulse.

If ventricular fibrillation/pulseless ventricular tachycardia persists:

3. Perform CPR.
4. Continue with Step 6 in section A, _Unmonitored Cardiac Arrest_ under _Ventricular Fibrillation/ Pulseless Ventricular Tachycardia,_ p. 212.

Notes

_____

_____

_____

_____

_____

_____

Postventricular Fibrillation/Pulseless Ventricular Tachycardia Termination

If ventricular fibrillation/pulseless ventricular tachycardia is terminated:

1. Perform CPR until the patient's pulse is palpable and the systolic blood pressure is 90 to 100 mm Hg or greater.

If a symptomatic postdefibrillation bradycardia or tachycardia is present:

2. Refer to the appropriate symptomatic bradycardia or tachycardia treatment protocol to revert the heart rate to normal.

If hypotension is present (systolic blood pressure less than 90 mm Hg) in the absence of pulmonary edema:

3. Consider the administration of fluid boluses of 250 to 500 mL of **normal saline** while monitoring the pulse and blood pressure and auscultating the lungs for pulmonary edema. Repeat the fluid boluses if a hemodynamic response is observed.

If hypotension persists and signs and symptoms of shock are present:

Systolic blood pressure less than 70 mm Hg:
◆ Start an IV infusion of **norepinephrine** at an initial rate of 0.5 to 1.0 μg/min, and adjust the rate of infusion up to 8 to 30 μg/min to increase the systolic blood pressure to 70 to 100 mm Hg.

NOTE: The infusion of norepinephrine may be replaced by an infusion of dopamine at this point.

OR

Systolic blood pressure 70 to 100 mm Hg:
◆ Start an IV infusion of **dopamine** at an initial rate of 2.5 to 5.0 μg/kg/min, and adjust the rate of infusion up to 20 μg/kg/min to increase the systolic blood pressure to 90 to 100 mm Hg or greater.

If hypotension is present (systolic blood pressure less than 90 mm Hg) in the presence of pulmonary edema and signs and symptoms of shock are absent:

4. Administer an IV infusion of **dobutamine** at an initial rate of 2 μg/kg/min, and adjust the rate of infusion up to 20 μg/kg/min to increase the systolic blood pressure to over 100 mm Hg.

If severe pulmonary edema is present and the patient is not hypotensive (systolic blood pressure greater than 90 mm Hg):

5. Place the patient in a semireclining or full upright position, with the legs dependent if possible.

AND

Administer 0.4 mg **nitroglycerin** by sublingual tablet or lingual aerosol and repeat every 5 to 10 minutes as needed, or by dermal application of 1 to 1.5 inches of nitroglycerin ointment.

AND/OR

Administer 1 to 3 mg of **morphine** IV slowly.

AND

Administer a dose of 40 to 80 mg (0.5 to 1.0 mg/kg) of **furosemide** IV slowly over 4 to 5 minutes.

If ventricular fibrillation/pulseless ventricular tachycardia recurs:

6. Deliver an unsynchronized shock immediately at the energy level at which termination of ventricular fibrillation/pulseless ventricular tachycardia was previously effective, and check the patient's ECG rhythm and pulse.

If ventricular fibrillation/pulseless ventricular tachycardia persists:

7. Consider the administration of a supplementary dose of **amiodarone,** if appropriate:

◆ Administer a dose of 150 to 300 mg of amiodarone IV rapidly followed by a 20-mL flush of IV fluid and, if necessary, administer one or two supplemental doses of 150 mg of amiodarone, each followed by a 20-mL flush of IV fluid.

◆ Continue CPR for 30 to 60 seconds after each administration to circulate the drug.

◆ Deliver an unsynchronized shock (360 J) and check the patient's ECG rhythm and pulse; repeat every 3 to 5 minutes after administration of amiodarone.

Notes

_____
_____
_____
_____
_____
_____
_____
_____
_____
_____
_____

Ventricular Asystole

Clinical Significance

Ventricular asystole is a life-threatening arrhythmia resulting in the absence of ventricular contractions, cardiac output, and a pulse. At the moment ventricular asystole occurs in a person with an adequate circulation, cardiac output stops and clinical death occurs. Biological death follows within 10 minutes unless ventricular asystole is reversed.

Indications for Treatment

Treatment of ventricular asystole is indicated immediately.

◆ TREATMENT

A. Unmonitored Cardiac Arrest

If the cardiac arrest is witnessed by the resuscitation team, or if cardiac arrest occurred before the arrival of the team and the patient's ECG is not being monitored, the following procedures should be performed:

Rescuer One:

1. Assess the patient's responsiveness.
2. Check the patient's ABCs.
3. Perform CPR until the defibrillator paddles or defibrillation pads are applied.

Rescuer Two:

1. Apply the defibrillator paddles or defibrillation pads and, if necessary, ECG leads to the patient.
2. Determine the ECG rhythm on the ECG monitor.
3. Verify cardiac arrest by checking the patient's pulse.

If ventricular asystole is present, confirm ventricular asystole in two ECG leads if possible, or by using the defibrillator monitor and repositioning the defibrillator paddles 90°, because fine ventricular fibrillation may mimic ventricular asystole.

---

4. Consider the treatment protocol for section A, *Unmonitored Cardiac Arrest* under *Ventricular Fibrillation/Pulseless Ventricular Tachycardia* (p. 211) and deliver three unsynchronized shocks **only** if ventricular asystole cannot be definitely confirmed.
5. Consider immediate TCP if the cardiac arrest was witnessed and of short duration.
6. Continue CPR.
7. Intubate the patient.
8. Ventilate with high-concentration oxygen.

9. Establish an IV line and attach ECG electrodes to the patient if not already done so.

10. Administer 1 mg of **epinephrine** (10 mL of a 1:10,000 solution of epinephrine) IV followed by a 20-mL flush of IV fluid, and repeat every 3 to 5 minutes during resuscitation.

    NOTE: If an IV line cannot be established, administer 2.0 to 2.5 mg of epinephrine diluted with 10 mL of normal saline via the tracheal tube, if one is in place, followed by three to four forceful ventilations.

    ◆ After each dose of epinephrine continue CPR for 30 to 60 seconds to circulate the drug, and then check the patient's ECG rhythm and pulse.

    If ventricular asystole persists:

11. Administer a 1-mg bolus of **atropine** IV rapidly followed by a 20-mL flush of IV fluid. Repeat every 3 to 5 minutes up to a total dose of 3 mg (0.04 mg/kg) of atropine.

    ◆ After each dose of atropine, continue CPR for 30 to 60 seconds to circulate the drug and then check the patient's ECG rhythm and pulse.

    If preexisting hyperkalemia, metabolic acidosis, or tricyclic antidepressant overdose is present:

12. Administer a 1-mEq/kg bolus of **sodium bicarbonate** and repeat 0.5-mEq/kg boluses of sodium bicarbonate IV every 10 minutes as needed, based on blood gas analyses.

    ◆ After each dose of sodium bicarbonate, continue CPR for 30 to 60 seconds to circulate the alkalization agent and then check the patient's ECG rhythm and pulse.

    If ventricular asystole persists:

13. Continue administration of epinephrine and atropine and CPR until ventricular asystole is terminated or a physician orders an end to the resuscitative efforts.

Notes

_____

_____

_____

_____

_____

_____

_____

_____

_____

_____

B. Monitored Cardiac Arrest

If the patient's ECG is being monitored and ventricular asystole occurs:

1. Verify cardiac arrest by checking the patient's pulse while checking the patient's ECG rhythm on the ECG monitor.

_____

If ventricular asystole is present, confirm ventricular asystole in two ECG leads if possible, or by using the defibrillator monitor and repositioning the defibrillator paddles 90°, because fine ventricular fibrillation may mimic ventricular asystole.

_____

2. Consider the treatment protocol for section A, *Unmonitored Cardiac Arrest* under *Ventricular Fibrillation/Pulseless Ventricular Tachycardia* (p. 211), and deliver three unsynchronized shocks if ventricular asystole cannot be definitely confirmed.
3. Consider immediate TCP.
4. Perform CPR.
5. Continue with Step 7 in section A, *Unmonitored Cardiac Arrest* under *Ventricular Asystole* (p. 212).

Notes

_____

_____

_____

_____

_____

_____

Pulseless Electrical Activity

Clinical Significance

Pulseless electrical activity—the absence of a detectable pulse and blood pressure in the presence of electrical activity of the heart as evidenced by some type of an ECG rhythm other than ventricular fibrillation or ventricular tachycardia—is a life-threatening condition. At the moment pulseless electrical activity occurs in a person with an adequate circulation, cardiac output ceases and clinical death occurs. Biological death follows within 10 minutes unless pulseless electrical activity is reversed.

Pulseless electrical activity is commonly the result of either:

◆ Complete absence of ventricular contractions (electromechanical dissociation [EMD]).

OR

A marked decrease in cardiac output because of (a) hypovolemia, (b) obstruction to blood flow, or (c) dysfunction of the myocardium or electrical conduction system or both from a variety of causes, resulting in ventricular contractions too weak to produce a detectable pulse and blood pressure (pseudoelectromechanical dissociation).

The ECG rhythms encountered in pulseless electrical activity include:

◆ Organized electrical activity with narrow QRS complexes as typically seen with EMD.
◆ Wide-QRS-complex arrhythmias, such as idioventricular rhythms and ventricular escape rhythms, which are more commonly seen in pseudoelectromechanical dissociation.
◆ Marked bradyarrhythmias.

Pulseless electrical activity can occur in the following conditions:

◆ Hypovolemia from acute blood loss (hemorrhagic shock secondary to trauma or other causes, such as ruptured abdominal aortic aneurysm or gastrointestinal hemorrhage) or from anaphylaxis-related vasodilation
◆ Obstruction of blood flow to or from the heart (tension pneumothorax or severe pulmonary embolization)
◆ Cardiac tamponade
◆ Cardiac rupture
◆ Massive acute MI
◆ Following cardiac defibrillation (postdefibrillation idioventricular rhythms)
◆ Hypoxemia
◆ Severe acidosis
◆ Excessive vagal tone or loss of sympathetic tone
◆ Digitalis toxicity
◆ Hyperkalemia
◆ Drug overdose from tricyclic antidepressants, β-blockers, and calcium channel blockers
◆ Hypothermia

Whenever CPR is unsuccessful in producing a palpable peripheral or carotid pulse or other evidence of perfusion, pulseless electrical activity must be suspected.

Indications for Treatment

Treatment of pulseless electrical activity is indicated immediately.

◆ TREATMENT

A. Unmonitored Cardiac Arrest

If the cardiac arrest is witnessed by the resuscitation team or if cardiac arrest occurred before the arrival of the team and the patient's ECG is not being monitored, the following procedures should be performed:

Rescuer One:
1. Assess the patient's responsiveness.
2. Check the patient's ABCs.
3. Perform CPR until the defibrillator paddles or defibrillation pads are applied.

Rescuer Two:
1. Apply the defibrillator paddles or defibrillation pads and, if necessary, ECG leads to the patient.
2. Determine the ECG rhythm on the ECG monitor.
3. Verify cardiac arrest by checking the patient's pulse.

If pulseless electrical activity is present:
4. Continue CPR.
5. Intubate the patient.
6. Ventilate with high-concentration oxygen.
7. Attempt to determine the cause of pulseless electrical activity and treat it, if possible:
◆ Hypoxemia
◆ Tension pneumothorax
◆ Loss of sympathetic tone or excessive vagal tone
◆ Hypovolemia
◆ Severe acidosis
◆ Hyperkalemia
◆ Drug overdose from tricyclic antidepressants, β-blockers, and calcium channel blockers
◆ Digitalis toxicity
◆ Hypothermia
◆ Severe pulmonary embolization
◆ Cardiac tamponade
◆ Myocardial rupture
8. If tension pneumothorax is suspected, perform needle decompression of the thorax immediately.
9. Establish an IV line.

If pulseless electrical activity persists:
10. Administer 1 mg of **epinephrine** (10 mL of a 1:10,000 solution of epinephrine) IV followed by a 20-mL flush of IV fluid, and repeat every 3 to 5 minutes during resuscitation.

NOTE: If an IV line cannot be established, administer 2.0 to 2.5 mg of epinephrine diluted with 10 mL of normal saline via the tracheal tube, if one is in place, followed by three to four forceful ventilations.
◆ After each dose of epinephrine, continue CPR for 30 to 60 seconds to circulate the drug, and then check the patient's ECG rhythm and pulse.

If pulseless electrical activity persists and the rate of the QRS complexes is about 80 per minute or less:
11. Administer a 1-mg bolus of **atropine** IV rapidly followed by a 20-mL flush of IV fluid. Repeat every 3 to 5 minutes up to a total dose of 3 mg (0.04 mg/kg) of atropine.
◆ After each dose of atropine, continue CPR for 30 to 60 seconds to circulate the drug, and then check the patient's ECG rhythm and pulse.

If pulseless electrical activity persists and hypovolemia is suspected:

12. Consider the administration of fluid boluses of 250 to 500 mL of **normal saline** while monitoring the patient's ECG rhythm and pulse. Repeat the fluid boluses, especially if a hemodynamic response is observed.
    ◆ Continue CPR.

If preexisting hyperkalemia, metabolic acidosis, or tricyclic antidepressant overdose is present:

13. Administer a 1-mEq/kg bolus of **sodium bicarbonate,** and repeat 0.5-mEq/kg boluses of sodium bicarbonate IV every 10 minutes as needed, based on blood gas analyses.
    ◆ After each dose of sodium bicarbonate, continue CPR for 30 to 60 seconds to circulate the alkalization agent, and then check the patient's ECG rhythm and pulse.

Notes

_____

_____

_____

_____

_____

_____

_____

_____

_____

_____

_____

_____

_____

B. Monitored Cardiac Arrest

If the patient's ECG is being monitored and pulseless electrical activity occurs:

1. Verify cardiac arrest by checking the patient's pulse while checking the patient's ECG rhythm on the ECG monitor.

If pulseless electrical activity is present:

2. Consider immediate TCP.
3. Perform CPR.
4. Continue with Step 5 in section A, *Unmonitored Cardiac Arrest* under *Pulseless Electrical Activity,* p. 212.

Notes

_____

_____

_____

_____

_____

_____

_____

_____

_____

SUMMARY OF ARRHYTHMIA TREATMENT

PART I

Bradycardias

Sinus Bradycardia
Sinus Arrest/Sinoatrial (SA) Exit Block
Second-Degree, Type I AV Block (Wenckebach)
Second-Degree, 2:1 and Advanced AV Block With Narrow QRS Complexes
Third-Degree AV Block With Narrow QRS Complexes

Symptomatic bradycardia:
1. Oxygen
2. Atropine sulfate
   AND/OR
   Transcutaneous pacing
3. Dopamine hydrochloride or epinephrine
4. Transvenous pacemaker

Junctional Escape Rhythm
Ventricular Escape Rhythm
Second-Degree, Type II AV Block
Second-Degree, 2:1 and Advanced AV Block With Wide QRS Complexes
Third-Degree AV Block With Wide QRS Complexes

Symptomatic bradycardia:
1. Oxygen
2. Transcutaneous pacing
3. Dopamine hydrochloride or epinephrine
4. Transvenous pacemaker

Tachycardias

Sinus Tachycardia
Atrial Tachycardia With Block

1. No specific treatment
2. Treat underlying cause
3. Discontinue any responsible drugs

Narrow-QRS-Complex Tachycardia of Unknown Origin (With Pulse)

Patient hemodynamically stable:
1. Oxygen
2. Vagal maneuvers
3. Adenosine
4. Determine if arrhythmia is:
   ◆ Paroxysmal supraventricular tachycardia (PSVT)
   ◆ Atrial tachycardia without block
   ◆ Junctional tachycardia

Atrial Tachycardia Without Block

Patient hemodynamically stable:
1. Oxygen
2. Diltiazem, β-blocker (esmolol, atenolol, or metoprolol), or amiodarone

Patient hemodynamically unstable:
1. Oxygen
2. Amiodarone or diltiazem

Paroxysmal Supraventricular Tachycardia (PSVT) With Narrow QRS Complexes

Patient hemodynamically stable:
1. Oxygen
2. Vagal maneuvers
3. Adenosine, diltiazem, or β-blocker (esmolol, atenolol, or metoprolol)
4. Digoxin
5. DC cardioversion

Patient hemodynamically unstable:
1. Oxygen
2. Vagal maneuvers
3. Digoxin
4. Amiodarone or diltiazem

Junctional Tachycardia

Patient hemodynamically stable:
1. Oxygen
2. Amiodarone or β-blocker (esmolol, atenolol, or metoprolol)

Patient hemodynamically unstable:
1. Oxygen
2. Amiodarone

Atrial Flutter/Atrial Fibrillation (Without Wolff-Parkinson-White Syndrome or Ventricular Preexcitation)

Treatment to Control the Heart Rate
Patient hemodynamically stable:
1. Oxygen
2. β-blocker (esmolol, atenolol, or metoprolol) or diltiazem
3. Digoxin

Patient hemodynamically unstable:
1. Oxygen
2. Digoxin
3. Diltiazem or, if duration of atrial fibrillation <48 hr, amiodarone

Treatment to Convert the Rhythm
Atrial Fibrillation <48 Hours and Atrial Flutter of Any Duration
Patient hemodynamically stable:
1. Oxygen
2. Ibutilide, amiodarone, or procainamide
3. DC cardioversion

Patient hemodynamically unstable:
1. Oxygen
2. DC cardioversion
   OR
3. Amiodarone

Atrial Fibrillation >48 Hours or of Unknown Duration

Patient hemodynamically stable:
1. Oxygen
2. β-blocker (esmolol, atenolol, or metoprolol) or diltiazem
3. Digoxin
4. Delay DC cardioversion until the patient is anticoagulated and atrial thrombi are excluded

Patient hemodynamically unstable:
1. Oxygen
2. Diltiazem
3. Digoxin
4. Delay DC cardioversion until the patient is anticoagulated and atrial thrombi are excluded

---

Atrial Flutter/Atrial Fibrillation (With Wolff-Parkinson-White Syndrome or Ventricular Preexcitation)

Treatment to Control the Heart Rate and/or Convert the Rhythm

Atrial Fibrillation <48 Hours and Atrial Flutter of Any Duration

Patient hemodynamically stable:
1. Oxygen
2. Amiodarone or procainamide
3. DC cardioversion

Patient hemodynamically unstable:
1. Oxygen
2. DC cardioversion
   OR
3. Amiodarone

Atrial Fibrillation >48 Hours or of Unknown Duration

Patient hemodynamically stable or unstable:
1. Oxygen
2. Amiodarone, with extreme caution
3. Delay DC cardioversion until patient is anticoagulated and atrial thrombi are excluded

Wide-QRS-Complex Tachycardia of Unknown Origin (With Pulse)

Patient hemodynamically stable:
1. Oxygen
2. DC cardioversion
   OR
3. Procainamide or amiodarone

Patient hemodynamically unstable:
1. Oxygen
2. DC cardioversion
   OR
3. Amiodarone

Ventricular Tachycardia (VT), Monomorphic (With Pulse)

Patient hemodynamically stable:
1. Oxygen
2. DC cardioversion
   OR
3. Procainamide, amiodarone, or lidocaine

Patient hemodynamically unstable:
1. Oxygen
2. DC cardioversion
   OR
3. Amiodarone or lidocaine

Ventricular Tachycardia (VT), Polymorphic (With Pulse)—Normal Baseline QT Interval

Patient hemodynamically stable:
1. Oxygen
2. Correct any electrolyte imbalance
3. DC cardioversion
   OR
4. β-blocker (esmolol, atenolol, or metoprolol) (if ventricular tachycardia is associated with an acute coronary syndrome)
   OR
   Procainamide, amiodarone, or lidocaine

Patient hemodynamically unstable:
1. Oxygen
2. Correct any electrolyte imbalance
3. DC cardioversion
   OR
4. Amiodarone or lidocaine

Ventricular Tachycardia (VT), Polymorphic (With Pulse)—Prolonged Baseline QT Interval
Torsade de Pointes (TdP) (With Pulse)

Patient hemodynamically stable or unstable:
1. Oxygen
2. Correct any electrolyte imbalance
3. Magnesium sulfate
4. Transcutaneous overdrive pacing
                    AND
   β-blocker (esmolol, atenolol, or metoprolol)
5. Unsynchronized DC cardioversion

Premature Ectopic Beats

Premature Atrial Contractions (PACs)
Premature Junctional Contractions (PJCs)

1. Discontinue any stimulants and sympathomimetic drugs.
2. Withhold digitalis (if digitalis toxicity is suspected)

Premature Ventricular Contractions (PVCs)

1. Oxygen
2. Consider one of the following:
   ◆ β-blocker (esmolol, atenolol, or metoprolol) (if PVCs are associated with an acute coronary syndrome)
   ◆ Procainamide
   ◆ Amiodarone
   ◆ Lidocaine

PART II

Cardiac Arrest

Ventricular Asystole

Unmonitored/monitored cardiac arrest:
1. ABCs, CPR, oxygen
2. Consider transcutaneous pacing
3. Epinephrine
4. Atropine
5. Sodium bicarbonate (if hyperkalemia, metabolic acidosis, tricyclic antidepressant overdose, etc. is present)

Ventricular Fibrillation/Pulseless Ventricular Tachycardia (VF/VT)

Unmonitored/monitored cardiac arrest:
1. ABCs, CPR, oxygen
2. Defibrillation
3. Epinephrine or vasopressin
4. Amiodarone
5. Magnesium sulfate (if torsade de pointes is present and/or hypomagnesemia suspected)
6. Sodium bicarbonate (if hyperkalemia and/or metabolic acidosis are present)

Postventricular fibrillation/ventricular tachycardia termination:
1. Fluid boluses and norepinephrine or dopamine (if hypotension and/or shock are present)
                    OR
   Dobutamine (if hypotension and pulmonary edema are present)
2. Nitroglycerin, morphine, and furosemide (if pulmonary edema is present)
3. Defibrillation and amiodarone (if VF/VT recurs)

Pulseless Electrical Activity

Unmonitored/monitored cardiac arrest:
1. ABCs, CPR, oxygen
2. Consider transcutaneous pacing
3. Epinephrine
4. Atropine
5. Fluid boluses (if hypovolemia is suspected)
6. Sodium bicarbonate (if hyperkalemia, metabolic acidosis, tricyclic antidepressant overdose, etc. is present)
7. Treat underlying cause, if known

Drugs Used to Treat Arrhythmias

Drug	Class
Adenosine (Adenocard)	Antiarrhythmic agent
Amiodarone (Cordarone)	Antiarrhythmic agent
Atropine sulfate	Anticholinergic agent
β-blocker	β-adrenergic blocking agent
Atenolol (Tenormin), Esmolol HCL (Brevibloc), Metoprolol (Toprol, Lopressor)	
Diazepam (Valium)	Tranquilizer, amnesiac, sedative
Digoxin (Lanoxin)	Antiarrhythmic agent, inotropic agent, digitalis glycoside
Diltiazem (Cardizem)	Calcium channel blocker
Dobutamine (Dobutrex)	Adrenergic agent
Dopamine (Intropin)	Adrenergic (sympathomimetic) agent
Epinephrine (Adrenalin chloride)	Adrenergic (sympathomimetic) agent
Furosemide (Lasix)	Diuretic
Ibutilide (Corvert)	Antiarrhythmic agent
Lidocaine (Xylocaine)	Antiarrhythmic agent
Magnesium sulfate	Electrolyte
Midazolam (Versed)	Sedative, tranquilizer, amnesiac
Morphine sulfate	Narcotic, analgesic
Nitroglycerin (Nitrostat, Nitrol, Tridil, etc.)	Antianginal agent, vasodilator
Norepinephrine (Levophed)	Adrenergic (sympathomimetic) agent
Procainamide (Pronestyl)	Antiarrhythmic agent
Sodium bicarbonate	Alkalinizing agent
Vasopressin	Vasoconstrictor

ARRHYTHMIA TREATMENT ALGORITHMS

Part I

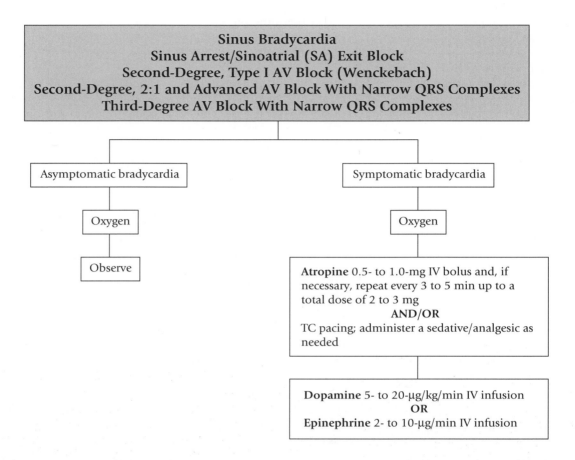

Sinus Bradycardia
Sinus Arrest/Sinoatrial (SA) Exit Block
Second-Degree, Type I AV Block (Wenckebach)
Second-Degree, 2:1 and Advanced AV Block With Narrow QRS Complexes
Third-Degree AV Block With Narrow QRS Complexes

Asymptomatic bradycardia

Oxygen

Observe

Symptomatic bradycardia

Oxygen

Atropine 0.5- to 1.0-mg IV bolus and, if necessary, repeat every 3 to 5 min up to a total dose of 2 to 3 mg
AND/OR
TC pacing; administer a sedative/analgesic as needed

Dopamine 5- to 20-µg/kg/min IV infusion
OR
Epinephrine 2- to 10-µg/min IV infusion

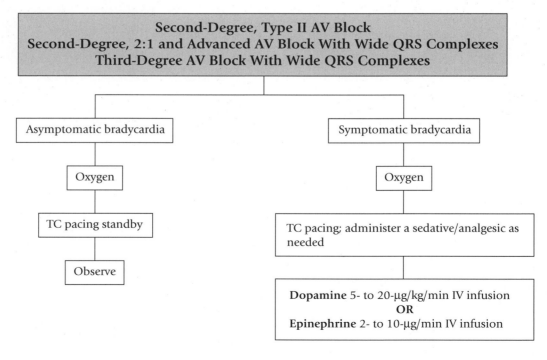

Second-Degree, Type II AV Block
Second-Degree, 2:1 and Advanced AV Block With Wide QRS Complexes
Third-Degree AV Block With Wide QRS Complexes

Asymptomatic bradycardia

Oxygen

TC pacing standby

Observe

Symptomatic bradycardia

Oxygen

TC pacing; administer a sedative/analgesic as needed

Dopamine 5- to 20-µg/kg/min IV infusion
OR
Epinephrine 2- to 10-µg/min IV infusion

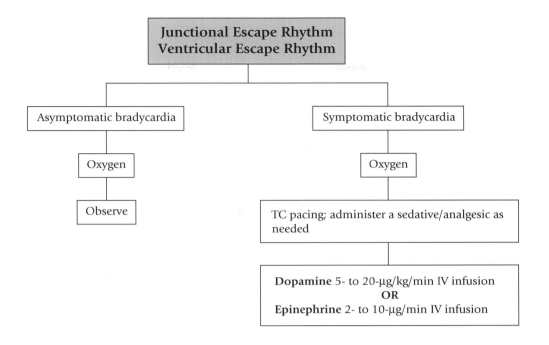

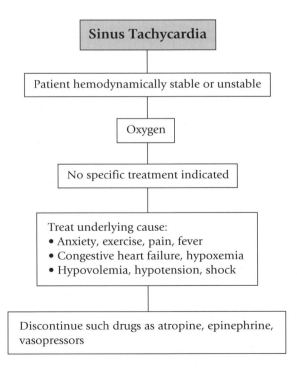

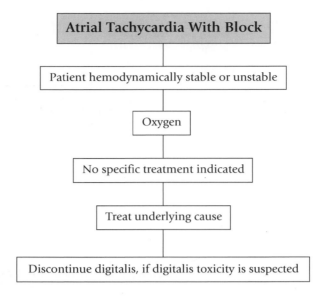

Atrial Tachycardia With Block

Patient hemodynamically stable or unstable

Oxygen

No specific treatment indicated

Treat underlying cause

Discontinue digitalis, if digitalis toxicity is suspected

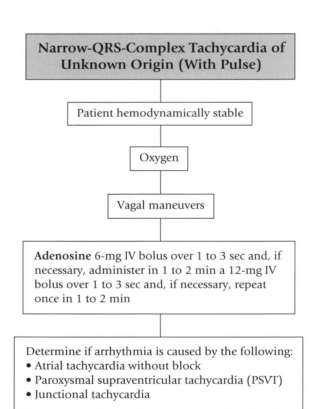

Narrow-QRS-Complex Tachycardia of Unknown Origin (With Pulse)

Patient hemodynamically stable

Oxygen

Vagal maneuvers

Adenosine 6-mg IV bolus over 1 to 3 sec and, if necessary, administer in 1 to 2 min a 12-mg IV bolus over 1 to 3 sec and, if necessary, repeat once in 1 to 2 min

Determine if arrhythmia is caused by the following:
• Atrial tachycardia without block
• Paroxysmal supraventricular tachycardia (PSVT)
• Junctional tachycardia

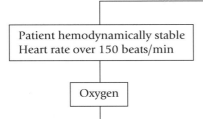

Atrial Tachycardia Without Block

Patient hemodynamically stable
Heart rate over 150 beats/min

Oxygen

Diltiazem 20-mg (0.25-mg/kg) IV bolus over 2 min and, if necessary, administer in 15 min a 25-mg (0.35-mg/kg) IV bolus over 2 min, followed by an IV infusion at a rate of 5 to 15 mg/h

OR

One of the following **β-blockers:**

- **Esmolol** 0.5-mg/kg IV bolus over 1 min, followed by an IV infusion at a rate of 0.05 mg/kg/min; repeat the IV bolus twice, 5 min between each bolus, while increasing the rate of the IV infusion 0.05 mg/kg/min after each bolus; then, if necessary, increase the IV infusion by 0.05 mg/kg/min every 5 min to a maximum of 0.30 mg/kg/min
- **Atenolol** 5 mg IV over 5 min and repeat in 10 min for a total dose of 10 mg
- **Metoprolol** 5 mg IV over 2 to 5 min and repeat every 5 min up to a total dose of 15 mg

OR

Amiodarone 150-mg IV infusion over 10 min, followed by a 1-mg/min IV infusion

Patient hemodynamically unstable
Heart rate over 150 beats/min or less

Oxygen

Amiodarone 150-mg IV infusion over 10 min, followed by a 1-mg/min IV infusion

OR

Diltiazem 20-mg (0.25-mg/kg) IV bolus over 2 min and, if necessary, administer in 15 min a 25-mg (0.35-mg/kg) IV bolus over 2 min, followed by an IV infusion at a rate of 5 to 15 mg/h

Paroxysmal Supraventricular Tachycardia (PSVT) With Narrow QRS Complexes (Without Wolff-Parkinson-White Syndrome or Ventricular Preexcitation)

Patient hemodynamically stable
Heart rate over 150 beats/min

Oxygen

Vagal maneuvers

Adenosine 6-mg IV bolus over 1 to 3 sec and, if necessary, administer in 1 to 2 min a 12-mg IV bolus over 1 to 3 sec and, if necessary, repeat once in 1 to 2 min

Diltiazem 20-mg (0.25-mg/kg) IV bolus over 2 min and, if necessary, administer in 15 min a 25-mg (0.35-mg/kg) IV bolus over 2 min, followed by an IV infusion at a rate of 5 to 15 mg/h
OR
One of the following β-blockers:
- **Esmolol** 0.5-mg/kg IV bolus over 1 min, followed by an IV infusion at a rate of 0.05 mg/kg/min; repeat the IV bolus twice, 5 min between each bolus, while increasing the rate of the IV infusion 0.05 mg/kg/min after each bolus; then, if necessary, increase the IV infusion by 0.05 mg/kg/min every 5 min to a maximum of 0.30 mg/kg/min
- **Atenolol** 5 mg IV over 5 min and repeat in 10 min for a total dose of 10 mg
- **Metoprolol** 5 mg IV over 2 to 5 min and repeat every 5 min up to a total dose of 15 mg

Digoxin 0.5 mg IV over 5 min

Synchronized shock 50-100 J and repeat as necessary at 100 J, 200 J, 300 J, etc.; administer a sedative/analgesic before cardioversion

Patient hemodynamically unstable
Heart rate over 150 beats/min or less

Oxygen

Vagal maneuvers

Digoxin 0.5 mg IV over 5 min

Amiodarone 150-mg IV infusion over 10 min, followed by a 1-mg/min IV infusion
OR
Diltiazem 20-mg (0.25-mg/kg) IV bolus over 2 min and, if necessary, administer in 15 min a 25-mg (0.35-mg/kg) IV bolus over 2 min, followed by an IV infusion at a rate of 5 to 15 mg/h

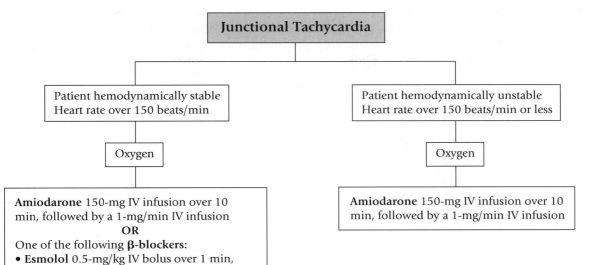

Junctional Tachycardia

Patient hemodynamically stable
Heart rate over 150 beats/min

Oxygen

Amiodarone 150-mg IV infusion over 10 min, followed by a 1-mg/min IV infusion
OR
One of the following **β-blockers:**
- **Esmolol** 0.5-mg/kg IV bolus over 1 min, followed by an IV infusion at a rate of 0.05 mg/kg/min; repeat the IV bolus twice, 5 min between each bolus, while increasing the rate of the IV infusion 0.05 mg/kg/min after each bolus; then, if necessary, increase the IV infusion by 0.05 mg/kg/min every 5 min to a maximum of 0.30 mg/kg/min
- **Atenolol** 5 mg IV over 5 min and repeat in 10 min for a total dose of 10 mg
- **Metoprolol** 5 mg IV over 2 to 5 min and repeat every 5 min up to a total dose of 15 mg

Patient hemodynamically unstable
Heart rate over 150 beats/min or less

Oxygen

Amiodarone 150-mg IV infusion over 10 min, followed by a 1-mg/min IV infusion

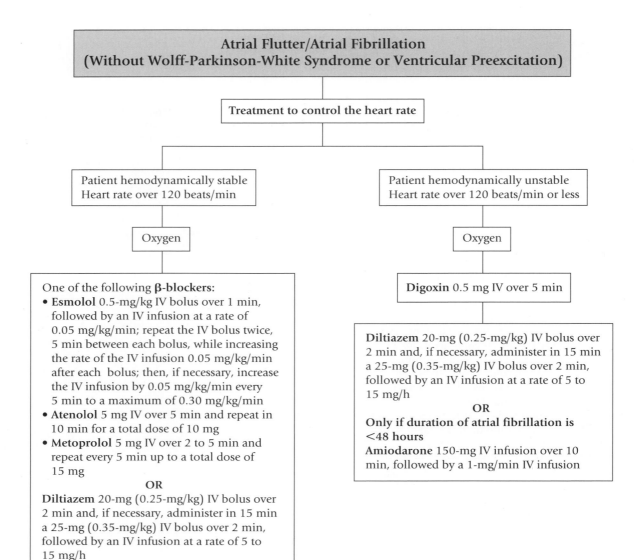

Atrial Flutter/Atrial Fibrillation
(Without Wolff-Parkinson-White Syndrome or Ventricular Preexcitation)

Treatment to control the heart rate

Patient hemodynamically stable
Heart rate over 120 beats/min

Patient hemodynamically unstable
Heart rate over 120 beats/min or less

Oxygen

Oxygen

Digoxin 0.5 mg IV over 5 min

One of the following **β-blockers:**
- **Esmolol** 0.5-mg/kg IV bolus over 1 min, followed by an IV infusion at a rate of 0.05 mg/kg/min; repeat the IV bolus twice, 5 min between each bolus, while increasing the rate of the IV infusion 0.05 mg/kg/min after each bolus; then, if necessary, increase the IV infusion by 0.05 mg/kg/min every 5 min to a maximum of 0.30 mg/kg/min
- **Atenolol** 5 mg IV over 5 min and repeat in 10 min for a total dose of 10 mg
- **Metoprolol** 5 mg IV over 2 to 5 min and repeat every 5 min up to a total dose of 15 mg

OR

Diltiazem 20-mg (0.25-mg/kg) IV bolus over 2 min and, if necessary, administer in 15 min a 25-mg (0.35-mg/kg) IV bolus over 2 min, followed by an IV infusion at a rate of 5 to 15 mg/h

Diltiazem 20-mg (0.25-mg/kg) IV bolus over 2 min and, if necessary, administer in 15 min a 25-mg (0.35-mg/kg) IV bolus over 2 min, followed by an IV infusion at a rate of 5 to 15 mg/h

OR

Only if duration of atrial fibrillation is <48 hours
Amiodarone 150-mg IV infusion over 10 min, followed by a 1-mg/min IV infusion

Digoxin 0.5 mg IV over 5 min

**Atrial Flutter/Atrial Fibrillation
(Without Wolff-Parkinson-White Syndrome or Ventricular Preexcitation)**

Treatment to convert the rhythm: atrial fibrillation
<48 hours and atrial flutter of any duration

Patient hemodynamically stable
Heart rate over 120 beats/min

Patient hemodynamically unstable
Heart rate over 120 beats/min or less

Oxygen

Oxygen

Ibutilide
• If patient's weight ≥60 kg (≥132 lb),
  ibutilide 1.0 mg IV over 10 min and repeat
  10 min after first infusion, if necessary
• If patient's weight <60 kg (<132 lb),
  ibutilide 0.1 mg/kg IV over 10 min and repeat
  10 min after first infusion, if necessary
  OR
Amiodarone 150-mg IV infusion over 10 min,
followed by a 1-mg/min IV infusion
  OR
Procainamide 20- to 30-mg/min IV infusion up
to a total dose of 17 mg/kg

Synchronized shock 50-100 J for atrial flutter
and 100-200 J for atrial fibrillation; repeat as
necessary at 100 J, 200 J, 300 J, etc.; administer
a sedative/analgesic before cardioversion
  OR
Amiodarone 150-mg IV infusion over 10 min,
followed by a 1-mg/min IV infusion

Synchronized shock 50-100 J for atrial flutter
and 100-200 J for atrial fibrillation; repeat as
necessary at 100 J, 200 J, 300 J, etc.; administer
a sedative/analgesic before cardioversion

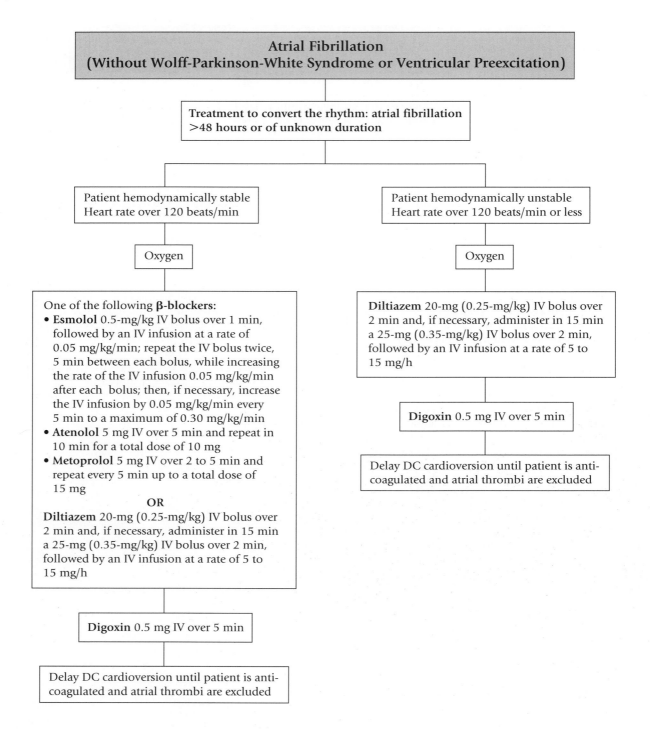

Atrial Fibrillation
(Without Wolff-Parkinson-White Syndrome or Ventricular Preexcitation)

Treatment to convert the rhythm: atrial fibrillation
>48 hours or of unknown duration

Patient hemodynamically stable
Heart rate over 120 beats/min

Patient hemodynamically unstable
Heart rate over 120 beats/min or less

Oxygen

Oxygen

One of the following β-blockers:
• **Esmolol** 0.5-mg/kg IV bolus over 1 min,
followed by an IV infusion at a rate of
0.05 mg/kg/min; repeat the IV bolus twice,
5 min between each bolus, while increasing
the rate of the IV infusion 0.05 mg/kg/min
after each bolus; then, if necessary, increase
the IV infusion by 0.05 mg/kg/min every
5 min to a maximum of 0.30 mg/kg/min
• **Atenolol** 5 mg IV over 5 min and repeat in
10 min for a total dose of 10 mg
• **Metoprolol** 5 mg IV over 2 to 5 min and
repeat every 5 min up to a total dose of
15 mg
        OR
Diltiazem 20-mg (0.25-mg/kg) IV bolus over
2 min and, if necessary, administer in 15 min
a 25-mg (0.35-mg/kg) IV bolus over 2 min,
followed by an IV infusion at a rate of 5 to
15 mg/h

Diltiazem 20-mg (0.25-mg/kg) IV bolus over
2 min and, if necessary, administer in 15 min
a 25-mg (0.35-mg/kg) IV bolus over 2 min,
followed by an IV infusion at a rate of 5 to
15 mg/h

Digoxin 0.5 mg IV over 5 min

Delay DC cardioversion until patient is anticoagulated and atrial thrombi are excluded

Digoxin 0.5 mg IV over 5 min

Delay DC cardioversion until patient is anticoagulated and atrial thrombi are excluded

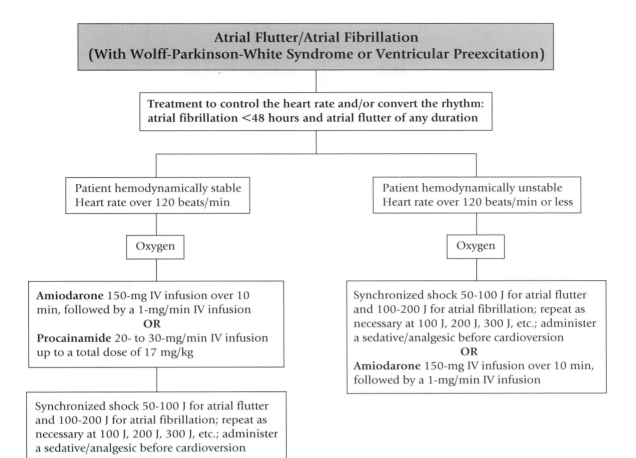

**Atrial Flutter/Atrial Fibrillation
(With Wolff-Parkinson-White Syndrome or Ventricular Preexcitation)**

Treatment to control the heart rate and/or convert the rhythm:
atrial fibrillation <48 hours and atrial flutter of any duration

Patient hemodynamically stable
Heart rate over 120 beats/min

Patient hemodynamically unstable
Heart rate over 120 beats/min or less

Oxygen

Oxygen

Amiodarone 150-mg IV infusion over 10
min, followed by a 1-mg/min IV infusion
OR
Procainamide 20- to 30-mg/min IV infusion
up to a total dose of 17 mg/kg

Synchronized shock 50-100 J for atrial flutter
and 100-200 J for atrial fibrillation; repeat as
necessary at 100 J, 200 J, 300 J, etc.; administer
a sedative/analgesic before cardioversion
OR
Amiodarone 150-mg IV infusion over 10 min,
followed by a 1-mg/min IV infusion

Synchronized shock 50-100 J for atrial flutter
and 100-200 J for atrial fibrillation; repeat as
necessary at 100 J, 200 J, 300 J, etc.; administer
a sedative/analgesic before cardioversion

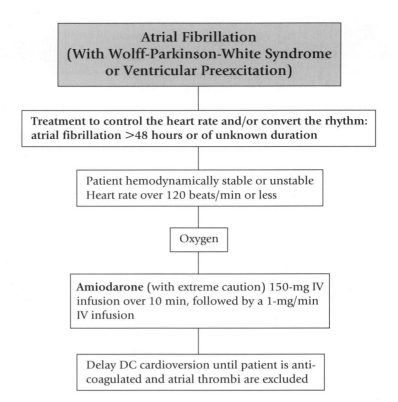

**Atrial Fibrillation
(With Wolff-Parkinson-White Syndrome
or Ventricular Preexcitation)**

Treatment to control the heart rate and/or convert the rhythm:
atrial fibrillation >48 hours or of unknown duration

Patient hemodynamically stable or unstable
Heart rate over 120 beats/min or less

Oxygen

Amiodarone (with extreme caution) 150-mg IV
infusion over 10 min, followed by a 1-mg/min
IV infusion

Delay DC cardioversion until patient is anticoagulated and atrial thrombi are excluded

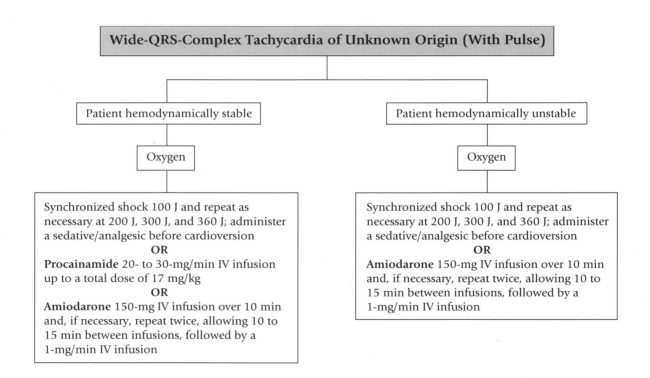

Wide-QRS-Complex Tachycardia of Unknown Origin (With Pulse)

Patient hemodynamically stable

Patient hemodynamically unstable

Oxygen

Oxygen

Synchronized shock 100 J and repeat as
necessary at 200 J, 300 J, and 360 J; administer
a sedative/analgesic before cardioversion
OR
Procainamide 20- to 30-mg/min IV infusion
up to a total dose of 17 mg/kg
OR
Amiodarone 150-mg IV infusion over 10 min
and, if necessary, repeat twice, allowing 10 to
15 min between infusions, followed by a
1-mg/min IV infusion

Synchronized shock 100 J and repeat as
necessary at 200 J, 300 J, and 360 J; administer
a sedative/analgesic before cardioversion
OR
Amiodarone 150-mg IV infusion over 10 min
and, if necessary, repeat twice, allowing 10 to
15 min between infusions, followed by a
1-mg/min IV infusion

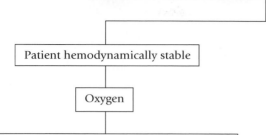

Ventricular Tachycardia (VT), Monomorphic (With Pulse)

Patient hemodynamically stable	Patient hemodynamically unstable
Oxygen	Oxygen

Patient hemodynamically stable / Oxygen:

Synchronized shock 100 J and repeat as necessary at 200 J, 300 J, and 360 J; administer a sedative/analgesic before cardioversion

OR

Procainamide 20- to 30-mg/min IV infusion up to a total dose of 17 mg/kg

OR

Amiodarone 150-mg IV infusion over 10 min and, if necessary, repeat twice, allowing 10 to 15 min between infusions, followed by a 1-mg/min IV infusion

OR

Lidocaine 75- to 100-mg (1.0- to 1.5-mg/kg) IV bolus slowly and, if necessary, repeat a 25- to 50-mg (0.5- to 0.75-mg/kg) IV bolus slowly every 5 to 10 min up to a total dose of 3 mg/kg

Patient hemodynamically unstable / Oxygen:

Synchronized shock 100 J and repeat as necessary at 200 J, 300 J, and 360 J; administer a sedative/analgesic before cardioversion

OR

Amiodarone 150-mg IV infusion over 10 min and, if necessary, repeat twice, allowing 10 to 15 min between infusions, followed by a 1-mg/min IV infusion

OR

Lidocaine 75- to 100-mg (1.0- to 1.5-mg/kg) IV bolus slowly and, if necessary, repeat a 25- to 50-mg (0.5- to 0.75-mg/kg) IV bolus slowly every 5 to 10 min up to a total dose of 3 mg/kg

Ventricular Tachycardia (VT), Polymorphic (With Pulse) Normal Baseline QT Interval

Patient hemodynamically stable

Oxygen

Synchronized shock 100 J and repeat as necessary at 200 J, 300 J, and 360 J; administer a sedative/analgesic before cardioversion

OR

One of the following β-blockers (especially if polymorphic VT is associated with an acute coronary syndrome):

- **Esmolol** 0.5-mg/kg IV bolus over 1 min, followed by an IV infusion at a rate of 0.05 mg/kg/min; repeat the bolus twice, 5 min between each bolus, while increasing the rate of the IV infusion 0.05 mg/kg/min after each bolus; then, if necessary, increase the IV infusion by 0.05 mg/kg/min every 5 min to a maximum of 0.30 mg/kg/min
- **Atenolol** 5 mg IV over 5 min and repeat in 10 min for a total dose of 10 mg
- **Metoprolol** 5 mg IV over 2 to 5 min and repeat every 5 min up to a total dose of 15 mg

OR

Procainamide 20- to 30-mg/min IV infusion up to a total dose of 17 mg/kg

OR

Amiodarone 150-mg IV infusion over 10 min and, if necessary, repeat twice, allowing 10 to 15 min between infusions, followed by a 1-mg/min IV infusion

OR

Lidocaine 75- to 100-mg (1.0- to 1.5-mg/kg) IV bolus slowly and, if necessary, repeat 25- to 50-mg (0.5- to 0.75-mg/kg) IV bolus slowly every 5 to 10 min up to a total dose of 3 mg/kg

Patient hemodynamically unstable

Oxygen

Synchronized shock 100 J and repeat as necessary at 200 J, 300 J, and 360 J; administer a sedative/analgesic before cardioversion

OR

Amiodarone 150-mg IV infusion over 10 min and, if necessary, repeat twice, allowing 10 to 15 min between infusions, followed by a 1-mg/min IV infusion

OR

Lidocaine 75- to 100-mg (1.0- to 1.5-mg/kg) IV bolus slowly and, if necessary, repeat a 25- to 50-mg (0.5- to 0.75-mg/kg) IV bolus slowly every 5 to 10 min up to a total dose of 3 mg/kg

**Ventricular Tachycardia (VT), Polymorphic
(With Pulse)
Prolonged Baseline QT Interval
Torsade de Pointes (TdP) (With Pulse)**

Patient hemodynamically stable or unstable

Oxygen

Magnesium sulfate 1- to 2-g IV infusion over
5 to 60 min, if indicated, followed by 0.5- to
1.0-g IV infusion over 1 h

TC overdrive pacing; administer a sedative/
analgesic before cardioversion
AND
Consider administration of one of the
following **β-blockers:**
• **Esmolol** 0.5-mg/kg IV bolus over 1 min,
  followed by an IV infusion at a rate of 0.05
  mg/kg/min; repeat the IV bolus twice, 5 min
  between each bolus, while increasing the
  rate of the IV infusion 0.05 mg/kg/min after
  each bolus; then, if necessary, increase the
  IV infusion by 0.05 mg/kg/min every 5 min
  to a maximum of 0.30 mg/kg/min
• **Atenolol** 5 mg IV over 5 min and repeat in
  10 min for a total dose of 10 mg
• **Metoprolol** 5 mg IV over 2 to 5 min and
  repeat every 5 min up to a total dose of
  15 mg

Discontinue such antiarrhythmic agents as the
following:
• Amiodarone, disopyramide
• Procainamide, quinidine, sotalol
• Any other agent that prolongs the QT
  interval (e.g., phenothiazines, tricyclic
  antidepressants, etc.)
AND
Correct any electrolyte imbalance

Unsynchronized shock 200 J and repeat as
necessary at 200-300 J and 360 J; administer a
sedative/analgesic before cardioversion

Premature Atrial Contractions (PACs)
Premature Junctional Contractions (PJCs)

Patient hemodynamically stable or unstable

Oxygen

Discontinue such drugs as stimulants, sympathomimetic drugs, digitalis (if digitalis toxicity is suspected)

Premature Ventricular Contractions (PVCs)

Patient hemodynamically stable or unstable

Oxygen

Consider one of the following:
- **β-blocker** (especially if the PVCs are associated with an acute coronary syndrome)
- **Procainamide,** if not contraindicated
- **Amiodarone**
- **Lidocaine**

Part II

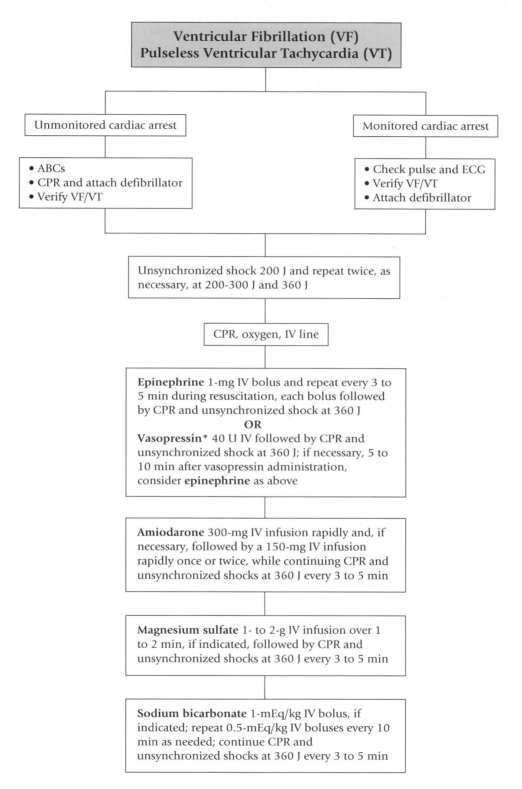

Ventricular Fibrillation (VF)
Pulseless Ventricular Tachycardia (VT)

Unmonitored cardiac arrest

- ABCs
- CPR and attach defibrillator
- Verify VF/VT

Monitored cardiac arrest

- Check pulse and ECG
- Verify VF/VT
- Attach defibrillator

Unsynchronized shock 200 J and repeat twice, as necessary, at 200-300 J and 360 J

CPR, oxygen, IV line

Epinephrine 1-mg IV bolus and repeat every 3 to 5 min during resuscitation, each bolus followed by CPR and unsynchronized shock at 360 J
OR
Vasopressin* 40 U IV followed by CPR and unsynchronized shock at 360 J; if necessary, 5 to 10 min after vasopressin administration, consider **epinephrine** as above

Amiodarone 300-mg IV infusion rapidly and, if necessary, followed by a 150-mg IV infusion rapidly once or twice, while continuing CPR and unsynchronized shocks at 360 J every 3 to 5 min

Magnesium sulfate 1- to 2-g IV infusion over 1 to 2 min, if indicated, followed by CPR and unsynchronized shocks at 360 J every 3 to 5 min

Sodium bicarbonate 1-mEq/kg IV bolus, if indicated; repeat 0.5-mEq/kg IV boluses every 10 min as needed; continue CPR and unsynchronized shocks at 360 J every 3 to 5 min

*At the time of publication of this book, vasopressin has not been approved for use in cardiac arrest in the United States.

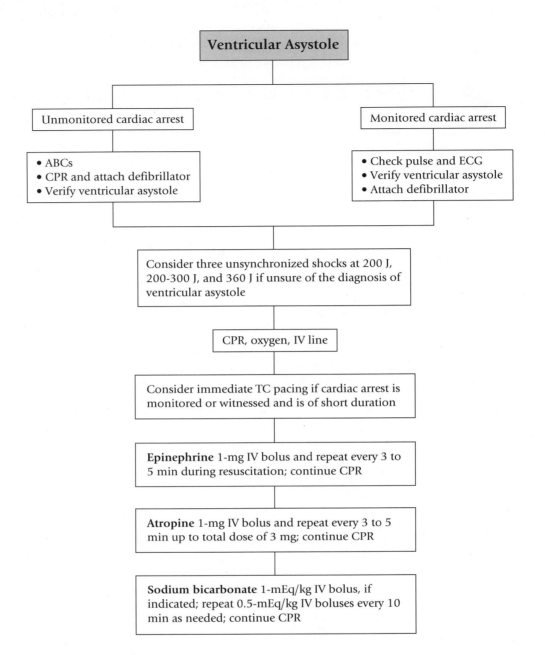

Ventricular Asystole

Unmonitored cardiac arrest

- ABCs
- CPR and attach defibrillator
- Verify ventricular asystole

Monitored cardiac arrest

- Check pulse and ECG
- Verify ventricular asystole
- Attach defibrillator

Consider three unsynchronized shocks at 200 J, 200-300 J, and 360 J if unsure of the diagnosis of ventricular asystole

CPR, oxygen, IV line

Consider immediate TC pacing if cardiac arrest is monitored or witnessed and is of short duration

Epinephrine 1-mg IV bolus and repeat every 3 to 5 min during resuscitation; continue CPR

Atropine 1-mg IV bolus and repeat every 3 to 5 min up to total dose of 3 mg; continue CPR

Sodium bicarbonate 1-mEq/kg IV bolus, if indicated; repeat 0.5-mEq/kg IV boluses every 10 min as needed; continue CPR

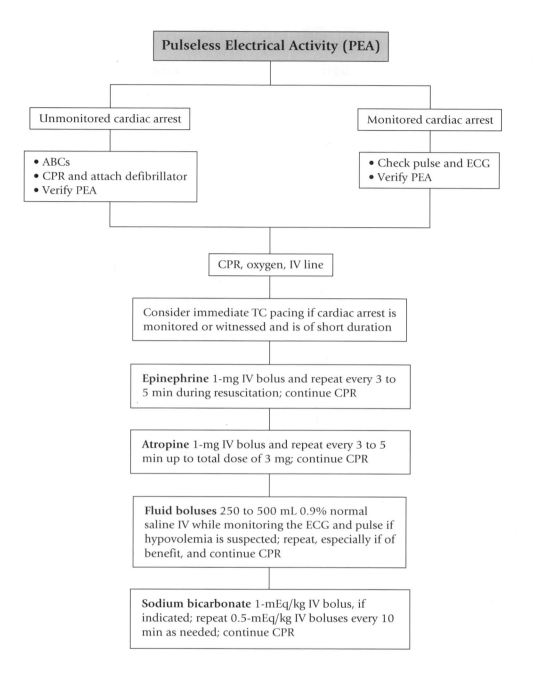

Pulseless Electrical Activity (PEA)

Unmonitored cardiac arrest
- ABCs
- CPR and attach defibrillator
- Verify PEA

Monitored cardiac arrest
- Check pulse and ECG
- Verify PEA

CPR, oxygen, IV line

Consider immediate TC pacing if cardiac arrest is monitored or witnessed and is of short duration

Epinephrine 1-mg IV bolus and repeat every 3 to 5 min during resuscitation; continue CPR

Atropine 1-mg IV bolus and repeat every 3 to 5 min up to total dose of 3 mg; continue CPR

Fluid boluses 250 to 500 mL 0.9% normal saline IV while monitoring the ECG and pulse if hypovolemia is suspected; repeat, especially if of benefit, and continue CPR

Sodium bicarbonate 1-mEq/kg IV bolus, if indicated; repeat 0.5-mEq/kg IV boluses every 10 min as needed; continue CPR

CHAPTER REVIEW QUESTIONS

1. In a patient with symptomatic bradycardia and an ECG showing a second-degree, type II AV block, you should administer oxygen, start an IV line, and administer or begin:
   A. an isoproterenol drip
   B. atropine
   C. transcutaneous pacing
   D. lidocaine

2. Patients with symptomatic sinus tachycardia should be treated with:
   A. diltiazem
   B. epinephrine
   C. dopamine
   D. appropriate treatment for the underlying cause of the tachycardia

3. If a patient is stable with an ECG showing PSVT after administering oxygen and starting an IV line, you should:
   A. attempt vagal maneuvers
   B. administer diltiazem
   C. administer adenosine
   D. administer Valium

4. Your patient presents with chest pain and signs and symptoms of an acute MI. His ECG shows atrial tachycardia without a block. After administering oxygen and starting an IV line you should immediately consider:
   A. transcutaneous pacing
   B. a loading dose of amiodarone
   C. a synchronized shock of 50 J
   D. an adenosine bolus

5. A patient with atrial fibrillation of less than 48 hours in duration, who is hemodynamically unstable and hypotensive, should be treated as follows:
   A. immediate DC cardioversion or amiodarone IV
   B. immediate DC cardioversion or amiodarone or a β-blocker IV
   C. immediate DC cardioversion or amiodarone or procainamide IV
   D. all of the above

6. Your patient is conscious and hemodynamically stable with a pulse and an ECG showing monomorphic ventricular tachycardia. After administering oxygen and starting an IV you should:
   A. start an infusion of procainamide
   B. administer a 150-mg loading dose of amiodarone IV
   C. deliver a synchronized shock of 100 J
   D. any one of the above

7. If your patient in question number 5 begins to complain of chest pain and then becomes pulseless, you should immediately:
   A. deliver an unsynchronized shock of 200 J
   B. administer a lidocaine bolus
   C. deliver a synchronized shock of 100 J
   D. begin transcutaneous pacing

8. Pulseless electrical activity may result from:
   A. electromechanical dissociation (EMD)
   B. hypovolemia
   C. cardiac rupture
   D. all of the above

9. In a cardiac arrest when you are having difficulty starting a peripheral IV line and your patient has just been defibrillated three times, you should:
   A. attempt a central IV line
   B. terminate the arrest
   C. administer epinephrine at 2 to 2.5 times the usual IV dose down the tracheal tube
   D. attempt an intraosseous line

10. If you suspect asystole, you should:
   A. confirm the arrhythmia in two ECG leads
   B. consider delivering three defibrillation shocks if asystole cannot be definitely confirmed
   C. consider transcutaneous pacing after confirming the presence of asystole
   D. all of the above

The 12-Lead Electrocardiogram

CHAPTER OUTLINE

The 12-Lead ECG Leads
Lead Axis
Frontal and Horizontal Planes
Standard (Bipolar) Limb Leads

Augmented (Unipolar) Leads
Precordial (Unipolar) Leads
Right-Sided Chest Leads
Facing Leads

CHAPTER OBJECTIVES

Upon completion of all or part of this chapter, you should be able to complete the following objectives:

1. List the leads of a 12-lead ECG and indicate which are unipolar and which are bipolar.
2. Define the following terms:
   Lead
   Lead axis
   Perpendicular axis
   Frontal and horizontal planes
3. Describe how the six limb leads of a 12-lead ECG are obtained.
4. Identify the sites of attachment of the electrodes for the six precordial leads of a 12-lead ECG on an anatomical drawing of the chest, and indicate over which region of the heart each electrode lies.
5. Explain how (1) the triaxial reference figures for the standard (bipolar) limb leads and the augmented (unipolar) leads, (2) the hexaxial reference figure, and (3) the precordial reference figure are derived.
6. Identify the right-sided chest leads, the sites of their attachment, and the indication for their use.
7. List the facing leads that view the following surfaces of the heart:
   Anterior
   Lateral
   Inferior (or diaphragmatic)
   Right ventricle

THE 12-LEAD ECG LEADS

> ### KEY DEFINITION
>
> *A 12-lead (or conventional) electrocardiogram (ECG) consists of the following:*
> - *Six limb or extremity leads*
>   - *Three standard (bipolar) limb leads: leads I, II, and III*
>   - *Three augmented (unipolar) leads: leads aVR, aVL, and aVF*
> - *Six precordial (unipolar) leads: leads V_1, V_2, V_3, V_4, V_5, and V_6*

Each lead of a 12-lead ECG (Figure 11-1) is obtained using a *positive ("sensing" or "probing") electrode* and a *negative electrode* to detect the electrical current generated by the depolarization and repolarization of the heart. An additional electrode, the *ground electrode,* is often attached to the right leg (or any other location on the body) to provide a path of least resistance for electrical interference in the body.

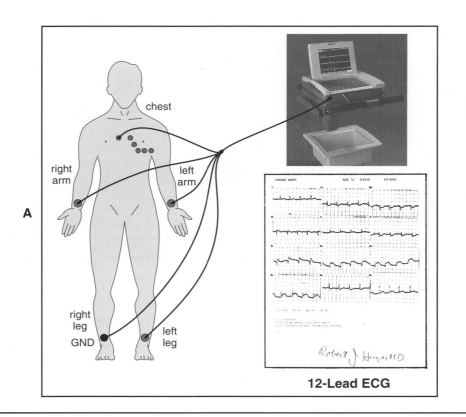

12-Lead ECG

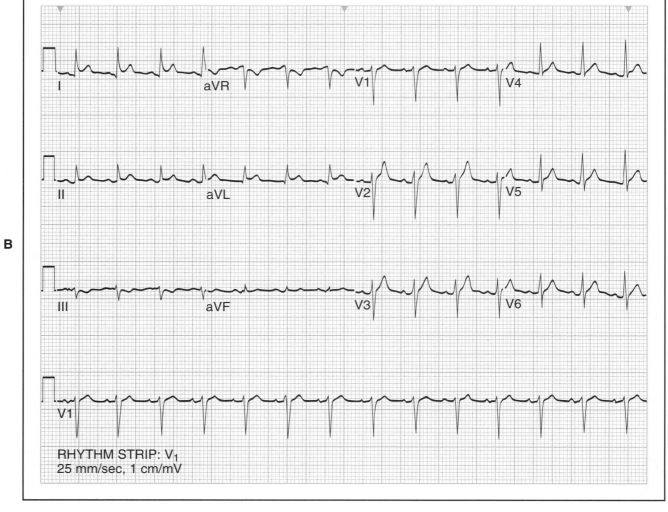

I aVR V1 V4

II aVL V2 V5

III aVF V3 V6

V1

RHYTHM STRIP: V₁
25 mm/sec, 1 cm/mV

Figure 11-1 **A,** The 12-lead ECG. **B,** 12-lead ECG printout with a lead V₁ rhythm strip.

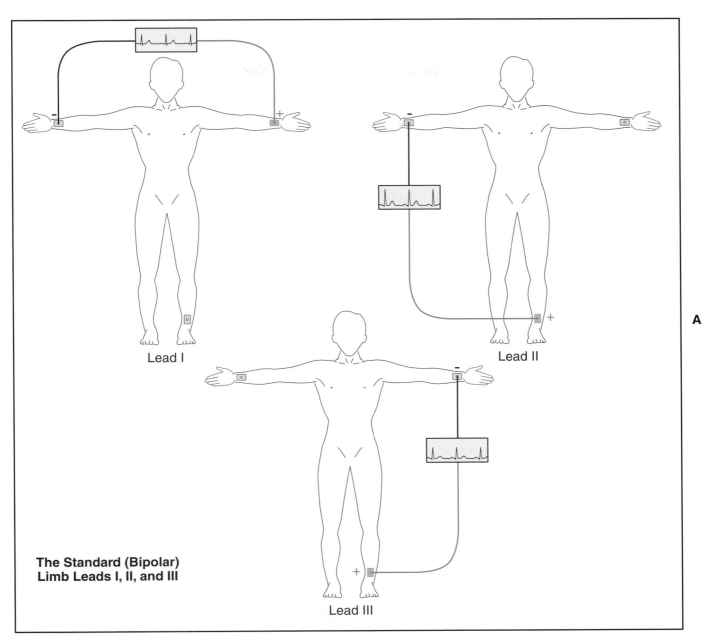

Figure 11-2 **A,** Standard limb leads.

Continued

The positive electrode can be attached to the extremities (right arm, left arm, or left leg) to obtain the six limb leads or to designated areas of the chest to obtain the six precordial leads. The negative electrode can be either a single electrode attached to an extremity or an "indifferent" zero reference point—the *central terminal*. The central terminal is created electronically within the circuitry of the ECG machine by combining two or three of the electrical currents obtained from electrodes attached to the right and left arms and left leg. (Which of the three limb electrodes are used to form the central terminal depends on the lead being viewed, as described below.) The central terminal is a common negative electrode with an electrical potential of essentially zero. It is hypothetically located in the heart, left of the interventricular septum and below the atrioventricular (AV) junction where the electrical center of the heart is located. It must be noted that a separate external negative electrode is not used when recording leads that utilize a central terminal.

The three bipolar limb leads—I, II, and III—detect the heart's electrical activity by using two electrodes, one positive and the other negative, attached to the extremities (Figure 11-2, *A*). A bipolar lead thus represents the difference in electrical potential (or voltage) between two electrodes.

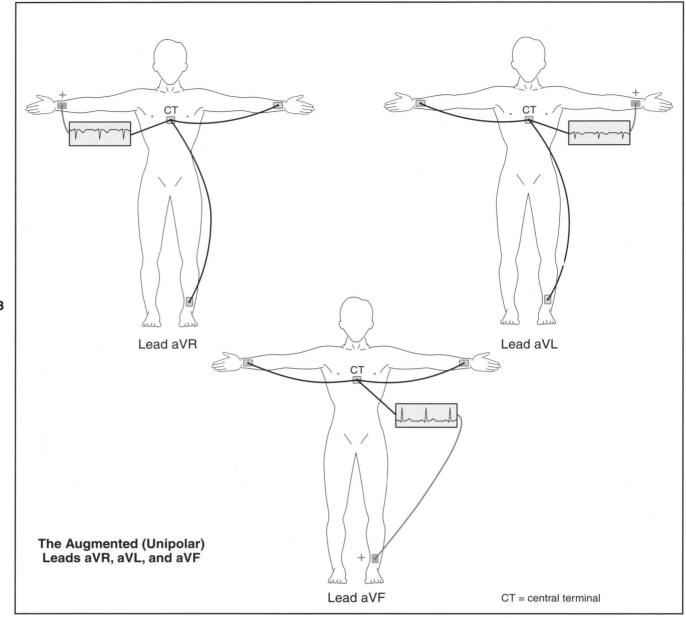

B

Lead aVR

Lead aVL

**The Augmented (Unipolar)
Leads aVR, aVL, and aVF**

Lead aVF

CT = central terminal

Figure 11-2, cont'd   B, Augmented leads.

The three unipolar augmented limb leads—aVR, aVL, and aVF—on the other hand, detect the electrical current generated by the heart by using a positive electrode attached to one of three extremities and the central terminal (Figure 11-2, B). The central terminal used in the augmented leads (the "a" in these leads stands for "augmented") is one obtained by combining the electrical currents from the two electrodes other than the one being used as the positive electrode. For example, when the patient's right arm electrode is used as the positive electrode, the central terminal is formed by joining the electrical currents obtained from the electrodes on the patient's left arm and left leg. A unipolar lead thus measures the difference in electrical potential between an electrode and the common terminal.

The six unipolar precordial leads—V_1, V_2, V_3, V_4, V_5, and V_6—detect the heart's electrical current using a positive electrode attached to one of six specified locations on the anterior chest wall and the central terminal (Figure 11-2, C). The central terminal used in the precordial leads, unlike that in the augmented limb leads, is obtained by combining the electrical

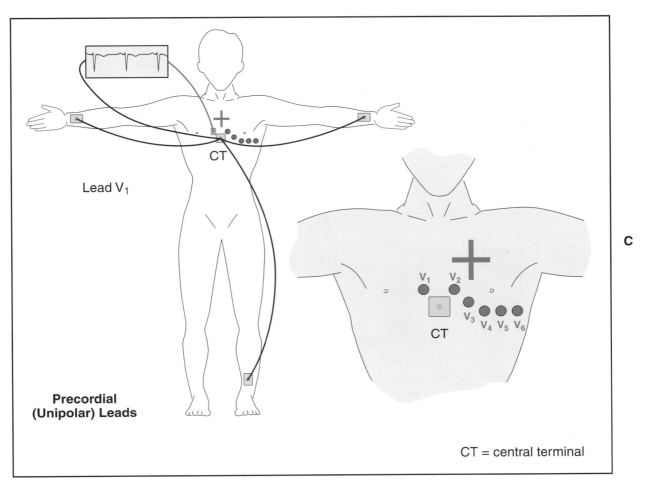

Figure 11-2, cont'd   C, Precordial leads.

currents from the electrodes attached to the right and left arms and left leg.

Notes

_____

_____

_____

_____

_____

LEAD AXIS

Each lead of the 12-lead ECG measures the difference in electrical potential between the positive and negative electrodes or central terminal (or poles). Thus each lead has a positive and negative pole.

A hypothetical line joining the poles of a lead is known as the axis of the lead (or lead axis) (Figure

11-3). The location of the positive and negative poles in a lead determines the orientation (or direction) of the axis of the lead. Thus a lead axis has a direction and polarity.

In addition, each lead axis has a perpendicular axis, or, simply, the *perpendicular*. It is usually depicted as a line intersecting or connecting with the lead axis at ±90 degrees (or a right angle), at its electrically "zero" point.

FRONTAL AND HORIZONTAL PLANES

The three standard limb leads (I, II, and III) and the three augmented leads (aVR, aVL, and aVF) measure the electrical activity of the heart in the two-dimensional *frontal plane* (i.e., viewed from the front of the patient's body) (Figure 11-4). The six precordial leads (V_1, V_2, V_3, V_4, V_5, and V_6) measure the electrical activity of the heart at a right angle to the frontal plane, the *horizontal plane*.

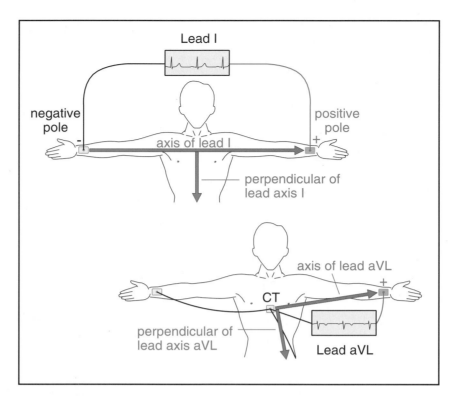

Figure 11-3 Axis of a lead and its perpendicular.

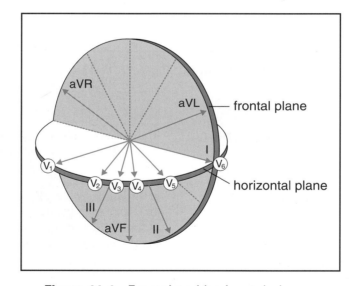

Figure 11-4 Frontal and horizontal planes.

STANDARD (BIPOLAR) LIMB LEADS

Each of the standard limb leads I, II, and III is obtained using a positive electrode attached to one of two extremities (left arm or left leg) and a single negative electrode attached to another extremity (right or left arm) (Figure 11-5). Thus each standard limb lead measures the difference in electrical potential between two extremity electrodes.

The electrodes are attached as follows to obtain the three standard limb leads:

◆ Lead I: The positive electrode is attached to the left arm and the negative electrode to the right arm
◆ Lead II: The positive electrode is attached to the left leg and the negative electrode to the right arm

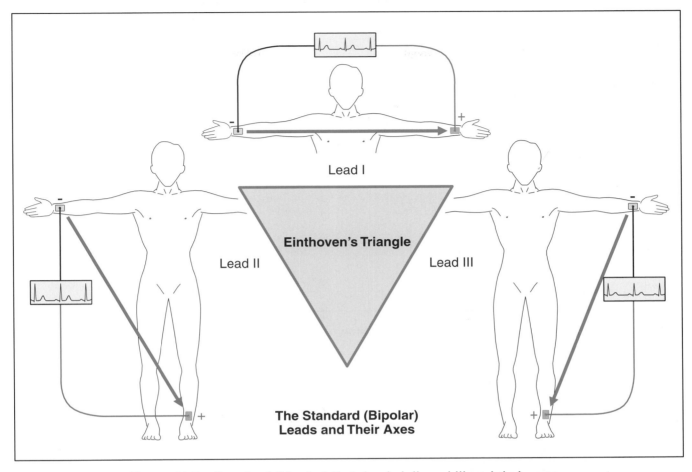

Lead I

Einthoven's Triangle

Lead II   Lead III

**The Standard (Bipolar)
Leads and Their Axes**

Figure 11-5 Standard (bipolar) limb leads I, II, and III and their axes.

◆ Lead III: The positive electrode is attached to the left leg and the negative electrode to the left arm

The lead axis for each standard limb lead is a line drawn between the two extremity electrodes, with one electrode designated as the negative pole and the other as the positive pole. The perpendicular divides the lead axis into a positive and a negative half.

The relationships of the standard limb leads are such that the sum of the electrical currents recorded in leads I and III equals the sum of the electrical current recorded in lead II. This is called *Einthoven's law,* named after the developer of three-lead electrocardiography.

Einthoven's law is expressed mathematically as follows:

$$\text{Lead I} + \text{Lead III} = \text{Lead II}$$

Because the positive electrodes of the three standard limb leads are electrically about the same distance from the zero reference point in the heart, an equilateral triangle (Einthoven's equilateral triangle) can be depicted in the body's frontal plane using the

three lead axes, with the heart and its zero reference point in the center (Figure 11-6). The three sides of the equilateral triangle can be shifted to the right, left, and down without changing the angle of their orientation until their midpoints intersect at the same point. This creates a standard limb lead triaxial reference figure, with each of the lead axes of the standard limb leads forming a 60-degree angle with its neighbors. The negative halves of the lead axes are usually depicted as dotted or dashed lines as shown in Figure 11-6.

AUGMENTED (UNIPOLAR) LEADS

The augmented leads aVR, aVL, and aVF are obtained using a positive electrode attached to one of three extremities (right arm, left arm, or right leg) and the central terminal obtained by connecting the other two extremity electrodes (Figure 11-7, *A*). Thus an augmented lead measures the difference in electrical potential between one of three extremity electrodes and the central terminal.

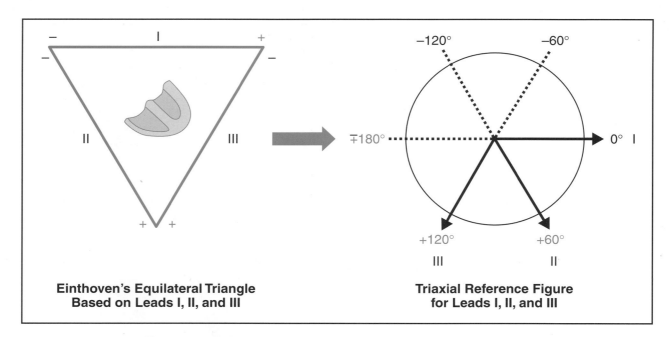

Figure 11-6 Einthoven's triangle and triaxial reference figure.

The three extremity electrodes are attached as follows to obtain the three augmented leads:

◆ Lead aVR: The positive electrode is attached to the right arm and the negative electrode to the central terminal (left arm and left leg)
◆ Lead aVL: The positive electrode is attached to the left arm and the negative electrode to the central terminal (right arm and left leg)
◆ Lead aVF: The positive electrode is attached to the left leg and the negative electrode to the central terminal (right and left arms)

It must be noted that originally the central terminal for these unipolar leads was obtained by connecting the right arm, left arm, and left leg together. Because this hookup resulted in a small electrical current and, consequently, small waves and complexes in the VR, VL, and VF leads (as they were originally called), the lead that was actually being taken was disconnected from the central terminal. Because this increased the electrical current (and size) of the waves and complexes in the ECG, the unipolar leads were renamed "augmented," thus the additional "a" in aVR, aVL, and aVF.

The lead axis for a particular augmented lead is a line drawn between the central terminal and its extremity electrode, with the central terminal designated as the negative pole and the extremity electrode as the positive pole. The augmented lead axis is usually depicted with its negative half extended as a dotted, dashed, or shaded line.

The positive electrodes of the three augmented leads, like those of the three standard limb leads, are also electrically equidistant from the zero reference point in the heart. The augmented lead triaxial reference figure (Figure 11-7, *B*) formed in the body's frontal plane by the axes of the three augmented leads is similar to that of the standard limb leads, with its lead axes 60 degrees apart but oriented around the zero reference point at slightly different angles.

When the triaxial reference figures of the standard limb leads and the augmented leads are superimposed, they form a hexaxial reference figure (Figure 11-8). Each augmented lead axis is perpendicular to a standard limb lead axis, so that each lead axis is spaced 30 degrees apart. The hexaxial reference figure's use in determining the major direction of the heart's electrical activity (e.g., the QRS axis) in the frontal plane will be discussed in Chapter 12.

PRECORDIAL (UNIPOLAR) LEADS

The precordial leads V_1, V_2, V_3, V_4, V_5, and V_6 are unipolar leads obtained by attaching the positive electrode to prescribed areas over the anterior chest wall (Figure 11-9, *A*) and the negative lead to the central terminal, which in this case is made by connecting all three extremity electrodes together: the right and left arm electrodes and the left leg electrode as shown in Figure 11-2, *C*. A precordial lead thus measures the difference in electrical potential between a chest electrode and the central terminal.

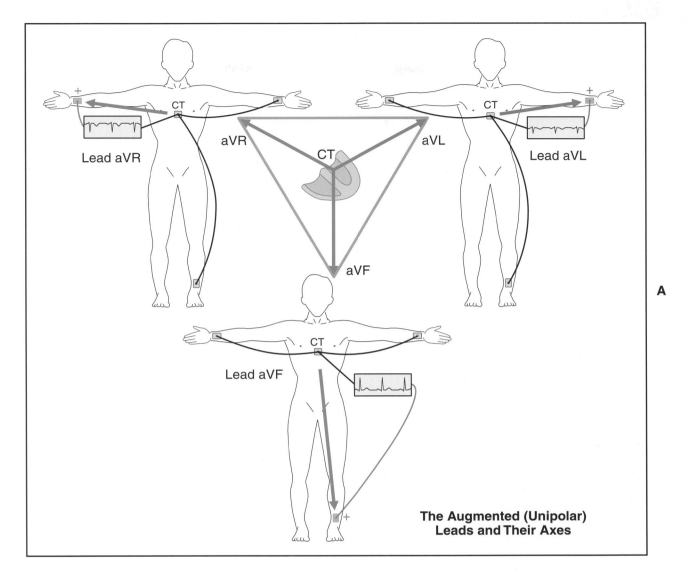

The Augmented (Unipolar)
Leads and Their Axes

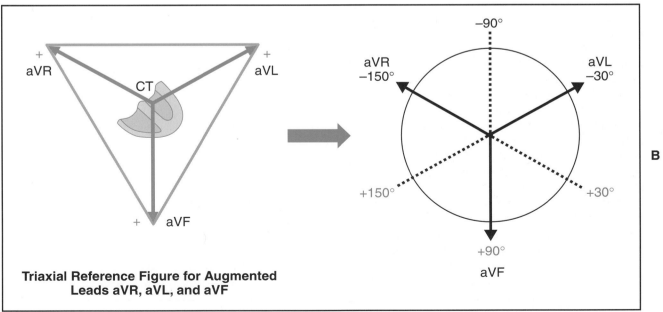

Triaxial Reference Figure for Augmented
Leads aVR, aVL, and aVF

Figure 11-7 **A,** Augmented leads aVR, aVL, and aVF and their axes.
B, Triaxial reference figure for the augmented leads.

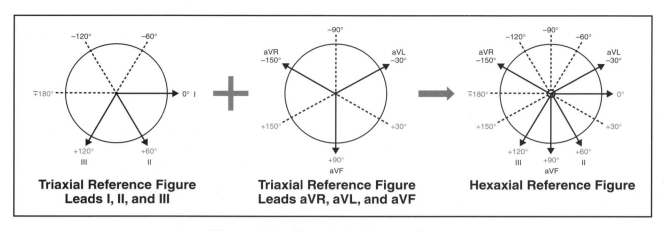

**Triaxial Reference Figure
Leads I, II, and III**

**Triaxial Reference Figure
Leads aVR, aVL, and aVF**

Hexaxial Reference Figure

Figure 11-8   Hexaxial reference figure.

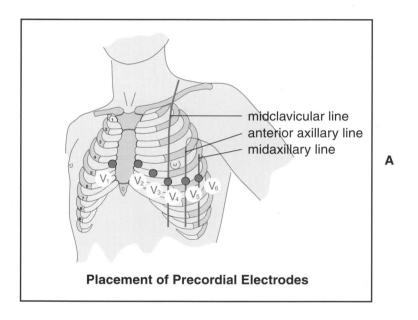

Placement of Precordial Electrodes

A

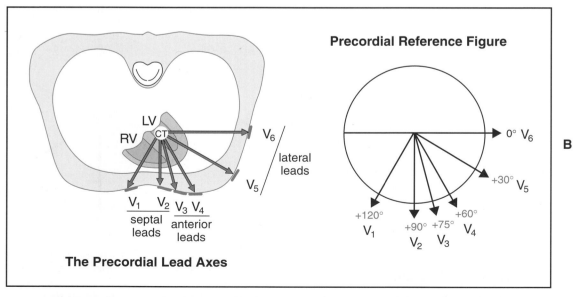

The Precordial Lead Axes

B

Figure 11-9   A, Placement of the precordial electrodes. **B,** Precordial lead axes and reference figure.

The individual chest electrodes are positioned across the anterior chest wall from right to left so that they overlie the right ventricle, the interventricular septum, and the anterior and lateral surfaces of the left ventricle. The placement of the positive chest electrodes is as follows:

◆ V_1: Right side of the sternum in the fourth intercostal space
◆ V_2: Left side of the sternum in the fourth intercostal space
◆ V_3: Midway between V_2 and V_4
◆ V_4: Left midclavicular line in the fifth intercostal space
◆ V_5: Left anterior axillary line at the same level as V_4
◆ V_6: Left midaxillary line at the same level as V_4

The chest electrodes for leads V_1 and V_2 (the right precordial [or septal] leads) overlie the right ventricle; the electrodes for leads V_3 and V_4 (the midprecordial [or anterior] leads) overlie the interventricular septum and part of the left ventricle; and those for leads V_5 and V_6 (the left precordial [or lateral] leads) overlie the rest of the left ventricle.

The lead axis for each precordial lead is drawn from the central terminal to the specific chest electrode, with the central terminal designated as the negative pole, and the chest electrode as the positive pole (Figure 11-9, *B*). A transverse (cross-sectional) outline of the chest wall showing the central terminal, the six chest electrodes, and the six precordial lead axes is called a *precordial reference figure*. It is used in plotting the heart's electrical activity in the body's horizontal plane.

RIGHT-SIDED CHEST LEADS

The precordial leads of the 12-lead ECG record the heart's electrical activity primarily over the left ventricle. To determine the electrical activity over the right ventricle, right-sided chest leads must be used. These leads—leads V_{2R}, V_{3R}, V_{4R}, V_{5R}, and V_{6R}—are obtained by attaching the positive chest electrodes to various locations on the right chest (Figure 11-10), similar to those used in the standard precordial leads, but on the opposite side of the chest. The placement of the positive right-sided chest electrodes is as follows:

◆ V_{2R}: Right side of the sternum in the fourth intercostal space
◆ V_{3R}: Midway between V_{2R} and V_{4R}
◆ V_{4R}: Right midclavicular line in the fifth intercostal space
◆ V_{5R}: Right anterior axillary line at the same level as V_{4R}
◆ V_{6R}: Right midaxillary line at the same level as V_{4R}

Right-sided chest leads are used to rule out a right ventricular myocardial infarction after the initial

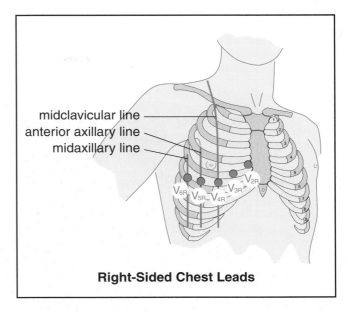

Right-Sided Chest Leads

Figure 11-10 Right-sided chest leads.

TABLE

11-1 Facing Leads

Facing Leads	Surface of the Heart Viewed
V_1-V_4	Anterior
I, aVL, V_5-V_6	Lateral
II, III, aVF	Inferior (or diaphragmatic)
V_{4R}	Right ventricle

finding of an inferior myocardial infarction. In the majority of instances, only one right-sided chest lead, lead V_{4R}, is needed to make the diagnosis.

FACING LEADS

A 12-lead ECG provides 12 different views of the electrical activity of the heart, each view looking from the outside of the chest toward the zero reference point within the chest (Table 11-1). Leads I and aVL and the precordial leads V_5 and V_6 view the lateral surface of the heart; leads II, III, and aVF view the inferior (diaphragmatic) surface; and leads V_1 through V_4 view the anterior surface of the heart. The right-sided precordial lead—lead V_{4R}—views the right ventricle. No leads face the posterior surface of the heart.

The leads that view specific surfaces of the heart are termed *facing* leads in this book (Figure 11-11). These include all of the leads except aVR, which faces the interior, endocardial surface of the ventricles.

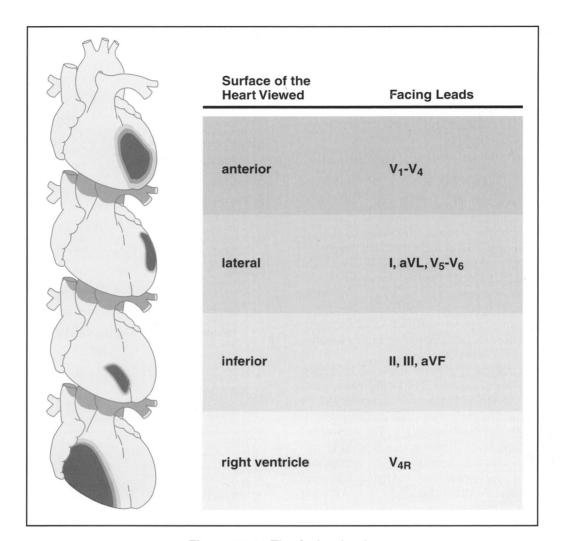

Surface of the Heart Viewed	Facing Leads
anterior	V_1-V_4
lateral	I, aVL, V_5-V_6
inferior	II, III, aVF
right ventricle	V_{4R}

Figure 11-11 The facing leads.

KEY POINT

It is important to know the facing leads in determining the location of an acute myocardial infarction!

Notes

CHAPTER REVIEW QUESTIONS

1. The electrode attached to the right leg is usually used as the _____ electrode.
   A. negative
   B. sensing
   C. probing
   D. ground

2. A _____ lead represents the difference in electrical potential between two electrodes.
   A. unipolar
   B. bipolar
   C. central
   D. terminal

3. In leads aVR, aVL, and aVF, the "a" stands for:
   A. atrial
   B. augmented
   C. arterial
   D. alternative

4. The relationships of the standard limb leads are such that the electrical currents of lead _____ + lead _____ = lead _____.
   A. I, II, III
   B. I, III, II
   C. II, III, I
   D. II, III, IV

5. To obtain lead aVL, the positive electrode is attached to the _____ arm and the other two electrodes to the _____, which, when combined, form the central terminal.
   A. left, right arm and left leg
   B. right, left arm and left leg
   C. left, right and left arms
   D. right, right and left legs

6. A _____ lead measures the difference in electrical potential between a chest electrode and the central terminal.
   A. unipolar, augmented
   B. precordial
   C. bipolar
   D. terminal

7. The placement of the V_4 positive chest electrode is:
   A. left side of the sternum in the fourth intercostal space
   B. midclavicular line in the fifth intercostal space
   C. in the anterior axillary line at the fifth intercostal space
   D. in the midaxillary line at the sixth intercostal space

8. The placement of the V_2 positive chest electrode is:
   A. midway between V_1 and V_3
   B. right side of the sternum in the fourth intercostal space
   C. anterior axillary line at the same level as V_1
   D. left side of the sternum in the fourth intercostal space

9. Correct placement of the V_{6R} positive right-sided chest electrodes is:
   A. right midclavicular line in the right fifth intercostal space
   B. midway between V_{2R} and V_{6R}
   C. right midaxillary line at the same level as V_{4R}
   D. on the right side of the sternum in the fourth intercostal space

10. The _____ surface of the heart is viewed by ECG leads II, III, and aVF.
    A. lateral
    B. anterior
    C. inferior
    D. posterior

CHAPTER OBJECTIVES

Upon completion of all or part of this chapter, you should be able to complete the following objectives:
1. Define the following terms:
   Vector
   Mean vector
   Biphasic deflection
   Equiphasic deflection
   Predominantly positive deflection
   Predominantly negative deflection
2. Define the following terms:
   Instantaneous electrical axis or vector
   Cardiac vector
   Mean QRS axis
   P axis
   T axis
3. Identify and label on a hexaxial figure (1) the 12 spokes of the hexaxial figure according to their polarity and degree and (2) the four quadrants.
4. Identify and label the lead axes of the six limb leads, their negative and positive poles, their direction in degrees, and their perpendiculars on a hexaxial figure in the frontal plane.
5. Define the following terms:
   Normal QRS axis
   Left axis deviation (LAD)
   Right axis deviation (RAD)
   Indeterminate axis (IND)
6. List the cardiac and pulmonary causes of left and right axis deviation.
7. List three major reasons for determining the QRS axis in an emergency situation.
8. List six important points to remember in the process of determining the QRS axis using leads I, II, and aVF.
9. List the basic steps in determining the QRS axis using leads I, II, III, and aVF.

ELECTRICAL AXES AND VECTORS

The electrical current generated by the depolarization or repolarization of the atria or ventricles at any given moment is called an *instantaneous cardiac vector* (Figure 12-1). It is commonly visualized graphically as an arrow that has magnitude, direction, and polarity (Figure 12-2). The length of the shaft of the arrow represents the magnitude of the electrical current; the orientation or position of the arrow indicates the direction of flow of the electrical current; the tip of the arrow represents the positive pole of the electrical current, and the tail is the negative pole.

The sequence of instantaneous electrical currents produced by the depolarization of the ventricles during one cardiac cycle, for example, can be depicted as a series of cardiac vectors, each representing the mo-

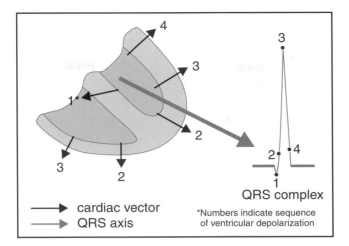

Figure 12-1   Cardiac vectors and the QRS axis.

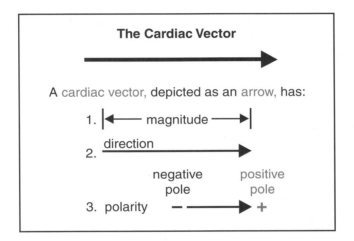

Figure 12-2   The cardiac vector.

ment-to-moment electrical current generated by depolarization of a small segment of the ventricular wall.

The initial cardiac vector represents the depolarization of the interventricular septum (1) and is directed from left to right. This is followed immediately by a sequence of vectors produced by the endocardial to epicardial depolarization of segments of the ventricular wall, beginning in the right and left ventricles in the apical region of the heart near the septum (2), continuing through the thin wall of the right ventricle and the thick lateral wall of the left ventricle (3), and ending in the lateral and posterior aspect of the left ventricle near its base (4).

The vectors arising in the right ventricle are directed mostly to the right when viewed in the frontal plane; those in the left ventricle are directed mostly to the left. The left ventricular vectors are larger and persist longer than those of the smaller right ventri-

cle, primarily because of the much greater thickness of the left ventricular wall.

The mean (or average) of all vectors that result from ventricular depolarization is a single large vector depicted as an arrow having magnitude and a direction—the *mean QRS axis* or, simply, the *QRS axis*. Normally, the QRS axis points to the left and downward, reflecting the dominance of the left ventricle over the right ventricle.

The mean of all vectors generated during the depolarization of the atria is the P axis; those generated during repolarization of the ventricles are the ST axis and T axis (Figure 12-3).

The P axis is rarely determined. The T axis is determined in certain conditions, such as myocardial ischemia and acute myocardial infarction, in which there is a significant shift in the direction of the T axis. Determination of the shift in the T axis helps to localize the affected area of the myocardium. The

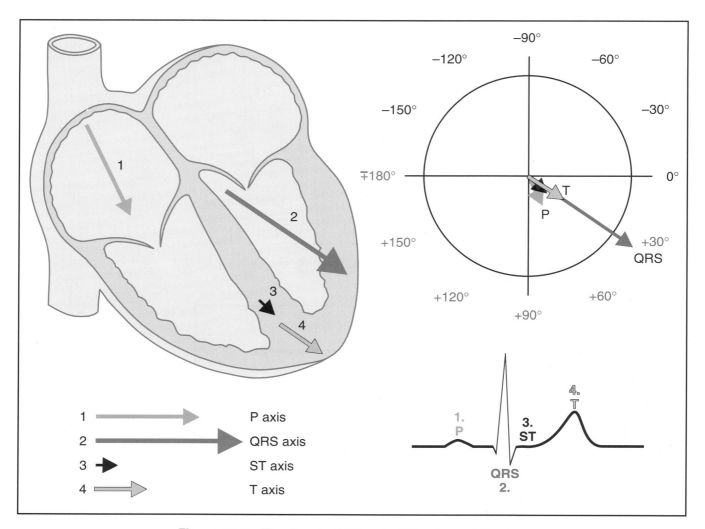

Figure 12-3   The P axis, QRS axis, ST axis, and T axis.

QRS axis is the most important and also the most frequently determined axis. Commonly, when the term *axis* is used alone, it refers to the QRS axis.

THE ELECTRICAL CURRENT, VECTORS, AND THE LEAD AXIS

An electrical current flowing parallel to the axis of a lead, the hypothetical line joining the negative and positive poles of a lead, produces either a positive or negative deflection on an electrocardiogram (ECG), depending on the direction of its flow. An electrical current flowing toward the positive pole produces a positive deflection on the ECG; one that flows toward the negative pole produces a negative deflection. The greater the magnitude of the electrical current, the larger the deflection, and vice versa. When the flow of electrical current is perpendicular to the axis of a

lead, no deflection is produced. Figure 12-4, *A* shows the relationship between the direction of flow of an electrical current, as represented by a vector, and the deflection it produces on an ECG.

When an electrical current flows in a direction that is somewhat between being parallel and perpendicular (i.e., oblique), the deflection is smaller than when the same electrical current flows parallel to the axis of a lead. The more parallel the electrical current is to the axis of the lead, the larger is the deflection; the more perpendicular, the smaller the deflection. This is true whether the electrical current is flowing toward or away from the positive pole (Figure 12-4, *B*).

When an electrical current flows partly toward and partly away from the positive pole, a bidirectional electrical current is present. It is represented by a single mean vector that is an average of all the positive and negative electrical currents (or vectors) present. Such an electrical current produces a biphasic deflec-

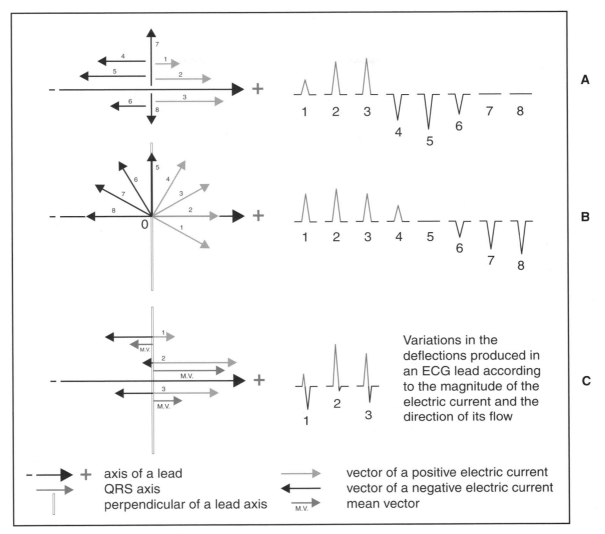

Figure 12-4   The axis of a lead, its perpendicular, and the direction of flow of electrical currents.

Continued

tion on the ECG, one that is partly positive and partly negative. The size of the components of the deflection depends on the magnitude of the individual electrical currents. If the mean (or average) direction of the biphasic deflection in an ECG is positive, no matter by how much, the deflection is predominantly positive; if the mean direction is negative, the deflection is predominantly negative.

Figure 12-4, *C* shows the relationship between a bidirectional electrical current, as represented by a mean vector, and the biphasic deflections on an ECG.

The more parallel the mean vector of a biphasic deflection is to the axis of the lead, the more positive is the biphasic deflection; the closer the orientation of the mean vector is to the perpendicular, the less positive is the biphasic deflection. When

the positive and negative deflections are equal in magnitude, an equiphasic deflection is present, and the sum of the deflections is zero. In this case, the mean vector is perpendicular to the lead axis (Figure 12-4, *D*).

It is important to understand the significance of the relationship between the predominant direction of the deflections of the QRS complexes in a given lead, the perpendicular of the related lead axis, and the QRS axis. A predominantly positive QRS complex in a given lead indicates that the positive pole of the vector of the QRS axis lies somewhere on the positive side of the perpendicular to that lead axis. Conversely, a predominantly negative QRS complex in a lead indicates that the positive pole of the vector of the QRS axis lies somewhere on the negative side of the perpendicular (Figure 12-4, *E*).

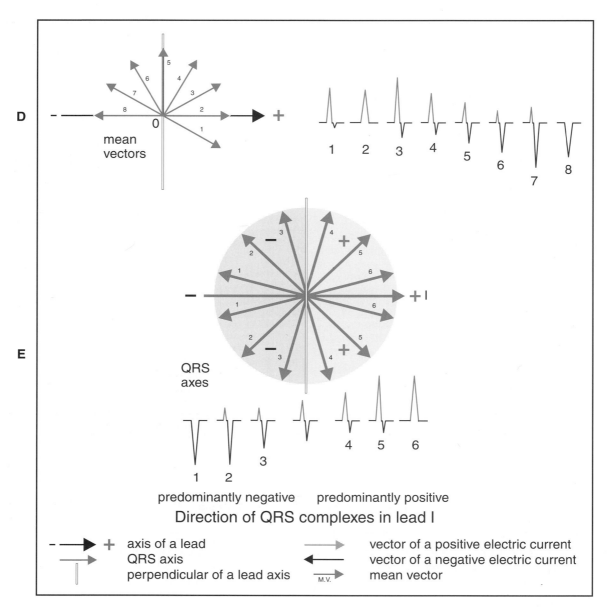

Figure 12-4, cont'd For legend see page 257.

Thus the perpendicular to an axis of a lead serves as a boundary between the predominantly positive and predominantly negative deflections of a QRS complex in any given lead.

THE HEXAXIAL REFERENCE FIGURE

The hexaxial reference figure, as noted earlier, is a composite of the two triaxial reference figures, formed by combining the axes of the three standard limb leads (I, II, III) and the three augmented leads (aVR, aVL, aVF) (Figure 12-5, *A*). The primary purpose of the hexaxial reference figure is to aid in the determination of the direction of the QRS axis in the frontal plane with some degree of precision.

Viewed from the front, the six lead axes are arranged like spokes within a wheel through a central point representing the potentially "zero" center of the heart. The axes of the leads are positioned within the wheel consistent with their actual direction and polarity in the frontal plane so that their positive and negative poles are spaced 30 degrees apart around the rim of the wheel.

Each positive and negative pole is assigned a degree number ranging from 0° to 180°. The poles around the rim of the upper half of the wheel of the

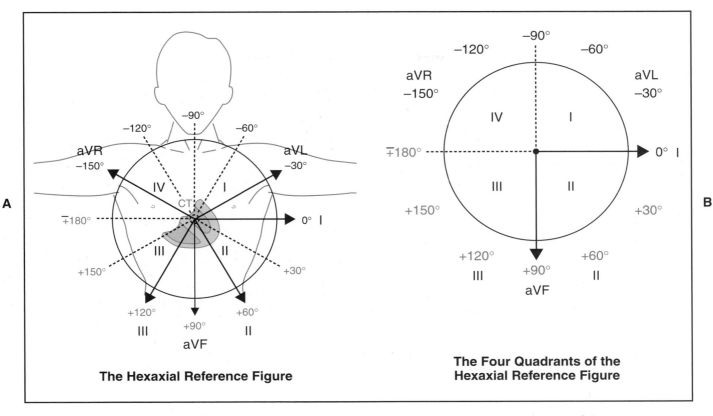

The Hexaxial Reference Figure

The Four Quadrants of the
Hexaxial Reference Figure

Figure 12-5 **A,** The hexaxial reference figure. **B,** The four quadrants of the hexaxial reference figure.

hexaxial reference figure are given negative degree numbers (−30°, −60°, −90°, −120°, −150°, and −180°); those around the lower half of the rim are given positive degree numbers (+30°, +60°, +90°, +120°, +150°, and +180°). The negative and positive degrees should not be confused with the negative and positive poles of the lead axes.

The positive and negative poles of the axes of the three standard limb leads and the three augmented leads are assigned the following degree numbers:

Standard Leads	−Pole	+Pole
Lead I	±180°	0°
Lead II	−120°	+60°
Lead III	−60°	+120°

Augmented Leads	−Pole	+Pole
Lead aVR	+30°	−150°
Lead aVL	+150°	−30°
Lead aVF	−90°	+90°

The hexaxial reference figure is divided into four quadrants by the bisection of lead axes I and aVF (Figure 12-5, *B*). Although there are several different

ways to designate the quadrants, the following designation is used in this book:

Quadrant	Number
0° to −90°	I
0° to +90°	II
+90° to ±180°	III
−90° to ±180°	IV

In some texts, the degree numbers in quadrant IV used here (i.e., −90°, −120°, −150°, and ±180°) are replaced by +270° (−90°), +240°, +210°, and +180°, respectively.

The perpendiculars of the lead axes have the same attributes as those of the lead axes with which they coincide (i.e., their coincident leads) (Figure 12-6). For example, the perpendicular to the axis of lead II, which coincides with the axis of lead aVL, has one pole at −30° and the other at +150°.

Table 12-1 summarizes the location of the negative and positive poles of the lead axes and their perpendiculars.

THE QRS AXIS

The normal QRS axis, as determined using the hexaxial reference figure, lies between −30° and +90°

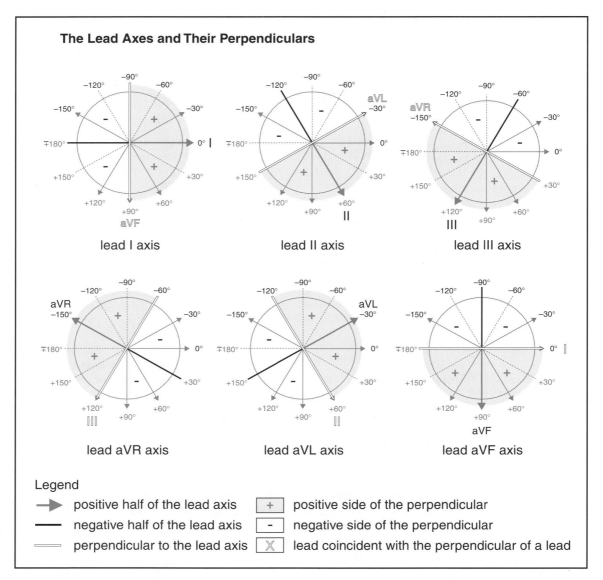

Figure 12-6 The lead axes and their perpendiculars.

TABLE

12-1 Negative and Positive Poles of the Lead Axes and Their Perpendiculars

Lead	Location of Lead Axis Poles −Pole	+Pole	Location of the Poles of the Perpendicular (and its coincident lead axis)
I	±180°	0°	−90°, +90° (aVF)
II	−120°	+60°	+150°, −30° (aVL)
III	−60°	+120°	+30°, −150° (aVR)
aVR	+30°	−150°	−60°, +120° (III)
aVL	+150°	−30°	−120°, +60° (II)
aVF	−90°	+90°	±180°, 0° (I)

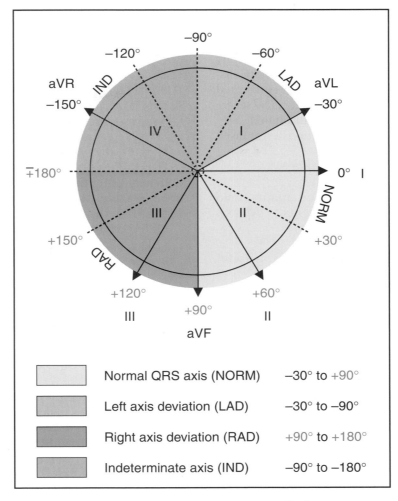

Figure 12-7 Normal and abnormal QRS axes.

Normal QRS axis (NORM)	−30° to +90°
Left axis deviation (LAD)	−30° to −90°
Right axis deviation (RAD)	+90° to +180°
Indeterminate axis (IND)	−90° to −180°

in the frontal plane (Figure 12-7). A change or "shift" in the direction of the QRS axis from normal to one between −30° and −90° is considered *left axis deviation (LAD)*; a shift of the QRS axis to one between +90° and ±180° is *right axis deviation (RAD)*. A QRS axis rarely falls between −90° and ±180°. If it does, extreme RAD or an *indeterminate axis (IND)* is present.

A QRS complex with LAD (i.e., a QRS axis greater than −30°) is always abnormal. A QRS complex with RAD (i.e., a QRS axis greater than +90°) may or may not be abnormal, depending on the age and body build of the patient. RAD of up to +120° or more may be present in newborns and infants, with RAD up to about +110° present in young adults with long, narrow chests and vertical hearts.

In the majority of adults, however, RAD is seldom present without some cardiac or pulmonary disorder.

For this reason, such a disorder should be suspected whenever RAD is present in adults.

In general, the causes of abnormal shift of the QRS axis to the left or right are (1) ventricular enlargement and hypertrophy and (2) bundle branch and fascicular block (see Chapters 13 and 14).

LAD (QRS axis greater then −30°) occurs in adults in the following cardiac disorders:

◆ Left ventricular enlargement and hypertrophy caused by systemic hypertension, aortic stenosis, ischemic heart disease, or other disorders affecting the left ventricle
◆ Left bundle branch block and left anterior fascicular block
◆ Premature ventricular contractions (PVCs) and ventricular tachycardia (VT) of right ventricular origin
◆ Inferior myocardial infarction (late)

RAD (QRS axis greater than +90°) occurs in adults with the following cardiac and pulmonary disorders:

◆ Right ventricular enlargement and hypertrophy secondary to chronic obstructive pulmonary disease (COPD), pulmonary embolism, congenital heart disease, and other disorders that cause severe pulmonary hypertension or cor pulmonale

◆ Right bundle branch block and left posterior fascicular block

◆ PVCs and VT of left ventricular origin

◆ Lateral myocardial infarction (late)

◆ Normal variant in the newborn and infants (QRS axis up to +120°) and young adults (QRS axis up to +110°)

◆ Dextrocardia

The determination of the QRS axis may be useful in the following emergency situations:

◆ In acute myocardial infarction to determine if an acute left anterior or posterior fascicular block is present

◆ In acute pulmonary embolism to determine if right ventricular stretching and enlargement and subsequent acute right bundle branch block are present

◆ In tachycardia with wide QRS complexes to differentiate between a tachycardia arising in the ventricles (ventricular ectopy) and one arising in the sinoatrial (SA) node, atria, or atrioventricular (AV) junction, with wide QRS complexes caused by a preexisting intraventricular conduction disturbance (such as a bundle branch block), aberrant ventricular conduction, or ventricular preexcitation

Determination of the QRS Axis

Several methods are used to determine the QRS axis. The most accurate method is by plotting leads I and III (or leads I and II) on a triaxial reference grid and calculating the axis by angulation. This method is somewhat time consuming and not adaptable to emergency situations. It is easier and quicker to approximate the QRS axes in the frontal plane using the hexaxial reference figure as follows:

◆ First, determine the net positivity or negativity of the QRS complexes in certain limb leads (i.e., whether the QRS complexes are predominantly positive or negative)

◆ Then, by using this information and knowing the perpendiculars to these leads, determine the approximate QRS axis on the hexaxial reference figure

Lead I is usually evaluated first, then lead II. Between the two, it can be determined whether the QRS axis is normal or LAD or RAD is present. Depending on the findings at this point, one or more of the other leads (i.e., leads III, aVF, aVR, and, rarely, aVL) are evaluated to determine the location of the QRS axis with greater accuracy if necessary. The next section depicts the basics of determining the QRS axis using the hexaxial reference figure. Several specific methods for determining the QRS axis are presented in Appendix A, *Methods of Determining the QRS Axis.*

Important points to remember in determining the QRS axis using the hexaxial reference figure are outlined in Table 12-2 and include the following:

1. Lead II in the presence of a predominantly positive QRS complex in lead I helps to determine whether LAD is present (Figure 12-8)
   a. A predominantly positive QRS complex in lead II indicates a normal QRS axis (−30° to +90° degrees = Normal)
   b. A predominantly negative QRS complex in lead II indicates an LAD (−30° to –90° = LAD)

2. Lead aVF, in the presence of a predominantly positive QRS complex in lead I, helps to determine whether the QRS axis lies in quadrant I or II (Figure 12-9)
   a. A predominantly positive QRS complex in lead aVF indicates that the QRS axis is in quadrant II (0° to +90° = Normal)
   b. A predominantly negative QRS complex in lead aVF indicates that the QRS axis is in quadrant I (0° to −90° = partly Normal, partly LAD)

3. Lead aVF, in the presence of a predominantly negative QRS complex in lead I, helps to determine whether the QRS axis lies in quadrant III or IV (Figure 12-10)
   a. A predominantly positive QRS complex in lead aVF indicates that the QRS axis is in quadrant III (+90° to ±180° = RAD)
   b. A predominantly negative QRS complex in lead aVF indicates that the QRS axis is in quadrant IV (−90° to ±180° = IND)

Other important points to remember include the following:

1. Lead II is the single lead that holds the clue in detecting LAD because its perpendicular coincides with the positive pole of the axis of lead aVL (−30°)

2. A predominantly positive QRS complex in lead I excludes RAD

3. A predominantly negative QRS complex in lead I and a predominantly positive QRS complex in lead aVR indicate a RAD (>+120°)

4. A QRS axis between −90° and ±180° (quadrant IV) indicating IND is rare except in ventricular ectopy

TABLE

12-2 Basic Points to Remember in Determining the QRS Axis

	Leads				
I	II	aVF	QRS axis range	Quadrant	Axis
Positive	Positive		−30° to +90°		Normal
Positive	Negative		−30° to −90°		LAD
Positive		Positive	0° to +90°	II	Normal
Positive		Negative	0° to −90°	I	LAD, Normal
Negative		Positive	+90° to ±180°	III	RAD
Negative		Negative	−90° to ±180°	IV	IND

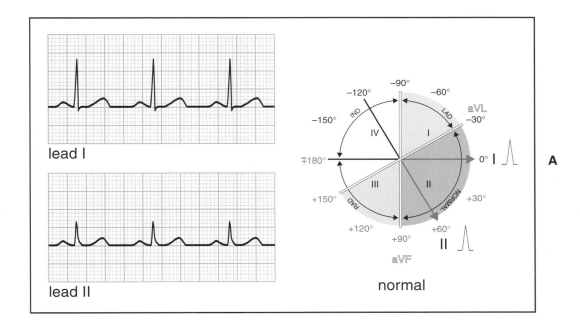

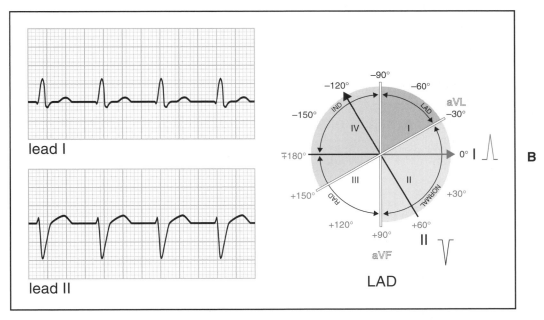

Figure 12-8 **A,** Normal QRS axis. **B,** Left axis deviation.

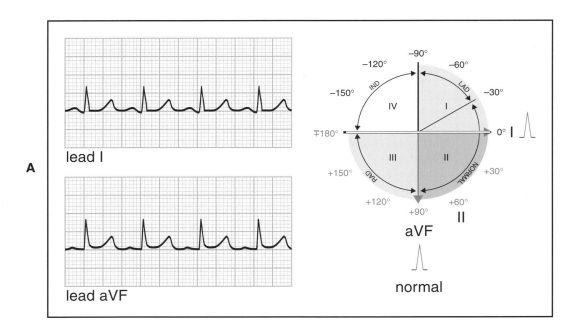

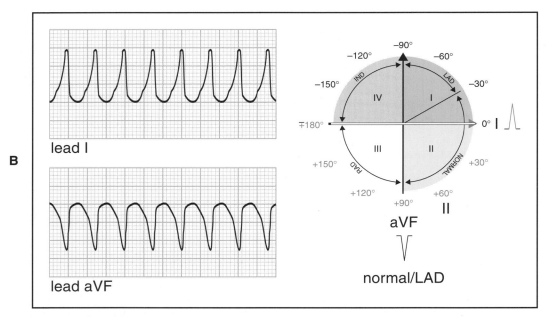

Figure 12-9 **A,** Normal QRS axis. **B,** Partially normal and partially left axis deviation.

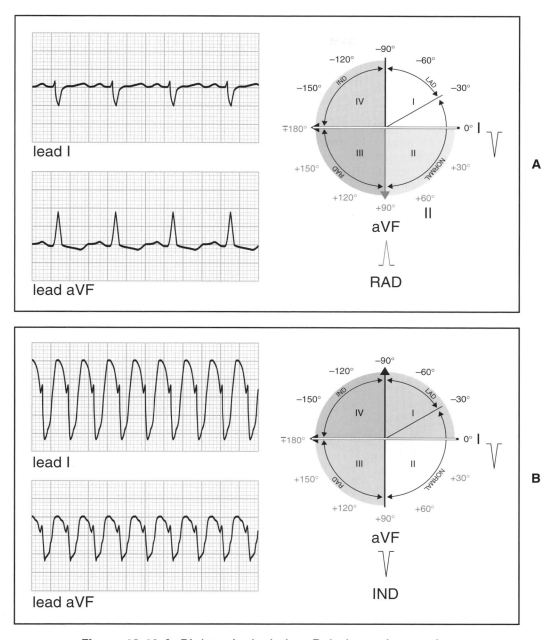

Figure 12-10 A, Right axis deviation. **B,** Indeterminate axis.

Basic Steps in Determining the QRS Axis

There are three basic steps in determining the QRS axis:

◆ STEP 1

◆ Determine the net positivity or negativity of the QRS complexes in lead I.

A. If the QRS complexes are predominantly *positive* in lead I, the QRS axis lies between −90° and +90° (i.e., in quadrant I or II). The QRS axis may be between –30° and +90° (normal QRS axis) or between –30° and –90° (LAD).

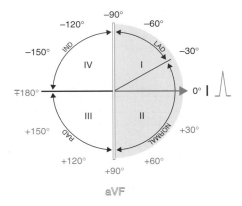

aVF

B. If the QRS complexes are predominantly *negative* in lead I, the QRS axis is greater than +90° (lying between +90° and −90°), indicating right axis deviation. Most likely, the QRS axis lies in quadrant III and, rarely, in quadrant IV.

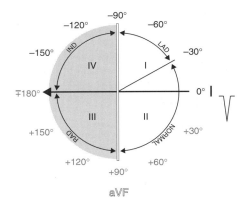

aVF

NOTE: If the QRS complexes are predominately *positive* in lead I, proceed to *Step 2*. If the QRS complexes are predominantly *negative* in lead I, proceed to *Step 3*.

KEY POINT

The steps used in determining the QRS axis outlined here may be modified according to the specific method used in determining the QRS axis or to local protocol.

Leads					Location of QRS Axis
I	II	aVF	III	aVR	
+	+	+	+		+30° to +90°
+	+	+	−		0° to +30°
+	+	−	−		0° to −30°
+	−	−	−		−30° to −90°
−	+	+	+	−	+90° to +120°
−	+	+	+	+	+120° to +150°
−	−	−	−		−90° to −150°

Equiphasic Leads						Location of QRS Axis
I	II	aVF	III	aVR	aVL	
±	−	−	−	+		−90
+	−	−	−	±		−60
+	±	−	−	−		−30
+	+	±	−	−		0
+	+	+	±	−		+30
+	+	+	+	−	±	+60
±	+	+	+	−		+90
−	+	+	+	±		+120
−	±	+	+	+		+150
−	−	±	+	+		±180
−	−	−	±	+		−150
−	−	−	−	+	±	−120

+, Predominantly positive.
−, Predominantly negative.
±, Equiphasic.

◆ STEP 2

If the QRS complexes are predominantly *positive* in lead I:

◆ Determine the net positivity or negativity of the QRS complexes in one or more of the following three leads (II, aVF, and III):

Lead II

A. If the QRS complexes are predominantly *positive* in lead II, the QRS axis is between −30° and +90° (normal QRS axis).

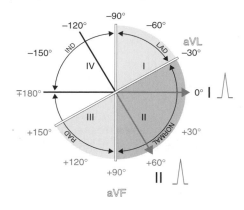

B. If the QRS complexes are predominantly *negative* in lead II, the QRS axis is between −30° and –90° (left axis deviation).

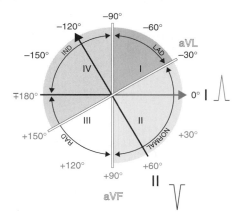

Lead aVF

C. If the QRS complexes are predominantly *positive* in lead aVF, the QRS axis is between 0° and +90° (quadrant II).

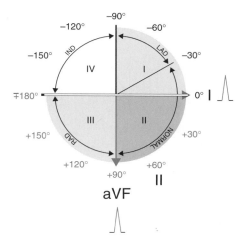

D. If the QRS complexes are predominantly *negative* in lead aVF, the QRS axis is between 0° and −90° (quadrant I).

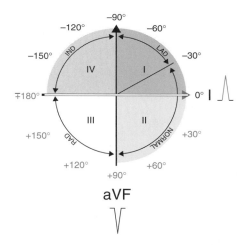

Lead III

E. If the QRS complexes are predominantly *positive* in lead III, the QRS axis is between +30° and +90°.

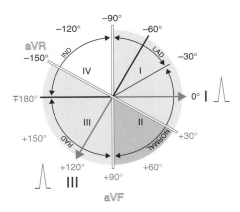

F. If the QRS complexes are predominantly *negative* in lead III, the QRS axis is between +30° and −90°.

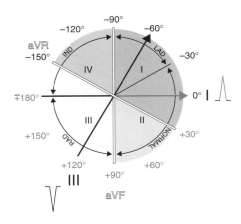

◆ STEP 3

If the QRS complexes are predominantly *negative* in lead I:

◆ Determine the net positivity or negativity of the QRS complexes in one or more of the following four leads (II, aVF, III, and aVR):

Lead II

A. If the QRS complexes are predominantly *positive* in lead II, the QRS axis is between +90° and +150°.

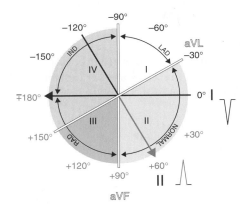

B. If the QRS complexes are predominantly *negative* in lead II, the QRS axis is greater than +150°.

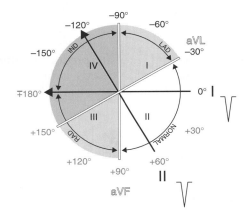

Lead aVF

C. If the QRS complexes are predominantly *positive* in lead aVF, the QRS axis is between +90° and +180° (quadrant III).

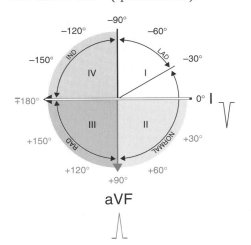

D. If the QRS complexes are predominantly *nega-tive* in lead aVF, the QRS axis is between −90° and −180° (quadrant IV).

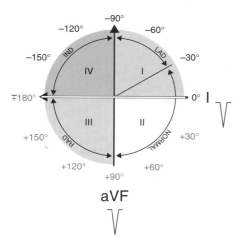

Lead III

E. If the QRS complexes are predominantly *posi-tive* in lead III, the QRS axis is between +90° and −150°.

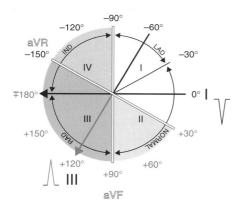

F. If the QRS complexes are predominantly *nega-tive* in lead III, the QRS axis is between −90° and −150°.

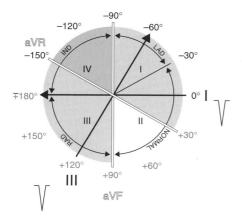

Lead aVR

G. If the QRS complexes are predominantly *posi-tive* in lead aVR, the QRS axis is greater than +120° (severe right axis deviation).

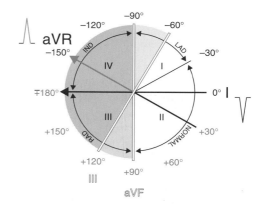

H. If the QRS complexes are predominantly *negative* in lead aVR, the QRS axis is between +90° and +120° (mild to moderate right axis deviation).

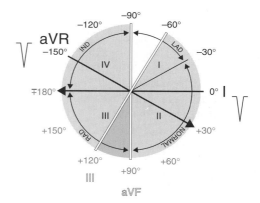

Notes

_____

_____

_____

_____

_____

_____

_____

_____

_____

_____

_____

_____

CHAPTER REVIEW QUESTIONS

1. The mean of all vectors generated during the depolarization of the atria is the _____ axis.
   A. P
   B. QRS
   C. ST
   D. T

2. An electrical current flowing toward the positive pole of a lead produces a(n) _____ on the ECG.
   A. elongated deflection
   B. parallel deflection
   C. positive deflection
   D. negative deflection

3. The more parallel the electrical current is to the axis of the lead, the _____ the deflection.
   A. more oblique
   B. larger
   C. smaller
   D. more regular

4. A predominantly positive QRS complex in a given lead indicates that the _____ pole of the vector of the QRS axis lies somewhere on the _____ side of the perpendicular axis.
   A. positive, positive
   B. positive, negative
   C. negative, negative
   D. negative, positive

5. A QRS complex with right axis deviation is:
   A. greater than $-90°$
   B. always abnormal
   C. greater than $+90°$
   D. greater than $-30°$

6. Left axis deviation with a QRS axis greater than $-30°$ occurs in adults with the following cardiac condition(s):
   A. hypertension
   B. aortic stenosis
   C. ischemic heart disease
   D. all of the above

7. Right axis deviation occurs in adults with which of the following disorders?
   A. dextrocardia
   B. right ventricular hypertrophy
   C. both of the above
   D. neither of the above

8. Patients who have right ventricular enlargement and hypertrophy secondary to pulmonary embolism, COPD, or cor pulmonale may most likely have an axis deviation of:
   A. greater than $+90°$
   B. between 0 and $+90°$
   C. between 0 and $-60°$
   D. greater than $-60°$

9. The determination of the QRS axis may be useful in which of the following emergency situations?
   A. acute myocardial infarction
   B. acute pulmonary embolism
   C. tachycardia with wide QRS complexes
   D. all of the above

10. If the QRS complexes are predominantly positive in leads I and aVF, the QRS axis is between:
    A. $-30°$ and $+90°$
    B. $0°$ and $+90°$
    C. $0°$ and $-90°$
    D. $+30°$ and $+90°$

CHAPTER OUTLINE

CHAPTER OBJECTIVES

Upon completion of all or part of this chapter, you
should be able to complete the following objectives:
1. Name and identify the atrioventricular (AV) node and
   the parts of the electrical conduction system within
   the ventricles on an anatomical drawing.
2. Name the artery or arteries that supply the following
   structures of the electrical conduction system:
   Interventricular septum
       Posterior portion
       Anterior portion
       Middle portion

AV node
Bundle of His
    Proximal part
    Distal part
Right bundle branch
    Proximal part
    Distal part
Left bundle branch
    Main stem
    Left anterior fascicle
    Left posterior fascicle

ANATOMY AND PHYSIOLOGY OF THE ELECTRICAL CONDUCTION SYSTEM

Anatomy of the Electrical Conduction System

The electrical conduction system located below the atrioventricular (AV) node and within the ventricles—the His-Purkinje system of the ventricles—consists of the bundle of His, the right and left bundle branches, and the Purkinje network, the terminal portion of the electrical conduction system composed of extremely fine Purkinje fibers (Figure 13-1).

The long, thin, round right bundle branch runs down the right side of the interventricular septum to conduct the electrical impulses to the right ventricle. The left bundle branch, which consists of a short, thick, flat left common bundle branch (or main stem) and two main divisions—the left anterior and posterior fascicles—conducts the electrical impulses to the left ventricle, including the interventricular septum. The relatively long, thin left anterior fascicle occupies the left side of the anterior wall of the interventricular septum. It conducts the electrical impulses from the main stem of the left bundle branch to the anterior and lateral walls of the left ventricle. The short, broad left posterior fascicle, which runs down the posterior wall of the interventricular septum, conducts the electrical impulses to the posterior wall of the left ventricle.

Blood Supply to the Electrical Conduction System

The anterior two thirds of the interventricular septum is supplied by the left anterior descending coronary artery of the left coronary artery; the posterior third of the septum is supplied by the posterior descending coronary artery. The posterior descending coronary artery arises from the right coronary artery in 85% to 90% of the hearts and from the left circumflex coronary artery of the left coronary artery in the other 10% to 15%.

The main blood supply of the AV node and proximal part of the bundle of His is the AV node artery (see Figure 13-1), which, like the posterior descending coronary artery, arises from the RCA in 85% to 90% of the hearts and, in the other 10% to 15%, from the left circumflex coronary artery.

In most hearts, the left anterior descending coronary artery, by way of its branches (particularly the septal perforator arteries), is the main blood supply to the distal part of the bundle of His, the entire right bundle branch (including the proximal and distal parts), the main stem of the left bundle branch, and the left anterior fascicle. Occasionally, the posterior descending coronary artery also supplies the distal part of the bundle of His, the proximal part of the right bundle branch, and the main stem of the left bundle branch.

The left posterior fascicle is supplied by both the left anterior descending coronary artery (anteriorly) and the posterior descending coronary artery (posteriorly).

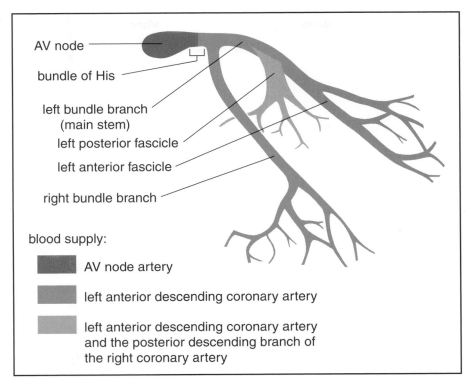

Figure 13-1 The electrical conduction system and its blood supply in most hearts.

TABLE

13-1   The Electrical Conduction System and Its Primary and Alternate Blood Supply

Electrical Conduction System	Primary Blood Supply	Alternate Blood Supply
AV node	AV node artery	None
Bundle of His		
Proximal	AV node artery	None
Distal	LAD	PDA
Right bundle branch		
Proximal	LAD	PDA
Distal	LAD	None
Left bundle branch		
Main stem	LAD	PDA
Left anterior fascicle	LAD	None
Left posterior fascicle	LAD and PDA	None

AV, Atrioventricular; *LAD,* left anterior descending artery by way of the septal perforator arteries; *PDA,* posterior descending coronary artery.

Table 13-1 summarizes the blood supply to the various parts of the electrical conduction system.

Physiology of the Electrical Conduction System

Normally, in a heart with an intact, viable interventricular septum, the electrical impulses progress through the right bundle branch and left bundle branch and its fascicles simultaneously (Figure 13-2), causing first the depolarization of the interventricular septum *(1)* and then the synchronous depolarization of the right and left ventricles *(2).* The electrical activity generated by the depolarization of the smaller right ventricle is buried in that generated by the left ventricle.

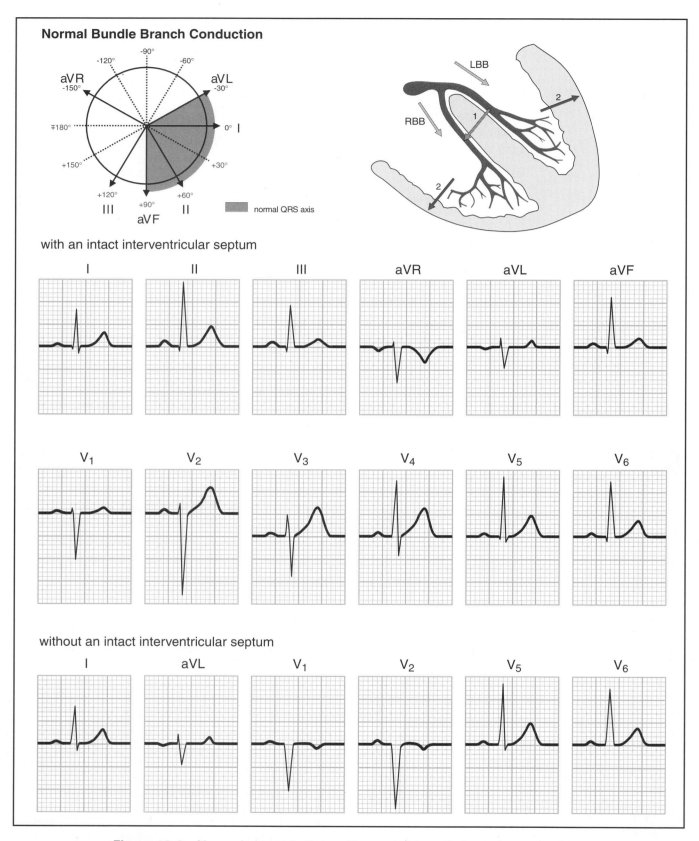

Figure 13-2 Normal sinus rhythm with normal bundle branch conduction.

> **KEY POINT**
>
> *An intact, viable interventricular septum is one that is capable of conducting an electrical impulse and depolarizing from left to right, producing an initial small q or r wave in the QRS complex, depending on the lead. An interventricular septum that is not intact or viable because of some form of heart disease, such as an anteroseptal myocardial infarction (MI), is unable to conduct an electrical impulse and depolarize normally. This results in the absence of a normal initial small q or r wave in the QRS complex.*

In a heart with normal bundle branch conduction but without an intact interventricular septum, depolarization of the nonviable interventricular septum does not occur as in *(2)*. The depolarization of the left and right ventricles, however, occurs as mentioned earlier in a heart with an intact septum.

Electrocardiograms (ECGs) typical of normal bundle branch conduction with and without an intact interventricular septum and their QRS axes are shown in Figure 13-2.

The time it takes for depolarization of the interventricular septum and the ventricle under a facing precordial lead, including the endocardial to epicardial depolarization of the ventricular wall, is commonly called the *ventricular activation time (VAT)* (Figure 13-3), or the *preintrinsicoid deflection*, the *intrinsicoid deflection time (IDT)*, the *duration of the intrinsicoid deflection*, or the *R peak time.*

The VAT is measured from the onset of the QRS complex to the peak of the last R wave in the QRS complex. Normally, it is less than 0.035 second in the right precordial leads V_1 and V_2 and less than 0.055 second in the left precordial leads V_5 and V_6. The rest of the QRS complex, from the peak of the R wave to the onset of the ST segment, or the *J point*, represents the final depolarization of the ventricles progressing away from the facing lead.

The downstroke of the R wave, which begins at the peak of the R wave and ends at the J point or tip of the following S wave, is called the *intrinsicoid deflection*. The VAT is prolonged in leads V_1 and V_2 in right bundle branch block (RBBB) and right ventricular hypertrophy and in leads V_5 and V_6 in left bundle branch block (LBBB) and left ventricular hypertrophy.

PATHOPHYSIOLOGY OF BUNDLE BRANCH AND FASCICULAR BLOCKS

The relatively thin right bundle branch is more vulnerable to disruption than the left bundle branch with its short, thick, wide main stem and widely spread fascicles. A relatively small lesion can disrupt the right bundle branch and cause a block, whereas a much more widespread lesion is necessary to block the less vulnerable main stem of the left bundle branch.

The left anterior fascicle of the left bundle branch, like the right bundle branch, is also thin and vulnerable to disruption. The left posterior fascicle, on the other hand, because it is short and thick and supplied by both the right coronary artery (via the posterior descending coronary artery) and the left anterior descending coronary artery, is rarely disrupted.

Right and left bundle branch block may be present in a heart with a normal, intact, and viable septum and in one whose septum has been damaged (e.g., by an anteroseptal MI).

Causes of Bundle Branch and Fascicular Blocks

Although bundle branch and fascicular blocks may be present on rare occasions in normal hearts, they are usually the result of heart disease. Common causes of bundle branch and fascicular blocks include the following:

◆ Ischemic heart disease affecting the interventricular septum within which the bundle branch or fascicle lies
◆ Acute MI; the relationship between the area of acute MI and the associated bundle branch and fascicular blocks are listed in Table 13-2 and expanded upon as follows:
  ◇ RBBB primarily occurs secondary to an anteroseptal MI and, rarely, to a right ventricular MI
  ◇ LBBB primarily occurs secondary to an anteroseptal and, rarely, to a right ventricular MI
  ◇ Left anterior fascicle block primarily occurs secondary to an anteroseptal MI
  ◇ Left posterior fascicle block is relatively rare in acute MI because both the left anterior descending coronary artery and the posterior descending coronary artery of the right coronary artery (or less commonly of the left circumflex artery) have to be occluded for left posterior fascicle block to occur, such as in an anteroseptal MI combined with a right ventricular or inferior MI.
◆ Idiopathic degenerative disease of the electrical conduction system with fibrosis and/or sclerosis and disruption of the conduction fibers (Lenegre's disease and Lev's disease)

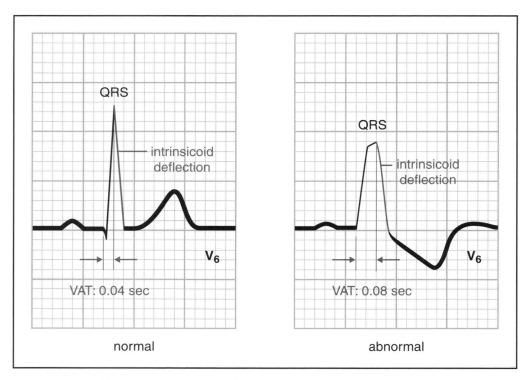

Figure 13-3 The ventricular activation time and intrinsicoid deflection.

TABLE

13-2 The Bundle Branch and Fascicular Blocks and the Acute Myocardial Infarctions That Usually Cause Them

Bundle Branch and Fascicular Block	Myocardial Infarction (Coronary Artery Involved)
Right bundle branch block	Anteroseptal (LAD)
	OR
	Right ventricular (RCA)
Left bundle branch block	Anteroseptal (LAD)
	OR
	Right ventricular (RCA)
Left anterior fascicular block	Anteroseptal (LAD)
Left posterior fascicular block	Anteroseptal (LAD)
	AND
	Right ventricular (RCA)
	OR
	Inferior (distal RCA or LCX)

LAD, Left anterior descending coronary artery; *LCX,* left circumflex coronary artery; *RCA,* right coronary artery.

◆ Cardiomyopathy, a primary disease of the myocardium affecting the bundle branches, often of unknown etiology

◆ Severe left ventricular hypertrophy (LVH) from whatever cause, such as hypertensive heart disease, may result in LBBB

◆ Aberrant ventricular conduction (or, simply, aberrancy) (i.e., the transient inability of the right or left bundle branch to conduct an electrical impulse normally. This may occur when an electrical impulse arrives at the bundle branch while it is still refractory after conducting a previous electri-

cal impulse, as in supraventricular premature contractions and tachycardias)
◆ Miscellaneous causes, acute or chronic, include the following:
  ◇ Acute congestive heart failure, acute pulmonary embolism or infarction, acute pericarditis or myocarditis
  ◇ Aortic valve disease, cardiac tumors, and syphilitic, rheumatic, and congenital heart disease
  ◇ Trauma, including cardiac catheterization, coronary angiography, and cardiac surgery
  ◇ Potassium overdose

Significance of Bundle Branch and Fascicular Blocks

A bundle branch or fascicular block by itself is not significant and requires no treatment. The underlying heart disease that produced the bundle branch or fascicular block usually determines the prognosis.

In general, a bundle branch or fascicular block complicating an acute anteroseptal MI indicates a more serious condition than an acute MI without one, presumably because of greater damage to the myocardium. The incidence of pump failure and life-threatening arrhythmias, such as sustained ventricular tachycardia and ventricular fibrillation, is much higher in patients with an acute MI complicated by a bundle branch block than in those who do not have such a complication. For this reason, the mortality rate in such patients is several times higher than in those with uncomplicated acute MI.

A bundle branch block may occasionally progress to a third-degree (complete) AV block in the setting of an acute MI, requiring temporary cardiac pacing. This is most likely to happen when a first- or second-degree AV block complicates a right or left bundle branch block occurring during the early stages of the infarction.

The progression of RBBB to complete AV block occurs twice as often as that of LBBB, especially when RBBB is associated with a fascicular block. The occurrence of a complete AV block in the setting of an acute MI is an ominous sign, indicating the involvement of both the left anterior descending coronary artery of the left coronary artery and the posterior descending artery of the right coronary artery. Complete AV block, in this instance, is usually transient, however, lasting about 1 to 2 weeks.

Left anterior and posterior fascicular blocks are usually benign and rarely progress to complete LBBB unless they are secondary to an acute MI. A left posterior fascicle block occurring with an RBBB, although rare, signifies a poor prognosis because occlusion of both the right coronary artery and the left

anterior descending coronary artery must occur for this to happen.

Treatment of Bundle Branch and Fascicular Blocks

Specific treatment is usually not indicated for a bundle branch or fascicular block if it is present alone and is not the result of an acute MI.

Temporary cardiac pacing is indicated for the treatment of a right or left bundle branch block under the following conditions:
◆ If a new right or left bundle branch block or an alternating bundle branch block (one in which an RBBB alternates with an LBBB) results from an acute MI
◆ If a bundle branch block is complicated by a fascicular block, a first- or second-degree AV block, or both, especially in the setting of an acute MI
◆ If a bundle branch block progresses to a complete AV block, especially in the setting of an acute MI

RIGHT BUNDLE BRANCH BLOCK

Pathophysiology of Right Bundle Branch Block

In RBBB (Figure 13-4), the electrical impulses are prevented from entering the right ventricle directly because of the disruption of conduction of the electrical impulses through the right bundle branch. RBBB may be present in a heart with a normally intact and viable interventricular septum or in one without an intact septum, as would result following an anteroseptal MI. The ECG characteristics of the two RBBBs differ significantly.

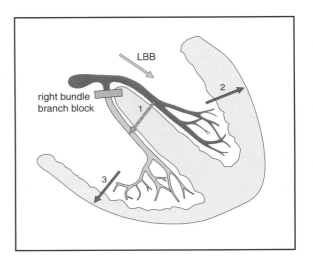

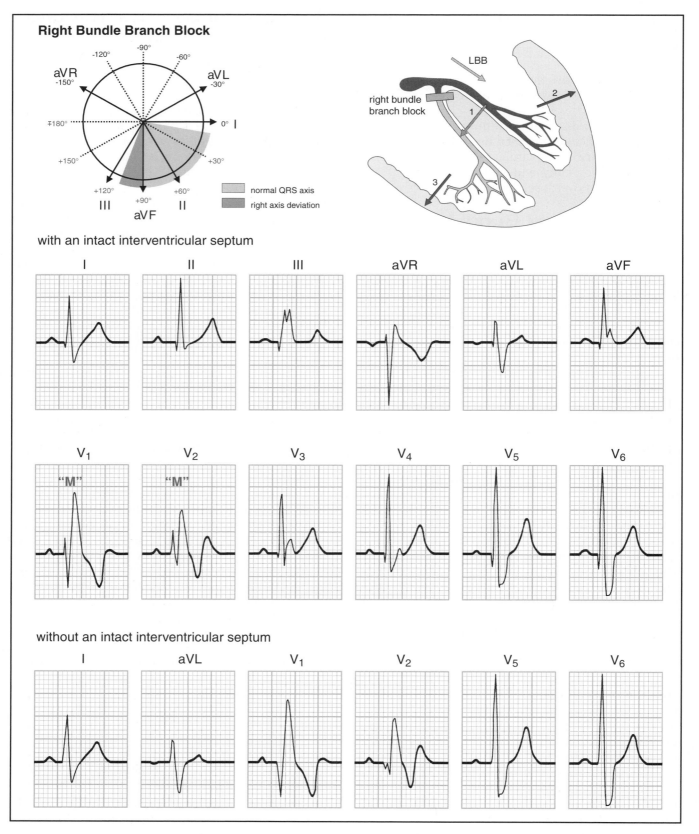

Figure 13-4 Right bundle branch block.

In RBBB with a normally intact and viable interventricular septum, the electrical impulses travel rapidly down the left bundle branch into the interventricular septum and left ventricle, as they normally do, while progressing slowly across the interventricular septum from left to right to enter the right ventricle after a short delay. Consequently, the interventricular septum and left ventricle depolarize in a normal way: first the septum from left to right *(1)* and then the left ventricle from right to left *(2)*. Following left ventricular depolarization, the right ventricle depolarizes in a normal direction, from left to right *(3)*.

The electrical forces generated by the depolarization of the right ventricle in RBBB occur after those of the interventricular septum and left ventricle and travel in a normal direction (i.e., anteriorly and to the right, toward lead V_1). Because of the delay in the depolarization of the right ventricle, the QRS complex is typically greater than 0.10 second in duration and bizarre in shape and appearance. When it is 0.12 second or greater in duration, it is said to be *complete*; between 0.10 and 0.11 second, it is *incomplete*. The term *RBBB* used alone signifies a *complete RBBB*.

In RBBB without an intact interventricular septum, depolarization of the nonviable interventricular septum does not occur. The depolarization of the left and right ventricles, however, occurs as it does in an RBBB with an intact septum.

Causes of Right Bundle Branch Block

RBBB may be present in healthy individuals with apparently normal hearts without any apparent cause. Common causes of chronic RBBB include the following:

◆ Coronary and hypertensive heart disease
◆ Cardiac tumors
◆ Cardiomyopathy and myocarditis
◆ Syphilitic, rheumatic, and congenital heart disease (atrial septal defect)
◆ Cardiac surgery
◆ Congenital RBBB
◆ Idiopathic degenerative disease of the electrical conduction system (i.e., Lenegre's and Lev's diseases)
◆ Aberrant ventricular conduction associated with supraventricular premature contractions and tachycardias (see Chapter 3)
 Common causes of acute RBBB include the following:
◆ Acute anteroseptal MI
◆ Acute pulmonary embolism or infarction
◆ Acute congestive heart failure
◆ Acute pericarditis or myocarditis

ECG Characteristics in Right Bundle Branch Block

◆ QRS COMPLEXES

Duration

The duration of the QRS complex in complete RBBB is 0.12 second or greater; in incomplete RBBB, the duration of the QRS complex is 0.10 to 0.11 second.

QRS Axis

The QRS axis may be normal or deviated to the right (i.e., right axis deviation, $>+90°$). If left axis deviation is present ($>-30°$), both RBBB and left anterior fascicle block are present.

Ventricular Activation Time

The VAT is prolonged beyond the upper normal limit of 0.035 second in the right precordial leads V_1 and V_2.

QRS Pattern in Right Bundle Branch Block With an Intact Interventricular Septum

In RBBB, the electrical forces of depolarization of the right ventricle occur abnormally late, following those of the interventricular septum and left ventricle. These right ventricular electrical forces are directed anteriorly and to the right and last more than 40 msec (0.04 sec), producing the typical late broad, or "terminal," R and S waves in various leads. The combined electrical forces of the left ventricle and delayed right ventricle produce the typical wide biphasic QRS complexes of RBBB.

◆ **Q waves:** Normal small septal q waves are present in leads I, aVL, and V_5-V_6, reflecting the normal depolarization of the interventricular septum.
◆ **R waves:** Small r waves are present in the right precordial leads V_1-V_2, reflecting the normal depolarization of the interventricular septum. Wide and slurred, tall "terminal" R waves are present in lead aVR and the right precordial leads V_1-V_2. This produces the classical triphasic rSR' pattern of RBBB (or the "M" or "rabbit ears" pattern) in leads V_1-V_2.
◆ **S waves:** Deep and slurred "terminal" S waves are present in leads I and aVL and the left precordial leads V_5-V_6. This produces the typical qRS pattern of RBBB in leads V_5-V_6.

QRS Pattern in Right Bundle Branch Block Without an Intact Interventricular Septum

In RBBB without an intact and viable interventricular septum, the initial normal depolarization of the interventricular septum does not occur. The result is the absence of initial small r waves in the precordial leads V_1-V_2 and septal q waves in leads I, aVL, and V_5-V_6. Consequently, the classical triphasic rSR' pattern of RBBB is replaced by a QSR pattern in V_1-V_2.

◆ ST SEGMENTS

ST segment depression may be present in leads V_1-V_3.

◆ T WAVES

T wave inversion may be present in leads V_1-V_3.

For a comparison of ECG characteristics of RBBB in leads I, V_1, and V_6 with an ECG with normal bundle branch conduction, see Figure 13-5.

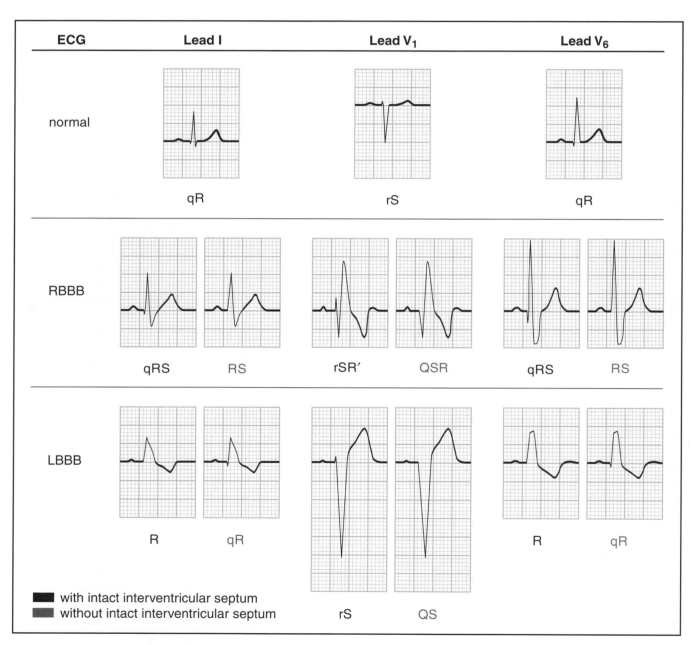

Figure 13-5 Comparison of leads I, V1, and V6 with normal conduction, right bundle branch block, and left bundle branch block.

Summary of the ECG Characteristics in Right Bundle Branch Block

With an Intact Interventricular Septum

Leads V_1-V_2

Wide QRS complex with a classic triphasic rSR′ pattern (the "M" or "rabbit ears" pattern)

◆ Initial small r wave (normal interventricular septal depolarization)

◆ Deep, slurred S wave (normal left ventricular depolarization)

◆ Late (terminal) tall R′ wave (delayed right ventricular depolarization)

ST segment depression

T wave inversion

Leads I, aVL, V_5-V_6

Wide QRS complex with a qRS pattern

◆ Initial small q wave (normal interventricular septal depolarization)

◆ Tall R wave (normal left ventricular depolarization)

◆ Late (terminal) deep, slurred S wave (delayed right ventricular depolarization)

QRS axis

Normal QRS axis or right axis deviation (+90° to ±110°).

Ventricular activation time

Prolonged beyond the upper normal limit of 0.035 second in the right precordial leads V_1 and V_2

Without an Intact Interventricular Septum

Leads V_1-V_2

Wide QRS complex with a QSR pattern.

◆ Absent initial small r wave (absent interventricular septal depolarization)

◆ Deep QS wave (normal left ventricular depolarization)

◆ Late (terminal) tall R wave (delayed right ventricular depolarization)

ST segment depression

T wave inversion

Leads I, aVL, V_5-V_6

Wide QRS complex with an RS pattern:

◆ Absent initial small q wave (absent interventricular septal depolarization)

◆ Tall R wave (normal left ventricular depolarization)

◆ Late (terminal) deep, slurred S wave (delayed right ventricular depolarization)

QRS axis

Normal QRS axis or right axis deviation (+90 to +110°).

Ventricular activation time

Prolonged beyond the upper normal limit of 0.035 second in the right precordial leads V_1 and V_2

Notes

_____

_____

_____

_____

_____

_____

_____

_____

_____

_____

_____

_____

_____

_____

LEFT BUNDLE BRANCH BLOCK

Pathophysiology of Left Bundle Branch Block

In LBBB (Figure 13-6), the electrical impulses are prevented from entering the left ventricle directly because of the disruption of conduction of the electrical impulses through the left bundle branch. Although LBBB may be present in a heart with a normally intact and viable interventricular septum, it usually occurs in hearts without an intact septum, as would result following an anteroseptal MI. The ECG characteristics of the two LBBBs differ somewhat.

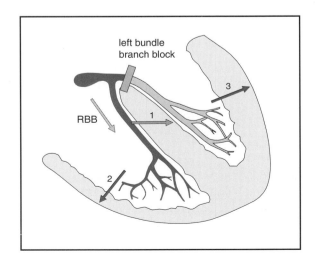

Left Bundle Branch Block

with an intact interventricular septum

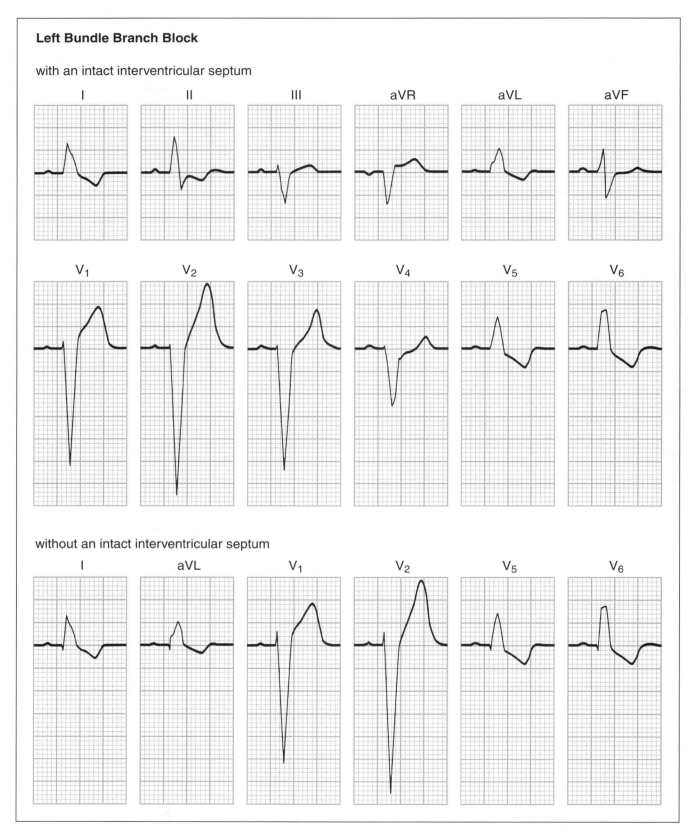

Figure 13-6 Left bundle branch block.

In LBBB with a normally intact and viable interventricular septum, the electrical impulses travel rapidly down the right bundle branch into the right ventricle, as they normally do, while progressing slowly across the interventricular septum from right to left into the left ventricle. Consequently, the interventricular septum depolarizes first in an abnormal way, from right to left *(1)*, and either anteriorly or posteriorly. This is followed by the depolarization of the right ventricle in a normal way, left to right *(2)*, and then depolarization of the left ventricle in a normal direction from right to left *(3)*.

The electrical forces generated by the depolarization of the left ventricle in LBBB occur after those of the interventricular septum and right ventricle and travel in a normal leftward direction, away from lead V_1.

Because the electrical impulses enter the left ventricle from the right via the interventricular septum instead of the left bundle branch, as they normally do, the depolarization of the left ventricle occurs slightly behind schedule, but in an essentially normal sequence.

Because of the delay in the depolarization of the left ventricle, the VAT is greater than 0.055 second and the QRS complex is typically greater than 0.10 second in duration and abnormal in shape and appearance. When the QRS complex is 0.12 second or greater in duration, the LBBB is said to be *complete*; when it is between 0.10 and 0.11 second, it is *incomplete*. The term *LBBB* used alone signifies a *complete LBB block*.

In LBBB without an intact interventricular septum, depolarization of the nonviable interventricular septum does not occur. The depolarization of the left and right ventricles, however, occurs as it does above in an LBBB with an intact septum.

Causes of Left Bundle Branch Block

LBBB, unlike RBBB, always indicates a diseased heart because it is an extremely unusual finding in healthy hearts. In general, LBBB is more common than is RBBB in elderly individuals with diseased hearts. Common causes of chronic LBBB include the following:

◆ Hypertensive heart disease (the most common cause) and coronary artery disease
◆ Cardiomyopathy and myocarditis
◆ Syphilitic, rheumatic, and congenital heart disease and aortic stenosis from whatever cause
◆ Cardiac tumors
◆ Idiopathic degenerative disease of the electrical conduction system (i.e., Lenegre's and Lev's diseases)
◆ Aberrant ventricular conduction associated with supraventricular premature contractions and tachycardias (see Chapter 3)

Common causes of acute LBBB include lowing:
◆ Acute anteroseptal MI
◆ Acute congestive heart failure
◆ Acute pericarditis or myocarditis
◆ Acute cardiac trauma
◆ Administration of such drugs as β-blockers, diltiazem and verapamil (rare)

ECG Characteristics in Left Bundle Branch Block

◆ QRS COMPLEXES

Duration

The duration of the QRS complex in complete LBBB is 0.12 second or greater; in incomplete LBBB, the duration of the QRS complex is 0.10 to 0.11 second.

QRS Axis

The QRS axis may be normal, but it is commonly deviated to the left (i.e., left axis deviation, $>-30°$).

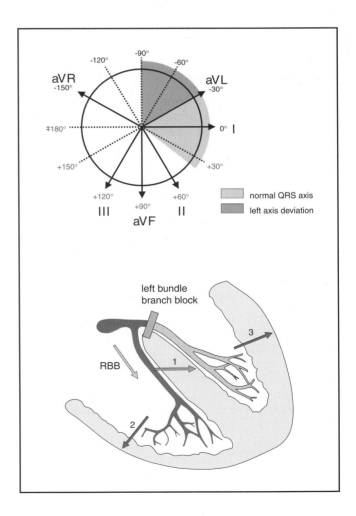

Ventricular Activation Time

The VAT is prolonged beyond the upper normal limit of 0.055 second in the left precordial leads V_5 and V_6.

QRS Pattern in Left Bundle Branch Block With an Intact Interventricular Septum

In LBBB, the electrical forces of depolarization of the left ventricle occur abnormally late, after those of the right ventricle. The electrical forces produced by the depolarization of the left ventricle are directed leftward and last more than 40 msec (0.04 sec), producing the typical broad R and S waves in the various leads. The combined electrical forces of the right ventricle and delayed left ventricle produce the typical wide monophasic QRS complexes of LBBB.

- **Q waves:** Septal q waves are absent in leads I and aVL and the left precordial leads V_5-V_6 where they normally occur. Their absence results from the depolarization of the interventricular septum in an abnormal direction, from right to left.
- **R waves:** Small to relatively tall, narrow R waves are present in leads V_1-V_3 when the interventricular septum depolarizes from right to left and anteriorly. This occurs in about two thirds of the LBBBs. These R waves in leads V_1-V_3 give the typical appearance of a "poor R-wave progression" across the precordial leads. In the other third of the LBBBs, where the interventricular septum depolarizes from right to left and posteriorly, R waves are absent in leads V_1-V_3.

  Tall, wide, slurred R waves are present in leads I and aVL and the left precordial leads V_5-V_6. These R waves may be notched, particularly near their peaks. The VAT is prolonged up to 0.07 second or more, particularly in lead aVL and the left precordial leads V_5-V_6.
- **S waves:** Deep, wide S waves are present in leads V_1-V_3, producing the typical rS or QS complexes. Because of these waves, an anteroseptal MI may be mistakenly diagnosed. S waves are absent in leads I and aVL and the left precordial leads V_5-V_6.

QRS Pattern in Left Bundle Branch Block Without an Intact Interventricular Septum

In LBBB without an intact interventricular septum, the initial depolarization of the septum from right to left does not occur. This leaves the initial electrical forces of right ventricular depolarization (from left to right) unopposed so that significant narrow r waves may be present in leads V_1 and V_2, with small q waves present in leads I and aVL and the left precordial leads V_5-V_6.

◆ ST SEGMENTS

ST segment depression is present in leads I and aVL and the left precordial leads V_5-V_6. ST segment elevation is present in leads V_1-V_3.

◆ T WAVES

T wave inversion is present in leads I and aVL and the left precordial leads V_5-V_6. T wave elevation is present in leads V_1-V_3.

For a comparison of ECG characteristics of LBBB in leads I, V_1m and V_6 with an ECG with normal bundle branch conduction, see Figure 13-5.

Notes

_____

_____

_____

_____

_____

_____

_____

_____

_____

_____

Summary of the ECG Characteristics in Left Bundle Branch Block

With an Intact Interventricular Septum
Leads V_1-V_3
Wide QRS complex with an rS or QS pattern
- Initial small r wave (abnormal interventricular septal depolarization from right to left and anteriorly)
- Deep, wide S wave (delayed, essentially normal left ventricular depolarization)

OR

- Absent R wave (abnormal interventricular septal depolarization from right to left and posteriorly)
- Deep, wide QS wave (delayed, essentially normal left ventricular depolarization)
- ST segment elevation
- T wave elevation

Leads I, aVL, V_5-V_6
Wide QRS complex with an R pattern
- Absent initial small q wave (absent normal interventricular septal depolarization from left to right)
- Tall, wide, slurred R wave with or without notching, and a prolonged VAT (delayed, essentially normal left ventricular depolarization)
- ST segment depression
- T wave inversion

QRS axis
Normal QRS axis or left axis deviation ($-30°$ to $-90°$)

Ventricular activation time

Prolonged beyond the upper normal limit of 0.055 second in the left precordial leads V_5 and V_6

Without an Intact Interventricular Septum

Leads V_1-V_2

Wide QRS complex with an rS pattern

◆ Small narrow r wave (unopposed normal right ventricular depolarization)

◆ Deep, wide S wave (delayed, essentially normal left ventricular depolarization)

◆ ST segment elevation

◆ T wave elevation

Leads I, aVL, V_5-V_6

Wide QRS complex with a qR pattern

◆ Small q wave (unopposed normal right ventricular depolarization)

◆ Tall, wide, slurred R wave with or without notching, and a prolonged VAT (delayed, essentially normal left ventricular depolarization)

◆ ST segment depression

◆ T wave inversion

QRS axis

Normal QRS axis or left axis deviation (–30° to –90°)

Ventricular activation time

Prolonged beyond the upper normal limit of 0.055 second in the left precordial leads V_5 and V_6

LEFT ANTERIOR FASCICULAR BLOCK (LEFT ANTERIOR HEMIBLOCK)

Pathophysiology of Left Anterior Fascicular Block

In left anterior fascicular block (Figure 13-7), the electrical impulses are prevented from entering the anterior and lateral walls of the left ventricle directly because of the disruption of conduction of the electrical impulses through the left anterior fascicle of the left bundle branch. The electrical impulses travel rapidly down the left posterior fascicle into the interventricular septum and posterior wall of the left ventricle and then, after a very slight delay, into the anterior and lateral walls of the left ventricle. At the same time, the electrical impulses travel down the right bundle branch into the right ventricle in a normal way.

The interventricular septum depolarizes first in a normal direction, from left to right *(1)*. This is followed by the depolarization of the right ventricle *(2)* and the posterior wall of the left ventricle *(2a)*, followed almost instantly by depolarization of the anterior and lateral walls of the left ventricle *(2b)*.

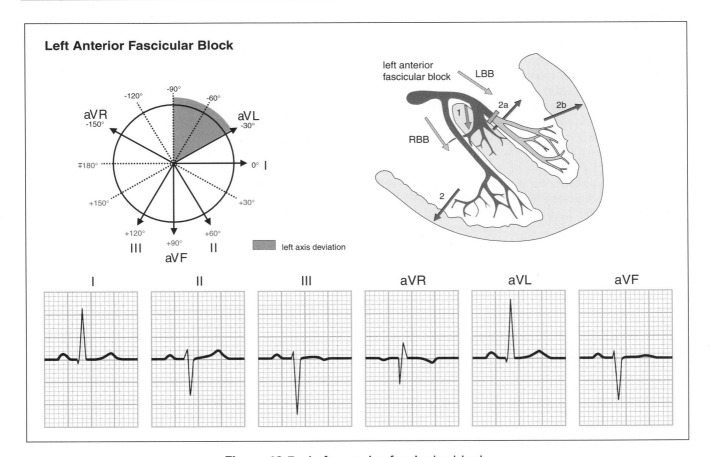

Figure 13-7 Left anterior fascicular block.

Because there is no appreciable delay between the depolarization of the posterior and anterolateral walls of the left ventricle, the QRS complex is of normal duration. The electrical forces generated by the slightly delayed depolarization of the anterior and lateral walls of the left ventricle travel in an upward and leftward direction, producing a marked left axis deviation.

Causes of Left Anterior Fascicular Block

The most common cause of left anterior fascicular block is acute anteroseptal MI. Left anterior fascicular block can occur alone or in combination with an RBBB.

ECG Characteristics in Left Anterior Fascicular Block

◆ QRS COMPLEXES

Duration

Normal, less than 0.10 second in duration.

QRS Axis

The QRS axis is typically deviated to the left (i.e., left axis deviation, −30° to −90°).

QRS Pattern

The QRS complexes appear normal without unusual notching or any delay in the VAT. The electrical forces of depolarization of the anterolateral area of the left ventricle, somewhat delayed by 40 msec (0.04 sec), are directed upward and leftward. The presence of an initial small q wave in lead I and an initial small r wave in lead III (q_1r_3 pattern) is an indication of a left anterior fascicular block.

◆ **Q waves:** Initial small q waves are present in leads I and aVL and absent in leads II, III, and aVF
◆ **R waves:** Initial small r waves are present in leads II, III, and aVF
◆ **S waves:** The S waves are typically deep and larger than the R waves in leads II, III, and aVF

KEY POINT

These findings relative to the QRS complexes are significant only in the absence of other causes of left axis deviation such as left ventricular hypertrophy and inferior (diaphragmatic) MI with Q waves in leads II, III, and aVF.

◆ ST SEGMENTS

Normal.

◆ T WAVES

Normal.

Notes

_____

_____

_____

LEFT POSTERIOR FASCICULAR BLOCK (LEFT POSTERIOR HEMIBLOCK)

Pathophysiology of Left Posterior Fascicular Block

In left posterior fascicular block (Figure 13-8), the electrical impulses are prevented from entering the interventricular septum and posterior wall of the left ventricle directly because of the disruption of conduction of the electrical impulses through the left posterior fascicle of the left bundle branch. The electrical impulses travel rapidly down the left anterior fascicle into the anterior and lateral walls of the left ventricle and then, after a very slight delay, into the posterior wall of the left ventricle. At the same time, the electrical impulses travel down the right bundle branch into the right ventricle in a normal way and into the interventricular septum.

The interventricular septum depolarizes first in an abnormal direction, from right to left (1). This is followed by the depolarization of the right ventricle (2) and the anterior and lateral walls of the left ventricle (2a), followed almost instantly by depolarization of the posterior wall of the left ventricle (2b).

Because there is no appreciable delay between the depolarization of the anterolateral and posterior walls of the left ventricle, the QRS complex is of normal duration. The electrical forces generated by the slightly delayed depolarization of the posterior wall of the left ventricle travel in a downward and rightward direction, producing a marked right axis deviation.

Causes of Left Posterior Fascicular Block

Left posterior fascicular block is rare, but it can occur in an acute anteroseptal MI involving the left anterior descending artery in combination with either an acute right ventricular or inferior MI where the pos-

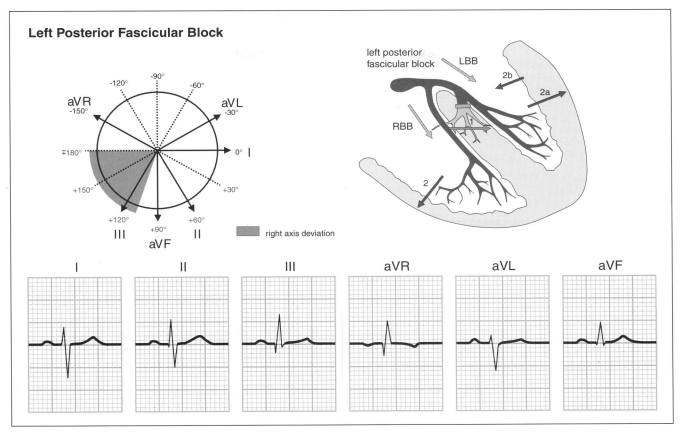

Figure 13-8 Left posterior fascicular block.

terior descending artery is also involved. The posterior descending artery most commonly arises from the right coronary artery but can arise occasionally from the left circumflex coronary artery. Left posterior fascicular block can occur alone or in combination with an RBBB.

ECG Characteristics in Left Posterior Fascicular Block

◆ QRS COMPLEXES

Duration

Normal, less than 0.10 second in duration.

QRS Axis

The QRS axis is typically deviated to the right (i.e., right axis deviation, +110° to +180°).

QRS Pattern

The QRS complexes appear normal without unusual notching or any delay in the VAT. The electrical forces of depolarization of the posterior part of the left ventricle, somewhat delayed by 40 msec (0.04 sec), are directed downward and rightward. The presence of

an initial small q wave in lead III and an initial small r wave in lead I (q_3r_1 pattern) is an indication of a left posterior fascicular block.

◆ **Q waves:** Initial small q waves are present in leads II, III, and aVF and absent in leads I, aVL, and V_5-V_6
◆ **R waves:** Initial small r waves are present in leads I and aVL, and tall R waves are present in leads II, III, and aVF
◆ **S waves:** Deep S waves are present in leads I and aVL

KEY POINT

These findings relative to the QRS complexes are significant only in the absence of other causes of right axis deviation, including the following:

◆ Right ventricular hypertrophy
◆ Pulmonary embolism and/or infarction
◆ Anterolateral MI with Q waves in leads I, aVL, and V_5-V_6
◆ Chronic obstructive pulmonary disease (COPD)

◆ **ST SEGMENTS**

Normal.

◆ **T WAVES**

Normal.

_____

_____

_____

CHAPTER REVIEW QUESTIONS

1. The time from the onset of the QRS complex to the peak of the R wave in the QRS complex is called:
   A. the ventricular activation time
   B. the preintrinsicoid deflection
   C. all of the above
   D. none of the above

2. The anterior portion of the septum is supplied with blood from the:
   A. posterior descending coronary artery
   B. AV nodal artery
   C. left anterior descending coronary artery
   D. right coronary artery

3. The main blood supply of the AV node and proximal part of the bundle of His is the AV node artery, which arises from the _____ in the majority of hearts.
   A. circumflex coronary artery
   B. right coronary artery
   C. posterior descending coronary artery
   D. none of the above

4. Common causes of bundle branch and fascicular blocks are:
   A. ischemic heart disease
   B. idiopathic degenerative disease of the electrical conduction system
   C. severe left ventricular hypertrophy
   D. all of the above

5. In the setting of an acute MI, a right bundle branch block occurs primarily in a(n):
   A. anteroseptal MI
   B. lateral MI
   C. posterior MI
   D. inferior MI

6. In patients with acute MI with a bundle branch block, _____ than in those not complicated by a bundle branch block.
   A. the incidence of pump failure and ventricular arrhythmias is much higher

   B. a temporary transcutaneous pacemaker is less frequently indicated
   C. the incidence of ventricular fibrillation is lower
   D. the incidence of supraventricular tachycardia is higher

7. Common causes of chronic right bundle branch block are:
   A. congestive heart failure, stroke, and seizures
   B. hyperventilation, acute MI, and diabetes
   C. myocarditis, cardiomyopathy, and cardiac surgery
   D. none of the above

8. In a right bundle branch block with an intact interventricular septum, the QRS complex in lead V_1 is:
   A. wide with a tall R wave
   B. wide with a classic triphasic rSR' pattern
   C. narrow with a QRS pattern
   D. none of the above

9. When the electrical impulses are prevented from directly entering the anterior and lateral walls of the left ventricle, the condition is called a:
   A. left anterior fascicular block
   B. left lateral hemiblock
   C. left posterior fascicular block
   D. none of the above

10. The electrical impulses are prevented from entering the interventricular septum and posterior wall of the left ventricle directly when the patient has a:
    A. left anterior fascicular block
    B. right posterior hemiblock
    C. left posterior fascicular block
    D. left inferior hemiblock

CHAPTER

14 Miscellaneous Electrocardiogram Changes

CHAPTER OBJECTIVES

Upon completion of all or part of this chapter, you should be able to complete the following objectives:

1. Discuss the pathophysiology of atrial and ventricular dilatation and hypertrophy and list four examples of atrial and ventricular dilatation and four examples of atrial and ventricular hypertrophy or enlargement.
2. Discuss the pathophysiology of enlargement or hypertrophy of the following heart chambers and list the electrocardiogram (ECG) abnormalities characteristic of each:
   Right atrial enlargement
   Left atrial enlargement
   Right ventricular hypertrophy
   Left ventricular hypertrophy
3. Discuss the effect each of the following conditions has on the heart and list the ECG changes characteristic of each:
   Pericarditis
   Chronic obstructive pulmonary disease (COPD)
   Cor pulmonale
   Pulmonary embolism
4. List the characteristic ECG changes in the following serum electrolyte imbalances according to the serum

levels where applicable:
Hyperkalemia
Hypokalemia
Hypercalcemia
Hypocalcemia

5. List the excitatory and inhibitory effects of the following drugs on the heart and its electrical conduction system and the characteristic ECG changes that occur with each:
   Digitalis
   Procainamide
   Quinidine
6. Describe the ECG abnormalities characteristic of early repolarization and discuss the implications of diagnosing certain cardiac disorders when it is present.
7. Describe the ECG changes in hypothermia and when they occur.
8. Discuss the anatomical features and pathophysiology of the accessory conduction pathways, the ECG abnormalities characteristic of each, and the potential for misinterpretation of such ECG abnormalities.

CHAMBER ENLARGEMENT

◆ PATHOPHYSIOLOGY

Enlargement of the atria and ventricles often occurs when heart disease forces them to accommodate greater pressure and/or volume than they normally do. The term *enlargement* includes *dilatation* and *hypertrophy*.

Dilatation

Dilatation means the distension of an individual heart chamber; it may be acute or chronic. Acute dilatation is usually not associated with hypertrophy of the chamber wall, whereas chronic dilatation commonly is. Examples of acute chamber dilatation include the following:

◆ Left atrial dilatation in acute left heart failure
◆ Right atrial and ventricular dilatation in acute pulmonary edema and acute pulmonary embolism
Examples of chronic chamber dilatation include the following:
◆ Left ventricular dilatation in severe aortic valve stenosis or insufficiency
◆ Left atrial dilatation in severe mitral valve stenosis or insufficiency

Hypertrophy

Hypertrophy is a chronic condition of the heart characterized by an increase in the thickness of a chamber's myocardial wall secondary to the increase in the size of the muscle fibers. This is the usual response of the myocardium to an increase in its workload over time. *Commonly, dilatation of the chamber accompanies hypertrophy;* to what extent depends on the heart disease causing the hypertrophy. Examples of chamber hypertrophy include the following:

◆ Left ventricular hypertrophy in aortic valve stenosis or insufficiency and systemic hypertension
◆ Right ventricular hypertrophy in pulmonary valve stenosis and chronic obstructive pulmonary disease (COPD)
◆ Left atrial enlargement in mitral valve stenosis and insufficiency and left ventricular hypertrophy from whatever cause
◆ Right atrial enlargement in tricuspid valve stenosis and insufficiency and right ventricular hypertrophy from whatever cause

RIGHT ATRIAL ENLARGEMENT

◆ PATHOPHYSIOLOGY

Right atrial enlargement (right atrial dilatation and hypertrophy) (Figure 14-1) is usually caused by increased pressure and/or volume in the right atrium—

right atrial overload. It occurs in the following conditions:
◆ Pulmonary valve stenosis
◆ Tricuspid valve stenosis and insufficiency (relatively rare)
◆ Pulmonary hypertension from various causes, such as the following:
  ◇ COPD
  ◇ Status asthmaticus
  ◇ Pulmonary embolism
  ◇ Pulmonary edema
  ◇ Mitral valve stenosis or insufficiency
  ◇ Congenital heart disease
The result of right atrial enlargement is, typically, a tall, symmetrically peaked P wave—the *P pulmonale.*

◆ ECG CHARACTERISTICS

P Waves

Duration. The duration of the P waves is usually normal (0.10 second or less).

Shape. P waves characteristic of right atrial enlargement include the following:
◆ A typically tall and symmetrically peaked P wave—the P pulmonale, present in leads II, III, and aVF
◆ A sharply peaked biphasic P wave in leads V_1 and V_2

Direction. The direction of the P waves is positive (upright) in leads II, III, and aVF and biphasic in V_1 and V_2, with the initial deflection greater than the terminal deflection.

Amplitude. The amplitude of the P waves is 2.5 mm or greater in leads II, III, and aVF.

Notes

_____

_____

_____

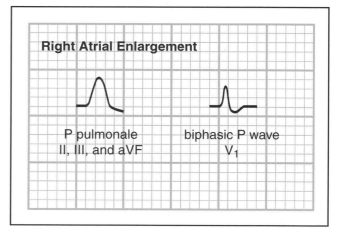

Figure 14-1 Right atrial enlargement.

LEFT ATRIAL ENLARGEMENT

◆ PATHOPHYSIOLOGY

Left atrial enlargement (left atrial dilatation and hypertrophy) (Figure14-2) is usually caused by increased pressure and/or volume in the left atrium—*left atrial overload*. It occurs in the following conditions:
◆ Mitral valve stenosis and insufficiency
◆ Acute myocardial infarction (MI)
◆ Left heart failure
◆ Left ventricular hypertrophy from various causes, such as the following:
    ◇ Aortic stenosis or insufficiency
    ◇ Systemic hypertension
    ◇ Hypertrophic cardiomyopathy
The result of left atrial enlargement is, typically, a wide, notched P wave—the *P mitrale*. Such P waves may also result from a delay or block of the progression of the electrical impulses through the interatrial conduction tract (Bachmann's bundle) between the right and left atria.

◆ ECG CHARACTERISTICS

P Waves

Duration. The duration of the P waves is usually greater than 0.10 second.

Shape. P waves characteristic of left atrial enlargement include the following:
◆ A broad positive (upright) P wave, 0.12 second or greater in duration, in any lead.
◆ A wide, notched P wave with two "humps" 0.04 second or more apart—the P mitrale. The first hump represents the depolarization of the right atrium; the second hump represents the depolarization of the enlarged left atrium. The P mitrale is usually present in leads I, II, and V_4-V_6.

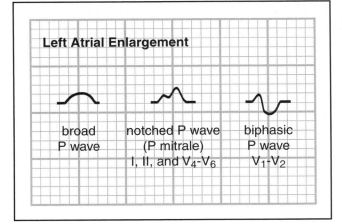

Figure 14-2   Left atrial enlargement.

◆ A biphasic P wave, greater than 0.10 second in total duration, with the terminal, negative component 1 mm (0.1 mV) or more deep and 1 mm (0.04 second) or more in duration (i.e., 1 small square or greater). The initial, positive (upright) component of the P wave represents the depolarization of the right atrium; the terminal, negative component represents the depolarization of the enlarged left atrium. Such biphasic P waves are commonly present in leads V_1-V_2.

Direction. The direction of the P waves is positive (upright) in leads I, II, and V_4-V_6 and biphasic in leads V_1-V_2. The P wave may be negative in leads III and aVF.

Amplitude. The amplitude of the P waves is usually normal (0.5 to 2.5 mm).

Notes

_____

_____

_____

_____

RIGHT VENTRICULAR HYPERTROPHY

◆ PATHOPHYSIOLOGY

Right ventricular hypertrophy (Figure14-3) is usually caused by increased pressure and/or volume in the right ventricle—*right ventricular overload*. It occurs in the following conditions:
◆ Pulmonary valve stenosis and other congenital heart defects (e.g., atrial and ventricular septal defects)
◆ Tricuspid valve insufficiency (relatively rare)
◆ Pulmonary hypertension from various causes, such as the following:
    ◇ COPD
    ◇ Status asthmaticus
    ◇ Pulmonary embolism
    ◇ Pulmonary edema
    ◇ Mitral valve stenosis or insufficiency
Right ventricular hypertrophy produces abnormally large rightward electrical forces that travel toward lead V_1 and away from the left precordial leads V_5-V_6. The sequence of depolarization of the ventricles, however, remains normal.

◆ ECG CHARACTERISTICS

P Waves

Changes indicative of right atrial enlargement are present (i.e., tall, symmetrically peaked P waves [P pulmonale] in leads II, III, and aVF and sharply peaked biphasic P waves in leads V_1 and V_2).

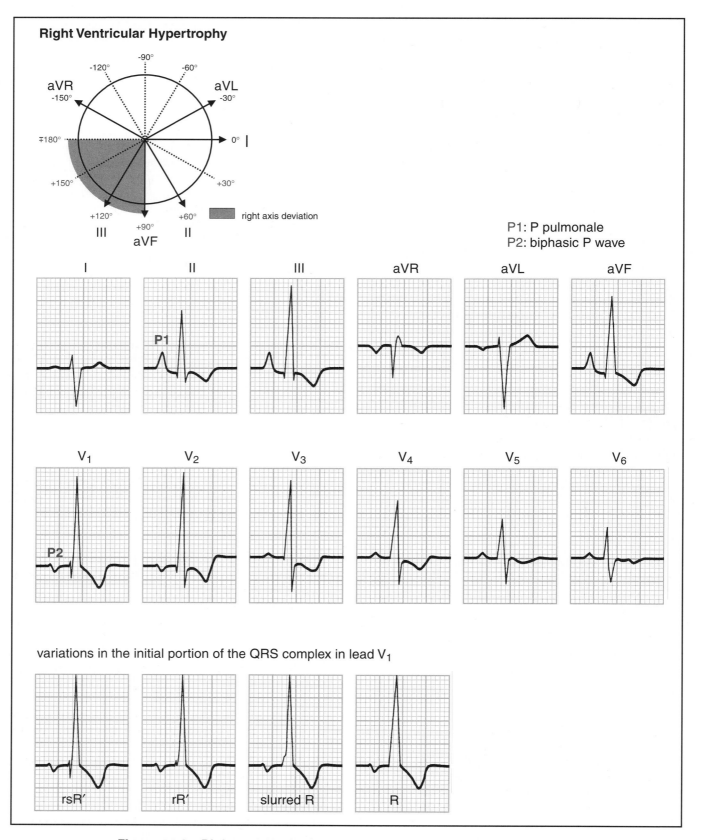

Figure 14-3 Right ventricular hypertrophy with right atrial enlargement.

QRS Complexes

Duration. The duration of the QRS complexes is 0.10 second or less.

QRS axis. A right axis deviation of +90° or more is usually present: $\geq +110°$ in adults and $\geq +120°$ in the young.

Ventricular activation time. The ventricular activation time (VAT) is prolonged beyond the upper normal limit of 0.035 second in the right precordial leads V_1 and V_2.

QRS pattern.
- **Q waves:** Q waves may be present in leads II, III, and aVF.
- **R waves:** Tall R waves are present in leads II, III, and V_1. The R waves are usually 7 mm or more (≥ 0.7 mV) in height in lead V_1. They are equal to or greater than the S waves in depth in this lead. Relatively tall R waves are also present in the adjacent precordial leads V_2-V_3.
- **S waves:** Relatively deeper than normal S waves are present in lead I and the left precordial leads V_4-V_6. In lead V_6, the depth of the S waves may be greater than the height of the R waves.

KEY POINT

Tall R waves equal to or greater than the S waves in lead V_1 may also be present in acute posterior MI and in counterclockwise rotation of the heart.

ST Segments

"Downsloping" ST segment depression of 1 mm or more may be present in leads II, III, aVF, and V_1 and sometimes in leads V_2 and V_3.

T Waves

T wave inversion is often present in leads II, III, aVF, and V_1 and sometimes in leads V_2 and V_3.

KEY POINT

The downsloping ST segment depression and the T wave inversion together form the "strain" pattern characteristic of long-standing right ventricular hypertrophy. This pattern gives the so-called "hockey stick" appearance to the QRS-ST-T complex.

Notes

_____

_____

_____

LEFT VENTRICULAR HYPERTROPHY

◆ PATHOPHYSIOLOGY

Left ventricular hypertrophy (Figure 14-4) is usually caused by increased pressure and/or volume in the left ventricle—*left ventricular overload.* It occurs in the following conditions:
- Mitral insufficiency
- Aortic stenosis or insufficiency
- Systemic hypertension
- Acute MI
- Hypertrophic cardiomyopathy

Left ventricular hypertrophy produces abnormally large leftward electrical forces that travel toward the left precordial leads V_5-V_6 and away from lead V_1. The sequence of depolarization of the ventricles, however, remains normal.

◆ ECG CHARACTERISTICS

P Waves

Changes indicative of left atrial enlargement are present (i.e., wide, notched P waves [P mitrale] in leads I, II, and V_4 and V_6 and biphasic P waves in leads V_1 and V_2).

QRS Complexes

Duration. The duration of the QRS complexes is 0.10 second or less.

QRS axis. The QRS axis is usually normal, but it may be deviated to the left (i.e., left axis deviation of $> -30°$).

Ventricular activation time. The VAT is prolonged beyond the upper normal limit of 0.04 to 0.05 second or more in the left precordial leads V_5 and V_6.

QRS pattern.
- **R waves:** Tall R waves are present in leads I and aVL and the left precordial leads V_5-V_6. The following criteria concerning the amplitude (or voltage) of the R wave in various leads are often used to diagnose left ventricular hypertrophy:
  ◇ An R wave of 20 mm (2.0 mV)* or more in lead I
  ◇ An R wave of 11 mm (1.1 mV) or more in lead aVL

---

*10 mm = 1.0 mV.

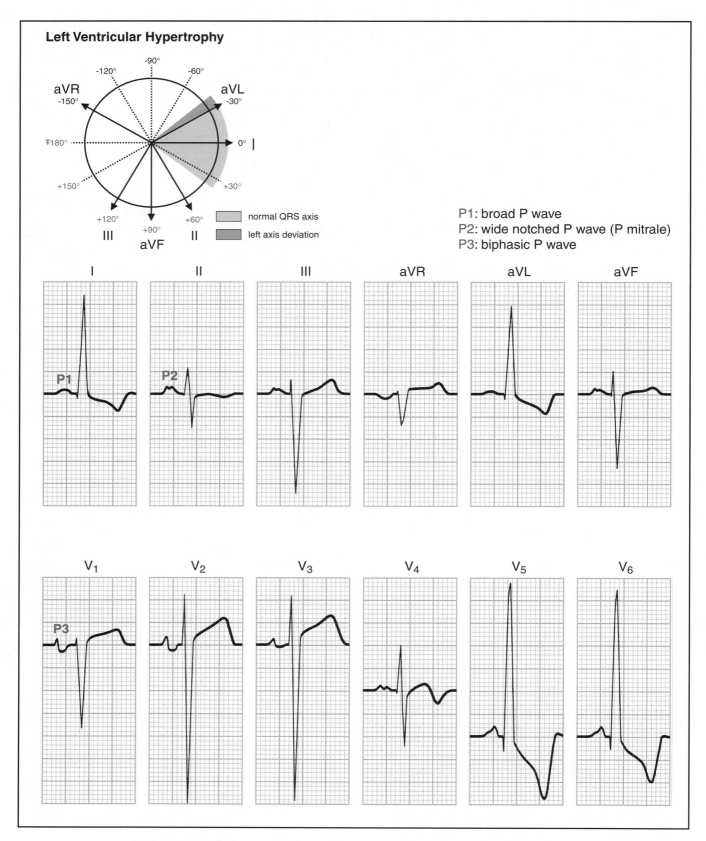

Figure 14-4 Left ventricular hypertrophy with left atrial enlargement.

◇ An R wave of 30 mm (3.0 mV) or more in lead V_5 or V_6

◆ **S waves:** Deep S waves are present in lead III and the right precordial leads V_1 and V_2. The following criteria concerning the depth (or voltage) of the S wave in various leads are often used to diagnose left ventricular hypertrophy:

◇ An S wave of 20 mm (2.0 mV) or more in lead III

◇ An S wave of 30 mm (3.0 mV) or more in lead V_1 or V_2

◆ **Sum of R and S waves:** The sum of the height of the R waves and the depth of the S waves (in mm or mV) in the leads in which these two waves are most prominent is often used to determine the presence of left ventricular hypertrophy. Left ventricular hypertrophy is considered to be present if any one of the following summations is exceeded:

◇ The sum of any R wave and any S wave in any of the limb leads I, II, or III is 20 mm (2.0 mV) or more

R (I, II, or III) + S (I, II, or III) = ≥20 mm (≥2.0 mV)

◇ The sum of the R wave in lead I and the S wave in lead III is 25 mm (2.5 mV) or more

R I + S III = ≥25 mm (≥2.5 mV)

◇ The sum of the S wave in lead V_1 or V_2 and the R wave in lead V_5 or V_6 is 35 mm (3.5 mV) or more

S V_1 (or S V_2) + R V_5 (or R V_6) = ≥35 mm (≥3.5 mV)

ST Segments

"Downsloping" ST segment depression of 1 mm or more is present in leads I, aVL, and V_5-V_6.

T Waves

T wave inversion is present in leads I, aVL, and V_5-V_6.

KEY POINT

The downsloping ST segment depression and the T wave inversion together form the "strain" pattern characteristic of long-standing left ventricular hypertrophy. This pattern gives the so-called "hockey stick" appearance to the QRS-ST-T complex. The strain pattern is less significant if the patient is taking digitalis, because this medication can also cause ST segment depression and T wave flattening and inversion.

◆ DIAGNOSIS OF LEFT VENTRICULAR HYPERTROPHY

Many criteria for the diagnosis of left ventricular hypertrophy exist. All are based on the three major ECG characteristics of left ventricular hypertrophy:

◆ Increased amplitude or depth of the R and S waves in specific limb and precordial leads

◆ QRS axis greater than −15°

◆ ST segment depression

An acceptable set of criteria for diagnosing left ventricular hypertrophy might include the following:

◆ Increased amplitude or depth of the R and S waves in any appropriate lead(s) satisfying the amplitude (or voltage) criteria of left ventricular hypertrophy, expressed in mm or mV (Table 14-1):

1. The amplitude of the R wave in lead I or the depth of the S wave in lead III of 20 mm (2.0 mV) or greater

OR

2. The sum of the S wave in lead V_1 or V_2 and the R wave in V_5 or V_6 of greater than 35 mm (3.5 mV)

◆ **AND,** one of the following:

1. QRS axis between −15° and −30° or greater than −30° (left axis deviation)

OR

2. ST segment depression of 1 mm in leads with an R wave having the amplitude (or voltage) criteria of left ventricular hypertrophy

Notes

_____

_____

_____

_____

_____

_____

PERICARDITIS

◆ PATHOPHYSIOLOGY

Pericarditis (Figure 14-5) is an inflammatory disease of the pericardium, directly involving the epicardium with deposition of inflammatory cells and a variable amount of serous, fibrous, purulent, or hemorrhagic exudate within the pericardial sac. Depending on the nature of the exudate, acute fibrinous pericarditis, pericardial effusion, cardiac tamponade, or constrictive pericarditis may develop. A variety of agents and conditions can cause acute pericarditis, including the following:

◆ Infectious agents (bacteria, viruses, tubercle bacilli, and mycotic agents)

TABLE 14-1 Criteria for Height or Depth of R and S Waves Used to Diagnose Left Ventricular Hypertropy

Wave	Lead: I	III	aVL	V_1 or V_2	V_5 or V_6
R Wave	≥ 20 mm		≥ 11 mm		≥ 30 mm
S Wave		≥ 20 mm		≥ 30 mm	

Summation
R (I, II, or III) + S (I, II, or III) = ≥ 20 mm (≥ 20 mV)
R I + S III = ≥ 25 mm (≥ 2.5 mV)
S V_1 or V_2 + R V_5 or V_6 = ≥ 35 mm (≥ 3.5 mV)

R-wave

I

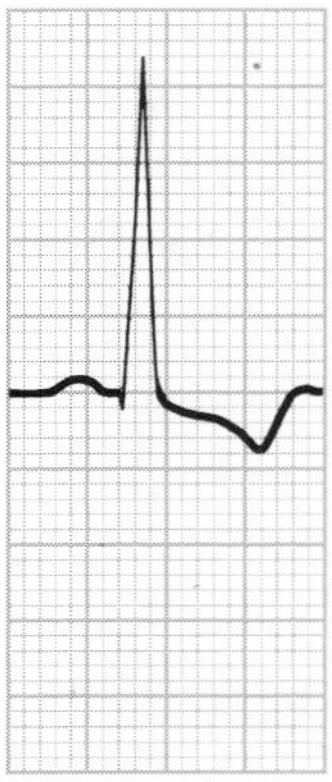

≥ 20 mm

or

aVL

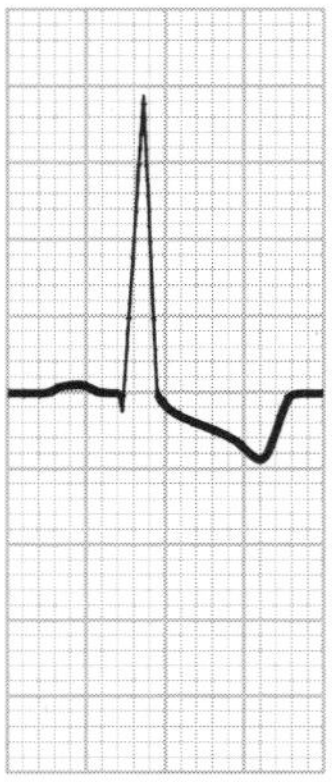

≥ 11 mm

or

V_5-V_6

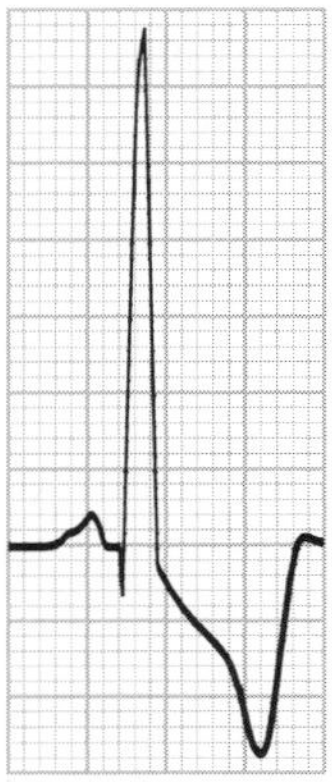

≥ 30 mm

S-wave

III

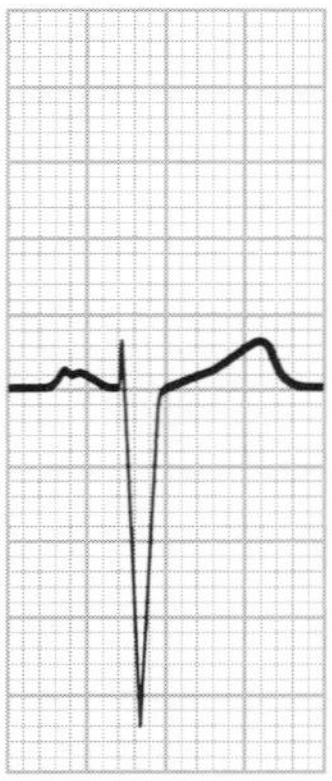

≥ 20 mm

or

V_1-V_2

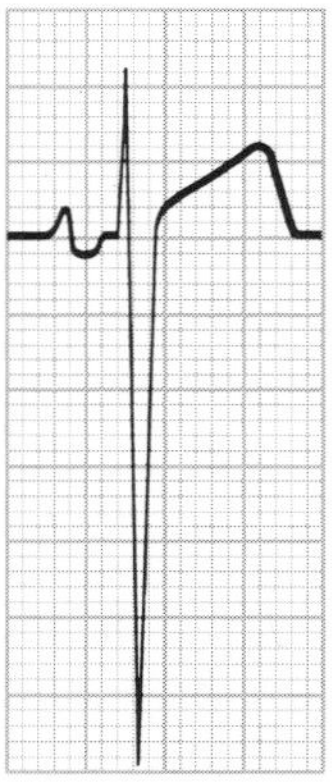

≥ 30 mm

Summation

R (I, II, III)

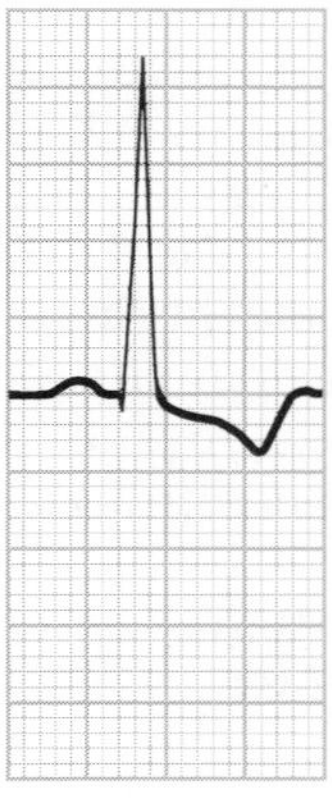

+

S (I, II, III)

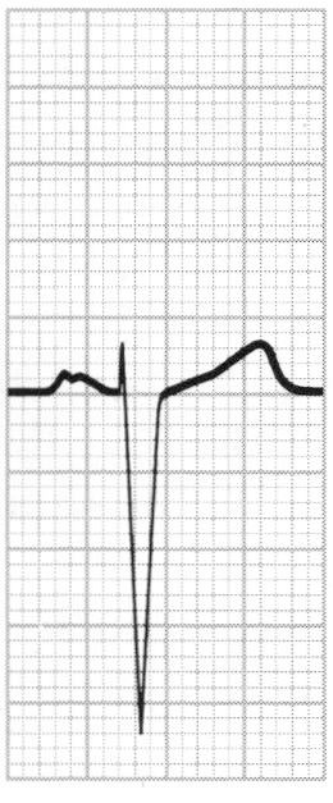

R + S = ≥ 20 mm

RI

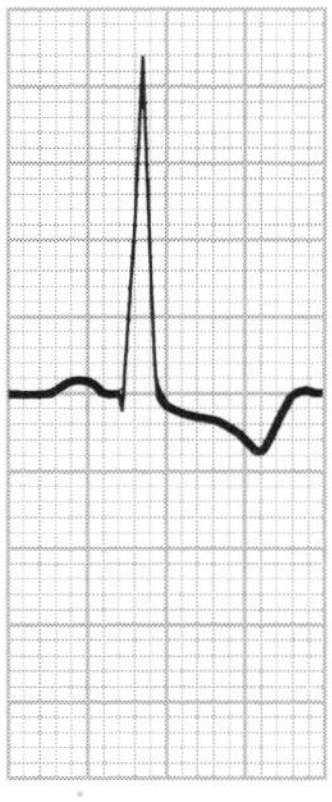

+

S III

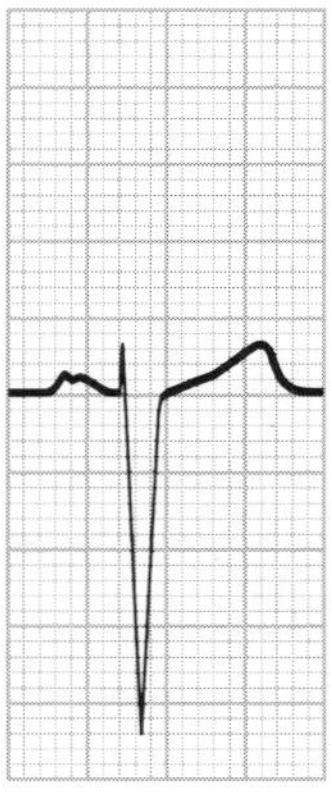

R + S = ≥ 25 mm

SV_1/V_2

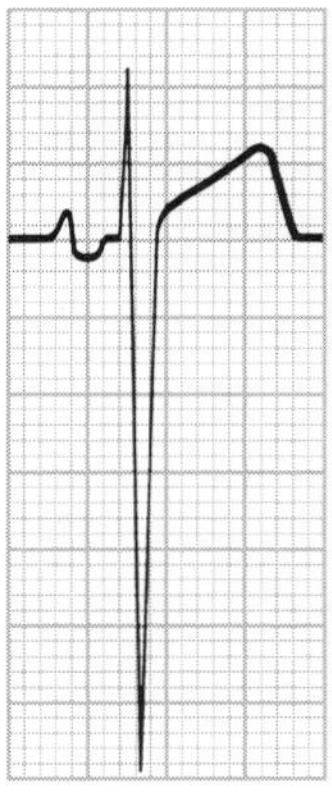

+

R V_5/V_6

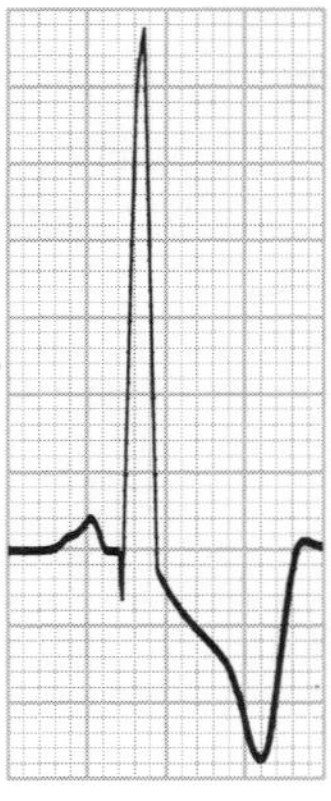

S + R = ≥ 35 mm

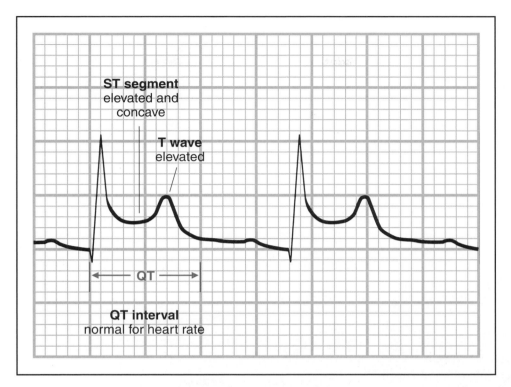

Figure 14-5   Pericarditis.

- Acute MI
- Trauma
- Connective tissue disorders
- Allergic and hypersensitivity diseases
- Metabolic disorders

Unlike acute MI, which pericarditis may mimic, pericarditis usually occurs in younger patients without cardiac risk factors who are not suspected of having coronary artery disease. The signs and symptoms of acute pericarditis include the following:

- Chest pain
- Dyspnea
- Tachycardia
- Fever
- Malaise
- Weakness
- Chills

The chest pain, which can mimic that of acute MI, is sharp and severe, with radiation to the neck, back, left shoulder, and, rarely, to the arm. Characteristically, it is present along the sternum, made worse by lying flat, and relieved by sitting or leaning forward. Often, the pain is pleuritic and made worse by breathing, especially during inspiration. Unlike the pain of acute MI, the pain may last for hours or even days.

A pericardial friction rub, resulting from the inflammation of the pericardial surface, is heard and even palpated along the lower left sternal border.

Characteristic ECG findings are present in 90% of the patients with acute pericarditis.

◆ ECG CHARACTERISTICS

QRS Complexes

Abnormal Q waves and QS complexes are absent. In pericarditis with pleural effusion, the QRS complexes are of low voltage. When pleural effusion becomes severe, cardiac tamponade may occur, causing the QRS complexes to alternate between normal and low amplitude, coincident with respiration (electrical alternans).

ST Segments

ST segment elevation is the primary ECG abnormality in acute pericarditis. Although the ST segments are somewhat concave, they appear quite similar to the elevated ST segments present in acute MI.

The ST segments are usually elevated in most, if not all, leads except leads aVR and V_1, because pericarditis usually affects the entire myocardial surface of the heart. In lead aVR, the ST segment is either normal or slightly depressed. This wide distribution of the ST segment elevation in pericarditis helps to differentiate it from acute MI in which there is a more limited distribution of ST segment elevation. Occasionally, pericarditis will be local-

TABLE

14-2   ST Segment Elevation

Location of Pericarditis	Leads With ST Segment Elevation
Anterior	V_2-V_4
Lateral	I, aVL, V_5-V_6
Inferior	II, III, aVF
Generalized	I, II, III, aVL, aVF, V_2-V_6

ized and therefore the ST segment elevation will only be seen in the leads reflecting the involved area. In this case, differentiating between pericarditis and an acute anterior, lateral, or inferior wall MI may be difficult. Reciprocal ST segment depression is usually not present. As the pericarditis resolves, the ST segments return back to the baseline (Table 14-2).

T Waves

The T waves remain elevated during the acute phase of pericarditis. As the pericarditis resolves, the T waves become inverted in the leads that had the ST segment elevation.

QT Intervals

The QT intervals are normal.

Notes

_____

_____

_____

_____

ELECTROLYTE IMBALANCE

Hyperkalemia

◆ PATHOPHYSIOLOGY

Hyperkalemia (Figure 14-6) is the excess of serum potassium above the normal levels of 3.5 to 5.0 milliequivalents per liter (mEq/L). The most common causes of hyperkalemia are kidney failure and certain diuretics (e.g., triamterene). Characteristic ECG changes occur at various levels of hyperkalemia. Sinus arrest may occur when the serum potassium level reaches about 7.5 mEq/L, and cardiac standstill or ventricular fibrillation may occur at about 10 to 12 mEq/L. Recognition of the early "peaking" of the T wave in hyperkalemia described below may be lifesaving.

◆ ECG CHARACTERISTICS

P Waves

The P waves begin to flatten out and become wider when the serum potassium level reaches about 6.5 mEq/L, and they disappear at 7.0 to 9.0 mEq/L.

PR Intervals

The PR intervals may be normal or prolonged, greater than 0.20 second. The PR interval is absent when the P waves disappear.

QRS Complexes

The QRS complexes begin to widen when the serum potassium level reaches about 6.0 to 6.5 mEq/L, becoming markedly slurred and abnormally widened beyond 0.12 second at 10 mEq/L. The QRS complexes may widen so that they "merge" with the following T waves, resulting in a "sine wave" QRS-ST-T pattern.

ST Segments

The ST segments disappear when the serum potassium level reaches about 6 mEq/L.

T Waves

The T waves become typically narrow, tall, and peaked when the serum potassium level reaches about 5.5 to 6.5 mEq/L. These T waves, described as tentlike, reach a height of at least 50% of the total height of the QRS complex. The earliest T wave changes are best seen in leads II, III, and V_2-V_6 in most cases.

Notes

_____

_____

_____

_____

_____

_____

_____

_____

_____

_____

_____

_____

_____

_____

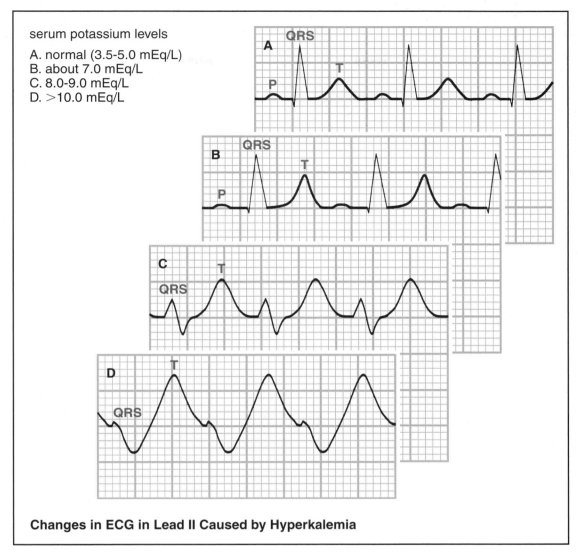

serum potassium levels

A. normal (3.5-5.0 mEq/L)
B. about 7.0 mEq/L
C. 8.0-9.0 mEq/L
D. >10.0 mEq/L

Changes in ECG in Lead II Caused by Hyperkalemia

Figure 14-6 Hyperkalemia.

Hypokalemia

◆ PATHOPHYSIOLOGY

Hypokalemia (Figure 14-7) is the deficiency of serum potassium below the normal levels of 3.5 to 5.0 mEq/L. The most common cause of hypokalemia is loss of potassium in body fluids through vomiting, gastric suction, and excessive use of diuretics. Hypokalemia may also result from low serum magnesium levels (hypomagnesemia). Incidentally, the ECG characteristics of hypomagnesemia resemble those of hypokalemia.

Symptoms of hypokalemia are polyuria in mild cases and muscle weakness in more severely affected patients. Digitalis in the presence of hypokalemia may precipitate serious ventricular arrhythmias, including the torsade de pointes form of ventricular tachycardia. The diagnosis of hypokalemia is often made by the characteristic ECG changes caused by low serum potassium. Characteristic ECG changes occur at various levels of hypokalemia.

◆ ECG CHARACTERISTICS

P Waves

The P waves become typically tall and symmetrically peaked with an amplitude of 2.5 mm or greater in leads II, III, and aVF in severe hypokalemia of about 2 mEq/L or less. Because these P waves resemble P pulmonale, they are called "pseudo P pulmonale."

QRS Complexes

The QRS complexes begin to widen when the serum potassium level drops to about 3.0 mEq/L.

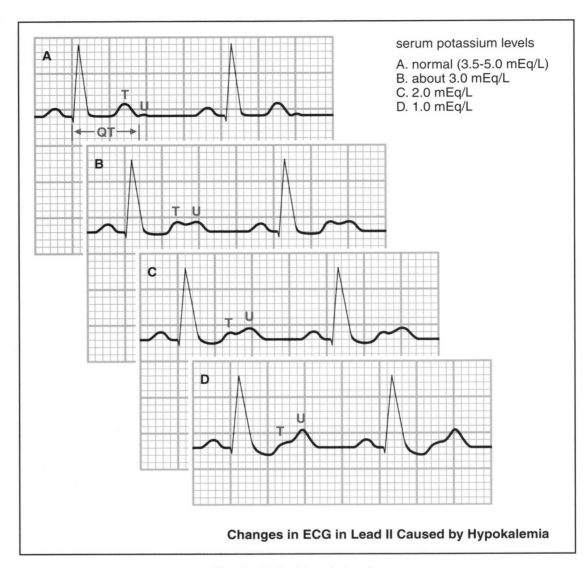

serum potassium levels

A. normal (3.5-5.0 mEq/L)
B. about 3.0 mEq/L
C. 2.0 mEq/L
D. 1.0 mEq/L

Changes in ECG in Lead II Caused by Hypokalemia

Figure 14-7 Hypokalemia.

ST Segments

The ST segments may become depressed by 1 mm or more.

T Waves

The T waves begin to flatten when the serum potassium level drops to about 3.0 mEq/L and continue to become smaller as the U waves increase in size. The T waves may either merge with the U waves or become inverted.

U Waves

The U waves begin to increase in size, becoming as tall as the T waves, when the serum potassium level drops to about 3.0 mEq/L; they become taller than the T waves at about 2 mEq/L. The U wave is considered to be "prominent" when it is equal to or taller than the T wave in the same lead. The U waves reach "giant" size and fuse with the T waves at 1 mEq/L.

QT Intervals

The QT intervals may appear to be prolonged when the U waves become prominent and fuse with the T waves.

Notes

_____

_____

_____

_____

_____

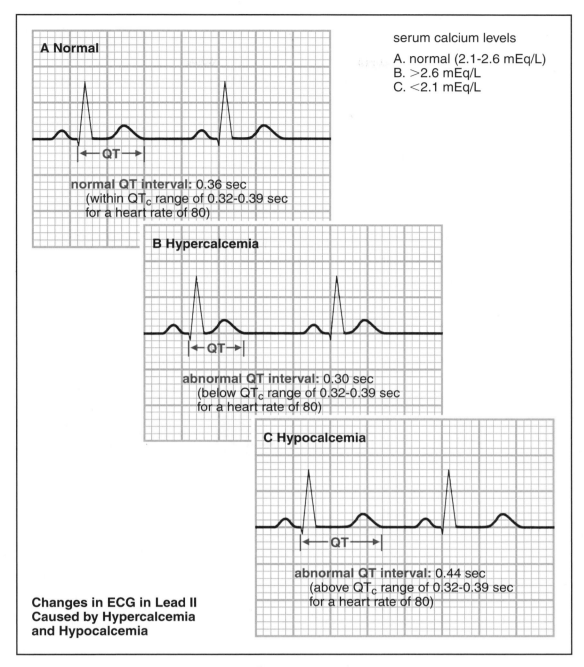

Figure 14-8 Hypercalcemia and hypocalcemia.

Hypercalcemia

◆ PATHOPHYSIOLOGY

Hypercalcemia (Figure 14-8, *B*) is the excess of serum calcium above the normal levels of 2.1 to 2.6 mEq/L (or 4.25 to 5.25 mg/100 mL). Common causes of hypercalcemia include the following:

◆ Adrenal insufficiency
◆ Hyperparathyroidism
◆ Immobilization
◆ Kidney failure
◆ Malignancy
◆ Sarcoidosis
◆ Thyrotoxicosis
◆ Vitamin A and D intoxication

Severe hypercalcemia is life threatening. Digitalis in the presence of hypercalcemia may precipitate serious arrhythmias.

◆ ECG CHARACTERISTICS

QT Intervals

The QT intervals are shorter than normal for the heart rate.

Notes

_____

_____

_____

Hypocalcemia

◆ PATHOPHYSIOLOGY

Hypocalcemia (Figure 14-8, *C*) is the shortage of serum calcium below the normal levels of 2.1 to 2.6 mEq/L (or 4.25 to 5.25 mg/100 mL). Common causes of hypocalcemia include the following:
◆ Chronic steatorrhea
◆ Diuretics (such as furosemide or ethacrynic acid)
◆ Hypomagnesemia (possibly because of release of parathyroid hormone)
◆ Osteomalacia in adults and rickets in children
◆ Hypoparathyroidism
◆ Pregnancy
◆ Respiratory alkalosis and hyperventilation

◆ ECG CHARACTERISTICS

ST Segments

The ST segments are prolonged.

QT Intervals

The QT intervals are prolonged beyond the normal limits for the heart rate because of the prolongation of the ST segments.

Notes

_____

_____

_____

_____

DRUG EFFECT

Digitalis

◆ PATHOPHYSIOLOGY

Digitalis administered within therapeutic range produces characteristic changes in the ECG (Figure 14-9). In addition, when given in excess, digitalis toxicity occurs, causing excitatory or inhibitory effects on the heart and its electrical conduction system.

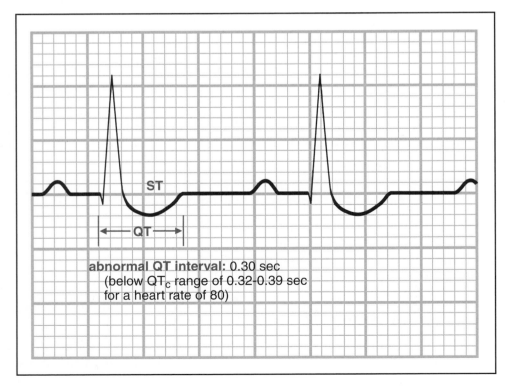

ST

QT

abnormal QT interval: 0.30 sec
(below QT$_c$ range of 0.32-0.39 sec
for a heart rate of 80)

Figure 14-9 Digitalis effect.

Excitatory effects include the following:
◆ Premature atrial contractions
◆ Atrial tachycardia with or without block
◆ Nonparoxysmal junctional tachycardia
◆ Premature ventricular contractions
◆ Ventricular tachycardia
◆ Ventricular fibrillation
Inhibitory effects include the following:
◆ Sinus bradycardia
◆ Sinoatrial (SA) exit block
◆ Atrioventricular (AV) block

◆ ECG CHARACTERISTICS

The ECG changes characteristic of a "digitalis effect" are as follows.

PR Intervals

The PR intervals are prolonged over 0.2 second.

ST Segments

The ST segments are depressed 1 mm or more in many of the leads, with a characteristic "scooped-out" appearance.

T Waves

The T waves may be flattened, inverted, or biphasic.

QT Intervals

The QT intervals are shorter than normal for the heart rate.

Notes

_____

_____

_____

_____

_____

_____

_____

Procainamide

◆ PATHOPHYSIOLOGY

Procainamide administered within therapeutic range produces characteristic changes in the ECG (Figure 14-10). In addition, when given in excess, procainamide toxicity occurs, causing excitatory or inhibitory effects on the heart and its electrical conduction system.

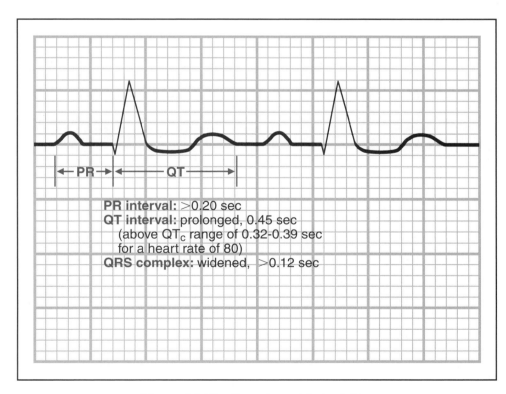

PR interval: >0.20 sec
QT interval: prolonged, 0.45 sec
    (above QT$_c$ range of 0.32-0.39 sec
    for a heart rate of 80)
QRS complex: widened, >0.12 sec

Figure 14-10 Procainamide toxicity.

Excitatory effects include the following:

◆ Premature ventricular contractions
◆ Ventricular tachycardia in the form of torsade de pointes (occurrence less common than in quinidine administration)
◆ Ventricular fibrillation
  Inhibitory effects include the following:
◆ Depression of myocardial contractility, which may cause hypotension and congestive heart failure
◆ AV block
◆ Ventricular asystole

◆ ECG CHARACTERISTICS

QRS Complexes

The duration of the QRS complexes may be increased beyond 0.12 second. QRS complex widening is a sign of toxicity. The R waves may be decreased in amplitude.

T Waves

The T waves may be decreased in amplitude. Occasionally the T waves may be widened and notched because of the appearance of a U wave.

PR Intervals

The PR intervals may be prolonged.

ST Segments

The ST segments may be depressed 1 mm or more.

QT Intervals

The QT intervals may occasionally be prolonged beyond the normal limits for the heart rate. Prolongation of the QT intervals is a sign of procainamide toxicity.

Notes

_____

_____

_____

_____

Quinidine

◆ PATHOPHYSIOLOGY

Quinidine administered within therapeutic range produces characteristic changes in the ECG (Figure 14-11). In addition, when given in excess, quinidine toxicity occurs, causing excitatory or inhibitory effects on the heart and its electrical conduction system.

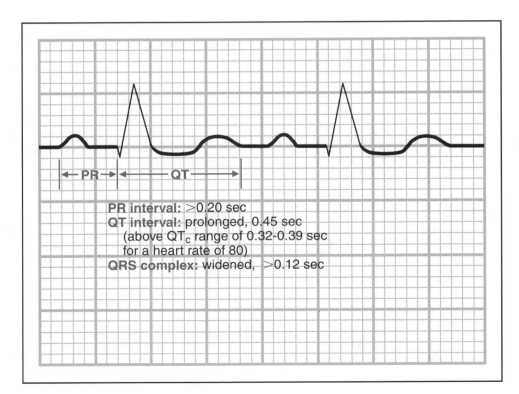

PR interval: >0.20 sec
QT interval: prolonged, 0.45 sec
  (above QT$_c$ range of 0.32-0.39 sec
  for a heart rate of 80)
QRS complex: widened, >0.12 sec

Figure 14-11 Quinidine toxicity.

Excitatory effects include the following:
- Premature ventricular contractions
- Ventricular tachycardia in the form of torsade de pointes (occurrence more common than in procainamide administration)
- Ventricular fibrillation
  Inhibitory effects include the following:
- Depression of myocardial contractility, which may cause hypotension and congestive heart failure
- SA exit block
- AV block
- Ventricular asystole

◆ ECG CHARACTERISTICS

P Waves

The P waves may be wide, often notched.

QRS Complexes

The duration of the QRS complexes may be increased beyond 0.12 second. QRS complex widening is a sign of toxicity.

T Waves

The T waves may be decreased in amplitude, wide, and notched, or they may be inverted. The notching is caused by the appearance of a U wave as the T wave widens.

PR Intervals

The PR intervals may be prolonged beyond normal.

ST Segments

The ST segments may be depressed 1 mm or more.

QT Intervals

The QT intervals may be prolonged beyond the normal limits for the heart rate. Prolongation of the QT intervals is a sign of quinidine toxicity.

Notes

_____

_____

_____

_____

_____

_____

_____

PULMONARY DISEASE

Chronic Obstructive Pulmonary Disease

◆ PATHOPHYSIOLOGY

Chronic obstructive pulmonary disease (COPD) (Figure 14-12) is a chronic disease of the lungs characterized by diffuse airway obstruction associated with varying degrees of chronic bronchitis and emphysema. The primary cause of COPD is prolonged heavy cigarette smoking. The lungs are typically overdistended and enlarged. A chronic productive cough and dyspnea on exertion are commonly present.

The following atrial arrhythmias frequently occur in COPD:
- Premature atrial contractions
- Wandering atrial pacemaker
- Multifocal atrial tachycardia
- Atrial flutter
- Atrial fibrillation

A typical ECG associated with COPD, characterized by a "P pulmonale" and precordial R waves of low voltage, is described here.

◆ ECG CHARACTERISTICS

P Waves

Changes indicative of right atrial enlargement are present (i.e., tall, symmetrically peaked P waves [P pulmonale] in leads II, III, and aVF and sharply peaked biphasic P waves in leads V_1 and V_2).

QRS Complexes

The QRS complexes are usually of low voltage. Poor R-wave progression across the precordium is usually present because of the increased volume of the thorax caused by overinflation of the lungs from emphysema.

QRS Axis

The QRS axis may be greater than +90°.

Notes

_____

_____

_____

_____

_____

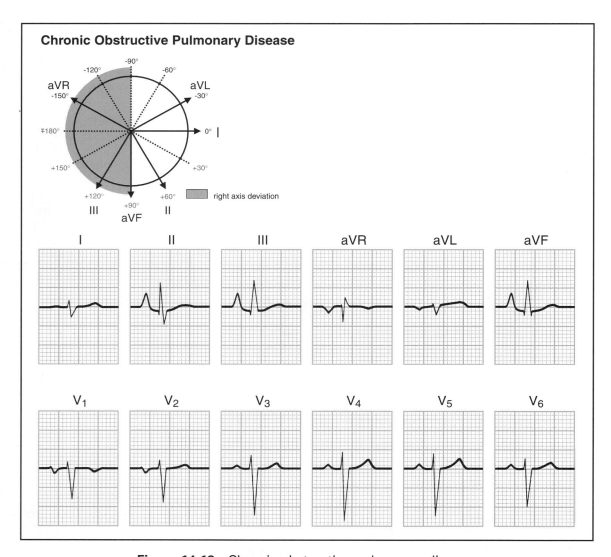

Figure 14-12 Chronic obstructive pulmonary disease.

Acute Pulmonary Embolism

◆ PATHOPHYSIOLOGY

Pulmonary embolism (Figure 14-13) occurs when a blood clot (thromboembolus) or other foreign matter (solid, liquid, or gaseous) lodges in a pulmonary artery and causes obstruction (occlusion) of blood flow to the lung segment supplied by the artery. The thromboemboli originate most commonly in the deep leg veins or the pelvic veins and infrequently in the veins of the upper extremities or in the right heart.

If the area of the pulmonary circulation affected by pulmonary embolization is small, the symptoms, if any, are minimal, such as sinus tachycardia and dyspnea. If pulmonary embolization shuts off a large part of the pulmonary circulation, it is con-sidered a massive pulmonary embolism. This results in hypoxemia and the following signs and symptoms.

Symptoms

- ◆ Sudden severe dyspnea
- ◆ Anxiety, restlessness, and apprehension
- ◆ Chilliness, dizziness, and mental confusion
- ◆ Nausea, vomiting, and abdominal pain (acute congestion of the liver caused by right-sided congestive heart failure)
- ◆ Precordial or substernal chest pain similar to that of acute MI

Signs

- ◆ Sinus tachycardia
- ◆ Tachypnea, cough, and wheezing

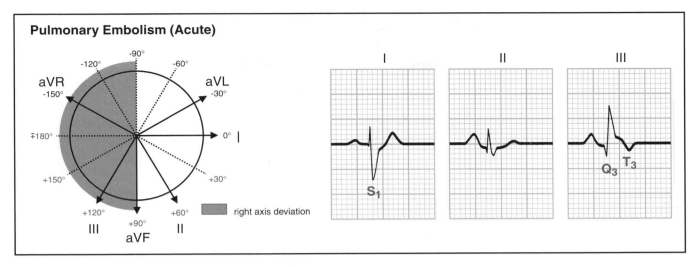

Figure 14-13   Pulmonary embolism.

◆ Cyanosis
◆ Distended neck veins (right-sided congestive heart failure)
◆ Forceful pulsation, seen and palpated, in the second left intercostal space with a systolic pulmonic murmur (dilated pulmonary artery)
◆ Hypotension, shock, and, rarely, cardiac arrest
    Because of the increased pressure in the pulmonary artery (pulmonary hypertension) caused by the major obstruction of blood flow through the pulmonary circulation, the right ventricle and atrium become distended, unable to function properly, leading to right heart failure. This condition is called *acute cor pulmonale.*

    In minimal pulmonary embolization, the ECG may be normal. However, in massive acute pulmonary embolization (acute cor pulmonale), the ECG shows a "P pulmonale" and a characteristic $S_1Q_3T_3$ pattern described below.

◆ ECG CHARACTERISTICS

P Waves

Changes indicative of right atrial enlargement are present (i.e., tall, symmetrically peaked P waves [P pulmonale] in leads II, III, and aVF and sharply peaked biphasic P waves in leads V_1 and V_2).

QRS Complexes

An S wave in lead I, a Q wave in lead III, and an inverted T wave in lead III (the $S_1Q_3T_3$ pattern) may occur acutely. In addition, a right bundle branch block may also occur.

QRS Axis

The QRS axis is greater than $+90°$.

ST Segments/T Waves

A right ventricular "strain" pattern may be present (inverted T waves in leads V_1-V_3).

Notes

_____

_____

_____

_____

_____

_____

_____

_____

Chronic Cor Pulmonale

◆ PATHOPHYSIOLOGY

Chronic cor pulmonale (Figure14-14) is the enlargement of the right ventricle (dilatation and/or hypertrophy) commonly accompanied by right heart failure. It is usually the end stage result of prolonged pulmonary hypertension that occurs with many diseases of the lung, including COPD and recurrent pulmonary embolization.

    Chronic cor pulmonale is often associated with atrial arrhythmias, including the following:
◆ Premature atrial contractions
◆ Wandering atrial pacemaker
◆ Multifocal atrial tachycardia
◆ Atrial flutter
◆ Atrial fibrillation

A typical ECG associated with chronic cor pulmonale, characterized by a "P pulmonale" and a classic right ventricle hypertrophy pattern, is described here.

◆ ECG CHARACTERISTICS

P Waves

Changes indicative of right atrial enlargement are present (i.e., tall, symmetrically peaked P waves [P pulmonale] in leads II, III, and aVF and sharply peaked biphasic P waves in leads V_1 and V_2).

QRS Complexes

Changes indicative of right ventricular hypertrophy are present.

QRS Axis

The QRS axis is greater than +90°.

ST Segments/T Waves

A right ventricular "strain" pattern is present (inverted T waves in leads V_1-V_3).

KEY POINT

The ECG in a small percentage of patients with chronic cor pulmonale, especially those with severe lung hyperinflation, shows S waves in leads I, II, and III (the S_1 S_2 S_3 pattern) along with a "P pulmonale" and a QRS axis in the –90° to –150° range. Patients with this type of ECG pattern have been shown to have a poor survival rate.

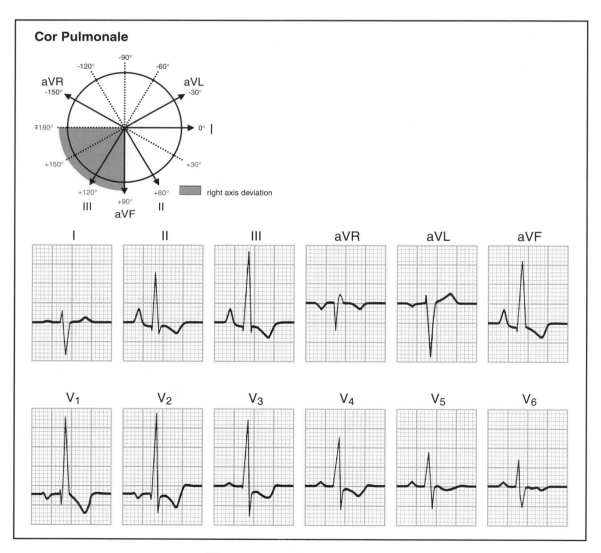

Figure 14-14 Cor pulmonale.

Notes

EARLY REPOLARIZATION

◆ PATHOPHYSIOLOGY

Early repolarization (Figure 14-15) is a term used to describe a form of myocardial repolarization in which the ST segment is elevated or depressed 1 to 3 mm above or below the baseline, respectively. The ST elevations are most commonly seen in leads I, II, and aVF and the precordial leads V_2-V_6. ST depression may be present in lead aVR. Early repolarization can occur in normal healthy people, commonly in young persons and sometimes in the elderly. The ST elevations can mimic the ECG pattern seen in acute MI and pericarditis.

The ST segment elevations present in early repolarization are similar to those seen during the early phase of acute anterior, lateral, and inferior MIs. However, there are no typical reciprocal ST depressions in the opposite leads. Unlike the elevated ST segments in early acute MI that later return to the baseline, these ST elevations persist. In addition, abnormally tall, peaked T waves seen in early acute MI, that later become inverted as the infarction progresses, and abnormal Q waves are absent in early repolarization.

The differentiation between the ST elevations of early repolarization and those seen in acute peri-

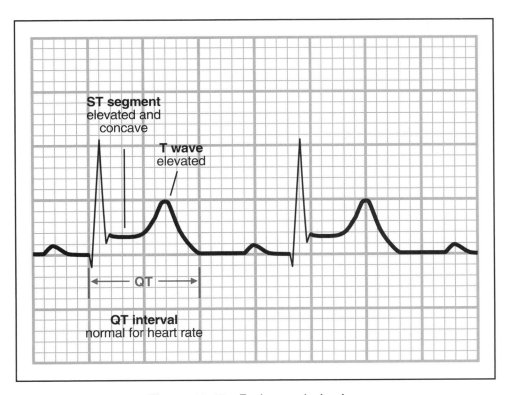

Figure 14-15   Early repolarization.

carditis is often difficult. The only clues are that early repolarization ST segments do not return to the baseline and that the T waves do not invert as they do over time in resolving pericarditis.

◆ ECG CHARACTERISTICS

QRS Complexes

Abnormal Q waves are usually absent.

ST Segments

The ST segments are elevated by about 1 to 3 mm or more in leads I, II, and aVF and the precordial leads V_2-V_6. The ST segment may be depressed in lead aVR.

T Waves

The T waves are usually normal.

Notes

_____

_____

_____

_____

HYPOTHERMIA

◆ PATHOPHYSIOLOGY

In the majority of hypothermic patients with a core body temperature of ≤95° F, a distinctive narrow, positive wave (Figure 14-16), the Osborn wave (also referred to as "the J wave," "the J deflection," or "the camel's hump"), occurs at the junction of the QRS complex and the ST segment—the QRS-ST junction. Associated ECG changes include prolonged PR and QT intervals and widening of the QRS complex.

Sinus bradycardia and junctional and ventricular arrhythmias also occur in hypothermia. The abnormal ECG changes and arrhythmias noted here are reversed after normalization of the body's temperature.

◆ ECG CHARACTERISTICS

PR Intervals

The PR intervals may occasionally be greater than 0.20 second.

QRS Complexes

The QRS complexes may occasionally be abnormally wide, greater than 0.12 second.

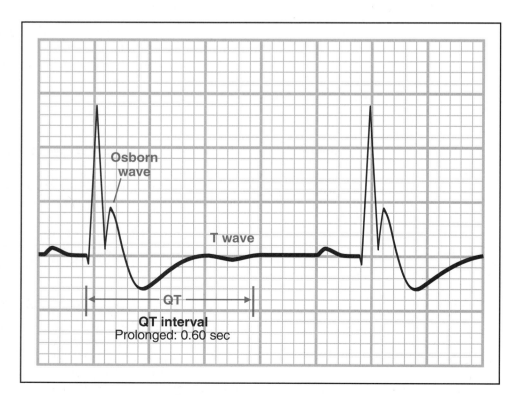

Figure 14-16 Hypothermia.

QT Interval

The corrected QT interval (QTc interval) may occasionally be prolonged.

Osborn Wave

An Osborn wave is present, typically in the leads facing the left ventricle. It is a narrow positive deflection that is closely attached to the end of the R or S wave of the QRS complex at the point where the QRS complex joins the ST segment—the J point.

Notes

_____

_____

_____

_____

_____

_____

_____

_____

_____

PREEXCITATION SYNDROMES

◆ PATHOPHYSIOLOGY

Preexcitation syndromes (Figure 14-17) occur when electrical impulses travel from the atria or AV junction into the ventricles through accessory conduction pathways, causing the ventricles to depolarize earlier than they normally would. Accessory conduction pathways are abnormal strands of myocardial fibers that conduct electrical impulses (1) from the atria to the ventricles or AV junction or (2) from the AV junction to the ventricles, bypassing various parts of the normal electrical conduction system (see Chapter 1). These pathways can not only conduct electrical impulses forward (anterograde), but most of them can also conduct the impulses backward (retrograde) as well, a potential set-up for reentry tachyarrhythmias, such as paroxysmal supraventricular tachycardias (PSVT).

The following are the three major accessory conduction pathways:

◆ **Accessory AV pathways (bundles of Kent).** These accessory tracts, located between the atria and ventricles, are responsible for accessory AV pathway conduction, also known as the *Wolff-Parkinson-*

White (WPW) conduction. These pathways conduct electrical impulses from the atria to the ventricles, bypassing the AV junction, producing premature depolarization of the ventricles—*ventricular preexcitation.* This results in a slurring of the onset of the QRS complex, the *delta wave.* When accessory AV pathway conduction is associated with episodes of PSVT, it is called the *Wolff-Parkinson-White syndrome.* During the tachycardia, the changes in the QRS complex characteristic of ventricular preexcitation described below disappear and the QRS complexes appear normal.

◆ **Atrio-His fibers (James fibers).** This accessory conduction pathway connects the atria with the lowermost part of the AV node, bypassing the slower conducting AV node. This results in *atrio-His preexcitation,* typified by an abnormally short PR interval. Because this type of accessory AV conduction does not conduct the electrical impulse directly into the ventricles, a delta wave is not produced.

◆ **Nodoventricular/fasciculoventricular fibers (Mahaim fibers).** These accessory conduction pathways provide bypass channels between the lower part of the AV node and the ventricles (the nodoventricular fibers) and between the bundle of His and the ventricles (the fasciculoventricular fibers), resulting in *nodoventricular* and *fasciculoventricular preexcitation.* Like ventricular preexcitation, this form of preexcitation also involves the conduction of the electrical impulse directly into the ventricles with premature depolarization of the ventricles, producing a delta wave. Because the AV node is not bypassed, the PR interval is usually normal.

◆ ECG CHARACTERISTICS

Ventricular Preexcitation (Accessory AV Pathways)

PR Intervals. The PR intervals are usually shortened to less than 0.12 second, between 0.09 and 0.12 second.

QRS Complexes. The duration of the QRS complexes are greater than 0.10 second and abnormally shaped, with a delta wave (the slurring of the onset of the QRS complex).

Atrio-His Preexcitation (Atrio-His Fibers)

PR Intervals. The PR intervals are usually shortened to less than 0.12 second.

QRS Complexes. The duration of the QRS complexes is normal, 0.10 second or less in adults and 0.08 second or less in children. A delta wave is not present.

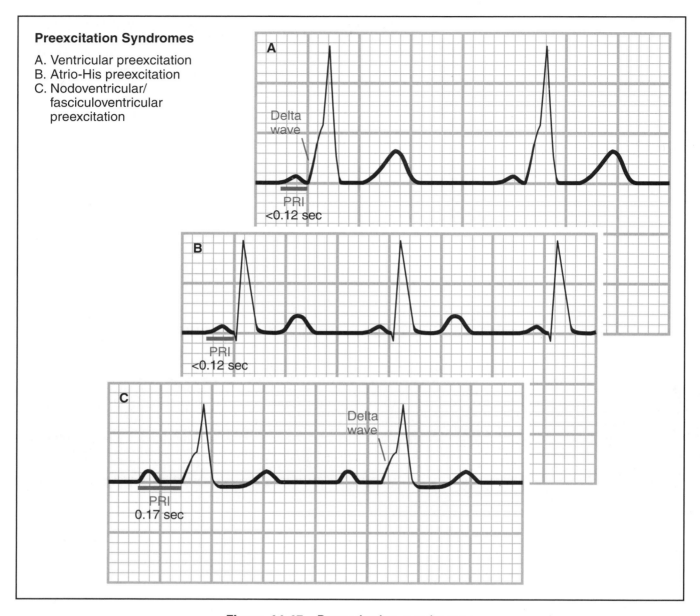

Figure 14-17 Preexcitation syndromes.

Nodoventricular/Fasciculoventricular Preexcitation (Nodoventricular/Fasciculoventricular Fibers)

PR Intervals. The PR intervals are usually normal, 0.12 second or greater.

QRS Complexes. The duration of the QRS complexes are greater than 0.10 second and abnormally shaped, with a delta wave (the slurring of the onset of the QRS complex) in both of these preexcitation syndromes.

◆ CLINICAL SIGNIFICANCE

Because of the wide and distorted QRS complexes associated with ventricular and nodoventricular/fasci-

culoventricular preexcitation, an ECG with such QRS complexes may be mistaken for a bundle branch block, ventricular hypertrophy, or MI. When the heart rate is rapid, the P waves are superimposed on the preceding T waves, causing, for example, a supraventricular tachycardia to resemble ventricular tachycardia.

Notes

_____

_____

_____

_____

_____

CHAPTER REVIEW QUESTIONS

1. A chronic condition of the heart characterized by an increase in the thickness of a chamber's myocardial wall secondary to the increase in the size of the muscle fibers is called:
   A. stenosis
   B. dilatation
   C. hypertrophy
   D. none of the above

2. A patient who has mitral valve insufficiency or left heart failure may have:
   A. right atrial and ventricular enlargement
   B. left atrial and ventricular enlargement
   C. right ventricular enlargement alone
   D. left ventricular enlargement alone

3. Left ventricular hypertrophy, a condition usually caused by increased pressure or volume in the left ventricle, is often found in:
   A. systemic hypertension and acute MI
   B. mitral insufficiency and hypertrophic cardiomyopathy
   C. aortic stenosis or insufficiency
   D. all of the above

4. The diagnosis of left ventricular hypertrophy is based on the ECG characteristics of increased amplitude or depth of the R and S waves in specific limb and precordial leads and:
   A. a QRS axis greater than $-15°$
   B. ST segment elevation
   C. all of the above
   D. none of the above

5. An inflammatory disease directly involving the epicardium with deposition of inflammatory cells and a variable amount of serous, fibrous, purulent, or hemorrhagic exudate within the sac surrounding the heart is called:
   A. pericarditis
   B. myocarditis
   C. cardiac tamponade
   D. none of the above

6. Signs and symptoms of the acute medical problems described in question number 5 include:
   A. chest pain and dyspnea
   B. chills and weakness
   C. fever and malaise
   D. all of the above

7. In a diffuse pericarditis (i.e., one that is not localized), the ST segments are elevated in:
   A. the precordial leads V_1 through V_4
   B. leads aVR, aVL, and aVF
   C. all leads except aVR and V_1
   D. the biphasic leads only

8. An excess serum potassium above the normal levels of 3.5 to 5.0 mEq/L is called:
   A. hypernatremia
   B. hypercalcemia
   C. hypercarbia
   D. hyperkalemia

9. The ECG changes that occur at various levels of excess serum potassium are:
   A. the QRS complexes widen and the T waves become tall
   B. The ST segments disappear and the T waves become peaked
   C. the PR intervals become prolonged and a "sine wave" QRS-ST-T pattern appears
   D. all of the above may occur

10. A medication normally prescribed to heart patients, which when taken in excess causes depression of myocardial contractility, AV block, ventricular asystole, and PVCs, is:
    A. digitalis
    B. procainamide
    C. Lasix
    D. verapamil

11. The ECG changes in acute pulmonary embolism include:
    A. a right ventricular "strain" pattern in leads V_5 and V_6
    B. an $S_3Q_1T_3$ pattern in leads I and III
    C. a QRS axis of greater than $+90°$
    D. all of the above

12. ECG changes indicative of right atrial enlargement and right ventricular hypertrophy and a QRS axis of greater than $+90°$ are characteristic of:
    A. chronic mitral insufficiency
    B. chronic cor pulmonale
    C. chronic obstructive pulmonary disease (COPD)
    D. all of the above

13. All but one of the following are typical of the ECG in early repolarization:
    A. the ST elevation typically occurs in leads II, III, aVR, and precordial leads V_2-V_6
    B. the ST elevation resembles that of acute MI and pericarditis
    C. abnormally tall, peaked T waves and abnormal Q waves are absent
    D. the ST elevations persist and do not return to the baseline as in a resolving acute MI

Continued

14. The Osborn wave is a sign of:
    A. pericarditis
    B. hypothermia
    C. hyperthermia
    D. ventricular preexcitation

15. A delta wave indicates the following:
    A. a preexcitation syndrome is present
    B. the QRS complex is greater than 0.10 second in duration
    C. accessory AV pathway conduction is present
    D. all of the above

16. Abnormal conduction of an electrical impulse through an accessory AV pathway results in the following:
    A. a normal PR interval and a delta wave
    B. an abnormally short PR interval and a normal QRS complex
    C. a Wolff-Parkinson-White syndrome
    D. an abnormally short PR interval and a delta wave

CHAPTER 15

Myocardial Ischemia, Injury, and Infarction

CHAPTER OUTLINE

CHAPTER OBJECTIVES

Upon completion of all or part of this chapter, you should be able to complete the following objectives:

1. Name and identify the right and left coronary arteries and their branches on an anatomical drawing of the coronary circulation.
2. Given a list of the arteries of the coronary circulation and a list of the regions of the heart, match the arteries with the regions of the heart they supply.
3. List the high risk factors for cardiovascular disease.
4. Describe the sequence of pathologic changes in the evolution of coronary atherosclerosis and the formation of a thrombus.
5. List the causes of myocardial ischemia, injury, and infarction.
6. Define *myocardial ischemia, myocardial injury,* and *myocardial infarction* and indicate which are reversible and which are not.
7. List and define the five coronary syndromes.
8. Define the following terms:
   Thrombolysis
   Transmural infarction
   Subendocardial infarction

9. On a drawing of an acute myocardial infarction, identify the zones of ischemia, injury, and infarction (necrosis).
10. Identify nine anatomic locations in the heart where acute myocardial infarctions occur and list the coronary arteries that supply these areas.
11. Describe the sequence of changes in the myocardium that occurs during the four phases of evolution of an acute anterior wall transmural myocardial infarction, including the timing and duration of each phase and sequence.
12. Define "facing" and "opposite" ECG leads.
13. Describe the changes in the Q, R, and T waves and ST segments in facing and opposite ECG leads in myocardial ischemia, injury, and necrosis and when they appear following the onset of an acute myocardial infarction.
14. Give the theoretical explanations for the following changes in the T waves associated with an acute myocardial infarction:
    Inverted T waves over ischemic tissue
    Tall and peaked T waves over ischemic tissue
    Inverted T waves over necrotic tissue

15. Describe the T wave changes in a typical transmural myocardial infarction and those in a subendocardial myocardial infarction.
16. Give the measurements characteristic of an abnormally elevated or depressed ST segment.
17. Explain the theory behind ST segment elevation in acute myocardial infarction, namely, the current of injury.
18. Name three cardiac conditions, other than acute myocardial infarction, in which ST segment elevation occurs.
19. List the three kinds of sloping of the ST segment found in ST depression associated with myocardial ischemia.
20. Name three cardiac conditions, other than myocardial ischemia, in which ST segment depression occurs.
21. Define "septal" q and r waves, and indicate in which leads they normally appear.
22. Discuss the following with regard to abnormal Q waves:
    Diagnostic characteristics
    Significance of appearance in the ECG
    Q-wave and non-Q-wave myocardial infarctions
    Time of appearance following the onset of an acute myocardial infarction
    "Window" theory
23. Describe the following:
    A Q wave
    A QS wave; a QS complex
    A QR complex; a Qr complex
24. Discuss the significance of abnormal Q waves appearing in the following leads:
    aVR
    aVL
    aVF
    III
    V_1
25. Discuss the significance of abnormal Q waves when they occur in the presence of the following conditions:
    ST segment elevation and T wave inversion
    Left or right bundle branch block
    Left anterior or left posterior fascicular block
    Left ventricular hypertrophy

26. Explain why a Q-wave myocardial infarction cannot be classified solely as a transmural myocardial infarction and why a non-Q-wave myocardial infarction cannot be classified as a nontransmural myocardial infarction.
27. Describe the typical changes in the Q, R, and T waves and ST segments present with each of the four phases in the evolution of the following:
    Q-wave (transmural) infarction
    Non-Q-wave (subendocardial) infarction
28. Review the pathophysiologic changes in the ventricular wall with respect to the associated ECG changes that occur during each of the four phases of a transmural myocardial infarction.
29. Name the facing and opposite ECG leads used in the diagnosis of the following acute myocardial infarctions:
    Septal MI
    Anterior (localized) MI
    Anteroseptal MI
    Lateral MI
    Anterolateral MI
    Extensive anterior MI
    Inferior MI
    Posterior MI
    Right ventricular MI
30. Name the potential complications of acute myocardial infarctions that involve the following regions of the heart:
    Septum
    Anterior LV wall
    Lateral LV wall
    Inferior LV wall
    Posterior LV wall
    Right ventricular and inferior LV wall

CORONARY CIRCULATION

The coronary circulation (Table 15-1 and Figure 15-1) consists of the *left* and *right coronary arteries.* The left coronary artery arises from the base of the aorta just above the left coronary cusp of the aortic valve. The right coronary artery arises from the aorta just above the right aortic coronary cusp.

Left Coronary Artery

The left coronary artery consists of the *left main coronary artery,* a short main stem of about 2 to 10 mm in length, that usually divides into two equal major branches, the *left anterior descending coronary artery* and the *left circumflex coronary artery.* Sometimes, a third major branch, the *diagonal (or intermediate) coronary artery,* arises from the left main coronary artery instead of from the left anterior descending coronary artery.

AUTHOR'S NOTE

The term *artery(ies)* is used interchangeably with the term *branch(es)* in this chapter.

Coronary Artery	Region Supplied
Left Coronary Artery	
Left anterior descending	
Diagonal	Anterolateral wall of the left ventricle
Septal perforator	Anterior two thirds of the interventricular septum
Right ventricular	Anterior wall of the right ventricle
Left circumflex	
SA node (40%-60%)*	SA node
Left atrial circumflex	Left atrium
Anterolateral marginal	Anterolateral wall of the left ventricle
Posterolateral marginal	Posterolateral wall of the left ventricle
Distal left circumflex	Posterior wall of the left ventricle
Posterior descending (10%-15%)	Posterior one third of the interventricular septum
AV node (10%-15%)	AV node
	Proximal bundle of His
Posterior left ventricular (10%-15%)	Inferior wall of the left ventricle
Right Coronary Artery	
Conus	Upper anterior wall of the right ventricle
SA node (50%-60%)	SA node
Anterior right ventricular	Anterolateral wall of the right ventricle
Right atrial	Right atrium
Acute marginal	Lateral wall of the right ventricle
Posterior descending (85%-90%)	Posterior one third of the interventricular septum
AV node (85%-90%)	AV node
	Proximal bundle of His
Posterior left ventricular (85%-90%)	Inferior wall of the left ventricle

AV, Atrioventricular; *SA*, sinoatrial.

*The percentage figures indicate in what percentage of hearts the indicated coronary artery is present.

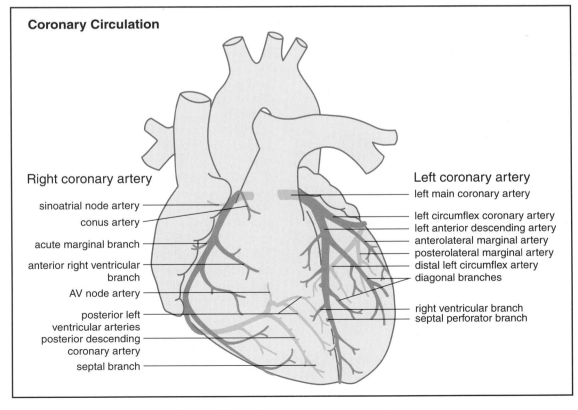

Coronary Circulation

Right coronary artery

- sinoatrial node artery
- conus artery
- acute marginal branch
- anterior right ventricular branch
- AV node artery
- posterior left ventricular arteries
- posterior descending coronary artery
- septal branch

Left coronary artery

- left main coronary artery
- left circumflex coronary artery
- left anterior descending artery
- anterolateral marginal artery
- posterolateral marginal artery
- distal left circumflex artery
- diagonal branches
- right ventricular branch
- septal perforator branch

Figure 15-1   The coronary circulation.

The left anterior descending coronary artery travels anteriorly and downward within the interventricular groove over the interventricular septum and circles the apex of the heart to end behind it. The left anterior descending coronary artery gives rise to at least one and often up to six diagonal branches, three to five septal perforator branches, and, sometimes, one or more right ventricular branches.

The diagonal arteries, the first of which may originate from the left main coronary artery, course over the anterior and lateral surface of the left ventricle between the left anterior descending coronary artery and the anterolateral marginal branch of the left circumflex coronary artery. The septal perforator arteries arise at a right angle from the left anterior descending coronary artery and run directly into the interventricular septum. The right ventricular arteries course over the anterior surface of the right ventricle.

The left circumflex coronary artery arises from the left main coronary artery at an obtuse angle and runs posteriorly along the left atrioventricular (AV) groove to end in back of the left ventricle in about 85% to 90% of hearts. In the remaining 10% to 15%, the left circumflex coronary artery continues along the AV groove to become the posterior left ventricular arteries. When this occurs, the left circumflex coronary artery usually continues farther to enter the posterior interventricular groove to become the posterior descending coronary artery while giving rise to the AV node artery.

The left circumflex coronary artery gives rise to the sinoatrial (SA) node artery in 40% to 50% of the hearts, one or two left atrial circumflex branches, the left obtuse marginal branches (the large anterolateral marginal artery and one or more smaller posterolateral marginal arteries), and the distal left circumflex artery. A left coronary artery with a circumflex coronary artery that gives rise to both the posterior left ventricular arteries and the posterior descending coronary artery is considered to be a "dominant" left coronary artery.

The anterolateral marginal artery runs over the anterolateral surface of the left ventricular wall toward the apex, lateral to the diagonal branches of the left anterior descending coronary artery. The posterolateral marginal arteries run down the posterolateral wall of the left ventricle, and the distal left circumflex artery runs down the left AV groove. When present, the posterior left ventricular arteries course over the inferior (or diaphragmatic) wall of the left ventricle; the posterior descending coronary artery runs down the posterior interventricular groove.

Right Coronary Artery

The right coronary artery travels downward and then posteriorly in the right AV groove, giving off the conus artery, the SA node artery in 50% to 60% of hearts, several anterior right ventricular branches, the right atrial branch, and the acute marginal branch.

In 85% to 90% of hearts, it also gives rise to the AV node artery and the posterior descending coronary artery (with its septal branches), which runs down the posterior interventricular groove, and, then, continuing into the left AV groove, the right coronary artery terminates as the posterior left ventricular arteries. A right coronary artery that gives rise to both the posterior descending coronary artery and the posterior left ventricular arteries is considered to be a "dominant" right coronary artery.

Summary

The left anterior descending coronary artery supplies the anterior two thirds of the interventricular septum, most of the right and left bundle branches, the anterior (apical) and lateral wall of the left ventricle, and, sometimes, the anterior wall of the right ventricle.

The left circumflex coronary artery supplies the left atrial wall, the lateral and posterior wall of the left ventricle, and, in 40% to 50% of hearts, the SA node. In 10% to 15% of hearts, when the posterior left ventricular, AV node, and posterior descending coronary arteries arise from the left circumflex artery, the left circumflex artery also supplies the inferior (diaphragmatic) wall of the left ventricle, the AV node, the proximal bundle of His, and the posterior (inferior) one third of the interventricular septum. When this occurs, the entire interventricular septum is supplied by the left coronary artery.

The right coronary artery supplies the right atrial and ventricular wall; the AV node, the proximal bundle of His, the posterior one third of the interventricular septum, and the inferior (diaphragmatic) wall of the left ventricle in 85% to 90% of hearts; and the SA node in 50% to 60% of hearts.

CORONARY ARTERY DISEASE

Coronary artery disease is the leading cause of death in the United States and in most of the rest of the world. High risk factors for cardiovascular disease include the following:

◆ Family history (heredity)
◆ Gender (male)
◆ Race
◆ Age
◆ Cigarette smoking
◆ Diabetes mellitus
◆ Hypertension

- Elevated cholesterol blood levels
- Elevated triglyceride blood levels
- Elevated homocysteine blood levels
- Obesity
- Lack of exercise
- Stress
- Cocaine use

Coronary atherosclerosis, a form of arteriosclerosis (hardening of the arteries), is the primary disease process involved in coronary artery disease. It is responsible for the formation of atheromatous plaques in large and medium-sized coronary arteries, often followed by plaque disruption, thrombosis, and coronary artery occlusion. The consequence of coronary atherosclerosis is a group of clinical syndromes, the "acute coronary syndromes," that include *unstable angina, myocardial infarction (MI),* and *sudden ischemic cardiac death.*

Pathophysiology of Coronary Atherosclerosis

The first phase in the evolution of coronary atherosclerosis is the appearance of *atheromatous plaques* within the inner layer of the coronary arteries (Figure 15-2). The atheromatous plaques begin with the migration of low-density lipoproteins (LDL) from the plasma into the intima, where they evolve into small clumps of lipid-filled foam cells seen as yellow dots or streaks on the intimal surface of the artery. These progress over time to large plaques consisting of a soft gruel-like lipid- and cholesterol-rich atheromatous core and an external fibrous cap composed primarily of smooth muscle cells and collagen. The volume and composition of the atheromatous core and the thickness of the fibrous cap vary from plaque to plaque even in the same coronary artery. Atheromatous plaques may remain stable for years without causing any symptoms or becoming involved with thrombi.

The second phase in the evolution of coronary atherosclerosis is the formation of a *thrombus* on the surface of the plaque after its erosion or in the plaque itself after rupture of the fibrous cap, often with an extension of the thrombus into the arterial lumen. Generally, a plaque does not rupture until its core becomes highly saturated with lipids. The rupture of the fibrous cap is at least three times more common then the erosion and denudation of the plaque surface.

Erosion is the process by which the endothelial cover of the plaque is torn away, exposing the plaque itself (denudation). A platelet-rich thrombus immediately forms on the denuded surface of the plaque, increasing the size of the plaque.

Rupture (disruption) of the fibrous cap is most likely to occur at its shoulder, the area of the cap where it connects with the normal arterial wall. The

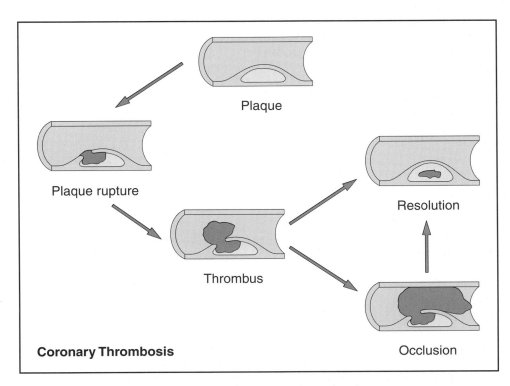

Figure 15-2   Coronary thrombosis.

cause of the rupture may be one or more of the following:

◆ Progressive weakening and/or thinning of the fibrous wall at one point
◆ Sudden surges in blood pressure, heart rate, or blood flow (as seen with emotional stress, heavy physical exertion in otherwise sedentary people, or the process of getting up in the morning)
◆ Vasospasm of the coronary artery at the site of the plaque
◆ Repetitive flexion of the artery at the site of the plaque

After rupture of the fibrous cap, blood enters the plaque and, on mixing with the atheromatous lipid-rich gruel, which appears to greatly enhance thrombus formation, immediately produces a thrombus rich in platelets and fibrin with some red cells. The thrombus may not extend beyond the plaque, causing no further occlusion. However, if the thrombus continues to grow, it may extend beyond the fibrous cap into the arterial lumen, as it often does, partially or completely occluding it. As the thrombus grows into the lumen, it becomes rich in fibrin. Sometimes clumps of platelets break off the distal end of the main thrombus and flow downstream, clogging arteries, arterioles, and even capillaries.

Once the thrombus is formed, it may spontaneously disintegrate, partially or completely (spontaneous thrombolysis), undergo further rethrombosis and enlarge, or undergo organization by connective tissue into a fibrotic lesion.

A stable atheromatous plaque that results in significant coronary artery stenosis is the main cause of stable angina and silent ischemia. This results from the inability of the stenotic artery to increase its delivery of blood to the myocardium whenever the myocardial oxygen demand is increased for whatever reason. On the other hand, sudden rupture of a plaque with thrombus formation, and subsequent partial or complete obstruction of the arterial lumen with an abrupt decrease in blood flow, is the common cause of unstable angina, MI, and sudden ischemic cardiac death.

Myocardial Ischemia, Injury, and Infarction

Myocardial ischemia, injury, and infarction result from the failure of local coronary arteries to supply sufficient oxygenated blood to the myocardial tissue they supply to meet the tissue's need for oxygen (ischemia). This can result from a variety of causes (Figure 15-3), including the following:

◆ Occlusion (or obstruction) of an already severely narrowed atherosclerotic coronary artery by a blood clot (coronary thrombosis) after rupture of an atherosclerotic plaque, with hemorrhage within the plaque extending into the arterial lumen. Acute increase in arterial pressure or heart rate such as associated with physical exertion or emotional stress commonly precedes the rupture of an atherosclerotic plaque. Coronary artery spasm and hypercoagulability of the blood predispose to plaque rupture and thrombus formation. Coronary thrombosis after plaque rupture is the most common cause of MI, occurring in about 90% of acute MIs.
◆ Coronary artery spasm caused by constriction of smooth muscle in the wall of the coronary artery. Generally, the spasm occurs at the site of narrowing from coronary atherosclerosis. As noted above, coronary artery spasm often accompanies or is the cause of plaque rupture that results in coronary thrombosis.

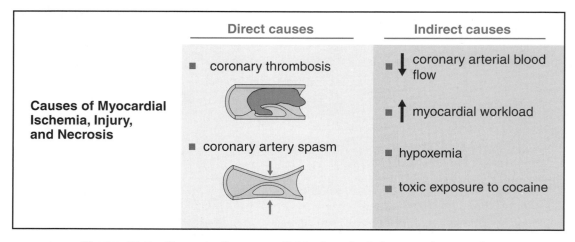

Figure 15-3 Causes of myocardial ischemia, injury, and necrosis.

◆ Decreased coronary arterial blood flow for whatever reason other than coronary artery occlusion or spasm, such as an arrhythmia, pulmonary embolism, or hypotension or shock from any cause (e.g., chest trauma and aortic dissection).

◆ Increased myocardial workload from unaccustomed effort, emotional stress, unrelieved fatigue, or increased blood volume (volume overload) imposed on a heart with atherosclerotic coronary arteries.

◆ Decreased level of oxygen in the blood delivered to the myocardium because of hypoxemia from acute respiratory failure.

◆ Toxic exposure to cocaine.

◆ MYOCARDIAL ISCHEMIA

Myocardial ischemia is present the moment there is a decrease or complete absence of blood supply to myocardial tissue. This immediately results in the lack of oxygen (anoxia) within the cardiac cells. For a short time after the onset of anoxia, certain reversible ischemic changes usually occur in the internal structure of the affected cells because of the lack of oxygen. These ischemic changes cause a delay in the depolarization and repolarization of the cells. Mild or moderate anoxia can be tolerated for a short time by the cardiac cells without greatly affecting their function. There may be some loss in the ability of the myocardial cells to contract and of the specialized cells of the electrical conduction system to generate or conduct electrical impulses. Upon the return of adequate blood flow and reoxygenation, these cells usually return to a normal or near normal condition.

◆ MYOCARDIAL INJURY

If ischemia is severe or prolonged, the anoxic cardiac cells sustain moderate to severe *myocardial injury* and stop functioning normally, unable to contract or generate or conduct electrical impulses

properly. At this stage, the damage to the cells still remains reversible so that the injured cells remain viable and salvageable for some time. As in ischemic cells, injured cells may also return to normal or near normal after the return of adequate blood flow and reoxygenation.

◆ MYOCARDIAL INFARCTION

If severe myocardial ischemia continues because of a continued complete absence of blood supply, the anoxic cardiac cells eventually sustain irreversible injury and die, becoming electrically inert. At the moment of cellular death, necrosis is present, and *myocardial infarction* occurs. Necrotic cells DO NOT return to normal upon revascularization or reoxygenation.

ACUTE CORONARY SYNDROMES

The term *acute coronary syndromes* includes a variety of cardiac conditions ranging from silent ischemia, stable angina, unstable angina, acute MI, to sudden cardiac death.

Silent Ischemia

The appearance of ST segment depression with or without T wave inversion on the electrocardiogram (ECG) during exertion and less commonly at rest without chest pain indicates silent subendocardial ischemia. This condition is considered to be stable if it recurs after the same degree of exertion. The cause is an atheromatous plaque producing significant coronary artery stenosis.

Stable Angina

Exertion-induced angina (Canadian Cardiovascular Society Angina Classification [CCSC] class II or III) (Table 15-2), that characteristically remains unchanged from episode to episode after the same

TABLE

15-2   Classification of Exertion-Induced Angina

Class	Activity Evoking Angina	Limits to Normal Activity
I	Prolonged exertion	None
II	Walking >2 blocks	Slight
III	Walking <2 blocks	Marked
IV	Minimal or at rest	Severe

amount of exertion is considered *stable angina.* It is the result of a stable atheromatous plaque causing significant coronary artery stenosis. The ECG usually shows ST segment depression with or without T wave inversion during angina, indicating subendocardial ischemia.

Unstable Angina

Unstable angina is considered to be present if one or more of the following occurs:

◆ A new onset of exertional angina of CCSC class III or IV
◆ An increase of existing angina to CCSC class III or IV
◆ The appearance of post-MI angina
◆ The appearance of angina at rest (usually prolonged for 20 minutes or longer)

The cause of unstable angina is usually the rupture of a plaque followed by the formation of a thrombus that partially occludes the lumen of the coronary artery for the first time or increases the existing stenosis or, in some instances, completely occludes the lumen for about 10 to 20 minutes followed by partial spontaneous thrombolysis. Unstable angina may also be caused by erosion of an existing plaque followed by thrombus formation. First-time partial occlusion of the coronary artery results in a new onset of exertional angina, an increase in an existing stenosis results in an increase in the angina and the appearance of post-MI angina, and a temporary total obstruction results in angina at rest. The ECG usually shows ST segment depression with or without T wave inversion during angina, indicating subendocardial ischemia.

It must be noted that a new onset of angina or an increase of existing angina denoting instability may also occur under certain circumstances in which an imbalance between oxygen demand and supply suddenly arises without being necessarily caused by an increase in the degree of the stenotic lesion within an atherosclerotic coronary artery. These circumstances include the following:

◆ Tachycardia from any cause, such as tachyarrhythmias, congestive heart failure, anemia, fever, hypoxia, hypotension, or shock
◆ Bradyarrhythmia
◆ Increased myocardial workload from unaccustomed effort, emotional stress, unrelieved fatigue, or increased blood volume (volume overload)
◆ Decreased level of oxygen in the blood delivered to the myocardium because of hypoxemia from acute respiratory failure
◆ Toxic exposure to cocaine, causing vasoconstriction

The ECG under these circumstances also usually shows ST segment depression with or without T wave inversion during angina, indicating subendocardial ischemia.

Acute Myocardial Infarction

Acute MI is the result of a plaque rupture followed by the formation of a large thrombus that partially or completely occludes the lumen of a coronary artery, resulting in myocardial ischemia, injury, and necrosis. It is accompanied by prolonged anterior chest pain in the majority of patients. The ECG initially shows ST segment and T wave changes, often followed by Q waves several hours later, indicating myocardial necrosis.

Sudden Cardiac Death

Ventricular tachycardia or fibrillation is the most common cause of sudden cardiac death, being responsible for about 80% of such deaths. Asystole or electromechanical dissociation is the cause in the rest. These lethal arrhythmias are most likely the result of the myocardial ischemia and injury that follows the rupture of a plaque and consequent thrombotic occlusion of a coronary artery.

ACUTE MYOCARDIAL INFARCTION

Myocardial infarction usually follows the occlusion of an atherosclerotic epicardial coronary artery by a thrombus—*coronary thrombosis.* This process, as described earlier, involves an intricate interaction between the rupture of an atherosclerotic plaque lining the coronary artery (often accompanied by vasospasm of the coronary artery smooth muscle), platelet activation, and formation of an occluding thrombus (see Figure 15-2).

Angiographic studies of the coronary arteries performed within the first few hours after the onset of symptoms of acute MI show that about 90% of the coronary artery occlusions are the result of thrombi. The incidence and degree of thrombus-related coronary artery occlusion, as shown by angiographic and autopsy studies, appears to diminish with time, primarily because of recanalization of the occluded coronary artery from spontaneous disintegration of the blood clot (thrombolysis).

After the occlusion of a coronary artery, the myocardium evolves through various stages and degrees of severity of impairment, beginning with myocardial ischemia, then progressing through myocardial injury, both of which are reversible, and ending with myocardial infarction, the stage of tissue necrosis, an irreversible condition. Along the way, characteristic changes in the ECG reflect the changes in the myocardium. This will be described later.

Typically, an MI at its height consists of a central area of dead, necrotic tissue—the *zone of infarction (or necrosis)*, surrounded immediately by a layer of injured myocardial tissue—*the zone of injury*, and then by an outer layer of ischemic tissue—*the zone of ischemia.*

An acute MI may be either transmural or nontransmural. A *transmural infarction* is one in which the zone of infarction involves the entire or almost entire thickness of the ventricular wall, including both the subendocardial and subepicardial areas of the myocardium. A *nontransmural infarction*, on the other hand, is one in which the zone of infarction only involves a part of the ventricular wall, usually the inner, subendocardial area of the myocardium (Figure 15-4).

Anatomic Locations of Myocardial Infarctions

The site of the MI depends on which coronary artery is occluded (Figure 15-5). Table 15-3 lists the locations of the MI and the coronary artery or arteries most likely occluded to produce them. Because the distribution of the coronary arteries varies from person to person, the arteries occluded in any specific MI may differ from the ones listed in the table.

The Four Phases of a Transmural Myocardial Infarction

The evolution and resolution of a typical transmural MI can be divided into four phases, depending on the stage and severity of involvement of the myocardium. The transmural MI usually begins in the subendocardium, presumably because this area has the highest myocardial oxygen demand and the least supply of blood. The infarct then progresses outward in a wave front pattern until it involves the entire myocardium. While the necrosis is progressing from the endocardium to the epicardium, the acute MI is said to be *"evolving."*

◆ PHASE 1

Within the first 2 hours after coronary artery occlusion the following sequence of changes occurs in the myocardium supplied by the occluded artery (Figure 15-6, *A*):
1. Within seconds of the coronary artery occlusion, extensive myocardial ischemia occurs.
2. During the first 20 to 40 minutes (average, 30 minutes) after the onset of the MI, reversible myocardial injury appears in the subendocardium.

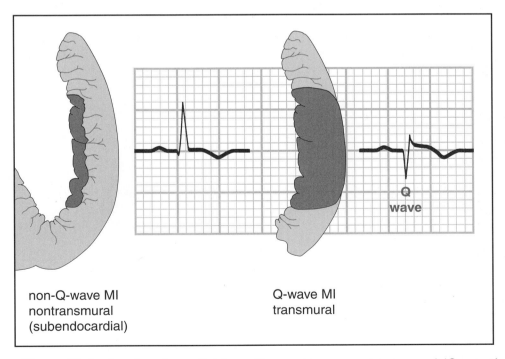

non-Q-wave MI
nontransmural
(subendocardial)

Q-wave MI
transmural

Figure 15-4 A subendocardial (non-Q-wave) versus a transmural (Q-wave) myocardial infarction.

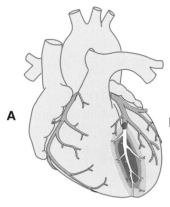

A

left anterior descending
septal perforator branches

septal MI

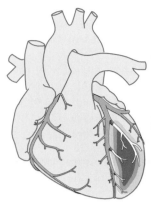

B

left anterior descending
diagonal branches

localized anterior MI

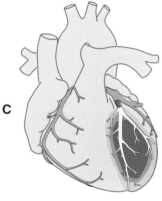

C

left anterior descending
septal perforator branches
diagonal branches

anteroseptal MI

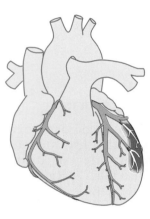

D

left anterior descending
diagonal branches
left circumflex
anterolateral marginal
branch

lateral MI

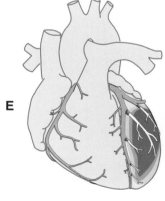

E

left anterior descending
diagonal branches
left circumflex
anterolateral marginal
branch

anterolateral MI

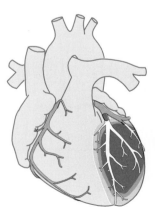

F

left anterior descending
left circumflex
anterolateral marginal
branch

extensive anterior MI

Figure 15-5 Location of myocardial infarction in relation to the coronary arteries occluded.

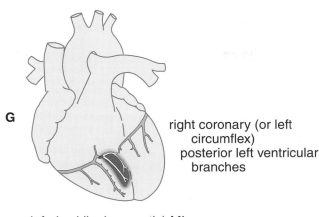

G

right coronary (or left
circumflex)
posterior left ventricular
branches

inferior (diaphragmatic) MI

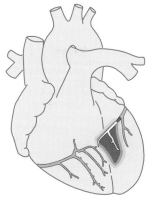

H

distal left circumflex
and/or
posterolateral marginal
branch

posterior MI

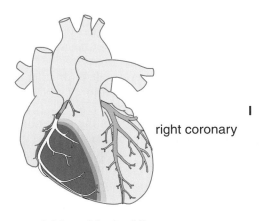

I

right coronary

right ventricular MI

Figure 15-5, cont'd

3. About 30 minutes after the interruption of blood flow, irreversible myocardial necrosis (infarction) occurs in the subendocardium as myocardial injury begins to spread toward the epicardium.
4. By 1 hour after the onset, myocardial necrosis has spread through over one third of the myocardium.
5. By 2 hours after the onset, myocardial necrosis has spread through about half of the myocardium.

◆ **PHASE 2**

Between the second and twenty-fourth hour after the occlusion, the evolution of the MI is completed in the following sequence (Figure 15-6, *B*):
1. By 3 hours, about two thirds of the myocardial cells within the affected myocardium become necrotic.
2. By 6 hours, only a small percentage of the cells remain viable. For all practical purposes, the evolu-

tion of the transmural MI is complete at this point.
3. By 24 hours, the progression of myocardial necrosis to the epicardium is usually complete.

◆ **PHASE 3**

After the first day, during the next 24 to 72 hours, little or no ischemic or injured myocardial cells remain because all cells have either died or recovered. Acute inflammation with edema and cellular infiltration begins within the necrotic tissue during this phase.

◆ **PHASE 4**

During the second week, inflammation continues, followed by proliferation of connective tissue during the third week. Healing with replacement of the necrotic tissue with fibrous connective tissue is generally complete by the seventh week.

15-3 Anatomic Locations of Myocardial Infarctions in Relation to the Coronary Arteries Occluded

Location of Infarction	Site of Coronary Artery Occlusion
Anterior MI	
Septal MI (Figure 15-5, *A*)	Left anterior descending coronary artery beyond the first diagonal branch, involving the septal perforator arteries
Anterior (localized) MI (Figure 15-5, *B*)	Diagonal arteries of the left anterior descending coronary artery
Anteroseptal MI (Figure 15-5, *C*)	Left anterior descending coronary artery involving both the septal perforator and diagonal arteries
Lateral MI (Figure 15-5, *D*)	Laterally-located diagonal arteries of the left anterior descending coronary artery and/or the anterolateral marginal artery of the left circumflex coronary artery
Anterolateral MI (Figure 15-5, *E*)	Diagonal arteries of the left anterior descending coronary artery alone or in conjunction with the anterolateral marginal artery of the left circumflex coronary artery
Extensive anterior MI (Figure 15-5, *F*)	Left anterior descending coronary artery alone or in conjunction with the anterolateral marginal artery of the left circumflex coronary artery
Inferior (diaphragmatic) MI (Figure 15-5, *G*)	(1) Posterior left ventricular arteries of the right coronary artery or, less commonly, of the left circumflex coronary artery of the left coronary artery or (2) the right coronary artery before the branching of the posterior descending, AV node, and posterior left ventricular arteries
Posterior MI (Figure 15-5, *H*)	Distal left circumflex artery and/or posterolateral marginal artery of the circumflex coronary artery
Right ventricular MI with inferior (diaphragmatic) MI (Figure 15-5, *I*)	Right coronary artery

MI, Myocardial infarction.

Table 15-4 summarizes the four phases of evolution of an acute transmural MI.

ECG Changes in Acute Myocardial Infarction

The ECG in an evolving acute MI, with its varying mix of myocardial ischemia, injury, and necrosis, is characterized by changes in three components of the ECG—the T wave, ST segment, and Q wave. The changes in the ECG ascribed to myocardial ischemia, injury, and necrosis include the following:

◆ *Myocardial ischemia:* Symmetrical T wave inversion or elevation and ST segment elevation or depression
◆ *Myocardial injury:* ST segment elevation or depression
◆ *Myocardial necrosis:* Abnormal Q waves

The nature of these ECG changes and the leads in which they appear will depend on (1) the anatomical location of the acute MI in the ventricles (anterior, posterior, inferior, or right ventricular) and (2) the extent of the involvement of the myocardial wall (transmural or nontransmural). The changes that acute MIs produce in the T waves, ST segments, and Q waves are summarized in Table 15-5 and described in detail in the following sections.

It is important to note here that the leads that record the electrical forces in acute MI through electrodes that view the exterior or epicardial surface of the area of the myocardium involved by myocardial ischemia, injury, and infarction are termed *"facing" leads* in this book. The leads that record the electrical forces through electrodes that view the epicardial surface of the uninvolved myocardium directly opposite the involved myocardium are termed *"opposite" (or reciprocal) leads.*

◆ ABNORMAL T WAVES

Abnormal T waves indicating myocardial ischemia usually appear within seconds of the onset of an acute MI. These ischemic T waves, which appear over the zone of ischemia in the facing leads, are primarily caused by a delay or change in direction in repo-

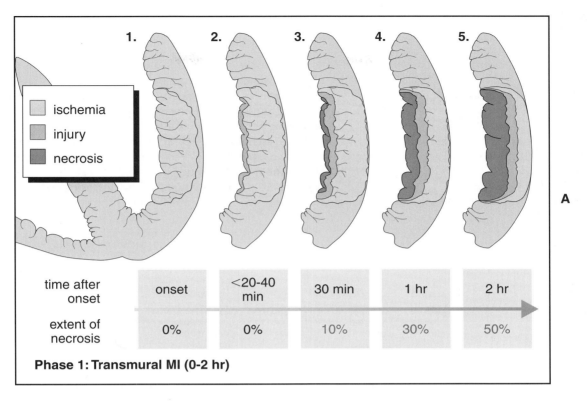

Phase 1: Transmural MI (0-2 hr)

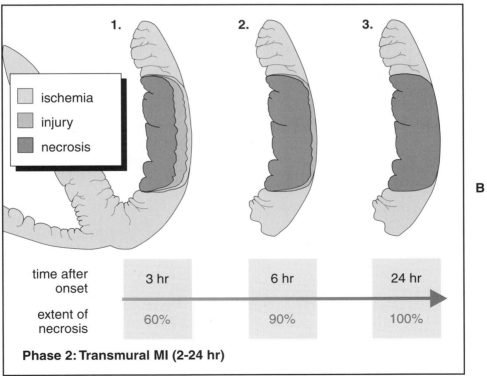

Phase 2: Transmural MI (2-24 hr)

Figure 15-6   The first two early phases of an acute myocardial infarction.
A, Phase 1. **B,** Phase 2.

TABLE

15-4 The Four Phases of Evolution of an Acute Transmural Myocardial Infarction

Phase	Time After Onset of Acute MI	Pathophysiology
1	0 to 2 hours (first few hours)	Extensive myocardial ischemia and injury occur with about 50% of the myocardium becoming necrotic
2	2 to 24 hours (first day)	The evolution of the MI is complete with about two thirds of the myocardium becoming necrotic by 3 hours and most of the rest becoming necrotic by 6 hours
3	24 to 72 hours (second to third day)	Little or no ischemic or injured myocardial cells remain because all cells have either died or recovered; acute inflammation begins within the necrotic tissue
4	2 to 8 weeks	Fibrous tissue completely replaces the necrotic tissue

MI, Myocardial infarction.

TABLE

15-5 ECG Changes in Acute Q-Wave Myocardial Infarction

Stage of Acute MI	Severity of Process	Changes in Facing ECG Leads	Reciprocal Changes in Opposite ECG Leads	Appearance of ECG Changes After Onset of Acute MI
Ischemia	Reversible	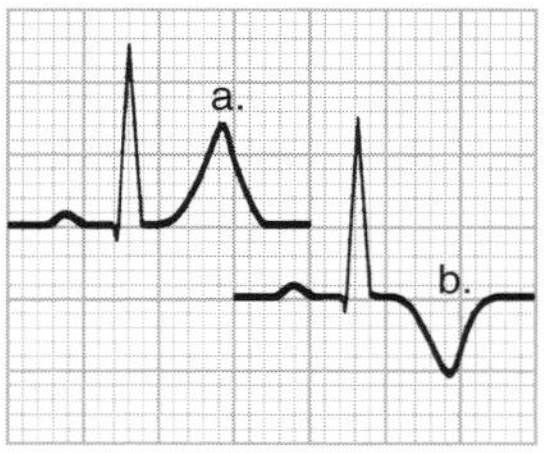 Tall, peaked (a) or inverted (b) T waves	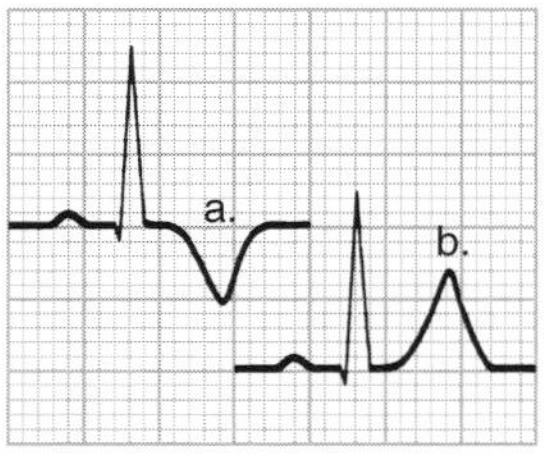 Inverted (a) or tall, peaked (b) T waves	Within seconds of onset
Ischemia, injury	Reversible	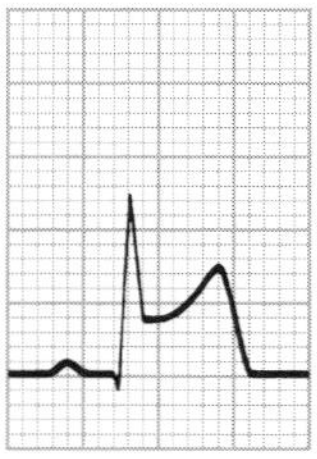 Elevated ST segments	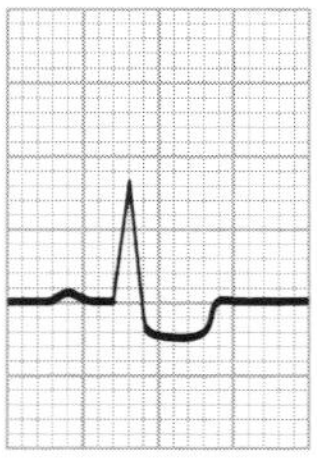 Depressed ST segments	Within minutes of onset
Necrosis	Irreversible	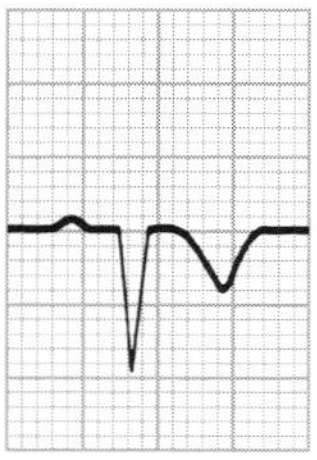 Abnormal Q waves and QS complexes	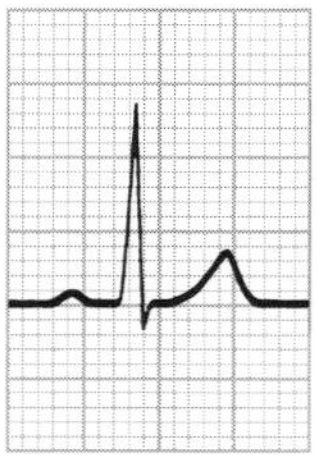 Tall R waves	In about 2 hours after onset

MI, Myocardial infarction.

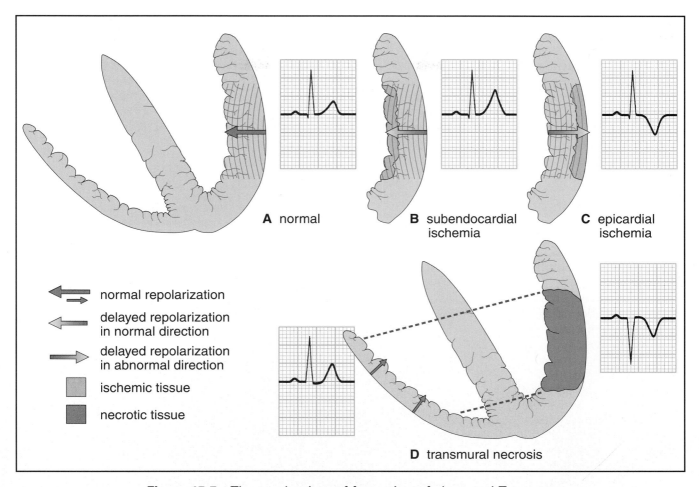

A normal

B subendocardial ischemia

C epicardial ischemia

⬅ normal repolarization

⬅ delayed repolarization in normal direction

➡ delayed repolarization in abnormal direction

▨ ischemic tissue

▨ necrotic tissue

D transmural necrosis

Figure 15-7 The mechanism of formation of abnormal T waves.

larization of the myocardium because of anoxia (Figure 15-7). They may be abnormally tall and peaked or deeply inverted. In addition, the QT intervals associated with the ischemic T waves are usually prolonged.

Whether the ischemic T waves are upright or inverted depends on where the ischemia is, subendocardial or subepicardial, respectively. In normal hearts, repolarization begins at the epicardium and progresses toward the endocardium, producing a positive T wave.

In subendocardial ischemia, there is a delay in repolarization of the subendocardial cardiac cells. Repolarization progresses in the normal direction from the epicardium to the endocardium but is slowed when it reaches the ischemic subendocardial area. This produces a prolonged QT interval and a symmetrically positive tall, peaked T wave.

In subepicardial ischemia, on the other hand, there is a delay in the repolarization in the subepicardial cardiac cells. Because of this, repolarization begins at the endocardium and progresses in a reverse direction,

from the endocardium to the epicardium, slowing when it reaches the ischemic subepicardial area. This produces a prolonged QT interval and a symmetrically negative deep T wave.

Abnormal ischemic T waves are often associated with depression or elevation of the ST segment, another manifestation of myocardial ischemia. Ischemic T waves and associated ST segment changes revert to normal quickly after an anginal attack. Those present in acute MI secondary to myocardial ischemia may disappear more gradually or not at all as healing proceeds.

Abnormal, deeply inverted T waves also appear in association with abnormal Q waves over the zone of necrosis in the later phases of acute MI. These T waves are deeply inverted, mirror images of the upright T waves normally generated in the opposite ventricular wall, being produced the same way as abnormal Q waves, described later.

In a typical transmural MI (Table 15-6), in leads that normally show positive T waves, the ischemic T waves are prolonged, abnormally tall, symmetrical, and peaked. Occasionally, the T waves become extremely tall—the so-called *hyperacute T waves*, appearing for only a short time at the onset. Almost immediately after the onset of ischemia, the ST segments become elevated, resulting in the typical ST-T complex elevation seen during the early ischemic phase of a typical transmural infarction. This ST-T complex pattern continues through the injury phase into the necrotic phase, at which time abnormal Q waves begin to appear. As the infarction evolves, the T waves revert to normal and then become deeply inverted in about 24 hours. Such an MI with Q waves is referred to as a *Q-wave MI*.

In a typical subendocardial MI, the T waves that follow the onset of infarction appear isoelectric, biphasic, or inverted. They are usually associated with depressed ST segments resembling those seen with angina pec-

TABLE

15-6   Changes in the Facing ECG Leads During the Four Phases of a Transmural, Q-Wave Myocardial Infarction

Phase of Infarction	Q Waves	R Waves	ST Segments	T Waves	ECG
Phase 1 (0 to 2 hours) Onset of extensive ischemia occurs immediately, subendocardial injury occurs within 20 to 40 minutes, and subendocardial necrosis occurs in about 30 minutes; necrosis extends to about half of the myocardial wall by 2 hours	Unchanged	Unchanged or abnormally tall	Onset of elevation	Amplitude increases; peaking may occur	
Phase 2 (2 to 24 hours) Transmural infarction is considered complete by 6 hours as necrosis involves about 90% of the myocardial wall; the rest of the necrosis occurs by the end of phase 2	Width and depth begin to increase	Amplitude begins to decrease	Maximum elevation	Amplitude and peaking lessen; T waves still positive	
Phase 3 (24 to 72 hours) Little or no ischemia or injury remains as healing begins	Reach maximum size	Absent	Return to baseline	Become maximally inverted	
Phase 4 (2 to 8 weeks) Replacement of the necrotic tissue by fibrous tissue	Q waves persist	May return partially	Usually normal	Slight inversion	

toris. Unlike the ST-T complexes associated with angina, which quickly revert to normal after an anginal attack, these abnormal ST-T complexes return to normal more gradually, if at all, as healing proceeds. Q waves usually do not appear in subendocardial MI. An MI in which Q waves are absent is called a *non-Q-wave MI.*

◆ ABNORMAL ST SEGMENTS

Abnormal ST segments are present in myocardial infarction, indicating myocardial ischemia and injury, and in noninfarction-related myocardial ischemia from any cause. The ST segments may be elevated or depressed.

ST Segment Elevation

Abnormal ST segment elevation is an ECG sign of severe, extensive, usually transmural, myocardial ischemia and injury in the evolution of an acute Q-wave MI. It may also be seen less frequently in a non-Q-wave, subendocardial myocardial ischemia. An ST segment is considered to be elevated when it is ≥1 mm (≥0.1 mV) above the baseline, measured 0.04 second (1 small square) after the J point of the QRS complex.

ST elevation usually appears within minutes after the onset of infarction, initially indicating extensive myocardial ischemia and foreshadowing a progression first to myocardial injury within 20 to 40 minutes (average, 30 minutes) and then to significant

myocardial necrosis in about 2 hours and the development of abnormal Q waves. Such ST segments are elevated in the leads facing the zone of ischemia and injury and depressed in the opposite, reciprocal leads (Figure 15-8). ST segment elevation is often accompanied by an increase in the size of the R wave.

The cause of ST segment elevation in acute MI is the "current of injury," an electrical manifestation of the inability of cardiac cells "injured" by severe ischemia to maintain a normal resting membrane potential during diastole. After injury, leakage of negative intracellular ions across the cell membrane into the surrounding extracellular fluid occurs during diastole when the cells are in the resting polarized state. The outside of the injured cardiac cells becomes more negative as the inside becomes more positive. As a result, (1) the cells' resting membrane potential drops below its normal level of −90 mV to about −70 mV and (2) the exterior of the injured cardiac cells becomes relatively more negative than that of the surrounding normal cardiac cells.

The difference in potential between the injured and normal cardiac cells causes a downward displacement of the baseline of the ECG in the leads facing the injured cells during electrical diastole. Thus the T-Q interval in the ECG (the interval between the end of the T wave and the beginning of the QRS complex), shifts downward in the ECG leads facing the zone of injury. The electrical potentials generated by depolarization (the QRS com-

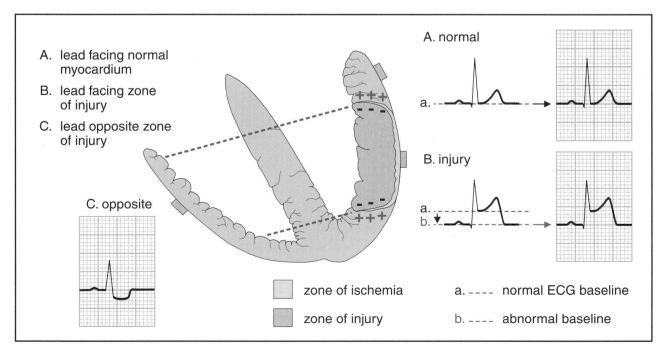

Figure 15-8 The mechanism of ST elevation in acute myocardial infarction.

plex) and repolarization (the ST segment and the T wave) of the injured cardiac cells during electrical systole are normal or slightly greater than normal. Because the amplifier circuit of the ECG machine maintains the baseline of each lead at the same level, a false impression is given that the ST segment and T wave, including the R wave, are elevated in the ECG leads facing the zone of injury and depressed in the opposite leads.

Following the ischemic and injury phases, as the MI progresses, the injured myocardial tissue turns necrotic and the current of injury disappears as the tissue becomes electrically inert. The ST segments become less elevated in the facing leads and finally return to the baseline. As this is occurring, the R waves begin to become smaller and disappear and significant Q waves and T wave inversion begin to appear in the facing leads.

Other causes of ST segment elevation that can be confused with that of acute MI include the following:

◆ **Coronary vasospasm.** Intense transmural myocardial ischemia brought on by vasospasm of a major coronary artery, often the left anterior descending coronary artery, Prinzmetal's angina, may mimic an acute MI electrocardiographically. Clinically, patients with Prinzmetal's angina have recurrent chest pain not related to exercise or other precipitating factors, often several times a day or night, and sometimes associated with significant arrhythmias.

◆ **Acute pericarditis.** The pain of acute pericarditis may mimic that of acute MI, but the younger age of the patient, who usually lacks the coronary risk factors, makes the diagnosis of acute MI unlikely. The pain of pericarditis is often pleuritic in nature, made worse on inspiration, and relieved by the patient sitting upright and leaning forward. The pleuritic pain, the presence of a pericardial friction rub, and the appearance of ST segment elevations in practically all of the ECG leads support the diagnosis of pericarditis. (See Pericarditis, p. 295.)

◆ **Ventricular aneurysm.**

◆ **Hyperkalemia** (see Hyperkalemia, p. 298.)

◆ **Early depolarization** (see Early Depolarization, p. 309.)

ST Segment Depression

ST segment depression is an ECG sign of subendocardial ischemia and injury. Similar to the criteria for ST elevation, an ST segment is considered to be depressed when it is ≥1 mm (≥0.1 mV) below the baseline, measured 0.04 second (1 small square) after the J point of the QRS complex.

ST depression usually appears within minutes after the onset of subendocardial non-Q-wave MI, during an anginal attack, or after exercise. ST depression may also be seen, but less frequently, in Q-wave MI. The ST segments are depressed in the leads facing the ischemic tissue and elevated in the opposite leads. Such abnormal ST segments are due to altered repolarization of the myocardium because of anoxia.

The ST segment depressions of subendocardial ischemia and injury have been classified as to the nature of the sloping of the segment (i.e., downsloping, horizontal, and upsloping) (Figure 15-9). The down-

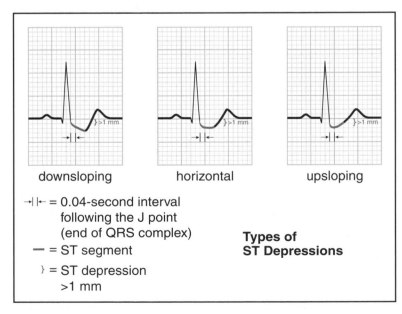

downsloping horizontal upsloping

→||← = 0.04-second interval
following the J point
(end of QRS complex)

— = ST segment

} = ST depression
>1 mm

Types of ST Depressions

Figure 15-9 Types of ST depression.

sloping of an ST segment is most specific for subendocardial ischemia and injury, as present in subendocardial infarction; horizontal sloping is of intermediate specificity; and upsloping is the least specific. However, regardless of the slope, an ST segment that is depressed ≥1 mm 0.04 second after the end of the QRS complex is significant. ST segment depression is often associated with ischemic biphasic or inverted T waves, another manifestation of myocardial ischemia.

ST segment depression quickly reverts to normal after an anginal attack or after exercise as myocardial ischemia is corrected. When associated with myocardial injury as present in acute MI, the ST depression may disappear more gradually or not at all as healing proceeds, becoming chronic.

Although ST segment depression is commonly associated with subendocardial ischemia and injury, other common causes include the followiong:

◆ Left and right ventricular hypertrophy
◆ Left and right bundle branch blocks
◆ Digitalis in therapeutic and toxic doses

◆ Q WAVES

A Q wave is the first negative deflection of the QRS complex. It may be normal (physiologic) or abnormal (pathologic) (Figure 15-10).

Normal Q Waves

Normal Q waves result from the normal depolarization of the interventricular septum from left to right. This relatively small electrical force is the first step in the depolarization of the ventricles. The electrical forces responsible for the normal Q wave are negative because they travel away from the leads in which they appear, being opposite in direction to the positive electrical forces producing the R wave. Because the interventricular septum is thin, the electrical forces are small and of short duration—within 0.04 second—and of low amplitude. The resultant "septal" q wave is less than 0.04 second wide and of a depth of less than 25% of the height of the succeeding R wave. Such small normal q waves are commonly present in the QRS complexes in leads I, II, III, aVL, aVF, V_5, and V_6.

Abnormal Q Waves

An abnormal Q wave is usually considered an ECG sign of irreversible myocardial necrosis in the evolution of an acute MI, specifically a Q-wave MI. A Q wave is considered abnormal if it is (0.04 second wide and has a depth of ≥25% of the height of the succeeding R wave.

Abnormal Q waves may begin to appear in about 2 hours (on the average between 8 to 12 hours) after the onset of the MI, reaching maximum size in about 24 to 48 hours. They typically appear in the facing leads directly over necrotic, infarcted myocardial tissue—the zone of infarction. Abnormal Q waves may persist indefinitely or disappear in months or years. Abnormal Q waves appear in less than 50% of patients with acute MI. As mentioned earlier, an MI in which abnormal Q waves are present is called a

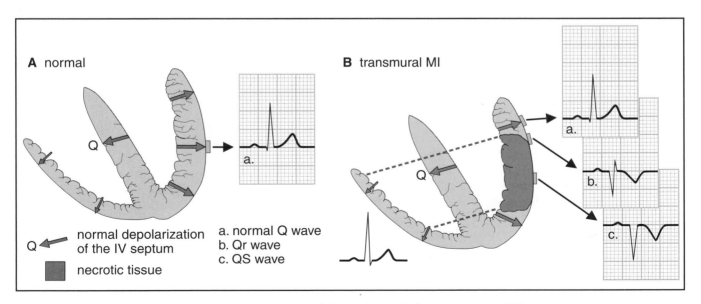

Figure 15-10 The mechanism of formation of Q waves and QS waves in acute myocardial infarction.

Q-wave MI; one in which abnormal Q waves are absent is a a *non-Q-wave MI.*

The cause of abnormal Q waves differs from that of normal Q waves. A popular theory of why Q waves occur is the "window" theory. Because infarcted myocardium cannot depolarize or repolarize, no electrical forces are generated, resulting in an electrically inert area. Thus infarcted myocardium can be considered a "window" through which the facing leads actually view the endocardium of the opposite noninfarcted ventricular wall, electrocardiographically speaking. Because depolarization progresses from the endocardium outward, the electrical forces generated by the wall opposite the infarct will be traveling away from the leads facing the infarct. Therefore these leads will detect the negative electrical forces generated by the opposite, noninfarcted ventricular wall as large negative abnormal Q waves. These abnormal Q waves can be looked on as mirror images of the R waves produced by the opposite ventricular wall.

The presence and size of the abnormal Q waves and the number of leads in which they occur depend on the size of the infarct, both on its depth (or thickness) and width. The larger the infarct (i.e., the larger the "window"), the larger the Q waves are and the greater the number of facing leads in which they appear. In general, the greater the depth of the infarct, the deeper are the Q waves; the wider the infarct, the wider the Q waves. A large abnormal Q wave with or without a succeeding R wave is often called a *QS wave.*

In contrast, the smaller the infarct, the smaller are the Q waves both in width and depth and the fewer the facing leads with Q waves. If the infarct is relatively small and nontransmural, such as a subendocardial MI, abnormal Q waves may be completely absent, resulting in a non-Q-wave MI. To complicate matters, abnormal Q waves may also be completely absent in a significant transmural MI.

The thickness of the myocardium of the opposite noninfarcted ventricular wall generally contributes to the size of the abnormal Q waves: the thicker the opposite myocardium, the larger the Q wave; the thinner the myocardium, the smaller the Q wave.

When the infarct is large, transmural, and entirely necrotic, the R waves completely disappear in the facing leads, resulting in a wide and deep QS complex. If enough viable cardiac cells capable of generating electrical forces survive within an infarct, if the infarct is nontransmural with viable cardiac cells between it and the epicardium, or if the facing lead overlies the boundary between an infarct and surrounding viable myocardium, an abnormal Q wave with an R wave will result. The size of the R wave will depend on the amount of viable cardiac cells lying under the facing electrode. A QR complex indicates a greater amount of viable cardiac tissue between the infarct and the facing electrode than does a Qr complex.

Another consequence of an electrically inert infarct is that the R waves in the opposite leads are larger than normal. The reason for this is that the positive electrical forces generated by the noninfarcted ventricular wall flowing toward the opposite leads are now unopposed by the negative, electrical forces that once were generated by the now infarcted wall and traveled away from the opposite leads.

The abnormal QS waves that occur in the right precordial leads V_1-V_2 within the first few hours of the onset of an acute anterior wall MI involving the interventricular septum result from the severe ischemia of the septum. The "septal" r waves normally produced by the left-to-right depolarization of the interventricular septum fail to occur, changing the normal rS pattern of the QRS complex in the right precordial leads to a QS complex.

Abnormal Q waves are *not* present in a 12-lead ECG in a posterior wall MI because there are no leads facing the infarct.

KEY POINT

Abnormal Q waves may be present in certain leads without being considered significant. An abnormal Q wave is commonly ignored in the following leads, especially if it occurs under certain circumstances.

◆ **Lead aVR.** An abnormal Q wave in lead aVR is usually ignored because the QRS complex in this lead normally consists of a large S wave.

◆ **Lead aVL.** A QS or a QR wave in lead aVL alone in which the QRS axis is greater than +60° (i.e., an electrically vertical heart) is usually ignored.

◆ **Lead aVF.** A QS or a QR wave in lead aVF alone is considered insignificant unless it is accompanied by abnormal Q waves, ST segment elevation, and abnormal T wave changes in one or both of the other inferior leads—leads II and III.

◆ **Lead III.** An abnormal Q wave in this lead by itself is considered insignificant, unless (1) it is accompanied by abnormal Q waves, ST segment elevation, and abnormal T wave changes in the other inferior leads (lead II or aVF or both) and (2) the abnormal Q wave in lead III is wider and deeper than those in leads II and aVF.

Acute Q-Wave and Non-Q-Wave Myocardial Infarctions

A Q-wave MI is identified as such by the presence of abnormal Q waves in the ECG taken within 24 hours after the onset of the infarction. The initial ECG in the majority of patients with Q-wave MI shows ST segment elevation and abnormally tall T waves in the facing ECG leads, whereas in the minority the initial ECG shows ST segment depression with or without T-wave inversion. Q-wave MIs occur in less than 50% of patients with a documented acute MI; the rest are non-Q-wave MIs.

A Q-wave MI commonly occurs after the total thrombotic occlusion of a coronary artery for at least a few hours, resulting in a complete shutdown of blood flow to the area of the myocardium supplied by the artery. This produces extensive myocardial necrosis of a segment of the myocardium usually extending from the endocardium to the epicardium, including both the subendocardial and subepicardial areas of the myocardium (i.e., a transmural MI).

However, it has been shown that abnormal Q waves may be absent in transmural infarctions for

whatever reason and present in nontransmural infarctions in which the myocardial necrosis does not extend from the endocardium to the epicardium.

The basis for identifying an acute MI as a non-Q-wave MI is the absence of abnormal Q waves in the ECG taken within 24 hours after the onset of the infarction. The ECG in the majority of patients with non-Q-wave MI initially shows ST segment depression, with or without T wave inversion in the facing ECG leads, indicating subendocardial ischemia and injury; in the rest of the patients, the ECG shows ST segment elevation and abnormally tall T waves, indicating transmural ischemia and injury.

A non-Q-wave MI may result in several different ways. In the majority of patients it occurs after incomplete thrombotic occlusion of a coronary artery that lasts about 1 hour or less because of (1) spontaneous thrombolysis or administration of thrombolytic agents or (2) cessation of vasoconstriction. In the rest of the patients it occurs because of the presence of collateral circulation supplying the myocardium normally perfused by the occluded artery, in which case the occlusion can last for more than 1 hour without developing a Q wave. In both instances, because myocardial necrosis is limited either to the subendocardial or midportion of the myocardium (i.e., a nontransmural infarct), the subepicardial myocardium is preserved, resulting in the absence of Q waves. As noted above, however, Q waves may be absent in transmural infarcts as well and present in nontransmural infarcts. *For this reason, a Q-wave MI cannot technically be classified solely as a transmural MI and a non-Q-wave MI cannot be classified solely as a subendocardial or nontransmural MI.*

◆ TYPICAL PATTERNS IN ACUTE Q-WAVE AND NON-Q-WAVE MYOCARDIAL INFARCTIONS

Acute Q-wave MI occurs in less than 50% of patients with acute infarction. In the rest, non-Q-wave MI is present, primarily as a subendocardial MI.

Acute Q-Wave Myocardial Infarction

In an acute Q-wave MI involving the entire thickness of the myocardial wall (transmural MI), the following typical pattern evolves. In the facing ECG leads (Table 15-6), within seconds of the onset of the acute MI, the initial ischemic stage produces tall, peaked T waves. This is followed within minutes by an elevation of the ST segments and often an increase in the size of the R waves during the ischemic/injury stage. Then, while the ST segments are still elevated, abnormal Q waves and QS complexes appear as necrosis

TABLE

15-7 Changes in the Facing ECG Leads During the Four Phases of a Subendocardial Non-Q-Wave Myocardial Infarction

Phase of Infarction	Q Waves	R Waves	ST Segments	T Waves	ECG
Phase 1 (0 to 2 hours) Onset of localized ischemia occurs immediately, subendocardial injury occurs within 20 to 40 minutes, and subendocardial necrosis occurs in about 30 minutes	Unchanged	Unchanged	Onset of depression	Amplitude may or may not increase slightly	
Phase 2 (2 to 24 hours) Subendocardial infarction is considered complete by 6 hours; generally, the necrosis involves only the inner parts of the myocardium, usually the subendocardial area, without extending to the epicardial surface	Unchanged	Amplitude may begin to decrease somewhat	May or may not return to normal	Inversion may occur	
Phase 3 (24 to 72 hours) Little or no ischemia or injury remains as healing begins	Unchanged	Unchanged	May or may not return to normal	Inversion may occur	
Phase 4 (2 to 8 weeks) Replacement of the infarcted tissue by fibrous tissue	Unchanged	Unchanged	May or may not return to normal	May or may not return to normal	

evolves. Finally, as the R waves become smaller and the ST segments return to the baseline, symmetrically deep inverted T waves appear.

In the opposite ECG leads, the ECG changes of evolving acute Q-wave MI differ considerably from those in the facing leads, for the most part being opposite in direction. These ECG changes, termed *reciprocal*, include depression of the ST segments, inverted or taller than normal T waves, and abnormally tall R waves, depending on the phase of infarction. Gener-

ally, Q waves do not appear in the opposite leads during an acute MI.

Acute Non-Q-Wave Myocardial Infarction

In an acute non-Q-wave MI involving the subendocardial area of the myocardial wall (nontransmural MI), the following typical pattern evolves. In the facing ECG leads (Table 15-7), within seconds of the onset of the acute MI, the initial ischemic stage produces isoelectric, biphasic, or inverted T waves. This is

15-8 The Facing and Opposite Leads Relative to the Various Sites of Acute Q-Wave Myocardial Infarction

Site of Infarction	Facing Leads	Opposite Leads
Anterior wall		
Septal	V_1-V_2	None
Anterior (localized)	V_3-V_4	None
Anteroseptal	V_1-V_4	None
Lateral	I, aVL, and V_5 or V_6	II, III, and aVF
Anterolateral	I, aVL, and V_3-V_6	II, III, and aVF
Extensive anterior	I, aVL, and V_1-V_6	II, III, and aVF
Inferior wall	II, III, and aVF	I and aVL
Posterior wall	None	V_1-V_4
Right ventricular	II, III, aVF, and V_{4R}	I and aVL

followed within minutes by depression of the ST segments during the ischemic/injury stage. Finally, as the ST segment returns to the baseline, symmetrically inverted T waves appear. Abnormal Q waves do not appear in non-Q-wave MI.

In the opposite ECG leads, the ECG changes of evolving acute non-Q-wave MI differ considerably from those in the facing leads, for the most part being opposite in direction. These reciprocal ECG changes include elevation of the ST segments and tall T waves.

Determining the Site of a Myocardial Infarction

The location of an acute Q-wave MI relates to the leads in which abnormal ST segment elevation and subsequent abnormal Q waves appear (i.e., the facing leads) (Table 15-8). For example, if ST segment elevation and abnormal Q waves appear in any or all of the leads I, aVL, and V_1-V_6, the MI is "anterior." If ST segment elevation and abnormal Q waves appear in leads II, III, and aVF, the MI is "inferior." If, in an inferior infarction, the ST segment in V_{4R} also becomes elevated, a "right ventricular" MI is present. Because there are no facing leads in a posterior MI, there are

no diagnostic ST segment elevation or abnormal Q waves present in the ECG leads. A posterior MI is diagnosed if reciprocal ECG changes of ST segment depression and tall R waves are present in leads V_1-V_4.

Complications of Acute Myocardial Infarction

The two major complications of acute MI are (1) myocardial dysfunction secondary to myocardial damage, resulting in right or left ventricular failure, and (2) the disruption of the electrical conduction system, resulting in various arrhythmias, AV blocks, or fascicular blocks. Which ventricle becomes dysfunctional and what types of arrhythmias or disruptions of the electrical conduction system develop depends on which coronary artery and related area of the heart is involved in the infarction. Table 15-9 details the relationship between the location of the infarction, the coronary arteries occluded, the ECG leads affected, and the complications that may be incurred. Because the distribution of the coronary arteries varies from person to person, and the location and degree of coronary artery occlusion varies from infarct to infarct, the type and extent of the complications will also vary from infarct to infarct.

TABLE

15-9 The Coronary Arteries Involved, the Facing Leads, and the Associated Potential Complications Relative to the Location of the Specific Acute Q-Wave Myocardial Infarctions

Location of the Infarction	Coronary Arteries Occluded	Facing ECG Leads	Potential Complications

Interventricular septum	Septal perforator arteries of the left anterior descending coronary artery	V_1-V_2 (ST↑)	*AV blocks:*
			  Second-degree, type II AV block[1]
			  Second-degree, 2:1 and advanced AV block[1]
			  Third-degree AV block[1]
			Bundle branch blocks:
			  RBBB
			  LBBB
			  LAFB
			  LPFB[3]

Anterior (localized) LV wall	Diagonal arteries of the left anterior descending coronary artery	V_3-V_4 (ST↑)	*LV dysfunction:*
			  CHF
			  Cardiogenic shock

Lateral LV wall	Diagonal arteries of the left anterior descending coronary artery and/or the anterolateral marginal artery of the left circumflex coronary artery	I, aVL, V_5-V_6 (ST↑)	*LV dysfunction:* CHF (moderate)

Inferior LV wall	Posterior left ventricular arteries of the right coronary artery or, less commonly, of the left circumflex coronary artery; the left posterior descending coronary artery and the AV node artery may also be involved	II, III, aVF (ST↑)	*LV dysfunction:*
			  CHF (mild, if any)
			AV blocks:
			  First-degree AV block[2]
			  Second-degree, type I AV block[2]
			  Second-degree, 2:1 and advanced AV block
			  Third-degree AV block[2]
			Bundle branch blocks:
			  LPFB[4]

CHF, Congestive heart failure; *LAFB,* left anterior fascicular block; *LBBB,* left bundle branch block; *LPFB,* left posterior fascicular block; *LV,* left ventricle; *RBBB,* right bundle branch block; *RV,* right ventricle;
[1] With abnormally wide QRS complexes.
[2] With normal QRS complexes.
[3] In conjunction with a right ventricular or inferior infarction.
[4] In conjunction with a septal infarction.

15-9 The Coronary Arteries Involved, the Facing Leads, and the Associated Potential Complications Relative to the Location of the Specific Acute Q-Wave Myocardial Infarctions—cont'd

Location of the Infarction	Coronary Arteries Occluded	Facing ECG Leads	Potential Complications
Posterior LV wall	Distal left circumflex artery and/or posterolateral marginal artery of the circumflex coronary artery	None Opposite leads: V_1-V_4 (ST↓)	*LV dysfunction:* CHF (mild, if any)
RV wall	Right coronary artery, including the SA node and AV node arteries, the posterior descending coronary artery, and the posterior left ventricular arteries	II, III, aVF, V_{4R} (ST↑)	*RV dysfunction:* Right heart failure *Arrhythmias:* Sinus arrest Sinus bradycardia Atrial premature beats Atrial flutter Atrial fibrillation *AV blocks:* First-degree AV block[2] Second-degree, type I AV block[2] Second-degree, 2:1 and advanced AV block[2] Third-degree AV block[2] *Bundle branch blocks:* RBBB LBBB LPFB[4]

CHAPTER REVIEW QUESTIONS

1. The artery that arises from the left main coronary artery at an obtuse angle and runs posteriorly along the left atrioventricular groove to end in back of the left ventricle is called the:
   A. septal perforator artery
   B. left circumflex coronary artery
   C. right ventricular artery
   D. left anterior descending coronary artery

2. The SA node is supplied with blood from:
   A. the left circumflex coronary artery
   B. the right coronary artery
   C. either of the above
   D. none of the above

3. Myocardial ischemia or infarction may be caused by:
   A. occlusion of an atherosclerotic coronary artery
   B. coronary artery spasm
   C. increased myocardial workload
   D. all of the above

4. An increase in existing angina from a CCSC class II to a class III indicates the following:
   A. the occurrence of an acute MI
   B. the appearance of angina at rest
   C. a decrease in the coronary artery stenosis
   D. the onset of unstable angina

5. The most common cause of acute MI is a(n):
   A. coronary thrombosis
   B. coronary artery spasm
   C. air embolism
   D. none of the above

6. Upon revascularization or reoxygenation, necrotic cells:
   A. return to normal or near normal function
   B. do not return to normal function
   C. usually take 24 hours to return to normal function
   D. revert to a previous state of injury

7. An MI in which the zone of infarction involves the entire full thickness of the ventricular wall, from the endocardium to the epicardial surface, is called a:
   A. nontransmural infarction
   B. necrotic infarction
   C. transmural infarction
   D. subendocardial infarction

8. By six hours after an acute transmural MI, the following can be said of the involved myocardium:
   A. only a small percentage of cells remain viable
   B. a large area of reversible myocardial injury is still present
   C. progression of the acute MI continues at a rapid pace
   D. none of the above

9. Inverted or tall peaked T waves in a facing lead during the early phase of an acute MI are an indication of:
   A. necrosis
   B. injury
   C. ischemia
   D. none of the above

10. The following is true of a Q-wave MI:
    A. a transmural MI is always present
    B. the classification is usually made hours after the onset of symptoms when Q waves appear
    C. an ST elevation is always present initially
    D. all of the above

11. The most likely cause of an inferior MI is an occlusion of the:
    A. left anterior descending artery
    B. anterolateral marginal artery
    C. posterior descending artery
    D. posterior left ventricular arteries

12. The ECG in an acute anteroseptal MI is characterized by ST segment elevation in the following facing leads:
    A. leads II, III, and aVF
    B. leads V_1-V_4
    C. leads I, aVL, and V_1-V_6
    D. leads V_5-V_6

Diagnostic ECG Changes in Specific Myocardial Infarctions

CHAPTER OBJECTIVES

Upon completion of all or part of this chapter, you should be able to complete the following objectives:

1. Name the coronary artery or arteries occluded and the region of the heart involved in the following acute myocardial infarctions (MIs):
   Septal MI
   Anterior (localized) MI
   Anteroseptal MI
   Lateral MI
   Anterolateral MI
   Extensive anterior MI
   Inferior MI
   Posterior MI
   Right ventricular MI
2. List the diagnostic changes in the Q waves, R waves, ST segments, and T waves in the facing and opposite ECG leads (where applicable) during the early and late phases of the following acute MIs:
   Septal MI
   Anterior (localized) MI
   Anteroseptal MI
   Lateral MI
   Anterolateral MI
   Extensive anterior MI

   Inferior MI
   Posterior MI
   Right ventricular MI
3. Name the potential complications of the following acute MIs:
   Septal MI
   Anterior (localized) MI
   Lateral MI
   Inferior MI
   Posterior MI
   Right ventricular MI
4. Identify the facing and opposite ECG leads that show the ST segment and T wave changes of early transmural Q-wave MIs in the following:
   Septal MI
   Anterior (localized) MI
   Anteroseptal MI
   Lateral MI
   Anterolateral MI
   Extensive anterior MI
   Inferior MI
   Posterior MI
   Right ventricular MI

The diagnostic features of the following specific Q-wave, transmural myocardial infarctions (MIs) will be presented in this section:

- Septal MI
- Anterior (localized) MI

- Anteroseptal MI
- Lateral MI
- Anterolateral MI
- Extensive anterior MI
- Inferior MI

◆ Posterior MI

◆ Right ventricular MI

Included in the diagnostic features of each of the specific MIs are the following:

◆ The coronary arteries involved and the site of occlusion of the coronary arteries

◆ The location of the infarct

◆ The changes in the electrocardiogram (ECG) in the facing and opposite leads

It should be noted that if the ECG being analyzed has changes consistent with both an anterolateral and an inferior MI, for example, then the patient has both an inferior and an anterolateral MI. This would also be true of an anterolateral and a posterior MI, an inferior and a posterior MI, and so forth.

The changes in the ECG presented for each specific MI are based on typical first-time infarcts and may not represent actual changes in a particular patient's ECG. The reasons for this include individual variations in the size, position in the chest, and rotation of the heart and in the distribution of the coronary artery circulation; the presence of bundle branch blocks, ventricular hypertrophy, and previous MIs; and coexisting drug- and electrolyte-related ECG changes.

Tables 16-10 and 16-11 at the end of the chapter summarize the diagnostic features of the specific Q-wave MIs and the potential complications associated with each one.

SEPTAL MYOCARDIAL INFARCTION

Coronary Arteries Involved and Site of Occlusion

The major coronary artery involved is the left coronary artery, specifically the following branches:

◆ The left anterior descending coronary artery beyond the first diagonal branch, involving the septal perforator arteries (Figure 16-1).

Location of Infarct

The septal MI involves (1) the anterior wall of the left ventricle overlying the interventricular septum and (2) the anterior two thirds of the interventricular septum.

ECG Changes (Table 16-1)

In facing leads V_1-V_2:

Early: Absence of normal "septal" r waves in the right precordial leads V_1-V_2, resulting in QS waves in these leads.

Absence of normal "septal" q waves where normally present (i.e., in leads I, II, III, aVF, and V_4-V_6).

TABLE

16-1 ECG Changes in Septal MI

	Q Waves (Abnormal Q Waves and QS Complexes)	R Waves (Abnormally Tall or Small)	ST Segments (Elevated or Depressed)	T Waves (Abnormally Tall or Inverted)
Early *Phase 1*				
First few hrs (0 to 2 hrs)	Absent "septal" q waves in I, II, III, aVF, and V_4-V_6 QS waves in V_1-V_2	Absent "septal" r waves in V_1-V_2	Elevated in V_1-V_2	Sometimes, abnormally tall with peaking in V_1-V_2
Phase 2				
First day (2 to 24 hrs)	Same as in Phase 1	Same as in Phase 1	Maximally elevated in V_1-V_2	Less tall, but generally still positive, in V_1-V_2
Late *Phase 3*				
Second and third day (24 to 72 hrs)	QS complexes in V_1-V_2	Same as in Phase 1	Return of the ST segments to the baseline throughout	T wave inversion in V_1-V_2

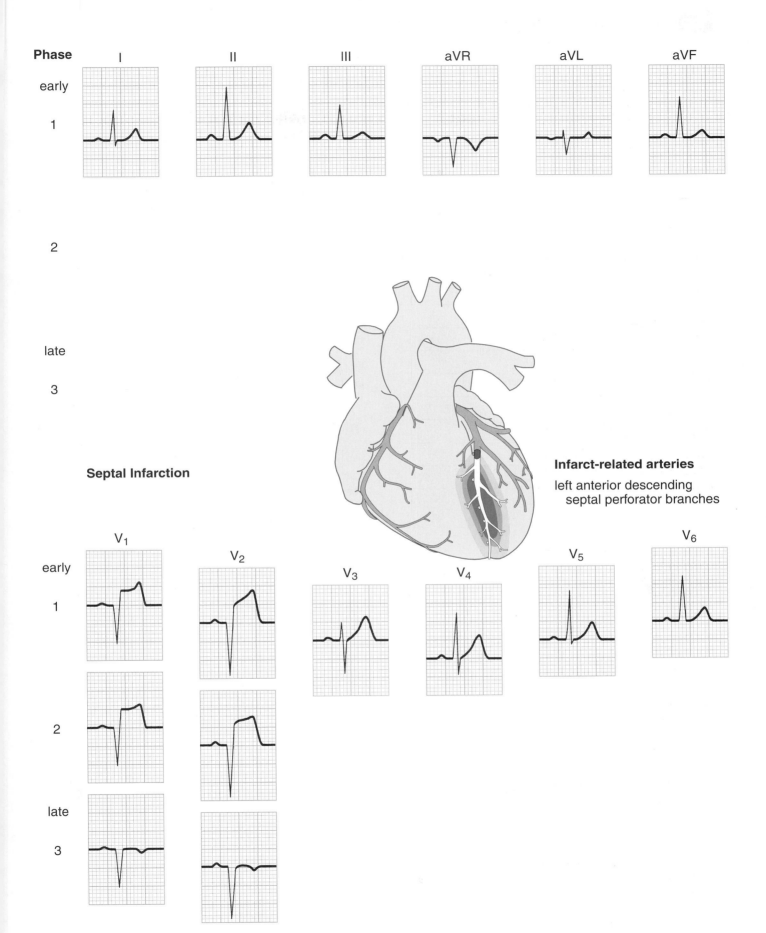

Figure 16-1   Septal MI.

ST segment elevation with tall T waves in leads V_1-V_2.
Late: QS complexes with T wave inversion in leads V_1-V_2.

In opposite leads II, III, and aVF:
Early: No significant ECG changes.
Late: No significant ECG changes.

Notes

_____
_____
_____
_____
_____
_____
_____
_____
_____
_____
_____

ANTERIOR (LOCALIZED) MYOCARDIAL INFARCTION

Coronary Arteries Involved and Site of Occlusion

The major coronary artery involved is the left coronary artery, specifically the following branches:
- The diagonal arteries of the left anterior descending coronary artery (Figure 16-2).

Location of Infarct

The anterior (localized) MI involves an area of the anterior wall of the left ventricle immediately to the left of the interventricular septum.

ECG Changes (Table 16-2)

In facing leads V_3-V_4:
Early: ST segment elevation with tall T waves and taller than normal R waves in the midprecordial leads V_3 and V_4.
Late: QS complexes with T wave inversion in leads V_3 and V_4.

In opposite leads II, III, and aVF:
Early: No significant ECG changes.
Late: No significant ECG changes.

TABLE
16-2 ECG Changes in Anterior (Localized) MI

	Q Waves (Abnormal Q Waves and QS Complexes)	R Waves (Abnormally Tall or Small)	ST Segments (Elevated or Depressed)	T Waves (Abnormally Tall or Inverted)
Early				
Phase 1				
First few hrs (0 to 2 hrs)	Normal Q waves	Normal or abnormally tall R waves in V_3-V_4	Elevated in V_3-V_4	Sometimes, abnormally tall with peaking in V_3-V_4
Phase 2				
First day (2 to 24 hrs)	Minimally abnormal in V_3-V_4	Minimally decreased in V_3-V_4	Maximally elevated in V_3-V_4	Less tall, but generally still positive, in V_3-V_4
Late				
Phase 3				
Second and third day (24 to 72 hrs)	QS complexes in V_3-V_4	Absent in V_3-V_4	Return of the ST segments to the baseline throughout	T wave inversion in V_3-V_4

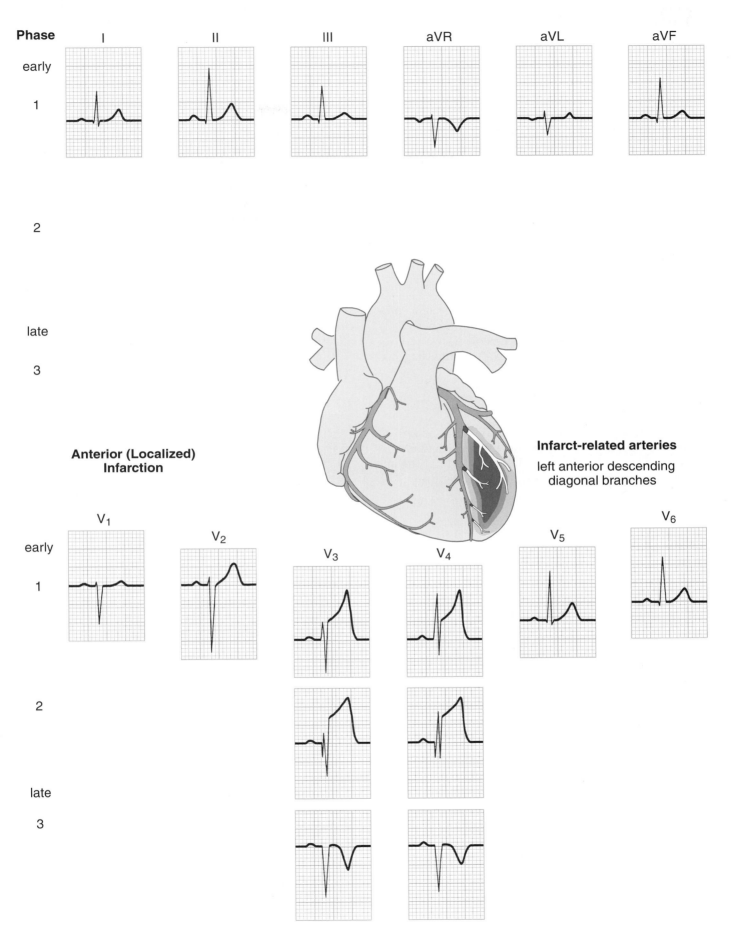

Figure 16-2 Anterior (localized) MI.

Notes

_____

_____

_____

_____

_____

ANTEROSEPTAL MYOCARDIAL INFARCTION

Coronary Arteries Involved and Site of Occlusion

The major coronary artery involved is the left coronary artery, specifically the following branches:
- ◆ The left anterior descending coronary artery involving both the septal perforator and diagonal arteries (Figure 16-3).

Location of Infarct

The anteroseptal MI involves (1) the anterior wall of the left ventricle overlying the interventricular septum and immediately to the left of it and (2) the anterior two thirds of the interventricular septum.

ECG Changes (Table 16-3)

In facing leads V_1-V_4:
Early: Absence of normal "septal" r waves in the right precordial leads V_1-V_2, resulting in QS waves in these leads.
Absence of normal "septal" q waves where normally present (i.e., in leads I, II, III, aVF, and V_4-V_6).
ST segment elevation with tall T waves in leads V_1-V_4 and taller than normal R waves in the midprecordial leads V_3-V_4.
Late: QS complexes with T wave inversion in leads V_1-V_4.
In opposite leads II, III, and aVF:
Early: No significant ECG changes.
Late: No significant ECG changes.

Notes

_____

_____

_____

_____

_____

_____

TABLE

16-3 ECG Changes in Anteroseptal MI

	Q Waves (Abnormal Q Waves and QS Complexes)	R Waves (Abnormally Tall or Small)	ST Segments (Elevated or Depressed)	T Waves (Abnormally Tall or Inverted)
Early _Phase 1_				
First few hrs (0 to 2 hrs)	Absent "septal" q waves in I, II, III, aVF, and V_4-V_6 QS waves in V_1-V_2	Absent "septal" r waves in V_1-V_2 Normal or abnormally tall R waves in V_3-V_4	Elevated in V_1-V_4	Sometimes, abnormally tall with peaking in V_1-V_4
Phase 2				
First day (2 to 24 hrs)	Same as in Phase 1	Absent "septal" r waves in V_1-V_2 Minimally decreased in V_3-V_4	Maximally elevated in V_1-V_4	Less tall, but generally still positive, in V_1-V_4
Late _Phase 3_				
Second and third day (24 to 72 hrs)	QS complexes in V_1-V_4	Absent in V_1-V_4	Return of the ST segments to the baseline throughout	T wave inversion in V_1-V_4

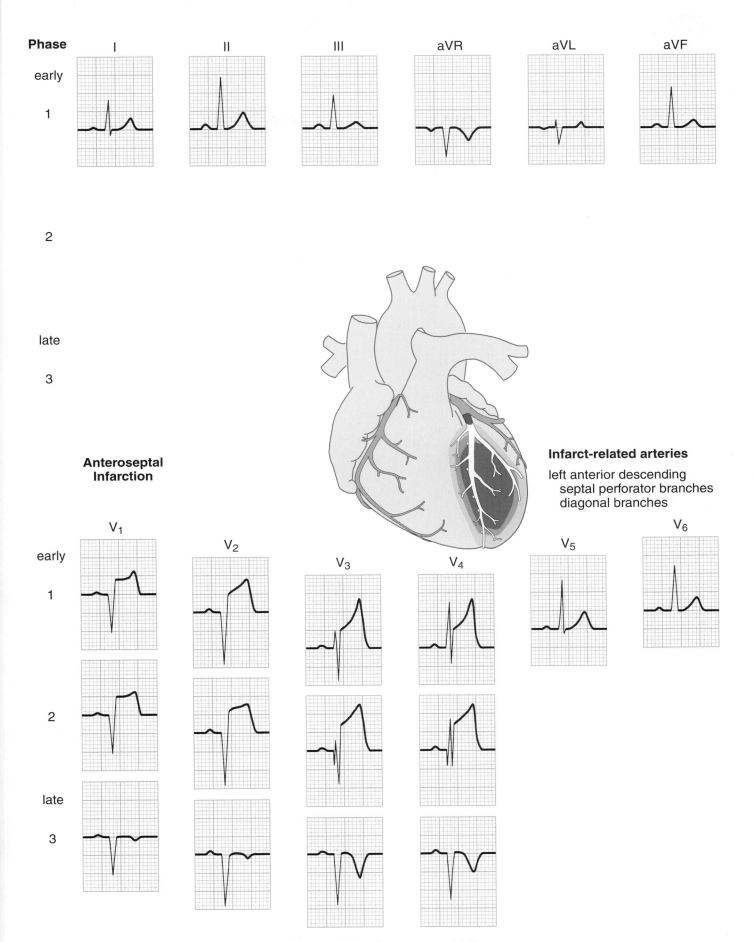

Figure 16-3 Anteroseptal MI.

LATERAL MYOCARDIAL INFARCTION

Coronary Arteries Involved and Site of Occlusion

The major artery involved is the left coronary artery, specifically the following branches:
- ◆ The laterally located diagonal arteries of the left anterior descending coronary artery and/or the anterolateral marginal artery of the left circumflex coronary artery (Figure 16-4).

Location of Infarct

The lateral MI involves the lateral wall of the left ventricle.

ECG Changes (Table 16-4)

In facing leads I, aVL, and V_5 or V_6 or both:

Early: ST segment elevation with tall T waves and taller than normal R waves in leads I, aVL, and the left precordial lead V_5 or V_6 or both.

Late: Abnormal Q waves and small R waves with T wave inversion in leads I, aVL, and V_5-V_6.

QS waves or complexes with T wave inversion in lead V_5 or V_6 or both.

In opposite leads II, III, and aVF:

Early: ST segment depression in leads II, III, and aVF.

Late: Abnormally tall T waves in leads II, III, and aVF.

Notes

_____

_____

_____

_____

_____

_____

_____

_____

_____

TABLE 16-4 ECG Changes in Lateral MI

	Q Waves (Abnormal Q Waves and QS Complexes)	R Waves (Abnormally Tall or Small)	ST Segments (Elevated or Depressed)	T Waves (Abnormally Tall or Inverted)
Early *Phase 1* First few hrs (0 to 2 hrs)	Normal Q waves	Normal or abnormally tall R waves in I, aVL, and V_5 or V_6 or both	Elevated in I, aVL, and V_5 or V_6 or both Depressed in II, III, and aVF	Sometimes, abnormally tall with peaking in I, aVL, and V_5 or V_6 or both
Phase 2 First day (2 to 24 hrs)	Minimally abnormal in I, aVL, and V_5 or V_6 or both	Minimally decreased in I, aVL, and V_5 or V_6 or both	Maximally elevated in I, aVL, and V_5 or V_6 or both Maximally depressed in II, III, and aVF	Less tall, but generally still positive, in I, aVL, and V_5 or V_6 or both
Late *Phase 3* Second and third day (24 to 72 hrs)	Significantly abnormal in I, aVL, and V_5-V_6 QS waves or complexes in V_5 or V_6 or both	Decreased or absent in V_5 or V_6 or both Small R waves in I and aVL	Return of the ST segments to the baseline throughout	T wave inversion in I, aVL, and V_5 or V_6 or both Tall T waves in II, III, and aVF

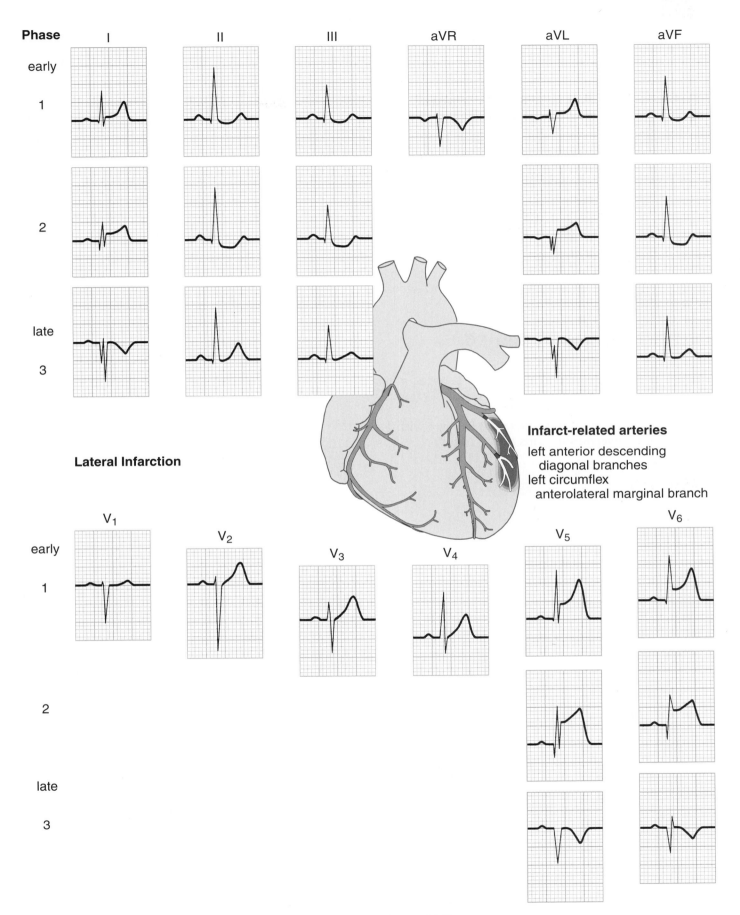

Figure 16-4 Lateral MI.

ANTEROLATERAL MYOCARDIAL INFARCTION

Coronary Arteries Involved and Site of Occlusion

The major artery involved is the left coronary artery, specifically the following branches:

♦ The diagonal arteries of the left anterior descending coronary artery alone or in conjunction with the anterolateral marginal artery of the left circumflex coronary artery (Figure 16-5).

Location of Infarct

The anterolateral MI involves the anterior and lateral wall of the left ventricle.

ECG Changes (Table 16-5)

In facing leads I, aVL, and V₃-V₆:

Early: ST segment elevation with tall T waves and taller than normal R waves in leads I, aVL, and the precordial leads V_3-V_6.

Late: Abnormal Q waves and small R waves with T wave inversion in leads I, aVL, and V_3-V_6.

QS waves or complexes with T wave inversion in leads V_3-V_5 and sometimes V_6.

In opposite leads II, III, and aVF:

Early: ST segment depression in leads II, III, and aVF.

Late: Abnormally tall T waves in leads II, III, and aVF.

Notes

_____

_____

_____

_____

_____

_____

_____

_____

_____

_____

_____

_____

TABLE

16-5 ECG Changes in Anterolateral MI

	Q Waves (Abnormal Q Waves and QS Complexes)	R Waves (Abnormally Tall or Small)	ST Segments (Elevated or Depressed)	T Waves (Abnormally Tall or Inverted)
Early *Phase 1* First few hrs (0 to 2 hrs)	Normal Q waves	Normal or abnormally tall R waves in I, aVL, and V_3-V_6	Elevated in I, aVL, and V_3-V_6 Depressed in II, III, and aVF	Sometimes, abnormally tall with peaking in I, aVL, and V_3-V_6
Phase 2 First day (2 to 24 hrs)	Minimally abnormal in I, aVL, and V_3-V_6	Minimally decreased in I, aVL, and V_3-V_6	Maximally elevated in I, aVL, and V_3-V_6 Maximally depressed in II, III, and aVF	Less tall, but generally still positive, in I, aVL, and V_3-V_6
Late *Phase 3* Second and third day (24 to 72 hrs)	Significantly abnormal in I, aVL, and V_3-V_6 QS waves or complexes in V_3-V_5 and sometimes V_6	Decreased or absent I and aVL Small R waves in I and aVL	Return of the ST in V_3-V_6 baseline throughout	T wave inversion in I, segments to the Tall T waves in II, III, and aVF

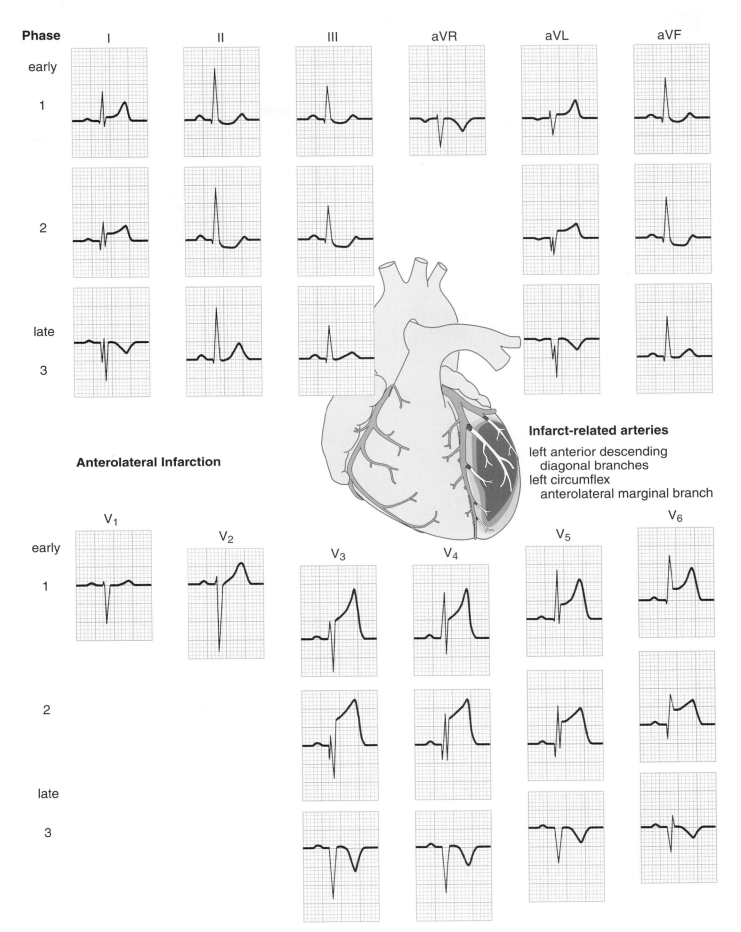

Figure 16-5 Anterolateral MI.

Phase — I, II, III, aVR, aVL, aVF
early — 1, 2, late — 3

Anterolateral Infarction

Infarct-related arteries
left anterior descending
  diagonal branches
left circumflex
  anterolateral marginal branch

V_1, V_2, V_3, V_4, V_5, V_6
early — 1, 2, late — 3

EXTENSIVE ANTERIOR MYOCARDIAL INFARCTION

Coronary Arteries Involved and Site of Occlusion

The major artery involved is the left coronary artery, specifically the following branches:

◆ The left anterior descending coronary artery alone or in conjunction with the anterolateral marginal artery of the left circumflex coronary artery (Figure 16-6).

Location of Infarct

The extensive anterior MI involves (1) the entire anterior and lateral wall of the left ventricle and (2) the anterior aspect of the interventricular septum.

ECG Changes (Table 16-6)

In facing leads I, aVL, and V_1-V_6:

Early: Absence of normal "septal" r waves in the right precordial leads V_1-V_2, resulting in QS complexes in these leads.

Absence of normal "septal" q waves where normally present (i.e., in leads I, II, III, aVF, and V_4-V_6).

ST segment elevation with tall T waves in leads I, aVL, and V_1-V_6 and taller than normal R waves in leads I, aVL, and V_3-V_6.

Late: Abnormal Q waves and small R waves with T wave inversion in leads I, aVL, and V_1-V_6.

QS waves or complexes with T wave inversion in leads V_1-V_5 and sometimes V_6.

In opposite leads II, III, and aVF:

Early: ST segment depression in leads II, III, and aVF.

Late: Abnormally tall T waves in leads II, III, and aVF.

Notes

_____

_____

_____

_____

_____

_____

TABLE

16-6 ECG Changes in Extensive Anterior MI

	Q Waves (Abnormal Q Waves and QS Complexes)	R Waves (Abnormally Tall or Small)	ST Segments (Elevated or Depressed)	T Waves (Abnormally Tall or Inverted)
Early *Phase 1* First few hrs (0 to 2 hrs)	Absent "septal" q waves in leads I, II, III, aVF, and V_4-V_6 QS waves in V_1-V_2	Absent "septal" r waves in V_1-V_2 Normal or abnormally tall R waves in I, aVL, and V_3-V_6	Elevated in I, aVL, and V_1-V_6 Depressed in II, III, and aVF	Sometimes, abnormally tall with peaking in I, aVL, and V_2-V_6
Phase 2 First day (2 to 24 hrs)	QS waves in V_1-V_2 Minimally abnormal in I, aVL, and V_3-V_6	Absent in V_1-V_2 Minimally decreased in I, aVL, and V_3-V_6	Maximally elevated in I, aVL, and V_1-V_6 Maximally depressed in II, III, and aVF	Less tall, but generally still positive, in I, aVL, and V_1-V_6
Late *Phase 3* Second and third day (24 to 72 hrs)	QS waves or complexes in V_1-V_5 and sometimes in V_6 Significantly abnormal in I, aVL, and V_1-V_6	Absent in V_1-V_2 Decreased or absent in V_3-V_5 and sometimes V_6 Small R waves in I and aVL	Return of the ST segments to the baseline throughout	T wave inversion in I, aVL, and V_1-V_6 Tall T waves in II, III, and aVF

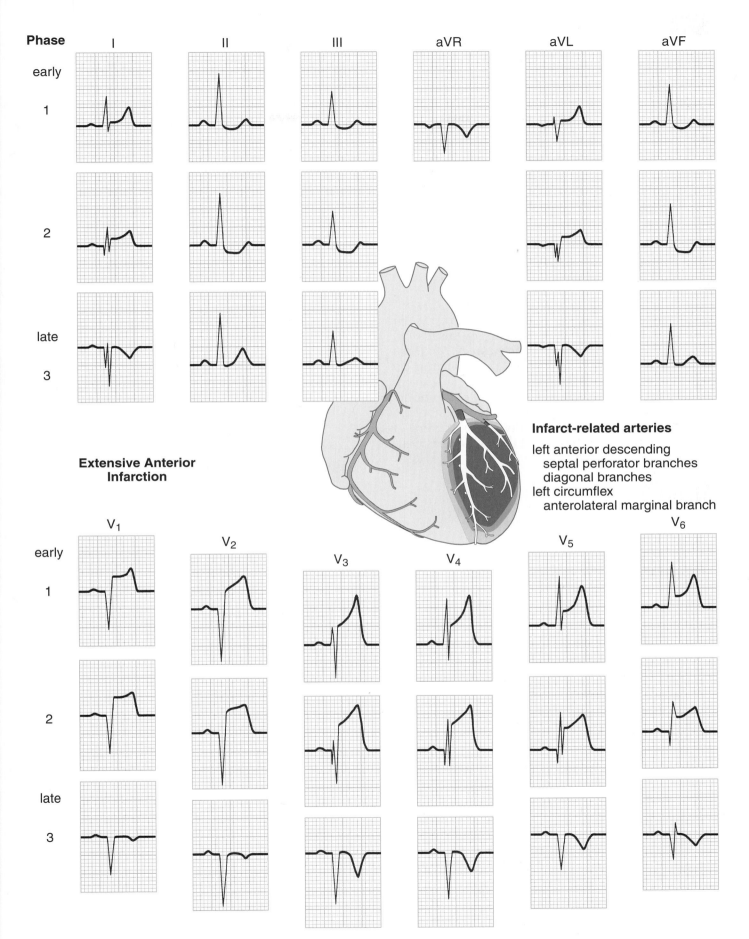

Figure 16-6 Extensive anterior MI.

INFERIOR MYOCARDIAL INFARCTION

Coronary Arteries Involved and Site of Occlusion

The major coronary arteries involved are the following:
- The posterior left ventricular arteries of the right coronary artery or, less commonly, of the left circumflex coronary artery of the left coronary artery. The posterior descending coronary artery and the atrioventricular (AV) node artery may also be involved (Figure 16-7).

Location of Infarct

The inferior MI involves the inferior wall of the left ventricle that rests on the diaphragm. For this reason, the inferior MI is also termed *diaphragmatic MI*. If the left circumflex artery is occluded, the infarction extends somewhat into the lateral wall of the left ventricle, causing an inferolateral MI. If the posterior descending coronary artery and the AV node artery are involved, the MI extends into the posterior third of the interventricular septum and the AV node as well.

ECG Changes (Table 16-7)

In facing leads II, III, and aVF:
Early: ST segment elevation with tall T waves and taller than normal R waves in leads II, III, and aVF.
Late: QS waves or complexes with T wave inversion in leads II, III, and aVF.
In opposite leads I and aVL:
Early: ST segment depression in leads I and aVL.
Late: Abnormally tall T waves in leads I and aVL.

Notes

_____

_____

_____

_____

_____

_____

_____

_____

TABLE

16-7   ECG Changes in Inferior MI

	Q Waves (Abnormal Q Waves and QS Complexes)	R Waves (Abnormally Tall or Small)	ST Segments (Elevated or Depressed)	T Waves (Abnormally Tall or Inverted)
Early *Phase 1* First few hrs (0 to 2 hrs)	Normal Q waves	Normal or abnormally tall R waves in II, III, and aVF	Elevated in II, III, and aVF Depressed in I and aVL	Sometimes, abnormally tall with peaking in II, III, and aVF
Phase 2 First day (2 to 24 hrs)	Minimally abnormal in II, III, and aVF	Minimally decreased in II, III, and aVF	Maximally elevated in II, III, and aVF Maximally depressed in I and aVL	Less tall, but generally still positive, in II, III, and aVF
Late *Phase 3* Second and third day (24 to 72 hrs)	QS waves or complexes in II, III, and aVF	Decreased or absent in II, III, and aVF	Return of the ST segments to the baseline throughout	T wave inversion in II, III, and aVF Tall T waves in I and aVL

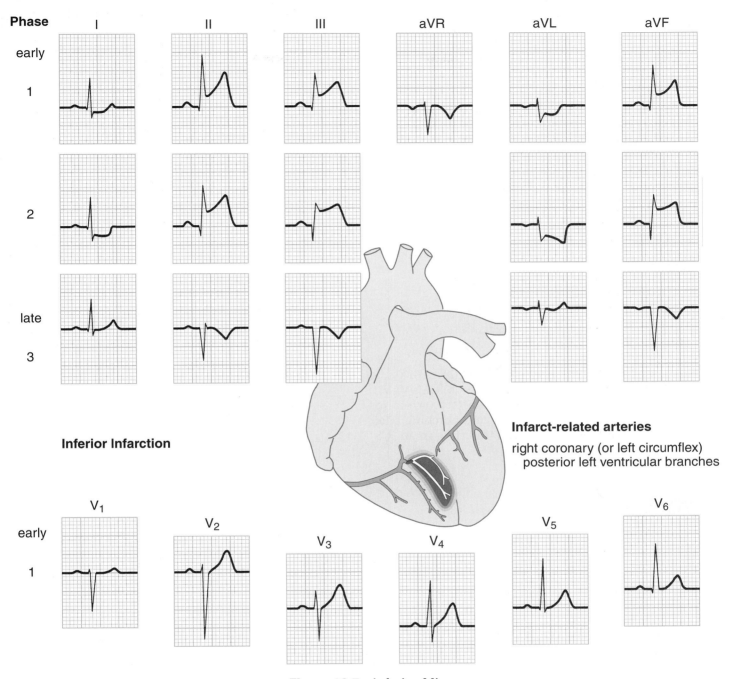

Inferior Infarction

Infarct-related arteries

right coronary (or left circumflex)
posterior left ventricular branches

Figure 16-7   Inferior MI.

POSTERIOR MYOCARDIAL INFARCTION

Coronary Arteries Involved and Site of Occlusion

The major coronary arteries involved are the following:
♦ The distal left circumflex artery and/or postero-lateral marginal artery of the left circumflex coronary artery (Figure 16-8).

Location of Infarct

The posterior MI involves the posterior wall of the left ventricle, located just below the left posterior AV groove and extending to the inferior wall of the left ventricle.

ECG Changes (Table 16-8)

Facing leads: There are no facing leads.
In opposite leads V_1-V_4:

Early: ST segment depression in leads V_1-V_4. The T wave is inverted in V_1 and sometimes in V_2.

Late: Large R waves with tall T waves in leads V_1-V_4. The R wave is tall and wide ($\geq$0.04 sec in width) in V_1 with slurring and notching. The S wave in V_1 is decreased, resulting in an R/S ratio of $\geq$1 in V_1.

Notes

TABLE

16-8 ECG Changes in Posterior MI

	Q Waves (Abnormal Q Waves and QS Complexes)	R Waves (Abnormally Tall or Small)	ST Segments (Elevated or Depressed)	T Waves (Abnormally Tall or Inverted)
Early *Phase 1*				
First few hrs (0 to 2 hrs)	Normal Q waves	Normal R waves	Depressed in V_1-V_4	Inverted in V_1 and sometimes in V_2
Phase 2				
First day (2 to 24 hrs)	Same as in Phase 1	Minimally increased in V_1-V_4	Maximally depressed in V_1-V_4	Same as Phase 1
Late *Phase 3*				
Second and third day (24 to 72 hrs)	Same as in Phase 1	Large R waves in V_1-V_4 with slurring and notching in V_1 S waves decreased in V_1 NOTE: In V_1, R/S ratio $\geq$1	Return of the ST segments to the baseline throughout	Tall T waves in V_1-V_4

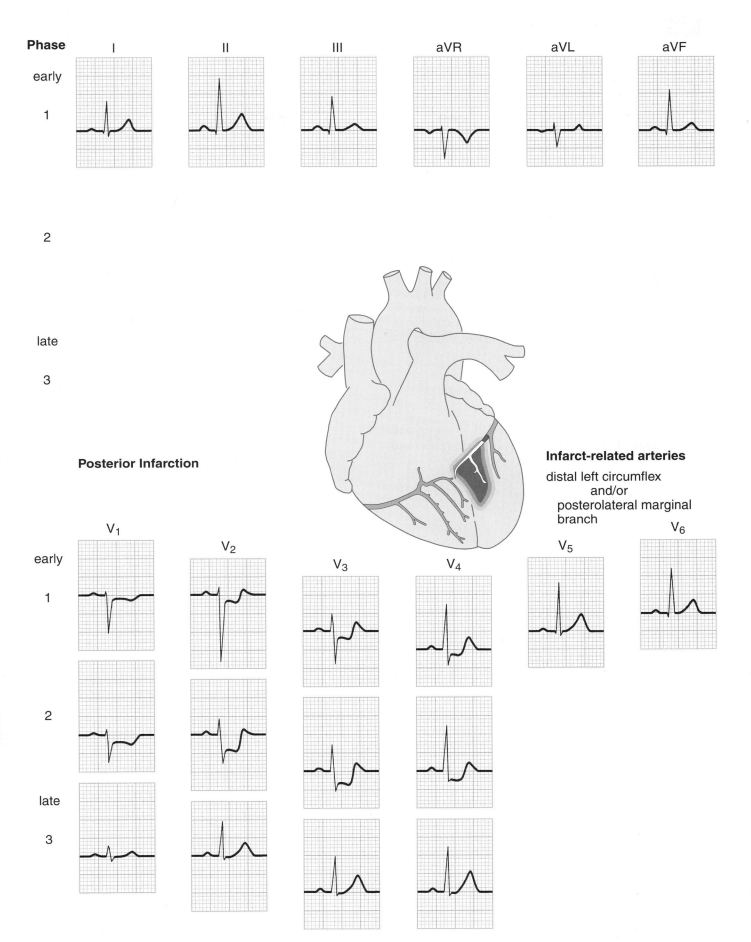

Figure 16-8 Posterior MI.

RIGHT VENTRICULAR MYOCARDIAL INFARCTION

Coronary Arteries Involved and Site of Occlusion

The major coronary artery involved is the following:
- The right coronary artery with its distal branches—the posterior left ventricular arteries, the posterior descending coronary artery, and the AV node artery (Figure 16-9).

Location of Infarct

The right ventricular MI involves the anterior, posterior, inferior, and lateral walls of the right ventricle, the posterior one third of the interventricular septum, the inferior wall of the left ventricle, and the AV node.

ECG Changes (Table 16-9)

In facing leads II, III, aVF, and V_{4R}:

Early: ST segment elevation with tall T waves and taller than normal R waves in leads II, III, and aVF.
ST segment elevation in V_{4R}.

Late: QS waves or complexes with T wave inversion in leads II, III, and aVF.
T wave inversion in V_{4R}.

In opposite leads I and aVL:
Early: ST segment depression in leads I and aVL.
Late: Abnormally tall T waves in leads I and aVL.

Notes

_____

_____

_____

_____

_____

_____

_____

_____

_____

_____

_____

_____

TABLE

16-9 ECG Changes in Right Ventricular MI

	Q Waves (Abnormal Q Waves and QS Complexes)	R Waves (Abnormally Tall or Small)	ST Segments (Elevated or Depressed)	T Waves (Abnormally Tall or Inverted)
Early *Phase 1* First few hrs (0 to 2 hrs)	Normal Q waves	Normal or abnormally tall R waves in II, III, and aVF	Elevated in II, III, aVF, and V_{4R} Depressed in I and aVL	Sometimes, abnormally tall with peaking in II, III, and aVF
Phase 2 First day (2 to 24 hrs)	Minimally abnormal in II, III, and aVF	Minimally decreased in II, III, and aVF	Maximally elevated in II, III, and aVF Elevated in V_{4R}, but may be normal Maximally depressed in I and aVL	Less tall, but generally still positive, in II, III, and aVF May be inverted in V_{4R}
Late *Phase 3* Second and third day (24 to 72 hrs)	QS waves or complexes in II, III, and aVF	Decreased or absent in II, III, and aVF	Return of the ST segments to the baseline throughout	T wave inversion in II, III, aVF, and V_{4R} Tall T waves in I and aVL

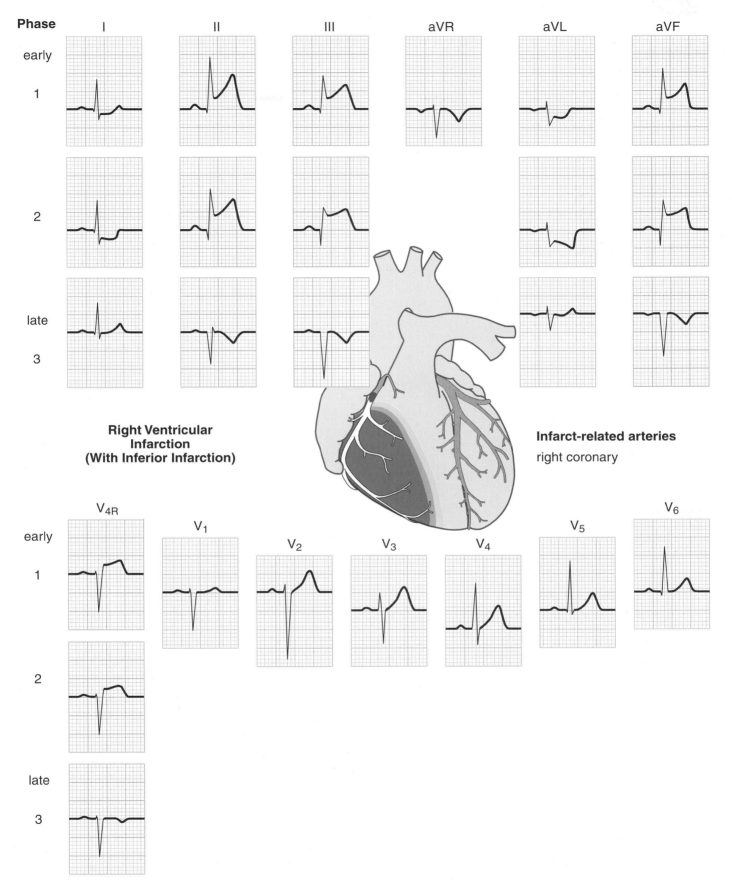

Figure 16-9 Right ventricular MI.

16-10 The Facing ECG Leads of Anterior, Inferior, and Right Ventricular MIs and Opposite ECG Leads of Posterior MI Showing the ST Segment and T Wave Changes in Early Acute Transmural Q-Wave Infarction

Infarction	I	II	III	aVR	aVL	aVF
Septal MI						
Anterior (localized) MI						
Anteroseptal MI						
Lateral MI						
Anterolateral MI						
Extensive Anterior MI Inferior MI						

V$_{R4}$	V$_1$	V$_2$	V$_3$	V$_4$	V$_5$	V$_6$

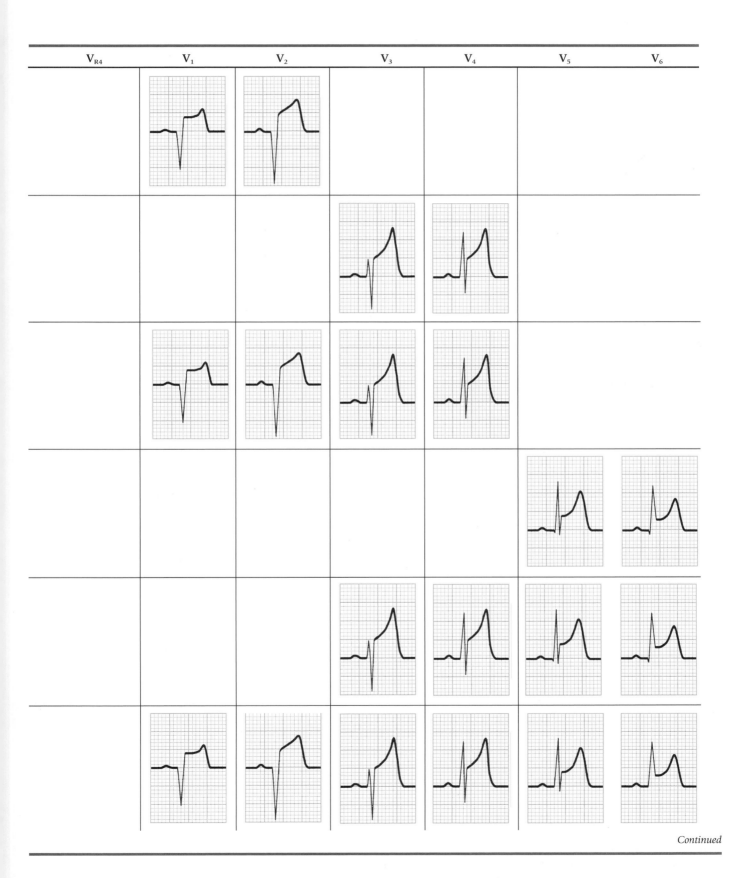

Continued

TABLE

16-10 The Facing ECG Leads of Anterior, Inferior, and Right Ventricular MIs and Opposite ECG Leads of Posterior MI Showing the ST Segment and T Wave Changes in Early Acute Transmural Q-Wave Infarction—cont'd

Infarction	I	II	III	aVR	aVL	aVF
Inferior MI						
Posterior MI						
Right Ventricular MI with Inferior MI						

V_{R4}	V₁	V₂	V₃	V₄	V₅	V₆

Infarction	Coronary Arteries Involved	Facing ECG Leads	Potential Complications
Septal MI	Septal perforator arteries of the left anterior descending coronary artery	V_1-V_2 (ST↑)	*AV blocks:* Second-degree, type II AV block[1] Second-degree, 2:1 and advanced AV block[1] Third-degree AV block[1] *Bundle branch blocks:* RBBB LBBB LAFB LPFB[3]
Anterior (localized) MI	Diagonal arteries of the left anterior descending coronary artery	V_3-V_4 (ST↑)	*LV dysfunction:* CHF Cardiogenic shock
Lateral MI	Diagonal arteries of the left anterior descending coronary artery and/or the anterolateral marginal artery of the left circumflex coronary artery	I, aVL, V_5-V_6 (ST↑)	*LV dysfunction:* CHF (moderate)
Inferior MI	Posterior left ventricular arteries of the right coronary artery or, less commonly, of the left circumflex coronary artery; the left posterior descending coronary artery and the AV node artery may also be involved	II, III, aVF (ST↑)	*LV dysfunction:* CHF (mild, if any) *AV blocks:* First-degree AV block[2] Second-degree, type I AV block[2] Second-degree, 2:1 and advanced AV block[2] Third-degree AV block[2] *Bundle branch blocks:* LPFB[4]
Posterior MI	Distal left circumflex artery and/or posterolateral marginal artery of the circumflex coronary artery	None Opposite leads: V_1-V_4 (ST↓)	*LV dysfunction:* CHF (mild, if any)
Right ventricular MI	Right coronary artery, including the SA node and AV node arteries, the posterior descending coronary artery, and the posterior left ventricular arteries	II, III, aVF, V_{4R} (ST↑)	*RV dysfunction:* Right heart failure *Arrhythmias:* Sinus arrest Sinus bradycardia Atrial premature beats Atrial flutter Atrial fibrillation *AV blocks:* First-degree AV block[2] Second-degree type I AV block[2] Second-degree, 2:1 and advanced AV block[2] Third-degree AV block[2] *Bundle branch blocks:* RBBB LBBB LPFB[4]

CHF, Congestive heart failure; *LAFB,* left anterior fascicular block; *LBBB,* left bundle branch block; *LPFB,* left posterior fascicular block; *LV,* left ventricular; *RBBB,* right bundle branch block; *RV,* right ventricular.

[1]With abnormally wide QRS complexes.
[2]With normal QRS complexes.
[3]In conjunction with a right ventricular or inferior infarction.
[4]In conjunction with a septal infarction.

CHAPTER REVIEW QUESTIONS

1. The type of MI presenting early with ST segment elevation, tall T waves, and taller than normal R waves in the midprecordial leads V_3 and V_4 and late with QS complexes and T wave inversion in leads V_3 and V_4 is a(n):
   A. septal MI
   B. anterior (localized) MI
   C. anteroseptal MI
   D. lateral MI

2. An MI presenting early with ST segment depression in leads II, III, and aVF and ST segment elevation, tall T waves, and taller than normal R waves in leads I, aVL, and the left precordial lead V_5 or V_6 or both indicates a(n) _____ MI.
   A. septal
   B. anterior (localized)
   C. anteroseptal
   D. lateral

3. The type of MI involving both the anterior wall of the left ventricle overlying the interventricular septum and the anterior two thirds of the interventricular septum is a(n):
   A. septal MI
   B. anterior (localized) MI
   C. anteroseptal MI
   D. lateral MI

4. The type of MI presenting late with QS complexes and T wave inversion in leads V_1-V_2 and absent normal "septal" q waves in leads II, III, and aVF is a(n) _____ MI.
   A. septal
   B. anterior (localized)
   C. anteroseptal
   D. lateral

5. The type of MI presenting early with ST segment elevation, tall T waves, and taller than normal R waves in leads I and aVL and the precordial leads V_3-V_6 and ST segment depression in leads II, III, and aVF is a(n):
   A. septal MI
   B. anterior (localized) MI
   C. anterolateral MI
   D. lateral MI

6. The type of MI presenting late with abnormal Q waves, small R waves, and T wave inversion in leads I and aVL and QS waves or complexes with T wave inversion in leads V_1-V_6 is a(n):
   A. septal MI
   B. anterior (localized) MI
   C. extensive anterior MI
   D. anterolateral MI

7. An MI involving the posterior left ventricular arteries of the right coronary artery or the left circumflex coronary artery of the left coronary artery is a(n):
   A. left ventricular MI
   B. posterior MI
   C. inferior MI
   D. anteroseptal MI

8. An MI that presents early with ST segment elevation, tall T waves, and taller than normal R waves in leads II, III, and aVF and ST segment depression in leads I and aVL is a(n):
   A. posterior MI
   B. inferior MI
   C. anteroseptal MI
   D. lateral MI

9. An MI that presents late with large R waves and tall T waves in leads V_1-V_4, an R wave ≥0. 04 second in width with slurring and notching in V_1, and an R/S ratio of ≥1 in V_1 is a(n):
   A. posterior MI
   B. inferior MI
   C. anteroseptal MI
   D. right ventricular MI

10. An MI that presents early with ST segment elevation, tall T waves, and taller than normal R waves in leads II, III, and aVF; ST segment elevation in V_{4R}; and ST segment depression in leads I and aVL is a(n):
    A. posterior MI
    B. inferior MI
    C. anteroseptal MI
    D. right ventricular MI with inferior myocardial infarction

CHAPTER 17

Signs and Symptoms of Acute Myocardial Infarction

CHAPTER OUTLINE

Diagnosis of Acute Myocardial Infarction
  Signs and Symptoms
  History and Physical Examination
Signs and Symptoms of Acute Myocardial
Infarction
  Symptoms of Acute Myocardial Infarction
  Signs of Acute Myocardial Infarction
Signs and Symptoms of Left Heart Failure
  Symptoms of Left Heart Failure
  Signs of Left Heart Failure

Signs of Right Heart Failure
Signs and Symptoms of Cardiogenic Shock
  Symptoms of Cardiogenic Shock
  Signs of Cardiogenic Shock
Signs of Cardiac Arrest
Summary of the Signs and Symptoms of Acute
Myocardial Infarction
  Symptoms in Acute Myocardial Infarction
  Signs in Acute Myocardial Infarction

CHAPTER OBJECTIVES

Upon completion of all or part of this chapter, you
should be able to complete the following:
1. Discuss the importance of the following in making a
   diagnosis of acute myocardial infarction (MI) in this
   early phase:
   Clinical evaluation
   ECG changes
   Serum cardiac markers
2. Define the following:
   Chief complaint
   Present illness
   Past cardiac history
3. List the specific symptoms commonly experienced by
   the patient during an acute MI and their causes under
   the following categories:
   General and neurological symptoms
   Cardiovascular symptoms
   Respiratory symptoms
   Gastrointestinal symptoms
4. Discuss the characteristics of the pain encountered in
   an acute MI according to:
   Frequency of occurrence
   Location and radiation

Quality, intensity, and duration
Relation to body movement
Associated emotional and psychological manifestations
Responsiveness to rest and/or nitroglycerin
5. List other conditions that can mimic the pain of acute
   MI.
6. Define dyspnea and its cause in acute MI and describe the three forms it may assume.
7. List the gastrointestinal symptoms commonly experienced in acute MI.
8. Describe the general appearance and neurological
   signs of a patient with acute MI.
9. Describe the characteristics of the following vital
   signs in acute MI, both normal and abnormal:
   Pulse: rate, rhythm, and force
   Respirations: rate, rhythm, depth, and character
   Blood pressure: systolic blood pressure
10. Describe the following parts of the body as they
    might appear in the acute MI, both normally or ab-
    normally:
    Skin
    Eyes

DIAGNOSIS OF ACUTE MYOCARDIAL INFARCTION

Diagnosis of acute myocardial infarction (MI), based solely on observation of specific symptoms and physical signs, is often tentative because only a small percentage (about 10%) of patients with chest pain when first seen have an acute MI. An electrocardiogram (ECG) is extremely useful as a diagnostic aid in detecting the presence of heart muscle ischemia and injury during the first half hour or so of acute MI. ECG changes include the appearance of T wave changes (the result of myocardial ischemia) and ST segment elevation or depression (the result of myocardial muscle ischemia and injury).

Serial ECGs obtained during the next few hours of an acute MI show the evolution of T wave changes and ST segment elevation or depression. ST elevation, the prime sign of myocardial injury, has been shown to appear in less than 50% of the patients suffering an acute MI. Q waves denoting myocardial necrosis, however, do not begin to appear until several hours or more into the acute MI, becoming fully developed 24 to 72 hours after the onset. Thus the clinical evaluation and the ST segment and T wave changes in the ECG are usually the only available data on which to base the diagnosis of an acute MI during the prehospital phase and the early minutes after admission to the emergency department (ED) and to initiate appropriate therapy. It should be noted that in a very small number of acute MIs, the only change is the sudden appearance of a complete left bundle branch block (LBBB).

The signs and symptoms of acute MI are described in this chapter. The ST segment and T wave changes in the early phase of acute MI are described in Chapters 15 and 16. These changes and the location of the infarct based on the leads in which the ECG changes appear are summarized below.

In the majority of Q-wave myocardial infarctions are the following:

◆ ST segment elevation of 0.1 mV or greater, measured 0.04 second (1 small square) after the J point, and abnormally tall peaked T waves in two or more contiguous facing leads:
  ◇ Anterior wall infarction: leads I, aVL, and V_1-V_6
  ◇ Inferior wall infarction: leads II, III, and aVF
  ◇ Right ventricular wall infarction: leads II, III, aVF, and V_{4R}
◆ ST depression of 0.1 mV or greater in two or more contiguous opposite leads:
  ◇ Posterior wall infarction: leads V_1-V_4

In the majority of non-Q-wave myocardial infarctions are the following:

◆ ST segment depression of 0.1 mV or greater and isoelectric, biphasic, or inverted T waves in two or more contiguous facing leads:
  ◇ Anterior wall infarction: leads I, aVL, and V_1-V_6
  ◇ Inferior wall infarction: leads II, III, and aVF

Upon admission to the ED, blood studies are routinely performed to determine whether certain proteins and enzymes released from damaged or necrotic myocardial tissue (or *serum cardiac markers*, as they are called) are abnormally elevated. These serum markers include the following:

◆ *Myoglobin.* Increase in myoglobin occurs with damage to both skeletal and cardiac muscle.
◆ *CK-MB (creatinine kinase MB isoenzyme).* CK-MB, unlike myoglobin, is more specific, increasing primarily after myocardial necrosis.
◆ *Troponin T and I (cTnT, cTnI).* The troponins, like CK-MB, are also myocardium specific, but they increase not only after myocardial necrosis but also after myocardial injury.

As shown in Figure 17-1, myoglobin is the first serum marker to become elevated after an acute MI, followed by the troponins and CK-MB. Because diagnostic levels of these serum enzymes do not appear immediately in the blood after an acute MI and their determination may take more than 20 minutes, these markers are usually not available during the early phase of acute MI to help in its diagnosis. Thus in most instances the diagnosis of acute MI at this stage is based solely on the clinical evaluation and the presence of ST segment elevation or depression on the initial ECGs, as noted above.

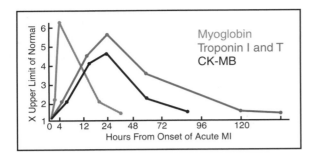

Figure 17-1 Time of appearance and degree of elevation of serum markers after the onset of acute myocardial infarction.

Other laboratory findings that may be present early in acute MI include the following:
◆ Elevated *serum C-reactive protein* and *serum amyloid*
◆ An elevated *white blood cell count (WBC)*, usually within 2 hours after the onset of infarction

Signs and Symptoms

Coronary artery disease (CAD) manifests itself by significant symptoms and signs. The symptoms and signs in acute MI vary, depending on the location and extent of the heart damage and the kind and degree of autonomic nervous system activity (sympathetic or parasympathetic) present.

A *symptom* is defined as an abnormal feeling of distress or an awareness of disturbances in bodily function experienced by the patient. The symptoms are obtained during the taking of the patient's history. Examples of symptoms of CAD are marked apprehension, chest pain (angina pectoris, pain of acute MI), dyspnea, palpitations, and nausea.

Signs are abnormalities of the patient's body structure and function that are detected by initial inspection of the patient and by the physical examination. Some examples of signs of CAD include tachycardia, distention of the neck veins, edema, and cyanosis.

History and Physical Examination

A patient's history includes information about his or her symptoms and any previous illness. It includes the chief complaint, present illness, and past cardiac history. The *chief complaint* is a short statement of the patient's major symptom requiring emergency medical care. The *present illness* is a more detailed description of the patient's chief complaint and includes the symptoms and their severity, duration, and relationship to precipitating causes, such as exercise, emotion, body position, and so forth.

Past cardiac history is a brief review of previous cardiovascular diseases and their treatment. This includes any history of previous MIs, angina pectoris, congestive heart failure (CHF), arrhythmias, syncope, hypertension, and so forth; previous hospitalizations; medications currently being taken; and any known allergies. The history may include any other information that medical control deems necessary.

Once an appropriate history is obtained or even while questioning the patient, a physical examination is performed to obtain the patient's physical signs, including the vital signs. These signs, in conjunction with the patient's history and the presence of abnormal ECG changes (ST segment elevation or depression and T wave changes) will help to determine the correct diagnosis and appropriate management.

SIGNS AND SYMPTOMS OF ACUTE MYOCARDIAL INFARCTION

The signs and symptoms of acute MI generally reflect the extent of myocardial damage and the severity of the complications that may be present (i.e., arrhythmias, mechanical pump failure, or cardiac rupture). Although pain is the most common symptom in acute MI, it is important to note that many of the following signs and symptoms may be present even in the absence of pain.

The symptoms of acute MI include the following:
◆ General and neurological symptoms
◆ Cardiovascular symptoms
◆ Respiratory symptoms
◆ Gastrointestinal symptoms

The signs of acute MI include the following:
◆ General appearance and neurological signs
◆ Vital signs (pulse, respirations, blood pressure)
◆ Appearance of the skin
◆ Appearance of the eyes
◆ Appearance of the veins
◆ Cardiovascular signs
◆ Respiratory signs
◆ Appearance of body tissues
◆ Appearance of the abdomen

Symptoms of Acute Myocardial Infarction

◆ GENERAL AND NEUROLOGICAL SYMPTOMS

General and neurological symptoms of acute MI include the following in varying degrees:
◆ Anxiety and apprehension
◆ Restlessness and agitation with a fear of impending death (or a sense of impending doom)

- Extreme fatigue and weakness
- Lightheadedness or dizziness
- Confusion, disorientation, or drowsiness
- Fainting or loss of consciousness (syncope)

When first seen, the patient with acute MI may appear fully alert and oriented. If the supply of oxygen to the brain becomes inadequate at any time because of (1) decreased cardiac output resulting from mechanical pump failure, myocardial rupture, or an arrhythmia or (2) hypoxemia from CHF, symptoms of cerebral anoxia rapidly appear. Commonly, the initial symptoms of cerebral anoxia are marked anxiety and apprehension, restlessness, and agitation, with a fear of impending death (or a sense of impending doom, as some would describe it) while the patient is still alert and oriented. Extreme fatigue or weakness and lightheadedness or dizziness are usually also present at this point when total body perfusion is inadequate.

If the brain becomes more anoxic, confusion, disorientation, and drowsiness follow. The patient may become faint and experience episodes of syncope in the presence of a severe tachycardia or bradycardia or an AV block. The final stages of oxygen deprivation are unconsciousness while still responsive to painful stimuli, followed by complete unresponsiveness, convulsions, and, eventually, death.

Hyperventilation, which may result in faintness, a sense of unreality, coldness or tingling of the extremities, spasms of the hands and feet (carpopedal spasm), and even loss of consciousness, often accompanies extreme anxiety states. This is known as the *hyperventilation syndrome.*

◆ CARDIOVASCULAR SYMPTOMS

Cardiovascular symptoms of acute MI include the following:
- Chest pain
- Palpitations (or "skipping of the heart")

Pain

Pain is the most conspicuous symptom of an acute MI. It appears in the majority (70% to 80%) of the patients with acute MI who are not in shock or cardiac arrest as a substernal (or retrosternal) constriction or crushing sensation. In the remaining 20% to 30% of patients, who most likely are experiencing their first attack, are elderly or diabetic, or are women, the pain of acute MI may be atypical or absent. When pain is absent, as it is in about 8% to 10% of the patients with acute MI, the MI is called *silent.* Even though pain may be atypical or absent in acute MI, other signs and symptoms are usually present to lead one to suspect acute MI.

The pain of acute MI results from the same factors that are responsible for angina pectoris (i.e., lack of oxygen to the myocardium and the accumulation of carbon dioxide and lactic acid). Although the pain of angina pectoris and the pain of acute MI often have similar characteristics, they can be differentiated from each other by an accurate and detailed history.

Unlike the pain of angina pectoris, which usually occurs after physical and emotional stress, the onset of pain in over half of those experiencing acute MI appears during rest. A smaller percentage of persons experience pain during activity, and a few are awakened from sleep by the pain. Often, many of the patients suffering their first acute MI (about 50%) have experienced recurrent warning attacks of anginal pain (preinfarction or prodromal angina) hours or days before the attack.

The pain of acute MI usually occurs in the middle or upper substernal area, the same as does angina pectoris, extending or radiating to any of the peripheral regions affected by angina pectoris, except that it is generally more intense and lasts longer. The pain of acute MI may radiate over the anterior chest and frequently to either of the shoulders and arms (usually the left), often extending down the medial aspect of the arm as far as the elbow, forearm, wrist, and, in some cases, the ring and little fingers. Less commonly, the pain radiates to the neck, jaw, and upper teeth; upper back, particularly between the scapulae; or the upper part of the abdomen in the midline (epigastrium). The pain may occasionally appear in these areas without first presenting substernally. About a third of the patients have substernal pain without radiation.

The pain of acute MI is typically terrifying for its victims, who describe it as constricting, compressing, crushing, bursting, oppressive, heavy, tight, squeezing, burning, aching, or a pressure or fullness. The pain of acute MI varies in intensity, often being severe and sometimes intolerable. At other times it may be mild in intensity, described as a dull substernal discomfort and easily ignored. If the pain radiates to the epigastrium, it may resemble that of indigestion. Rarely does the patient describe the chest pain as sharp, stabbing, or throbbing.

The pain is usually continuous after its crescendo-like appearance, varying sometimes in intensity. It does not move, nor does coughing, breathing, or changes in body position alter or alleviate it. In localizing the pain, the patient may place a clenched fist against his or her sternum. These patients may sometimes thrash about and beat their chests with their fists. Restlessness, anxiety, anguish, distress, apprehension, extreme fear, and a sense of impending doom often accompany the pain of acute MI. Signs and symptoms of serious complications, such as arrhythmias, cardiac arrest, CHF, or cardiogenic shock, all of which threaten the life of the patient, may also be present.

Although the pain of acute MI sometimes lasts only a few minutes and disappears spontaneously, it generally lasts longer than 30 minutes, commonly for an hour or longer. In most cases it can only be relieved by medication, such as meperidine or morphine sulfate. Nitroglycerin does not ease the pain of acute MI, as it does in angina pectoris. For example, if the pain of acute MI is associated with exertion, it can be confused with angina. If the pain is unresponsive to rest or three nitroglycerin tablets during the first 10 minutes after its onset, it is most likely due to an acute MI. A patient with chest pain having one or more of the characteristics of pain of acute MI listed below should be considered to have suffered an acute MI and managed accordingly, regardless of age, until proved otherwise.

- Location of the pain
- Description of the pain
- Radiation of the pain
- Relationship to body movement
- Duration of the pain
- Associated emotional and psychological manifestations
- Unresponsiveness to rest and/or nitroglycerin

Other conditions that mimic the pain of acute MI and should be ruled out include the following:

- Acute myocarditis
- Acute pericarditis
- Aortic dissection
- Spontaneous pneumothorax
- Pulmonary embolism

Palpitations

A regular heart beat interrupted by one or more extra beats (premature contractions) is a very common cardiac irregularity present in the majority of patients with acute MI. Such irregularities in heart beat are also commonly experienced by most people from time to time. This sensation occurs under the left breast or substernally and is described as palpitations, or "skipping of the heart." It is difficult to assess the significance of the palpitations in asymptomatic people. In persons with symptoms of CAD such as acute MI, however, palpitations may indicate the presence of a potentially life-threatening ventricular arrhythmia and impending cardiac arrest.

◆ RESPIRATORY SYMPTOMS

Respiratory symptoms of acute MI include the following:

- Shortness of breath (dyspnea), with or without a sensation of suffocation; a tight, constricted feeling in the chest; and even pain on breathing

- Wheezing
- Spasmodic coughing, productive of copious, frothy sputum that is frequently pink- or blood-tinged (hemoptysis)
- Choking

Dyspnea

Dyspnea, described as shortness of breath or difficulty in breathing, is commonly seen in acute MI, appearing gradually or suddenly. It is the primary symptom of left ventricular failure and is characterized by rapid, shallow, labored respirations. Dyspnea is always accompanied by an awareness of discomfort and, when it is severe, by extreme apprehension and agitation. A sensation of suffocation and a tight, constricting sensation in the chest and possibly pain on breathing may accompany dyspnea. Dyspnea occurs in pulmonary congestion and edema during exertion and even at rest. It may assume several forms, including dyspnea on exertion, orthopnea, and paroxysmal nocturnal dyspnea.

- *Dyspnea on exertion (DOE)* is usually the first noticeable symptom of left heart failure. It first appears after an exercise or effort, such as climbing two flights of stairs or walking a distance of two blocks, that previously did not produce shortness of breath.
- *Orthopnea* is severe dyspnea that is relieved only by the patient assuming a sitting or semireclining position or standing up.
- *Paroxysmal nocturnal dyspnea (PND)*, sometimes called "cardiac asthma," is characterized by sudden attacks of dyspnea, occurring at night, in a patient who may be asymptomatic during the day. The reason for this is the gradual redistribution of the blood and body fluids from the lower extremities into the lungs after the patient has been lying in bed for several hours. Because the left heart cannot cope with the increased volume of fluid presented to it, left heart failure and pulmonary congestion and edema follow, forcing the patient to sit up in bed or use extra pillows to breathe.

Cough

Cough accompanied by sputum, or a *productive cough*, is a common symptom in patients with pulmonary edema secondary to left heart failure. It is caused by excessive bronchial secretions arising from congested mucous membranes. The cough is often spasmodic and productive of copious, frothy sputum. Frequently the sputum is pink- or blood-tinged (hemoptysis), the result of hemorrhaging from congested bronchial mucosa. Wheezing and choking may accompany the cough.

◆ GASTROINTESTINAL SYMPTOMS

Gastrointestinal symptoms of acute MI include the following:

- ◆ Loss of appetite (anorexia)
- ◆ Nausea
- ◆ Vomiting
- ◆ Thirst
- ◆ Urge to defecate

Loss of appetite (anorexia) and nausea with or without vomiting are common in acute MI. These symptoms may also occur in CHF and after administration of certain cardiac drugs. The patient may misinterpret these gastrointestinal symptoms as being caused by "indigestion" and ignore them, especially if the pain of acute MI has radiated from the chest into the epigastric region. Thirst and the urge to defecate may also be present, especially if hypotension and shock occur.

Signs of Acute Myocardial Infarction

◆ GENERAL APPEARANCE AND NEUROLOGICAL SIGNS

General appearance and neurological signs of acute MI include the following:

- ◆ Fright
- ◆ Anxiety and apprehension
- ◆ Restlessness and agitation
- ◆ Disorientation and drowsiness
- ◆ Unconsciousness

The patient with acute MI may be alert and oriented, but frightened, anxious, and apprehensive, appearing restless, agitated, and in pain. If hypotension or shock occurs, the patient becomes confused and disoriented, then drowsy and unresponsive, and finally unconscious. At this point, the patient may convulse.

Unlike the patient with angina pectoris, who remains perfectly still during the attack of pain, the patient with acute MI may walk or thrash about and even beat his or her chest with his or her fists. A patient who has severe pulmonary congestion and edema is typically sitting up, struggling to breathe, and coughing up frothy sputum that is often tinged with blood.

◆ VITAL SIGNS

Box 17-1 lists the variations in vital signs that can be found in patients with acute MI. The patient's vital signs, which include the pulse, respirations, and blood pressure, vary, depending on the site and ex-

tent of the myocardial damage and on the degree of imbalance of the autonomic nervous system.

Pulse

Rate. In acute MI the pulse rate is usually rapid (greater than 100 beats per minute [tachycardia]) because of the predominance of sympathetic nervous system activity during acute MI or the presence of CHF, hypotension, or shock. It may, however, be normal (60 to 100 beats per minute) or even slow (less

---

BOX

17-1   Variations in Vital Signs in Patients With Acute Myocardial Infarction

Pulse
  Rate:
- • Normal (60 to 100/min)
- • Rapid (over 100/min [tachycardia])
- • Slow (less than 60/min [bradycardia])
  Rhythm:
- • Regular
- • Irregular
  Force:
- • Normal
- • Strong and full
- • Weak and thready

Respirations
  Rate:
- • Normal (12 to 16/min)
- • Rapid (over 16/min [tachypnea])
- • Slow (less than 12/min)
  Rhythm:
- • Regular
- • Irregular
  Depth:
- • Normal
- • Shallow
- • Deep
  Character:
- • Labored
- • Noisy, wheezing
- • Gasping
- • Periodic breathing (Cheyne-Stokes respiration)

Blood Pressure
  Systolic blood pressure:
- • Normal (90 to 140 mm Hg)
- • Elevated (above 140 mm Hg)
- • Low (less than 90 mm Hg)

than 60 beats per minute [bradycardia]) if the parasympathetic nervous system activity predominates or a slow arrhythmia is present.

Rhythm. The rhythm of the pulse in acute MI may be regular or irregular. An irregular pulse caused by numerous premature ventricular contractions (PVCs) or ventricular bigeminy may indicate a potentially life-threatening arrhythmia and impending cardiac arrest in a small percentage of patients.

The most common cause of gross pulse irregularity is chaotic beating of the atria (atrial fibrillation). This arrhythmia is characterized by variations in the force of contractions and pulsations in addition to a grossly irregular rhythm.

When any irregular heart rhythm is present, it is not uncommon to find that the radial pulse is slower than the pulse obtained over the cardiac apex. This discrepancy occurs because some of the cardiac contractions are weak and cannot produce a strong enough pulse wave to reach the radial artery. This is called a *pulse deficit.*

Force. The force of the pulse is related to the stroke volume and the pulse pressure (the difference between the systolic and diastolic pressures in mm Hg). The abnormally strong and full (bounding) pulse present during states of anxiety and excess emotion (increased sympathetic nervous system activity), strenuous exercise, and fever indicates a large stroke volume and a wide pulse pressure. The weak, thready pulse present in hypotension and shock and parasympathetic nervous system activity, on the other hand, indicates a low stroke volume and a narrow pulse pressure.

In acute MI, the pulse is often weak and thready, particularly in CHF, hypotension, and shock, but it may be normal or strong and full in the absence of any complication.

Respirations

The respirations in acute MI may vary depending on the presence or absence of anxiety and apprehension, CHF, hypotension, and shock. The rate of respirations may be normal, 12 to 16 per minute at rest (eupnea); slow, less than 12 per minute; or rapid, greater than 16 per minute (tachypnea). The rhythm of breathing may be regular or irregular. The depth of respirations may be normal, shallow, or deep. The respirations may appear quiet, labored and noisy, or gasping. Hyperpnea (rapid breathing accompanied by an increased depth of breathing) may be present. Usually, the respirations in acute MI are greater than 16 per minute (tachypnea) and shallow. In CHF, the respirations are typically rapid and shallow, often labored and noisy. In addition, the accessory muscles of respiration may be prominent during labored breathing.

Periodic breathing—*Cheyne-Stokes respiration*—is present when periods of increased rate and depth of breathing (hyperventilation) alternate with periods of absence of breathing (apnea). The periods of hyperventilation come on gradually, build up to a peak, and disappear gradually. Each period of hyperventilation and apnea lasts from about 15 to 60 seconds. This kind of breathing is caused by low levels of oxygen in the respiratory center of the brain, which can result from low cardiac output, CHF, brain tumors, diseased cerebral arteries, and stroke.

Blood Pressure

The blood pressure is usually elevated (greater than 140/90) initially in acute MI because of increased sympathetic nervous system activity. Later the blood pressure often returns to normal (about 120/80) or slightly below normal (less than 120/80 but greater than 90/60) unless hypotension or shock occurs, in which case the systolic blood pressure is less than 90 mm Hg. Initially, if excessive parasympathetic nervous activity is present initially or if the cardiac output is decreased because of significant mechanical pump failure, myocardial rupture, or an arrhythmia, the blood pressure will be low.

◆ APPEARANCE OF THE SKIN

The skin in acute MI may be:
◆ Pale, cold, sweaty, and clammy
◆ Cyanotic
◆ Mottled bluish-red
  The lips in acute MI may be:
◆ Pale
◆ Cyanotic
  The skin is usually pale, cold, and clammy in acute MI because of excessive sympathetic nervous system activity or because of hypotension and shock. Both result in the vasoconstriction of superficial blood vessels and marked stimulation of the sweat glands. In addition, profuse sweating (diaphoresis) may be present.

Often cyanosis of the skin, fingernail beds, and mucous membranes is present because of pulmonary congestion and edema. In the presence of both severe shock and cyanosis, the skin assumes a mottled bluish-red appearance. The lips are normal, pale, or cyanotic.

In general, cyanosis (the result of decreased oxygenation of arterial blood) is characterized by gray, slate blue, or purplish discoloration of the skin, mucous membranes, and nail beds. This sign is present in congenital heart disease, such lung diseases as emphysema and severe pneumonia, and any condition accompanied by low cardiac output (e.g., CHF, shock, and cardiac arrest).

◆ APPEARANCE OF THE EYES

The eyes in acute MI may be:
- Apprehensive and fearful
- Glassy with a lackluster, vacant, dull stare
- Ground-glass in appearance

The pupils in acute MI may be:
- Normal
- Dilated
- Constricted

The eyelids in acute MI may be:
- Normal
- Drooping

In acute MI, the eyes, pupils, and eyelids are usually normal unless hypotension, shock, or cardiac arrest is present. The pupils may be normal, dilated, or constricted. In hypotension and shock, the eyes may have an apprehensive and fearful look and appear glassy with a lackluster and vacant, dull stare. The eyelids may be drooping. The eyes of a patient who suffers a cardiac arrest assume a vacant, dull appearance immediately. Their surface takes on a ground-glass appearance as the eyelids begin to droop. The pupils start to dilate within 30 seconds after the cessation of blood flow to the brain and become fully dilated within 1.5 to 2 minutes.

◆ APPEARANCE OF THE VEINS

The veins in acute MI may be:
- Normal
- Distended and pulsating
- Collapsed

The veins of the neck may be normal, distended and pulsating, or collapsed. Generally, the patient's neck veins are assessed with the patient lying flat and propped up at a 45-degree angle. Distention of the neck veins typically occurs in right heart failure when the blood volume and venous pressure are significantly increased because of fluid retention within the body. The degree of distention depends on the severity of right-sided failure. In mild right heart failure, the neck veins are only slightly to moderately distended when the patient is lying flat. When the failure is severe, the jugular veins become markedly distended and pulsate even when the patient is sitting upright. The neck veins may also be slightly distended in left heart failure because of the increased pressure in the right atrium reflecting the increased pressure in the left atrium by way of the pulmonary circulation.

In hypotension and shock, by contrast, the neck veins are usually collapsed when the patient is sitting or propped up at a 45-degree angle. If right heart failure is also present in hypotension and shock, however, the neck veins may be distended and pulsating.

The superficial peripheral veins of the rest of the body may be normal or distended in right heart failure, or collapsed in hypotension and shock.

◆ CARDIOVASCULAR SIGNS

Cardiovascular signs in acute MI may include:
- Distant heart sounds
- A third heart sound (S_3) early in diastole
- A fourth heart sound (S_4) late in diastole
- A gallop rhythm
- A systolic murmur

Heart Sounds

The heart sounds after an acute MI are generally muffled, being described as "distant." A fourth heart sound (S_4), late in diastole just before the first heart sound, is often present. Its cause is usually a forceful atrial contraction and sudden distention of the incapacitated left ventricle with blood. A soft systolic murmur is also often present at the apex, the result of mitral regurgitation caused by disruption of the papillary muscles from myocardial injury. If left heart failure occurs after acute MI, an additional heart sound, the third heart sound (S_3), appears shortly after the second heart sound early in diastole. This sound results from the rapid filling of the weakened left ventricle during early diastole.

An S_3 or S_4 gallop rhythm exists when a third or fourth heart sound is present, respectively. When both a third and fourth heart sound are present, the rhythm is called a *quadruple gallop*. When the heart rate becomes very rapid in a quadruple gallop, the third and fourth heart sounds may come together, producing a "summation gallop."

◆ RESPIRATORY SIGNS

Respiratory signs in acute MI may include:
- Labored and noisy breathing
- Wheezing
- Dry coarse rattling in the throat
- Spasmodic coughing with expectoration of frothy, pink- or blood-tinged sputum (hemoptysis)
- Choking
- Dullness to percussion over both lungs, particularly at the bases, posteriorly
- Decreased (or absent) breath sounds, rales, wheezes, rhonchi, and loud gurgling or bubbling sounds at the bases of the lungs, up as high as the scapulae, on auscultation

Breath Sounds

The breath sounds produced by the flow of air through the pulmonary air passages may be normal, labored and noisy, decreased, or absent. In pulmonary congestion and edema the breath sounds on auscultation are usually slightly diminished or even absent at one or both bases of the lungs posteriorly. This results from the decrease or absence of flow of air through partially or completely obstructed air passages in the congested and edematous parts of the lungs.

Rales, Rhonchi, Coughing, and Wheezes

The passage of air through bronchi and bronchioles narrowed by edema and spasm and filled with fluid and foam produces abnormal respiratory sounds called *rales, rhonchi,* and *wheezes.* They vary in aural texture and intensity, depending on the size of the air passages involved and the degree of fluid accumulation. Rales may be "fine" or "course" according to their site of origin. They are very fine ("crepitant," "crackling," or "bubbling") when originating in the very small air passages, such as the bronchioles, and coarse ("gurgling") when originating in larger ones. Rales may also be dry or moist, according to the amount of moisture in the air passages. Rales are the most common signs in pulmonary edema after left heart failure and in pneumonia.

Rhonchi are bubbling or gurgling sounds that are generally louder and courser than rales. They usually originate in the larger air passages (i.e., the trachea and larger bronchi), most often because of partial lower airway obstruction by fluid. Very coarse gurgling or bubbling sounds are also produced in cavities containing fluid, as in severe pulmonary edema. Rhonchi occur in pulmonary edema, bronchitis, resolving pneumonia, emphysema, and pleural effusion. Dry, coarse rattling in the throat may also be present.

Spasmodic coughing with expectoration of frothy sputum, often pink- or blood-tinged (hemoptysis), and choking may be present. Wheezes are present when only narrowing of the bronchi and bronchioles is present without significant accumulation of fluid, as in pulmonary congestion and asthma. As with wheezing in asthma, they are heard best during exhalation.

Rales, rhonchi, and wheezes are heard best by auscultation (i.e., listening by using a stethoscope), although if they are loud enough they can be heard without a stethoscope. In patients with early left heart failure, fine, crepitant rales and wheezes are frequently heard at both bases of the lungs posteriorly and sometimes as high up as the scapulae; often, however, they are heard over only the right lung. As the edema progresses, becoming more severe, the rales become coarse and moist, and rhonchi and pos-

sibly loud gurgling or bubbling sounds may appear. These sounds may be present at one or both bases of the lungs only or up to the scapulae posteriorly or throughout the lungs and anteriorly as well. Rales can be elicited by having the patient breath deeply and forcefully through a wide-open mouth. They are best heard during inspiration, especially toward the end of deep breaths. Rhonchi can be heard during both exhalation and late inspiration over the bronchi and trachea.

Consolidation and Pleural Effusion

When a segment of the lung becomes completely filled with fluid, preventing air from entering, consolidation is present. Breath sounds and rales that were once there initially, disappear. The breath sounds may also be markedly decreased and even absent over one or both bases of the lungs posteriorly because of fluid in the pleural space (pleural effusion) caused by right heart failure. This results primarily because of compression of the lungs by the effusion. The areas of the lungs where the breath sounds decrease or disappear because of consolidation or pleural effusion lose their resonance and become dull to percussion. Thus dullness to percussion may be present over one or both lungs, particularly at the bases of the lungs posteriorly.

◆ APPEARANCE OF BODY TISSUES

The tissues of the body in acute MI may show the following:
- ◆ Pitting edema in front of the tibia (pretibial edema), over the lower part of the back over the spine (presacral edema), in the abdominal wall, and over the entire body (anasarca)

Edema

Edema is the accumulation of serous fluid in body tissue. It may be confined to one or more areas or exist throughout the body. When generalized, it is known as *anasarca.*

Some degree of edema is always present in right heart failure. Early in the course of fluid retention, weight gain is the only sign indicating the presence of increased body fluid. As failure increases, however, further fluid accumulates, producing noticeable swelling of the legs, especially the anterior lower leg in front of the tibia (pretibial edema) and feet and ankles (pedal edema), the lower part of the back over the spine (presacral edema), and abdominal wall. The skin usually becomes taut and shiny over the edematous tissue. When pressure is applied with a finger, a dent appears in the edematous tissue that does not disappear immediately upon withdrawal of pressure. This sign of peripheral edema is called *pitting edema*. This is in contrast to *nonpitting edema* that results from tissue swelling caused by trauma or inflammation.

◆ APPEARANCE OF THE ABDOMEN

The abdomen in acute MI may be:
- ◆ Swollen and distended (ascites) with engorged liver and spleen (hepatomegaly and splenomegaly)
- ◆ Tender in the right upper quadrant

If right heart failure remains unchecked, the liver and spleen become engorged with fluid and palpable (hepatomegaly, splenomegaly), and fluid accumulates in the abdominal cavity (ascites). If the engorgement and enlargement of the liver have been rapid, pain and tenderness on palpation may be present in the right upper quadrant of the abdomen over the liver.

SIGNS AND SYMPTOMS OF LEFT HEART FAILURE

The following are the signs and symptoms of left heart failure. Pulmonary congestion and edema are responsible for most of the respiratory signs and symptoms. When left heart failure complicates acute MI, the signs and symptoms of acute MI are also present.

Symptoms of Left Heart Failure

◆ GENERAL AND NEUROLOGICAL SYMPTOMS

Severe anxiety and apprehension, restlessness, and agitation are common. Confusion, disorientation, or drowsiness may also be present.

◆ RESPIRATORY SYMPTOMS

Dyspnea is common, often accompanied by a sensation of suffocation; a tight, constricted feeling in the chest; and even pain on breathing. Dyspnea may appear as *dyspnea on exertion (DOE), orthopnea,* or *paroxysmal nocturnal dyspnea (PND)*. Wheezing; spasmodic coughing, often productive of copious, frothy sputum, frequently pink- or blood-tinged (hemoptysis); and choking may also be present.

◆ GASTROINTESTINAL SYMPTOMS

"Indigestion" may be present.

Signs of Left Heart Failure

◆ GENERAL APPEARANCE AND NEUROLOGICAL SIGNS

The patient may be alert and oriented but extremely anxious and apprehensive, restless, agitated or confused, disoriented, or drowsy.

◆ VITAL SIGNS

Pulse

The pulse is usually rapid, over 100/min (tachycardia). The rhythm may be regular or irregular. The force of the pulse is usually normal or strong and full.

Respirations

The respiratory rate is typically greater than 16/min (tachypnea) and shallow, often labored and noisy. Accessory muscles of respiration may be prominent during breathing in severe pulmonary edema.

Blood Pressure

The systolic blood pressure is usually elevated (above 140 mm Hg).

◆ APPEARANCE OF THE SKIN

The skin is usually pale, cold, and clammy. Cyanosis of the skin, fingernail beds, and mucous membranes is present when pulmonary congestion and edema are severe.

◆ APPEARANCE OF THE VEINS

The neck veins may be moderately distended.

◆ CARDIOVASCULAR SIGNS

Usually a third heart sound (S_3) is present early in diastole, producing a gallop rhythm of the heart.

◆ RESPIRATORY SIGNS

Breathing is usually labored and noisy. Wheezing, dry, coarse rattling in the throat; spasmodic coughing with expectoration of frothy sputum, often pink- or blood-tinged (hemoptysis); and choking may be present. Dullness to percussion may be present over one or both lungs, particularly at the bases of the lungs posteriorly. On auscultation, the breath sounds may be normal, decreased, or absent. Rales, wheezes, rhonchi, and possibly loud gurgling or bubbling sounds may be present at one or both bases of the lungs only or up to the scapulae posteriorly or throughout the lungs.

SIGNS OF RIGHT HEART FAILURE

In right heart failure, in the absence of left heart failure, the following signs are present. If acute right ventricular MI is the cause of the right heart failure, the signs and symptoms of acute MI are also present. On the other hand, if the right heart failure is caused by severe left heart failure (the result of an acute anterior, posterior, or inferior MI), the signs and symptoms of left heart failure and acute MI are present as well.

◆ APPEARANCE OF THE VEINS

With the patient lying flat or propped up at a 45-degree angle, the jugular veins are distended and pulsating. In severe right heart failure and one caused by an acute right ventricular MI, the jugular veins become more distended during inspiration *(Kussmaul's sign)*. The superficial veins of the body are distended.

◆ RESPIRATORY SIGNS

The lungs are clear.

◆ BODY TISSUE EDEMA

Pitting edema in the lower extremities, particularly in the ankles and feet and in front of the tibia (pedal and pretibial edema), lower part of the back over the spine (presacral edema), and abdominal wall may be present. If the tissues of the entire body are edematous, anasarca is present.

◆ ABDOMINAL SIGNS

The liver and spleen may be engorged with fluid and swollen (hepatomegaly and splenomegaly). If they are, tenderness is present on palpation of the right upper quadrant of the abdomen because of the engorged tender liver. The abdominal cavity may also be distended with fluid (ascites).

SIGNS AND SYMPTOMS OF CARDIOGENIC SHOCK

The early and late signs and symptoms of cardiogenic shock, in addition to those of acute MI, are as follows.

Symptoms of Cardiogenic Shock

◆ EARLY

General and Neurological Symptoms

The patient may be extremely restless, anxious, and apprehensive. Extreme confusion, disorientation, and drowsiness may also be present.

Gastrointestinal Symptoms

Nausea, with or without vomiting, may be present. The patient may complain of thirst and have an urge to defecate.

◆ LATE

General and Neurological Symptoms

The patient is usually drowsy if not unconscious.

Signs of Cardiogenic Shock

◆ GENERAL APPEARANCE AND NEUROLOGICAL SIGNS

In early shock, the patient is restless, anxious, and apprehensive, or confused and disoriented. Terminally, the patient becomes drowsy and unresponsive and then loses consciousness.

◆ VITAL SIGNS

Pulse

In early shock, the pulse is rapid, usually over 100/min (sinus tachycardia is usually present). The rhythm may be regular or irregular. The pulse is typically weak and thready. Terminally, the pulse rate may become very slow (bradycardia) as the pulse becomes unpalpable.

Respirations

The respirations are usually rapid (greater than 16/min, often as high as 30 to 40/min) and labored, with the patient often gasping for air. Later the respirations become shallow, slow (less than 12/min), and irregular. Terminally, the patient may stop breathing (apnea).

Blood Pressure

In compensated cardiogenic shock, the systolic blood pressure is above 90 mm Hg and often normal. In decompensated cardiogenic shock, it is 90 mm Hg or less. In cases of known hypertension, however, if the systolic pressure drops to 100 mm Hg, or if the pressure suddenly drops by 30 mm Hg below the patient's previous level, decompensated cardiogenic shock is present.

◆ APPEARANCE OF THE SKIN

The skin is usually pale, cold, and clammy, and sometimes mottled red and cyanotic. The lips may be normal, pale, or cyanotic.

◆ APPEARANCE OF THE EYES

The eyes are glassy with a lackluster and vacant, dull stare. They may have an apprehensive and fearful look. The eyelids are drooping. The pupils are normal or dilated.

◆ APPEARANCE OF THE VEINS

The neck veins and superficial veins of the body may be collapsed, but if right heart failure is present, the neck veins may be distended and pulsating, with the superficial veins distended.

SIGNS OF CARDIAC ARREST

The signs of cardiac arrest are as follows.

◆ GENERAL APPEARANCE

The patient appears lifeless and deathlike. Transient convulsions may be present at the onset of cardiac arrest.

◆ VITAL SIGNS

Pulse

The pulse is absent immediately.

Respirations

The respirations are initially slow, becoming absent within 15 to 30 seconds of onset. While present, they may be gasping, noisy, or bubbling.

Blood Pressure

The blood pressure is absent at the onset.

◆ APPEARANCE OF THE SKIN

The skin becomes pale, cold, clammy, and cyanotic.

◆ APPEARANCE OF THE EYES

The eyes assume a dull, vacant stare as their surface becomes glazed, with a ground-glass or hazy appearance because of drying. The eyelids begin to droop. The pupils start dilating within 30 to 40 seconds and become fully dilated by 1.5 to 2 minutes.

◆ CARDIOVASCULAR SIGNS

The heart sounds are absent.

SUMMARY OF THE SIGNS AND SYMPTOMS OF ACUTE MYOCARDIAL INFARCTION

Pain is the most common symptom, appearing in 70% to 80% of the patients with acute MI who are not in shock or cardiac arrest. One or more of the following signs and symptoms frequently accompany the pain of acute MI, depending on the degree of mechanical pump failure present and whether an arrhythmia is present. It is important to note that many of these signs and symptoms may be present even in the absence of pain, as in a so-called *silent acute MI.* The finding of any one or more of the following symptoms should lead one to suspect acute MI, especially if the patient is middle-aged or older.

Symptoms in Acute Myocardial Infarction

◆ **General and neurological symptoms.** Anxiety and apprehension, extreme fatigue and weakness, restlessness, and agitation, with a fear of impending death (or a sense of impending doom) are common. Lightheadedness or dizziness, confusion, disorientation, drowsiness, or loss of consciousness may also be present.

◆ **Cardiovascular symptoms.** Chest pain and palpitations or "skipping of the heart" are usually present in the majority of the patients.

◆ **Respiratory symptoms.** Dyspnea is common, often accompanied by a sensation of suffocation; a tight, constricted feeling in the chest; and even pain on breathing. Wheezing; spasmodic coughing, often productive of copious, frothy sputum, frequently pink- or blood-tinged (hemoptysis); and choking may be present.

◆ **Gastrointestinal symptoms.** Nausea, with or without vomiting, and a loss of appetite (anorexia) are common. If gastrointestinal symptoms are present, and especially if the chest pain radiates to the epigastrium, the patient often misinterprets the symptoms as being those of indigestion and ignores them. Thirst and an urge to defecate may also be present.

Signs in Acute Myocardial Infarction

◆ **General appearance and neurological signs.** The patient may be alert and oriented initially but restless, anxious, and apprehensive or confused and disoriented. The patient may become drowsy and unresponsive and then lose consciousness and convulse.

- ◆ **Vital Signs**
  - ◇ **Pulse.** The pulse is usually rapid, over 100/min (tachycardia), but may be 60 to 100/min (normal) or less than 60/min (bradycardia). The rhythm may be regular or irregular. The force of the pulse may be normal, strong, and full, or if hypotension or shock is present, it may be weak and thready.
  - ◇ **Respirations.** The respirations are typically greater than 16/min (tachypnea) and shallow, but may be 12 to 16/min (normal, eupnea) or less. The rhythm of the respirations may be regular or irregular; their depth may be normal, shallow, or deep. The respirations may be labored and noisy or gasping. Hyperpnea may be present. The accessory muscles of respiration may be prominent during breathing if severe pulmonary congestion and edema are present.
  - ◇ **Blood pressure.** The systolic blood pressure may be normal, elevated (above 140 mm Hg), or low (less than 90 mm Hg) if hypotension or shock is present.
- ◆ **Skin.** The skin is usually pale, cold, sweaty, and clammy. Often, cyanosis of the skin, fingernail beds, and mucous membranes is present because of pulmonary congestion and edema. Skin is mottled bluish-red if shock is present. The lips may be normal in color, pale, or cyanotic.
- ◆ **Eyes.** The eyes appear normal, or if hypotension or shock is present they may appear glassy, with a lackluster and vacant, dull stare or a ground-glass appearance. They may have an apprehensive and fearful look. The eyelids may be drooping. The pupils may be normal or dilated.
- ◆ **Veins.** With the patient lying flat or propped up at a 45-degree angle, the neck veins may be normal, moderately distended (in left heart failure and mild right heart failure), markedly distended and pulsating (in severe right heart failure), or collapsed (in hypotension or shock). The superficial veins of the body may be normal, distended, or collapsed.
- ◆ **Cardiovascular signs.** The heart sounds are usually distant. A fourth heart sound (S_4) in late diastole and often a systolic murmur are present. If left heart failure complicates acute MI, a third heart sound (S_3) appears early in diastole. A gallop rhythm exists when a third or fourth heart sound or both are present.
- ◆ **Respiratory signs.** Breathing may be normal or labored and noisy. Wheezing; dry, coarse rattling in the throat; spasmodic coughing, with expectoration of frothy sputum, often pink- or blood-tinged (hemoptysis); and choking may be present. Dullness to percussion may be present over one or both lungs, particularly at the bases of the lungs posteriorly. On auscultation, the breath sounds may be normal, decreased, or absent. Rales, wheezes, rhonchi, and possibly loud gurgling or bubbling sounds may be present at one or both bases of the lungs only or up to the scapulae posteriorly or throughout the lungs.
- ◆ **Body tissue edema.** Pitting edema in the lower extremities, particularly in the ankles and feet and in front of the tibia (pedal and pretibial edema), lower part of the back over the spine (presacral edema), and abdominal wall may be present in right heart failure. If the tissues of the entire body are edematous, anasarca is present.
- ◆ **Abdomen.** The liver and spleen may be engorged with fluid and swollen (hepatomegaly and splenomegaly) and painful to palpation in severe right heart failure. The abdominal cavity may also be distended with fluid (ascites) in right heart failure.
- ◆ **Arrhythmias.** An arrhythmia may be present.

CHAPTER REVIEW QUESTIONS

1. The initial symptom of cerebral anoxia is commonly:
   A. marked anxiety
   B. agitation with a sense of impending doom
   C. extreme fatigue and weakness
   D. all of the above

2. The first noticeable symptom of left heart failure is usually:
   A. orthopnea
   B. chest pain
   C. dyspnea on exertion (DOE)
   D. all of the above

3. The patient with an acute MI might present with a pulse rate that is:
   A. normal
   B. rapid
   C. slow
   D. all of the above

4. A patient suffering from an acute MI usually presents with skin that is:
   A. pale, warm, and dry
   B. pale, cold, and clammy
   C. cyanotic, warm, and moist
   D. cyanotic, diaphoretic, and dry

5. Pupils start to dilate within _____ following cessation of blood flow to the brain and become fully dilated within ____.
   A. 30 seconds; 1.5 to 2 minutes
   B. 1 minute; 2 to 3 minutes
   C. 15 seconds; 1 minute
   D. 1 minute; 5 minutes

6. If left heart failure occurs after acute MI, which of the following heart sounds will most likely be present?
   A. S_4 late in diastole
   B. S_3 early in diastole
   C. a quadruple gallop
   D. a summation gallop

7. Generalized edema over the entire body is called:
   A. pretibial edema
   B. presacral edema
   C. predominate edema
   D. anasarca

8. An agitated patient presents with dyspnea on exertion, wheezing, and a cough productive of blood-tinged sputum. The vital signs are as follows: the pulse is 104 and regular, the respirations are 24 and shallow, and the blood pressure is 160/90 mm Hg. The neck veins are distended, and a gallop heart rhythm is noted. This patient is most likely suffering from:
   A. uncomplicated acute MI
   B. left heart failure
   C. right heart failure
   D. cardiogenic shock

9. A patient presents with distended jugular veins, pitting edema in the lower extremities, and abdominal tenderness in the right upper quadrant. The lungs are clear. This patient is most likely suffering from:
   A. uncomplicated acute MI
   B. right heart failure
   C. left heart failure
   D. cardiogenic shock

10. A patient presents with chest pain; confusion; mottled, cold, and clammy skin; and dilated pupils. The vital signs are as follows: the pulse is 112 and thready, the respirations are 32 and labored, and the blood pressure is 100/70 mm Hg. This patient is most likely suffering from:
    A. left heart failure
    B. right heart failure
    C. uncompensated cardiogenic shock
    D. compensated cardiogenic shock

CHAPTER OBJECTIVES

Upon completion of all or part of this chapter, you should be able to complete the following objectives:

1. List the blood and tissue components involved and their function in the following:
   Thrombus formation (thrombosis)
   Thrombolysis
2. Describe the following:
   The four phases of thrombus formation
   The three phases of thrombolysis
3. Identify the antithrombus drugs used in the management of acute myocardial infarction (MI), the drug category in which they belong, and their action.
4. Discuss the following protocols in the management of acute MI:
   Initial assessment and management of a patient with chest pain
   Initial treatment of suspected acute MI
   Reperfusion therapy
   Management of congestive heart failure (CHF) caused by left and right heart failure
   Management of cardiogenic shock

5. Discuss the rationale of using a checklist to determine a patient's eligibility for thrombolytic therapy.
6. Identify the absolute contraindications for the use of fibrinolytic agents.

THROMBUS FORMATION AND LYSIS

To understand the rationale for the treatment of acute myocardial infarction (MI), one must understand the basics of thrombus (blood clot) formation (coagulation) in the presence of damage to an atherosclerotic plaque within a coronary artery wall and of the eventual lysis (or dissolution) of the thrombus. Of the numerous factors necessary for thrombus formation and lysis normally present in the blood and connective tissue of the blood vessel wall, the following are considered the principal components (Table 18-1).

TABLE

18-1   Blood and Tissue Components Involved in Thrombus Formation and Lysis

Component	Function
Thrombus Formation	
Blood	
Platelets	
GP Ia	Binds platelets directly to collagen fibers
GP Ib	Binds platelets to von Willebrand factor
GP IIb/IIIa	Binds initially to von Willebrand factor, then to fibrinogen after platelet activation
Adenosine (ADP), serotonin, thromboxane A$_2$ (TxA$_2$)	Stimulates platelet aggregation
Prothrombin	Converts to thrombin when activated by tissue factor released from injured blood vessel walls; thrombin then converts fibrinogen to fibrin
Fibrinogen	Converts to fibrin when exposed to thrombin
Tissue	
von Willebrand factor	Binds to platelets' GP Ib and GP IIb/IIIa and to collagen fibers
Collagen fibers	Bind directly to platelets' GP Ia and to GP Ib and GP IIb/IIIa via von Willebrand factor
Tissue factor	Initiates the conversion of prothrombin to thrombin
Thrombolysis	
Blood	
Plasminogen	Converts to plasmin when activated by tissue plasminogen activator (tPA); plasmin then dissolves the fibrin (fibrinolysis), causing the thrombus to break apart (thrombolysis)
Tissue	
Tissue plasminogen activator (tPA)	Activates plasminogen to convert to plasmin

Blood Components

◆ PLATELETS

Platelets contain adhesive glycoproteins (GP) (or receptors) that bind with various components of connective tissue and blood to form thrombi. The major receptors and their function include the following:

- ◆ **GP Ia** binds the platelets directly to collagen fibers present in connective tissue
- ◆ **GP Ib** binds the platelets to von Willebrand factor
- ◆ **GP IIb/IIIa** binds the platelets to von Willebrand factor and, after the platelets are activated, to fibrinogen

Platelets also contain several substances that, when released after platelet activation, promote thrombus formation by stimulating platelet aggregation. These substances, among others, include the following:

- ◆ Adenosine diphosphate (ADP)
- ◆ Serotonin
- ◆ Thromboxane A$_2$ (TxA$_2$)

◆ PROTHROMBIN

Prothrombin is a plasma protein that, when activated by exposure of the blood to tissue factor released from damaged arterial wall tissue, converts to thrombin. Thrombin in turn converts fibrinogen to fibrin.

◆ FIBRINOGEN

Fibrinogen is a plasma protein that converts to fibrin, an elastic, threadlike filament, when exposed to thrombin.

◆ PLASMINOGEN

Plasminogen is a plasma glycoprotein that converts to an enzyme—plasmin—when activated by tissue-type plasminogen activator (tPA) normally present in the endothelium lining the blood vessels. Plasmin, in turn, dissolves the fibrin strands (fibrinolysis) binding the platelets together within a thrombus. Plasminogen normally attaches itself to fibrin during thrombus formation, making it instantly available for conversion to plasmin when needed.

Tissue Components

◆ VON WILLEBRAND FACTOR

Von Willebrand factor is a protein stored in the cells of the endothelium lining the arteries. When exposed to blood after an injury to the endothelial cells, von Willebrand factor immediately binds to the platelets (via GP Ib and GP IIb/IIIa), adhering them to the collagen fibers located beneath the endothelium in the intima.

◆ COLLAGEN FIBERS

Collagen fibers are the white protein fibers present within the intima of the arterial wall. After an injury and exposure to blood, the collagen fibers immediately bind to the platelets directly (via GP Ia) and indirectly through von Willebrand factor (via GP Ib and GP IIb/IIIa).

◆ TISSUE FACTOR

Tissue factor is a substance present in tissue, platelets, and leukocytes that, when released after injury, initiates the conversion of prothrombin to thrombin.

◆ TISSUE PLASMINOGEN ACTIVATOR

Tissue plasminogen factor (tPA) is a glycoprotein present primarily in the vascular endothelium that, when released into the plasma, activates plasminogen to convert to plasmin. Plasmin, in turn, dissolves fibrinogen and fibrin.

Phases of Thrombus Formation

Formation of a coronary artery thrombus consists of four phases: (1) platelet adhesion, (2) platelet activation, (3) platelet aggregation, and (4) thrombus formation (Figure 18-1).

◆ PHASE 1: PLATELET ADHESION

At the moment an atherosclerotic plaque becomes denuded or ruptures, the platelets are exposed to collagen fibers and von Willebrand factor present within the cap of the atherosclerotic plaque. The platelets'

GP 1a receptors bind with the collagen fibers directly, and the GP Ib and GP IIb/IIIa receptors bind with von Willebrand factor, which in turn also binds with the collagen fibers. The result is the adhesion of platelets to the collagen fibers within the plaque, forming a layer of platelets overlying the damaged plaque.

◆ PHASE 2: PLATELET ACTIVATION

Upon being bound to the collagen fibers the platelets become activated. The platelets change their shape from smooth ovals to tiny spheres while releasing adenosine diphosphate (ADP), serotonin, and thromboxane A_2 (TxA$_2$), substances that stimulate platelet aggregation. Platelet activation is also stimulated by the lipid-rich gruel within the atherosclerotic plaque. At the same time, the GP IIb/IIIa receptors are turned on to bind with fibrinogen. While this is going on, tissue factor is being released from the tissue and platelets.

◆ PHASE 3: PLATELET AGGREGATION

Once activated, the platelets bind to each other by means of fibrinogen, a cordlike structure that binds to the platelets' GP IIb/IIIa receptors. One fibrinogen can bind to two platelets, one at each end. Stimulated by ADP and TxA$_2$, the binding of fibrinogen to the GP IIb/IIIa receptors is greatly enhanced, resulting in a rapid growth of the platelet plug. By this time, the prothrombin in the vicinity of the damaged plaque has been converted to thrombin by the tissue factor.

◆ PHASE 4: THROMBUS FORMATION

At first, the platelet plug is rather unstable but becomes firmer as the fibrinogen between the platelets is replaced by stronger strands of fibrin. This occurs after prothrombin is converted to thrombin by tissue factor. Thrombin in turn converts fibrinogen to fibrin threads. Plasminogen usually becomes attached to the fibrin during its formation. As the thrombus grows, red cells and leukocytes (white cells) become entrapped in the platelet-fibrin mesh.

Phases of Thrombolysis

Normally, the breakdown of a thrombus—*thrombolysis*—occurs when the thrombus is no longer needed to maintain the integrity of the blood vessel wall.

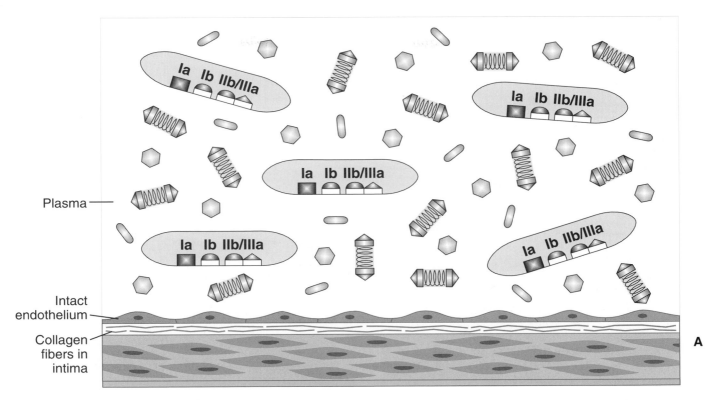

Pre-thrombus phase.

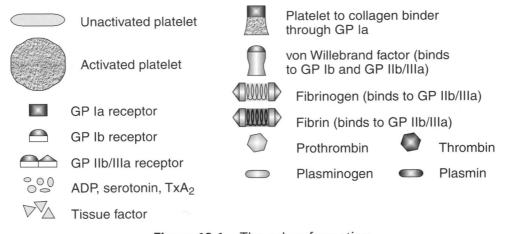

Figure 18-1   Thrombus formation.   *Continued*

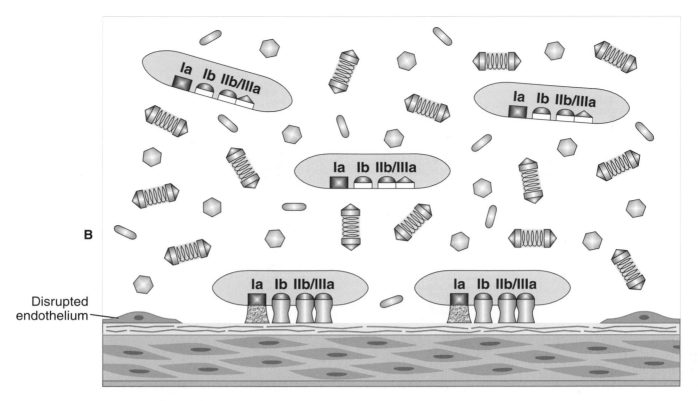

Phase 1. Platelet adhesion.
1. Following disruption of the endothelium, the platelets' GP Ia receptors bind directly to the collagen fibers, and the GP Ib and GP IIb/IIIa receptors bind to the von Willebrand factor (vWF), which in turn binds to the collagen fibers.

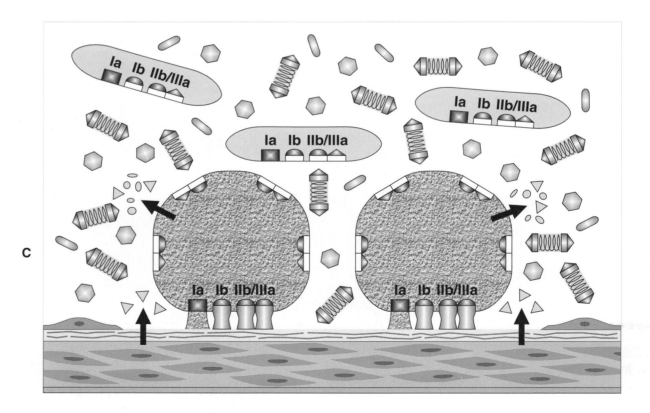

Phase 2. Platelet activation.
2. The platelets change their shape, becoming spherical, while releasing adenosine diphosphate (ADP), serotonin, and thrombaxine A$_2$ (TxA$_2$).
3. The GP IIb/IIIa receptors are turned on to bind to fibrinogen.
4. Tissue factor is released from the platelets and arterial wall tissue.

Figure 18-1, cont'd   Thrombus formation.

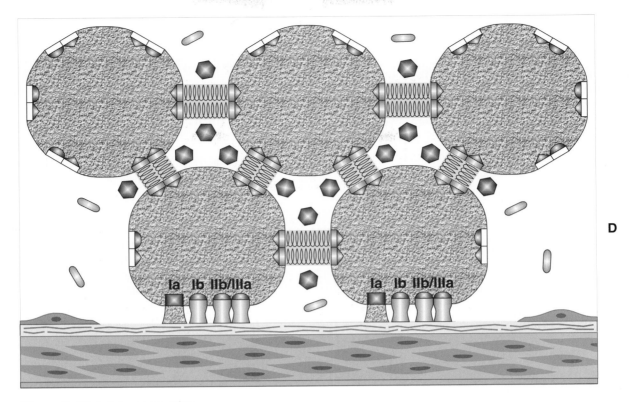

Phase 3. Platelet aggregation.
5. The platelets adhere to each other by means of fibrinogen, which binds to the platelets' GP IIb/IIIa receptors.
6. Prothrombin, present in the plasma, is converted to thrombin by the tissue factor.

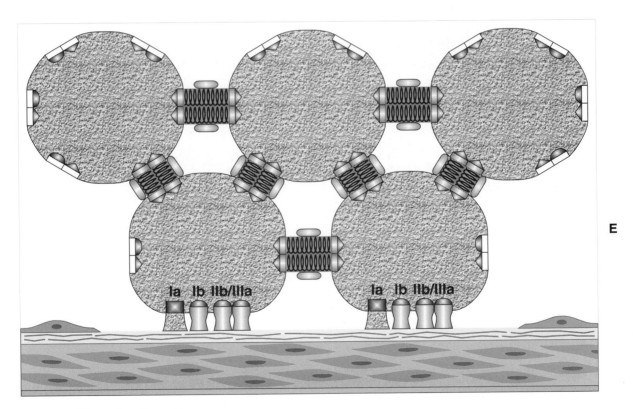

Phase 4. Thrombus formation.
7. The fibrinogen is converted to fibrin by the thrombin, strengthening the thrombus.
8. Plasminogen attaches itself to the fibrin.

Figure 18-1, cont'd   Thrombus formation.

Thrombolysis can also be initiated by the intravenous injection of thrombolytic agents such as alteplase, reteplase, and tenecteplase. Thrombolysis consists of three phases: (1) release of tPA, (2) plasmin formation, and (3) fibrinolysis (Figure 18-2).

◆ PHASE 1: RELEASE OF tPA

The tPA is released from the endothelium of the blood vessel wall into the plasma.

◆ PHASE 2: PLASMIN FORMATION

The tPA activates plasminogen attached to the fibrin strands within the thrombus, resulting in its conversion to plasmin.

◆ PHASE 3: FIBRINOLYSIS

Plasmin breaks down the fibrin into soluble fragments, causing the platelets to separate from each other and the thrombus to break apart.

GOALS IN THE MANAGEMENT OF ACUTE MYOCARDIAL INFARCTION

The primary goals in the management of acute MI are (1) to stop the formation of the thrombus, (2) to dissolve or lyse the thrombus already formed, and (3) to recanalize the occluded coronary artery. Ideally, the first two goals, the arrest of the formation of the thrombus and the beginning of its dissolution, should be initiated within the first 30 to 60

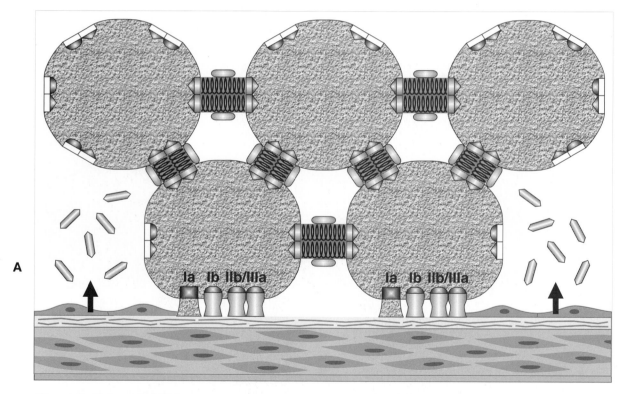

A

Phase 1. Release of tPA.
1. Tissue plasminogen activator (tPA) is released from the endothelium.

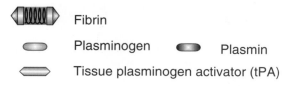

Fibrin

Plasminogen   Plasmin

Tissue plasminogen activator (tPA)

Figure 18-2   Thrombolysis.

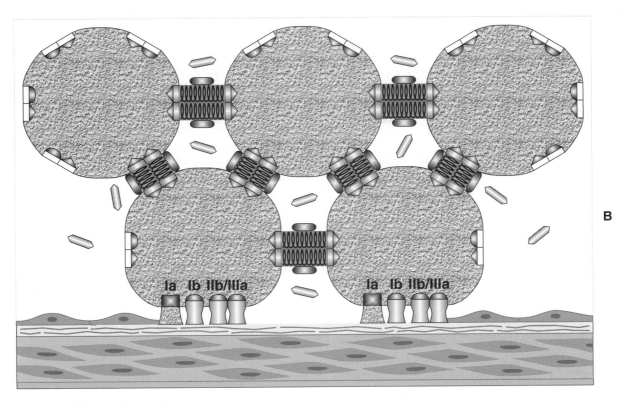

Phase 2. Plasmin formation.
2. Tissue plasminogen activator converts plasminogen to plasmin.

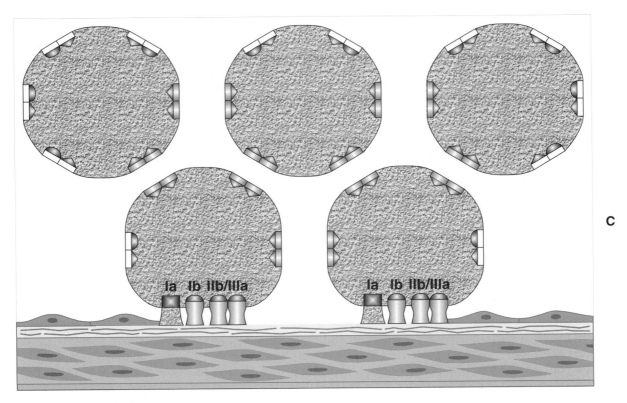

Phase 3. Fibrinolysis.
3. Plasmin lyses the fibrin, freeing the platelets and dissolving the thrombus.

Figure 18-2, cont'd   Thrombolysis.

minutes after the onset of infarction. The third goal, the recanalization of the coronary artery, if indicated, should be performed through percutaneous transluminal coronary angioplasty (PTCA) and/or coronary artery stenting as soon as possible after admission to the emergency department (ED), ideally within the first 30 minutes. The three goals in the management of an acute MI and the means to attain them are as follows:

1. Prevent the further expansion of the original thrombus and/or prevent the formation of a new thrombus. This is accomplished by the administration of the following drugs (Table 18-2):
   - An **antiplatelet agent,** such as **aspirin,** that inhibits TxA$_2$ formation and its release from the platelets, thus partially impeding platelet aggregation. It does not, however, interfere with the adhesion of platelets to the collagen fibers in the arterial wall.
   - An **anticoagulant,** such as **enoxaparin,** a low-molecular-weight (LMW) heparin, or **unfractionated heparin,** that blocks the conversion of prothrombin to thrombin and, in addition, inhibits the action of thrombin on fibrinogen, thus preventing the conversion of fibrinogen to fibrin threads.
   - A **platelet GP IIb/IIIa receptor inhibitor,** such as **abciximab** or **eptifibatide,** that blocks the GP IIb/IIIa receptors on activated platelets from binding to fibrinogen, thus inhibiting platelet adhesion and aggregation and further thrombus formation.
2. Dissolve or lyse the existing thrombus (thrombolysis) using a **thrombolytic agent,** such as **alte-**plase (t-PA), reteplase (r-PA), or **tenecteplase (TNK-tPA),** that converts plasminogen, normally present in the blood, to plasmin, an enzyme that dissolves fibrin within the thrombus, helping to break the thrombus apart (thrombolysis).
3. Enlarge the lumen of the occluded section of the affected coronary artery mechanically by means of one or more of the following catheter-based **percutaneous coronary interventions (PCI).**
   - **Percutaneous transluminal coronary angioplasty (PTCA).** The insertion of a balloon-tipped catheter into the occluded or narrowed coronary artery followed by the inflation of the balloon, thus fracturing the atherosclerotic plaque and dilating the arterial lumen. This procedure, also referred to as *balloon angioplasty,* is the most commonly performed invasive treatment for coronary artery occlusion. It is often followed by insertion of a coronary artery stent.
   - **Coronary artery stenting.** The insertion of a cylindrical wire sheath into the occluded or narrowed coronary artery, followed by the expansion of the sheath to fit snugly within the dilated lumen of the coronary artery. Stents may be used alone as a primary procedure or after balloon angioplasty.
   - **Directional coronary atherectomy (DCA).** The mechanical removal of a noncalcified thrombus through a catheter inserted in the occluded or narrowed coronary artery.
   - **Rotational atherectomy.** The use of a rotational, drill-like device to remove a calcified thrombus.

Emergency coronary artery bypass grafting (CABG) should be considered under the following

TABLE 18-2 Antithrombus Drugs Used in the Management of Acute Myocardial Infarction

Drug Category	Action	Drug
Antiplatelet agent	Inhibits thromboxane A$_2$ (TxA$_2$) formation and release from platelets, thereby inhibiting platelet aggregation	Aspirin
Anticoagulant	Blocks conversion of fibrinogen to fibrin by inhibiting the action of thrombin on fibrinogen	Low-molecular-weight heparin such as enoxaparin (Lovenox) Unfractionated heparin
GP IIb/IIIa receptor inhibitor	Inhibits platelet adhesion and aggregation by blocking the platelets' GP IIb/IIIa receptors	Abciximab (ReoPro) Eptifibatide (Integrilin)
Thrombolytic agent	Converts plasminogen to plasmin, which in turn dissolves the fibrin binding the platelets together	Alteplase (Activase) (t-PA) Reteplase (Retavase) (r-PA) Tenecteplase (TNKase) (TNK-tPA)

conditions if still within 4 to 6 hours of the onset of symptoms of acute MI:

◆ Reperfusion of the occluded coronary artery fails using the above percutaneous coronary interventions and the patient is hemodynamically unstable (i.e., in cardiogenic shock) or continues to have persistent chest pain

◆ The percutaneous coronary interventions listed above are contraindicated

◆ Multivessel coronary artery disease is present

MANAGEMENT OF ACUTE MYOCARDIAL INFARCTION*

A suspected acute MI must be regarded as an extreme emergency and be provided emergency medical care immediately, even before a full history is obtained and a physical examination is performed. The immediate management of an acute MI includes the following:

1. Administration of oxygen
2. Termination of arrhythmias
3. Relief of chest pain (nitroglycerin, morphine sulfate), apprehension and anxiety (diazepam), and nausea and vomiting (promethazine hydrochloride)
4. Prevention of any further thrombus formation by the administration of the following:
   ◆ An antiplatelet agent (aspirin)
   ◆ An anticoagulant (LMW heparin) or unfactionated heparin
   ◆ A GP IIb/IIIa receptor inhibitor (abciximab or eptifibatide)
5. Reopening of the thrombus-occluded artery, ideally, within the first 2 hours after coronary artery occlusion, by the administration of the following:
   ◆ A thrombolytic agent (alteplase, reteplase, or tenecteplase) followed by PCI (percutaneous transluminal angioplasty and/or coronary artery stenting), if necessary
6. Vasodilation of the coronary arteries (nitroglycerin)
7. Reduction of the heart rate, systemic arterial blood pressure, and myocardial contractility (β-blocker)
8. Alleviation of congestive heart failure (CHF) secondary to the following:

◆ Left heart failure (nitroglycerin, morphine sulfate, furosemide, digoxin)
◆ Right heart failure (IV fluid boluses, dobutamine)
9. Reversal of cardiogenic shock (norepinephrine, dopamine)

A. Initial Assessment and Management of a Patient With Chest Pain

◆ **PREHOSPITAL/EMERGENCY DEPARTMENT**

1. Establish and maintain an open airway.
2. Quickly assess the patient's ventilatory status.
3. Administer high-concentration oxygen
   AND
   Suction the airway as necessary.
4. Start monitoring the blood oxygen saturation by pulse oximetry.
5. Quickly assess the patient's circulatory status while obtaining the vital signs, including the level of consciousness, and repeat as the situation requires and circumstances permit.
6. Start an intravenous (IV) drip of 500 mL of 5% dextrose in water to keep the vein open. Do not use saline solutions because of the risk of precipitating or worsening any existing congestive heart failure.
7. Start monitoring the electrocardiogram (ECG) for significant ST segment elevations/depressions and arrhythmias.
8. Obtain a 12-lead ECG (plus lead V$_{4R}$, if indicated), using an ECG monitor with or without computerized ECG interpretation, and, if appropriate, transmit the 12-lead ECG and/or the computerized ECG interpretation to the base hospital for physician interpretation.
9. While performing the above, obtain a brief history and physical examination to determine the cause of the chest pain.

If the patient's history and physical examination are suggestive of an acute MI:

10. Obtain blood samples for determination of cardiac serum markers, C-reactive protein, etc.
11. Determine the patient's eligibility for reperfusion therapy using the checklist shown in Box 18-1 or one provided by medical control.
    AND
12. While completing steps 10 and 11, proceed immediately to section B, *Initial Treatment and Assessment of Suspected Acute Myocardial Infarction.*

---

*The management of acute MI presented in this section is based on the references cited in Chapter 10, *Clinical Significance and Treatment of Arrhythmias.* In addition, as the results of various on-going reperfusion trials are reported, section C, *Reperfusion Therapy,* should be updated accordingly.

BOX
18-1 Checklist to Determine a Patient's Eligibility for Thrombolytic Therapy

Initial Patient Assessment

Yes No
- ☐ ☐ Patient oriented, cooperative, and reliable
- ☐ ☐ Age between 30 and 74 years
- ☐ ☐ Pain typical of acute MI
- ☐ ☐ Pain onset between 30 minutes and 6 hours at time of patient assessment
- ☐ ☐ Continuation of pain after administration of nitroglycerin
- ☐ ☐ History of previous MI
- ☐ ☐ Hypertension: systolic blood pressure >180 mm Hg and/or diastolic blood pressure >110 mm Hg
- ☐ ☐ Current use of warfarin (Coumadin) or other "blood thinner"
- ☐ ☐ 12-lead ECG with significant ST segment and T wave changes
- ☐ ☐ Estimated time of arrival at ED _____

History

Yes No
- ☐ ☐ Recent (within 2-4 weeks) major surgery (e.g., intracranial or intraspinal surgery), obstetrical delivery, organ biopsy, or previous puncture of noncompressible blood vessels
- ☐ ☐ Recent (within 2-4 weeks) active internal bleeding (e.g., gastrointestinal or genitourinary bleeding)
- ☐ ☐ Recent (within 2-4 weeks) trauma (e.g., intracranial or intraspinal trauma) or cardiopulmonary resuscitation

- ☐ ☐ Pregnancy or active menstrual bleeding
- ☐ ☐ Hemostatic defects, including those secondary to severe hepatic or renal disease
- ☐ ☐ Known bleeding diathesis
- ☐ ☐ Significant hepatic dysfunction
- ☐ ☐ Diabetic hemorrhagic retinopathy, or other hemorrhagic ophthalmic conditions
- ☐ ☐ Any other condition in which bleeding may occur, especially if its management would be particularly difficult because of its location
- ☐ ☐ Severe uncontrollable hypertension
- ☐ ☐ Cerebrovascular disease, including cerebrovascular accident (CVA), seizure, cerebral aneurysm, intracranial neoplasm, or arteriovenous (AV) malformation
- ☐ ☐ Suspected aortic dissection or known aneurysm
- ☐ ☐ Suspected left heart thrombus secondary to atrial fibrillation associated with mitral stenosis
- ☐ ☐ Subacute bacterial endocarditis, septic thrombophlebitis, or an occluded AV cannula at a seriously infected site
- ☐ ☐ Pericarditis
- ☐ ☐ Cancer or other terminal disease

B. Initial Treatment and Assessment of Suspected Acute Myocardial Infarction

◆ PREHOSPITAL/EMERGENCY DEPARTMENT

1. Administer a **chewable aspirin** 160 to 325 mg. If chest pain is present:
2. Administer **nitroglycerin** 0.4 mg by sublingual tablet or lingual aerosol if the patient's systolic blood pressure is 90 mm Hg or greater and the pulse is 50 beats/min or greater. Administer with the patient sitting or lying down. If hypotension does not occur, repeat approximately every 5 minutes as necessary, for a total dose of three tablets or three lingual aerosol applications.

AND

If nitroglycerin is not effective after the third dose or the pain is severe:
- ◆ Administer **morphine sulfate** 1 to 3 mg IV slowly over 3 to 5 minutes and repeat in 5 to 30 minutes as necessary, up to a total dose of 25 to 30 mg.

If the patient is apprehensive and anxious but has little or no pain:
3. Administer **diazepam** 5 to 15 mg IV slowly. If nausea or vomiting is present:
4. Administer **promethazine hydrochloride** 12.5 to 25 mg IV.

BOX

18-2   Administration of
          Nitroglycerin, Morphine
          Sulfate, Diazepam, and
          Promethazine Hydrochloride

Administer nitroglycerin and morphine sulfate with caution to patients with possible right ventricular MI while monitoring their pulse and blood pressure.

In addition, the level of consciousness and respiratory status must also be monitored in *all* patients receiving morphine sulfate, diazepam, and/or promethazine hydrochloride.

5. Evaluate the ECG. If any of the following ECG changes are present, the ECG is diagnostic of an acute MI:
   ◆ ST-segment elevation of ≥1mm in two or more contiguous leads (indicative of an acute anterior, lateral, inferior, or right ventricular MI)
   ◆ ST-segment depression of ≥1mm with upright T waves in two or more contiguous precordial leads (indicative of an acute posterior MI)
   ◆ New or presumably new LBBB

Precautionary information about administration of the above drugs is listed in Box 18-2. If the ECG is diagnostic of an acute MI:
6. Administer a **β-blocker** if not contraindicated (Box 18-3).
   ◆ Administer 5 mg **atenolol** IV over 5 minutes and repeat in 10 minutes to a total dose of 10 mg.

                    OR

   Administer 5 mg **metoprolol** IV over 2 to 5 minutes and repeat every 5 minutes to a total dose of 15 mg.

                    AND

   Monitor the pulse, blood pressure, and ECG while administering the drug. Stop the administration of the β-blocker if the systolic blood pressure falls below 100 mm Hg.

If the following signs or symptoms are present:
◆ Persistent or recurring chest pain
◆ CHF associated with left ventricular failure
◆ Extensive anterior MI
◆ Hypertension
7. Administer intravenous **nitroglycerin** if not contraindicated.
   ◆ Administer a 12.5- to 25.0-μg bolus of nitroglycerin IV

                    AND

Start an IV infusion of nitroglycerin at a rate of 10 to 20 μg/min and increase the rate of infusion by 5 to 10 μg/min every 5 to 10 minutes until one of

BOX

18-3   Administration of β-Blockers

Beta blockers are contraindicated:
• If bradycardia (heart rate <60 bpm) is present
• If hypotension (systolic blood pressure <100 mm Hg) is present
• If PR interval is >0.24 second, or second- or third-degree AV block is present
• If severe congestive heart failure (CHF) (left and/or right heart failure) is present
• If bronchospasm or a history of asthma is present
• If severe chronic obstructive pulmonary disease (COPD) is present
• If intravenous calcium channel blockers have been administered within a few hours

The patient's blood pressure and pulse must be monitored frequently during and after the administration of a b-blocker.

If hypotension occurs with a β-blocker, place the patient in the Trendelenburg position and administer a vasopressor.

If bradycardia, AV block, or asystole occurs, refer to the appropriate treatment protocol.

the following occurs, at which time stop increasing the infusion rate and continue it at its current rate:
   ◆ The chest pain or the symptoms of congestive heart failure are relieved
   ◆ The mean arterial blood pressure drops by 10% in a normotensive patient
   ◆ The mean arterial blood pressure drops by 30% in a hypertensive patient
   ◆ The heart rate increases by 10 beats per minute, or
   ◆ The maximum infusion rate of 200 μg/min is reached

                    AND

If the mean arterial blood pressure drops below 80 mm Hg or the systolic blood pressure drops below 90 mm Hg at any time:
   ◆ Slow or temporarily stop the IV infusion of nitroglycerin

If acute MI is confirmed and no contraindications to reperfusion therapy are present (Box 18-4):
8. Proceed immediately to section C, *Reperfusion Therapy.*

If any arrhythmias, CHF, or cardiogenic shock are present initially or occur later, or if cardiac arrest occurs at any time:
9. Manage such complications of acute MI according to the following sections, as appropriate:
   ◆ Chapter 10, *Clinical Significance and Treatment of Arrhythmias.*

18-3 Tenecteplase Dosage Table

Patient Weight	<60 kg	60-<70 kg	70-<80 kg	80-<90 kg	≥90 kg
TNK-tPA (mg)	30 mg	35 mg	40 mg	45 mg	50 mg
Volume (mL)	(6 mL)	(7 mL)	(8 mL)	(9 mL)	(10 mL)

◆ Section D, *Management of Congestive Heart Failure.*
◆ Section E, *Management of Cardiogenic Shock*

C. Reperfusion Therapy

◆ PREHOSPITAL*/EMERGENCY DEPARTMENT

If acute MI is confirmed and no contraindications to reperfusion therapy are present:

1. Administer a **thrombolytic agent.**
   ◆ Administer a 10-U bolus of **reteplase** IV in 2 minutes and repeat in 30 minutes.
   OR
   ◆ Administer a 30- to 50-mg bolus of **tenecteplase** IV in 5 seconds based on the patient's weight as indicated in Table 18-3.

Contraindications and cautions for the use of fibrinolytic agents in the treatment of acute MI are listed in Box 18-4.

◆ EMERGENCY DEPARTMENT

2. Administer an **anticoagulant** such as **LMW heparin** or **unfractionated heparin.**
   ◆ Administer a 30-mg bolus of **enoxaparin** IV followed in 15 minutes by 1 mg/kg enoxaparin subcutaneously.
   OR
   Administer a 60-U/kg bolus of unfractionated heparin IV (maximum 4000-U bolus for patients ≥68 kg followed by a 12-U/kg/hr unfractionated heparin IV infusion (maximum 1000 U/hr for patients >70 kg) to maintain an aPTT of 50 to 70 seconds.
3. Consider the administration of a **GP IIb/IIIa receptor inhibitor.**
   ◆ Administer a 0.25-mg/kg bolus of **abciximab** IV.
   AND
   Start a 0.125-µg/kg/min IV infusion of abciximab.
   OR
   ◆ Administer a 180-µg/kg bolus of **eptifibatide** IV

*If the hospital protocols permit reperfusion therapy.

AND
   Start a 2-µg/kg/min IV infusion of eptifibatide.
   NOTE: If a GP IIb/IIIa receptor inhibitor is administered in combination with a thrombolytic agent, the dosage of the thrombolytic agent should be reduced to approximately half of that indicated above (e.g., 5-U bolus of reteplase IV initially; 15- to 25-mg bolus of tenectaplase IV).
   CAUTION: After the administration of any of the above, closely monitor the patient for any bleeding.
4. After reperfusion therapy, evaluate the patient for need of PCI (coronary artery angioplasty or stenting).

D. Management of Congestive Heart Failure

◆ LEFT HEART FAILURE SECONDARY TO LEFT VENTRICULAR MYOCARDIAL INFARCTION

Prehospital/Emergency Department

If the patient has signs and symptoms of CHF secondary to left heart failure, the result of left ventricular MI:

1. Place the patient in a semireclining or full upright position, if possible, while reassuring the patient and loosening any tight clothing.
2. Secure the airway and administer high-concentration oxygen.
3. Reassess the patient's vital signs, including the respiratory and circulatory status.
4. Administer a **vasodilator,** if the patient's systolic blood pressure is 90 mm Hg or greater and the heart rate is 50 beats/min or greater, to reduce pulmonary congestion and edema, if not administered earlier for pain.
   ◆ Administer **nitroglycerin** 0.4 mg by sublingual tablet or lingual aerosol, and repeat every 5 to 10 minutes as needed for a total of three appli-

18-4   Contraindications and Cautions for the Use of Thrombolytic Agents in Acute Myocardial Infarction

Absolute Contraindications

◆ Active internal bleeding (e.g., gastrointestinal or genitourinary)
◆ Previous hemorrhagic stroke at any time; other strokes or cerebrovascular events within the past year
◆ Recent intracranial or intraspinal surgery or trauma
◆ Known intracranial neoplasm, arteriovenous malformation, or cerebral aneurysm
◆ Severe uncontrolled hypertension during initial treatment and assessment ($\geq$180/110 mm Hg)
◆ Suspected aortic dissection

Cautions/Relative Contraindications

◆ Recent (within 2-4 weeks) major surgery (e.g., coronary artery bypass graft), obstetrical delivery, or organ biopsy
◆ Recent (within 2-4 weeks) trauma, including head trauma and cardiopulmonary resuscitation
◆ Previous puncture of noncompressible blood vessels
◆ Any other condition in which bleeding constitutes a significant hazard or would be particularly difficult to manage because of its location
◆ Known bleeding diathesis

◆ Current use of oral anticoagulants (e.g., warfarin sodium) with INR $\geq$2-3
◆ Diabetic hemorrhagic retinopathy or other hemorrhagic ophthalmic conditions
◆ History of recent (within 2-4 weeks) gastrointestinal, genitourinary, or other internal bleeding
◆ Active peptic ulcer
◆ Hemostatic defects, including those secondary to severe hepatic or renal disease
◆ History of chronic hypertension ($\geq$180/110 mm Hg)
◆ History of prior cerebrovascular accident, seizures, or cerebrovascular disease not covered above
◆ High likelihood of left heart thrombus if mitral stenosis with atrial fibrillation is present without anticoagulation
◆ Subacute bacterial endocarditis
◆ Acute pericarditis
◆ Aortic aneurysm
◆ Septic thrombophlebitis or occluded arteriovenous cannula at a seriously infected site
◆ Severe hepatic or renal dysfunction
◆ Pregnancy or menstrual bleeding
◆ Advanced age
◆ Cancer or other terminal disease

---

cations, or by dermal application of 1 to 1.5 inches of nitroglycerin ointment

AND/OR

Administer **morphine sulfate** 1 to 3 mg IV slowly over 3 to 5 minutes and repeat every 5 to 30 minutes as necessary, up to a total dose of 25 to 30 mg.

5. Administer a rapidly acting **diuretic** to reduce pulmonary congestion and edema.
   ◆ Administer **furosemide** 40 to 80 mg (0.5 to 1.0 mg/kg) IV slowly over 4 to 5 minutes
6. Administer a rapidly acting **digitalis preparation** to decrease the heart rate in atrial flutter and fibrillation with a rapid ventricular response and to improve myocardial function.
   ◆ Administer **digoxin** 0.5 mg IV over 5 minutes
7. Administer a **bronchodilator** to relieve respiratory distress, especially in the presence of wheezing.
   ◆ Administer **aminophylline** 250 to 500 mg IV (2 to 5 mg/kg diluted with 100 mL of 5% dextrose in water) slowly over 20 to 30 minutes
8. Administer an **antianxiety drug** to ease apprehension and anxiety.
   ◆ Administer **diazepam** 5 to 15 mg IV, or, prefer-

ably, a narcotic (i.e., **morphine sulfate** 1 to 3 mg IV slowly), if not administered earlier

Emergency Department

If sublingual or aerosol nitroglycerin or morphine sulfate is ineffective in relieving the signs and symptoms of congestive heart failure:

9. Administer **nitroglycerin** intravenously as in **Step 8** in section B, *Initial Treatment of Suspected Uncomplicated Acute Myocardial Infarction.*

◆ **RIGHT HEART FAILURE SECONDARY TO RIGHT VENTRICULAR MYOCARDIAL INFARCTION**

Prehospital/Emergency Department

If the patient has signs and symptoms of congestive right heart failure per se, as occurs in right ventricular MI, accompanied by hypotension:

1. Administer 250 to 500 mL of **normal saline** IV rapidly while monitoring the pulse and blood

pressure. Repeat up to a total of 1 to 2 L or until the systolic blood pressure increases to 90 mm Hg or more.

AND

If saline administration is ineffective in restoring cardiac output and elevating the systolic blood pressure to 90 to 100 mm Hg:

- Administer **dobutamine** 2 to 20 μg/kg per/min IV to increase the cardiac output and elevate and maintain the systolic blood pressure within normal limits.

CAUTION!

Administer nitroglycerin and morphine sulfate with caution to patients with possible right ventricular MI while monitoring their pulse and blood pressure.

E. Management of Cardiogenic Shock

◆ PREHOSPITAL/EMERGENCY DEPARTMENT

If the patient is or becomes unconscious and a gag reflex is absent:

1. Place the patient in a face-up position.
2. Secure the airway and ventilate the patient with high-concentration oxygen.

AND

If pulmonary congestion and edema are absent, elevate the patient's legs at approximately a 30-degree angle with the rest of the body to aid the blood flow to the brain. This means that in an adult of average size, the feet are elevated about 18 inches above the level of the patient's heart.

3. Assess the patient's circulatory status and vital signs, including the level of consciousness, and repeat as the situation requires and circumstances permit.

If the systolic blood pressure is 70 to 100 mm Hg or less:

4. Administer a **vasoconstrictive agent (norepinephrine)** or an **inotropic/vasoconstrictive agent (dopamine)** as follows:

Systolic blood pressure less than 70 mm Hg:

- Start an IV infusion of **norepinephrine** at an initial rate of 0.5 to 1.0 μg/min, and adjust the rate of infusion up to 8 to 30 μg/min to increase the systolic blood pressure to 70 to 100 mm Hg.

NOTE: The infusion of norepinephrine may be replaced by an infusion of dopamine at this point.

OR

Systolic blood pressure 70 to 100 mm Hg:

- Start an IV infusion of **dopamine** at an initial rate of 2.5 to 5.0 μg/kg/min and adjust the rate of infusion up to 20 μg/kg/min to increase the cardiac output and to elevate and maintain the systolic blood pressure within normal limits.

NOTE: When administering vasoconstrictive agents, the systolic blood pressure must be monitored frequently so that the systolic blood pressure stays within a certain range. The rate of administration of such agents is decreased if the systolic blood pressure rises above 100 mm Hg and increased if the systolic blood pressure drops below 90 mm Hg.

◆ EMERGENCY DEPARTMENT

If the shock condition continues for 1 hour in spite of maximum therapy, and if the patient cannot maintain an adequate blood pressure without a vasoconstrictor, the use of a mechanical device such as an intraaortic balloon pump to augment the vascular circulation is recommended.

Drugs Used to Treat Acute Myocardial Infarction

Drug	Class
Abciximab (ReoPro)	GP IIb/IIIa receptor inhibitor
Adenosine (Adenocard)	Antiarrhythmic agent
Alteplase (t-PA) (Activase)	Thrombolytic agent
Aminophylline	Bronchodilator
Amiodarone (Cordarone)	Antiarrhythmic agent
Aspirin	Antiplatelet agent
Atenolol (Tenormin)	β-adrenergic blocking agent
Atropine sulfate	Anticholinergic agent

β-Blocker
    Atenolol (Tenormin), Esmolol (Brevibloc),
      Metoprolol (Toprol, Lopressor)
	β-adrenergic blocking agent

Diazepam (Valium)	Tranquilizer, amnesiac, sedative
Digoxin (Lanoxin)	Antiarrhythmic agent, inotropic agent, digitalis glycoside
Diltiazem (Cardizem)	Calcium channel blocker
Dobutamine (Dobutrex)	Adrenergic agent
Dopamine (Intropin)	Adrenergic (sympathomimetic) agent
Enoxaparin (Lovenox)	Anticoagulant, LMW heparin
Eptifibatide (Integrilin)	GP IIb/IIIa receptor inhibitor
Epinephrine (Adrenalin chloride)	Adrenergic (sympathomimetic) agent
Esmolol (Brevibloc)	β-adrenergic blocking agent
Furosemide (Lasix)	Diuretic
Ibutilide (Corvert)	Antiarrhythmic agent
Lidocaine (Xylocaine)	Antiarrhythmic agent
Magnesium sulfate	Electrolyte
Metoprolol (Toprol, Lopressor)	β-adrenergic blocking agent
Midazolam (Versed)	Sedative, tranquilizer, amnesiac
Morphine sulfate	Narcotic, analgesic

Nitroglycerin (Nitrostat, Nitro-Bid IV,
  Nitrol, Tridil, etc.)
	Antianginal agent, vasodilator, coronary
	  vasodilator

Norepinephrine (Levophed)	Adrenergic (sympathomimetic) agent
Procainamide (Pronestyl)	Antiarrhythmic agent
Promethazine hydrochloride (Phenergan)	Antiemetic, antihistamine
Reteplase (r-PA) (Retavase)	Thrombolytic agent
Sodium bicarbonate	Alkalinizing agent
Tenecteplase (TNK-tPA) (TNKase)	Thrombolytic agent
Unfractionated heparin	Anticoagulant
Vasopressin	Vasoconstrictor

LMW, Low molecular weight.

ACUTE MYOCARDIAL INFARCTION MANAGEMENT ALGORITHMS

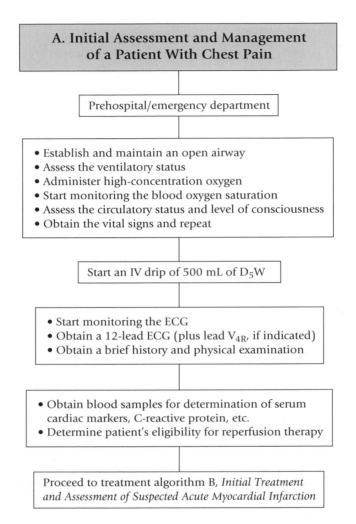

A. Initial Assessment and Management of a Patient With Chest Pain

Prehospital/emergency department

- Establish and maintain an open airway
- Assess the ventilatory status
- Administer high-concentration oxygen
- Start monitoring the blood oxygen saturation
- Assess the circulatory status and level of consciousness
- Obtain the vital signs and repeat

Start an IV drip of 500 mL of D_5W

- Start monitoring the ECG
- Obtain a 12-lead ECG (plus lead V_{4R}, if indicated)
- Obtain a brief history and physical examination

- Obtain blood samples for determination of serum cardiac markers, C-reactive protein, etc.
- Determine patient's eligibility for reperfusion therapy

Proceed to treatment algorithm B, *Initial Treatment and Assessment of Suspected Acute Myocardial Infarction*

B. Initial Treatment and Assessment of Suspected Acute Myocardial Infarction

Prehospital/emergency department

Chewable aspirin 160 to 325 mg
Nitroglycerin 0.4-mg sublingual tablet or lingual aerosol and repeat twice, 5 min apart, for pain
AND
Morphine sulfate 1 to 3 mg IV and repeat every 5 to 30 min (if nitroglycerin ineffective)

Diazepam 5 to 15 mg IV (if patient apprehensive/anxious)
Promethazine hydrochloride 12.5 to 25 mg IV (if patient nauseous/vomiting)

Evaluate the ECG for ST-segment elevation/depression and new or presumably new left bundle branch block

Atenolol 5 mg IV over 5 min and repeat in 10 min to a total dose of 10 mg (if ECG is diagnostic of an acute MI)
OR
Metoprolol 5 mg IV over 2 to 5 min and repeat every 5 min to a total dose of 15 mg

Nitroglycerin 12.5- to 25.0-μg IV bolus, followed by an IV infusion at a rate of 10 to 20 μg/min initially, then increasing the rate by 5 to 10 μg/min every 5 to 10 min as needed (if indicated and not contraindicated)

Proceed to treatment algorithm C, *Reperfusion Therapy* if acute MI is confirmed and no contraindications to reperfusion are present

Proceed to the following as appropriate:
• Chapter 10, *Clinical Significance and Treatment of Arrhythmias*
• Treatment algorithm D, *Management of Congestive Heart Failure*
• Treatment algorithm E, *Management of Cardiogenic Shock*

C. Reperfusion Therapy

Prehospital/emergency department

Reteplase 10-U IV bolus in 2 min; repeat once in 30 min

OR

Tenecteplase 30- to 50-mg IV bolus in 5 sec based on the patient's weight (see dosage table below)

NOTE: Reduce dosage of thrombolytic agent to half if administering in combination with a GP IIb/IIIa receptor inhibitor

Enoxaparin 30-mg IV bolus, followed in 15 min by 1 mg/kg enoxaparin subcutaneously

OR

Unfractionated heparin 60-U/kg IV bolus (maximum 4000-U bolus for patients ≥68 kg) followed by a 12-U/kg/hr unfractionated heparin IV infusion (maximum 1000 U/hr for patients >70 kg) to maintain an aPTT of 50 to 70 seconds

AND

Consider one of the following GP IIb/IIIa receptor inhibitors:

- **Abciximab** 0.25-mg/kg IV bolus, followed by an IV infusion at a rate of 0.125 µg/kg/min
- **Eptifibatide** 180-µg/kg IV bolus, followed by an IV infusion at a rate of 2 µg/kg/min

CAUTION: After the administration of any of the above, closely monitor the patient for any bleeding

After reperfusion therapy, evaluate the patient for need of percutaneous coronary intervention (coronary artery angioplasty or stenting)

Tenecteplase Dosage Table

Patient weight (kg)	TNK-tPA (volume)
<60	30 mg (6 mL)
60 to <70	35 mg (7 mL)
70 to <80	40 mg (8 mL)
80 to <90	45 mg (9 mL)
≥90	50 mg (10mL)

D. Management of Congestive Heart Failure

Left heart failure secondary to left ventricular myocardial infarction	Right heart failure secondary to right ventricular myocardial infarction

Prehospital/emergency department	Prehospital/emergency department

Left side:

- Place the patient in a semireclining or full upright position
- Secure the airway and administer high-concentration oxygen
- Reassess the vital signs, including the respiratory and circulatory status
- Prepare to administer the following drugs as appropriate, if not administered earlier

Nitroglycerin 0.4 mg by sublingual tablet or lingual aerosol and repeat twice, 5 min apart, or by dermal application of 1 to 1.5 inches of nitroglycerin ointment
AND/OR
Morphine sulfate 1 to 3 mg IV and repeat every 5 to 30 min as necessary

Furosemide 40 to 80 mg IV
Digoxin 0.5 mg IV

Aminophylline 250 to 500 mg IV (if patient in respiratory distress)
Diazepam 5 to 15 mg IV or **morphine sulfate** 1 to 3 mg IV, if not administered earlier (if patient apprehensive/anxious)

If nitroglycerin as administered above and/or morphine sulfate are ineffective:
Nitroglycerin 12.5- to 25.0-μg IV bolus, followed by an IV infusion at a rate of 10 to 20 μg/min initially, then increasing the rate by 5 to 10 μg/min every 5 to 10 min as needed

Right side:

Normal saline, 250 to 500 mL IV boluses rapidly; repeat up to a total of 1 to 2 L or until the systolic blood pressure increases to 90 mm Hg or more
AND
If saline administration is ineffective:
Dobutamine 2 to 20 μg/kg/min IV to increase and maintain the systolic blood pressure within normal limits

E. Management of Cardiogenic Shock

Prehospital/emergency department

- Place the patient in a face-up position, with legs elevated if pulmonary congestion and edema are absent
- Secure the airway and administer high-concentration oxygen
- Reassess the vital signs, including the respiratory and circulatory status

If the systolic blood pressure is less than 70 mm Hg initially:
- **Norepinephrine** 0.5 to 1.0 μg/min IV initially and increase to 8 to 30 μg/min to elevate the systolic blood pressure to 70 to 100 mm Hg

  OR

If the systolic blood pressure is 70 to 100 mm Hg initially:
- **Dopamine** 2.5 to 5.0 μg/kg/min IV initially and increase up to 20 μg/kg/min to elevate and maintain the systolic blood pressure within normal limits

If the shock condition continues for 1 hour in spite of maximum therapy, proceed with an intraaortic balloon pump

CHAPTER REVIEW QUESTIONS

1. A substance that enhances thrombus formation by stimulating platelet aggregation is:
   A. adenosine diphosphate
   B. serotonin
   C. thromboxane A$_2$
   D. all of the above

2. A plasma protein that eventually converts fibrinogen to fibrin is:
   A. tissue factor
   B. prothrombin
   C. plasminogen
   D. plasmapro

3. A glycoprotein that works to dissolve fibrinogen and fibrin is:
   A. von Willebrand factor
   B. GP Ia
   C. tPA
   D. prothrombin

4. The formation of a coronary artery thrombus consists of all of the following phases *except:*
   A. platelet adhesion
   B. platelet activation
   C. platelet aggregation
   D. fibrinolysis

5. Thrombolysis consists of all of the following phases *except:*
   A. release of tPA
   B. plasmin formation
   C. platelet aggregation
   D. fibrinolysis

6. All of the following drugs are used to prevent the expansion of an original thrombus or the formation of a new thrombus *except:*
   A. LMW heparin
   B. warfarin
   C. promethazine
   D. abciximab

7. The insertion of a balloon-tipped catheter into an occluded artery to fracture an atherosclerotic plaque and dilate the arterial lumen is called:
   A. percutaneous transluminal coronary angioplasty
   B. coronary artery stenting
   C. directional coronary atherectomy
   D. rotational atherectomy

8. The correct dosage of reteplase for thrombolytic therapy alone is:
   A. 10-U IV bolus in 5 minutes, repeated in 60 minutes
   B. 10-U IV bolus in 2 minutes, repeated in 30 minutes
   C. 20-U IV bolus in 3 minutes, repeated in 15 minutes
   D. 5-U IV bolus in 1 minute, repeated in 30 minutes

9. The correct dosage of tenectaplase for thrombolytic therapy alone is:
   A. 10-U IV bolus in 5 minutes, repeated in 60 minutes
   B. 30- to 40-U IV bolus in 2 minutes, repeated in 30 minutes
   C. 30- to 50-mg IV bolus in 5 minutes based on the patient's weight in 1 minute, repeated in 30 minutes
   D. 30- to 50-mg IV bolus in 5 seconds based on the patient's weight

10. A patient presents with jugular vein distention during inspiration and pitting edema in the lower extremities. The patient's systolic blood pressure is 70 mm Hg by palpation. Which of the following steps is indicated for management of this patient?
    A. 250 to 500 mL of normal saline rapidly
    B. Dobutamine 4 to 40 μg/kg/min IV
    C. Furosemide 0.5 to 1.0 mg/kg IV slowly
    D. Morphine sulphate 1 to 3 mg IV slowly

11. Which of the following drugs would be indicated for management of a patient with left heart failure secondary to left ventricular MI?
    A. digoxin 5 mg IV
    B. morphine sulfate 1 to 3 mg IV
    C. aminophylline 100 to 250 mg IV
    D. furosemide 20 to 40 mg IV

Methods of Determining the QRS Axis

APPENDIX OBJECTIVES

Upon completion of all or part of this appendix, you should be able to complete the following objectives:
1. Describe in detail the steps in determining the QRS axis using one or more of the following methods:
   The Two-Lead Method (Leads I and II)
   The Three-Lead Method (Leads I, II, and aVF)
   The Four-Lead Method (Leads I, II, III, and aVF)
   The Six-Lead Method (Leads I, II, III, aVR, aVL, and aVF)
   The "Perpendicular" Method

METHODS OF DETERMINING THE QRS AXIS

Various methods of determining the approximate position of the QRS axis in the frontal plane are available using the hexaxial reference figure. The methods presented in the following section are listed below.

Method A: The Two-Lead Method. This method uses leads I and II to make a rapid determination of whether the QRS axis is normal or abnormally deviated to the left or right. This is one of the fastest methods in determining the QRS axis. It is especially useful in the emergency situation to spot left axis de-viation because the perpendicular of lead II lies on the $-30°$ axis.

Method B: The Three-Lead Method. This method uses leads I, II, and aVF to make a rapid approximation of whether the QRS axis is normal or abnormally deviated to the left or right. The positivity or negativity of leads I and aVF are determined first to ascertain in which of the four quadrants the QRS axis lies. Then, determining the positivity or negativity of lead II helps to place the QRS axis in quadrant I or III within a 30° to 60° arc.

Method C: The Four-Lead Method. This method uses leads I, II, III, and aVF, and sometimes aVR in certain circumstances, to make a rapid determination of the QRS axis within a 30° arc.

Method D: The Six-Lead Method. This method uses leads I and aVF to determine in which quadrant the QRS axis lies. Then, depending on which quadrant the QRS axis lies in, leads II and aVR or leads III and aVL are used to determine the position of the QRS axis in the quadrant, within a 30° arc. This method is probably too slow for use in an emergency situation.

Method E: The "Perpendicular" Method. This method is a rapid determination of the QRS axis based on the perpendicular of a bipolar or unipolar limb lead with an equiphasic QRS complex, if one is present.

Method A: The Two-Lead Method

The two-lead method uses leads I and II to determine the general position of the QRS axis and to identify left axis deviation quickly.

Determine the net positivity or negativity of the QRS complexes in leads I and II.

If lead I is *positive* and:

A. Lead II is predominantly positive, the QRS axis is between −30° and +90°.

B. Lead II is equiphasic, the QRS axis is exactly −30°.

C. Lead II is predominantly negative, the QRS axis is between −30° and −90°.

If lead I is *negative* and:

D. Lead II is predominantly positive, the QRS axis is between +90° and +150°.

E. Lead II is equiphasic, the QRS axis is exactly +150°.

F. Lead II is predominantly negative, the QRS axis is greater than +150°.

Method A

Figure	Leads		Location of QRS Axis
	I	II	
A	+	+	−30° to +90°
B	+	±	−30°
C	+	−	−30° to −90°
D	−	+	+90° to +150°
E	−	±	+150°
F	−	−	>+150°

+, Predominantly positive; −, predominantly negative; ±, equiphasic.

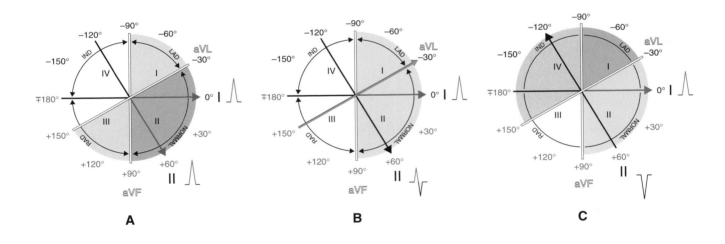

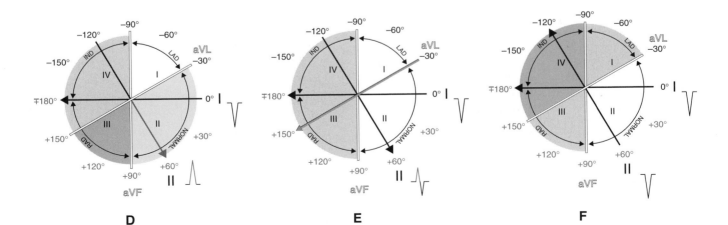

Method B: The Three-Lead Method

The three-lead method uses leads I, II, and aVF, and sometimes aVR in certain circumstances, to determine the general position of the QRS axis and to identify left and right axis deviation quickly.

Determine the net positivity or negativity of the QRS complexes in leads I, aVF, and II, in that order, and also aVR if lead I is negative.

If lead I is *positive* and:

A. Leads aVF and II are predominantly positive, the QRS axis is between 0° and +90°.

B. Lead aVF is predominantly negative and lead II is predominantly positive, the QRS axis is between 0° and −30°.

C. Lead aVF is predominantly negative and lead II is equiphasic, the QRS axis is exactly −30°.

D. Leads aVF and II are predominantly negative, the QRS axis is between −30° and −90°.

If Lead I is *equiphasic* and:

E. Leads aVF and II are predominantly negative, the QRS axis is exactly −90°.

F. Leads aVF and II are predominantly positive, the QRS axis is exactly +90°.

If Lead I is *negative* and:

G. 1. Leads aVF and II are predominantly positive, the QRS axis is between +90° and +150°.

Method B

Figure	Leads				Location of QRS Axis
	I	aVF	II	aVR	
A	+	+	+		0° to +90°
B	+	−	+		0° to −30°
C	+	−	±		−30°
D	+	−	−		−30° to −90°
E	±	−	−		−90°
F	±	+	+		+90°
G (1)	−	+	+		+90° to +150°
G (2)	−	+	+	+	+120° to +150°
H	−	+	±		+150°
I	−	−	−		−90° to −180°

+, Predominantly positive; −, predominantly negative; ±, equiphasic.

2. If, in addition, aVR is also predominantly positive, the QRS axis is between +120° and +150°.

H. Lead aVF is predominantly positive and lead II is equiphasic, the QRS axis is exactly +150°.

I. Leads aVF and II are predominantly negative, the QRS axis is between −90° and −180°.

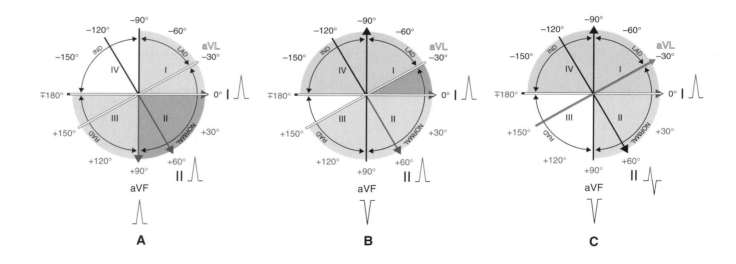

A   **B**   **C**

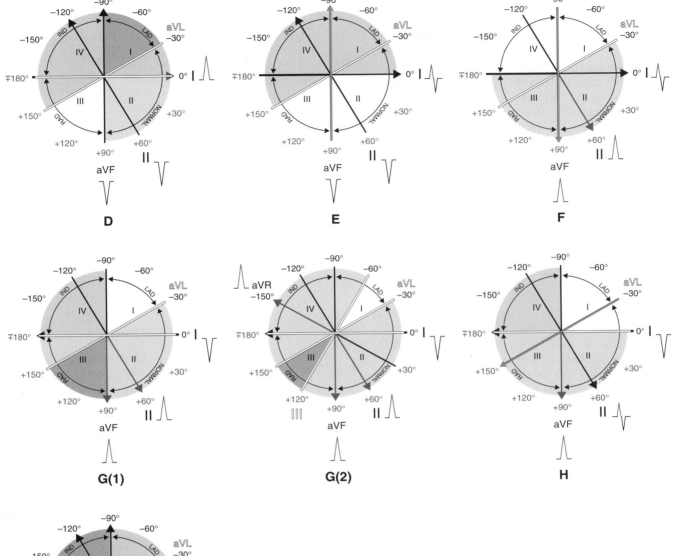

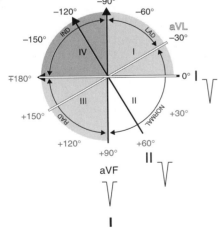

Method C: The Four-Lead Method

The four-lead method uses leads I, II, III, and aVF, and sometimes aVR in certain circumstances, to determine the QRS axis within 30°.

Determine the net positivity or negativity of the QRS complexes in leads I, III, aVF, and II, in that order, and also aVR if lead I is negative.

If lead I is *positive* and:

A. Leads III, aVF, and II are predominantly positive, the QRS axis is between +30° and +90°.

B. Lead III is predominantly negative and leads aVF and II are predominantly positive, the QRS axis is between 0° and +30°.

C. Leads III and aVF are predominantly negative and lead II is predominantly positive, the QRS axis is between 0° and −30°.

D. Leads III and aVF are predominantly negative and lead II is equiphasic, the QRS axis is exactly −30°.

E. Leads III, aVF, and II are predominantly negative, the QRS axis is between −30° and −90°.

If lead I is *equiphasic* and:

F. Leads III, aVF, and II are predominantly negative, the QRS axis is exactly −90°.

G. Leads III, aVF, and II are predominantly positive, the QRS axis is exactly +90°.

If lead I is *negative* and:

H. 1. Leads III, aVF, and II are predominantly positive, the QRS axis is between +90° and +150°.

2. If, in addition, aVR is also predominantly positive, the QRS axis is between +120° and +150°.

I. Leads III and aVF are predominantly positive and lead II is equiphasic, the QRS axis is exactly +150°.

J. Leads III, aVF, and II are predominantly negative, the QRS axis is between −90° and −150°.

Method C

| | Leads | | | | | |
Figure	I	III	aVF	II	aVR	Location of QRS Axis
A	+	+	+	+		+30° to +90°
B	+	−	+	+		0° to +30°
C	+	−	−	+		0° to −30°
D	+	−	−	±		−30°
E	+	−	−	−		−30° to −90°
F	±	−	−	−		−90°
G	±	+	+	+		+90°
H (1)	−	+	+	+		+90° to +150°
H (2)	−	+	+	+	+	+120° to +150°
I	−	+	+	±		+150°
J	−	−	−	−		−90° to −150°

+, Predominantly positive; −, predominantly negative; ±, equiphasic.

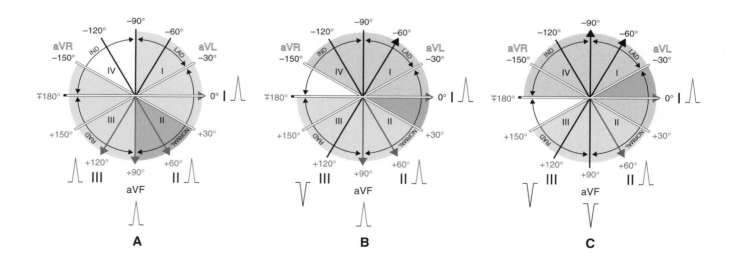

A **B** **C**

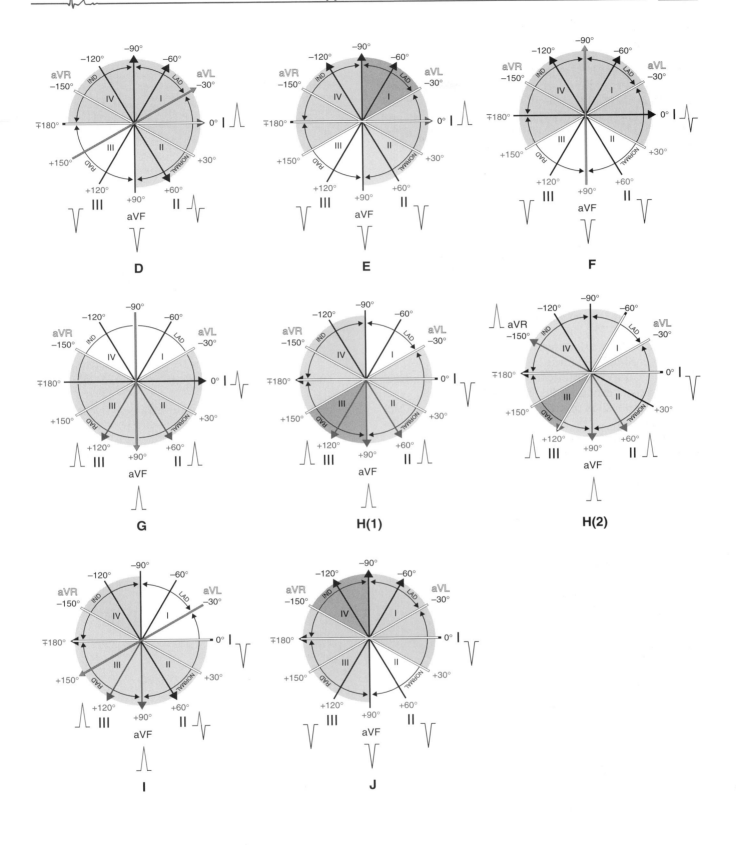

Method D: The Six-Lead Method

The two-step six-lead method uses leads I and aVF in step 1 to determine in which quadrant the QRS axis lies. Then, in step 2, depending on the quadrant initially determined, leads II and aVR or leads III and aVL are used to determine the 30° arc in which the QRS axis lies.

◆ **STEP 1**

Determine the quadrant in which the QRS axis lies.

Determine the net positivity and negativity of the QRS complexes in leads I and aVF.

If lead I is *positive* and:

1A. Lead aVF is predominantly positive, the QRS axis is in quadrant II (0° to +90°).

1B. Lead aVF is equiphasic, the QRS axis is exactly 0°.

1C. Lead aVF is predominantly negative, the QRS axis is in quadrant I (0° to −90°).

If lead I is *equiphasic* and:

1D. Lead aVF is predominantly positive, the QRS axis is exactly +90°.

1E. Lead aVF is predominantly negative, the QRS axis is exactly −90°.

Method D: Step 1, A-H

| | Leads | | Location | |
Figure	I	aVF	of QRS Axis	Quadrant
1A	+	+	0° to +90°	II
1B	+	±	0°	
1C	+	−	0° to −90°	I
1D	±	+	+90°	
1E	±	−	−90°	
1F	−	+	+90° to +180°	III
1G	−	±	±180°	
1H	−	−	−90° to −180°	IV

+, Predominantly positive; −, predominantly negative; ±, equiphasic.

If lead I is *negative* and:

1F. Lead aVF is predominantly positive, the QRS axis is in quadrant III (+90° to +180°).

1G. Lead aVF is equiphasic, the QRS axis is exactly ±180°.

1H. Lead aVF is predominantly negative, the QRS axis is in quadrant IV (−90° to −180°).

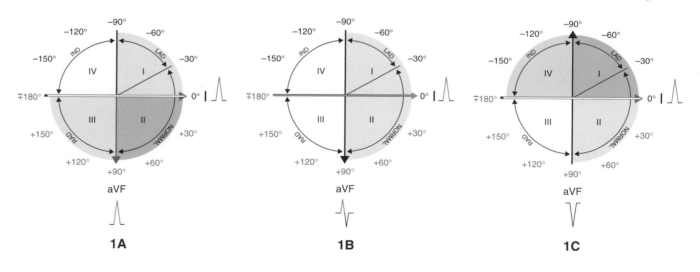

1A   1B   1C

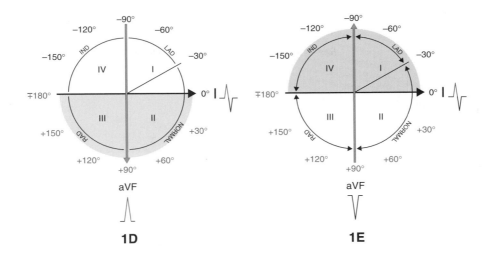

1D

1E

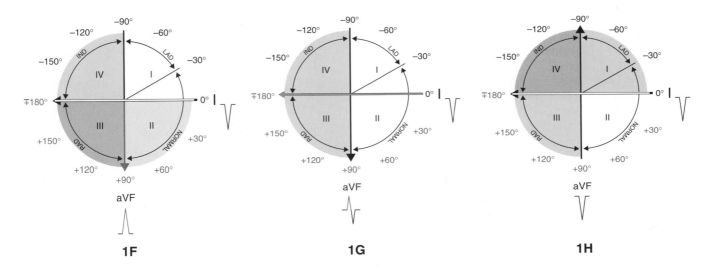

1F

1G

1H

◆ STEP 2

Determine the placement of the QRS axis in the quadrant in which it lies to within a 30° arc.

If the QRS axis lies in quadrant I (0° to −90°):

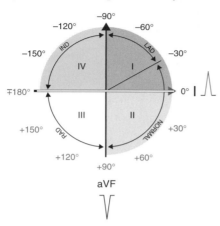

Determine the net positivity or negativity of the QRS complexes in leads II and aVR.

If lead II is *positive* and:

2A. Lead aVR is predominantly negative, the QRS axis is between 0° and −30°.

Method D: Step 2, A-E

Figure	Leads				Location of QRS Axis
	I	aVF	II	aVR	
2A	+	−	+	−	0° to −30°
2B	+	−	±		−30°
2C	+	−	−	−	−30° to −60°
2D	+	−	−	±	−60°
2E	+	−	−	+	−60° to −90°

+, Predominantly positive; −, predominantly negative; ±, equiphasic.

If lead II is *equiphasic:*

2B. The QRS axis is exactly −30°.

If lead II is *negative* and:

2C. Lead aVR is predominantly negative, the QRS axis is between −30° and −60°.

2D. Lead aVR is equiphasic, the QRS axis is exactly −60°.

2E. Lead aVR is predominantly positive, the QRS axis is between −60° and −90°.

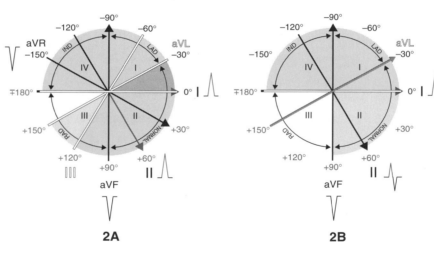

2A   **2B**

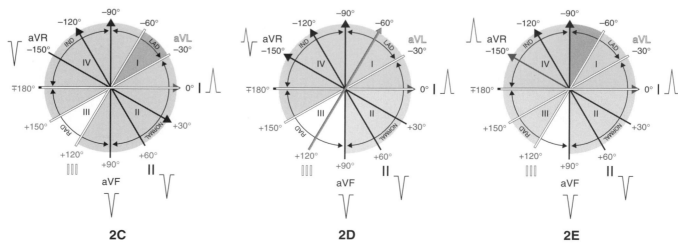

2C   **2D**   **2E**

If the QRS axis lies in quadrant II (0° to +90°):

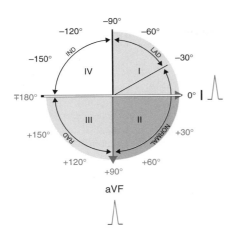

Method D: Step 2, F-J

Figure	Leads				Location of QRS Axis
	I	aVF	III	aVL	
2F	+	+	+	+	+30° to +60°
2G	+	+	+	±	+60°
2H	+	+	+	−	+60° to +90°
2I	+	+	±	+	+30°
2J	+	+	−	+	0° to +30°

+, Predominantly positive; −, predominantly negative; ±, equiphasic.

Determine the net positivity or negativity of the QRS complexes in leads III and aVL.
If lead III is *positive* and:
  2F. Lead aVL is predominantly positive, the QRS axis is between +30° and +60°.
  2G. Lead aVL is equiphasic, the QRS axis is exactly +60°.

  2H. Lead aVL is predominantly negative, the QRS axis is between +60° and +90°.
If lead III is *equiphasic* and:
  2I. Lead aVL is predominantly positive, the QRS axis is exactly +30°.
If Lead III is *negative* and:
  2J. Lead aVL is predominantly positive, the QRS axis is between 0° and +30°.

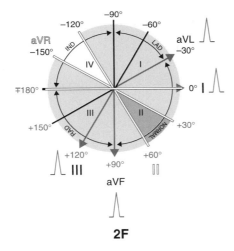

2F

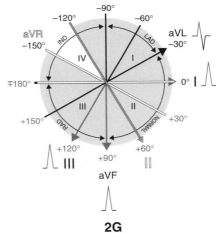

2G

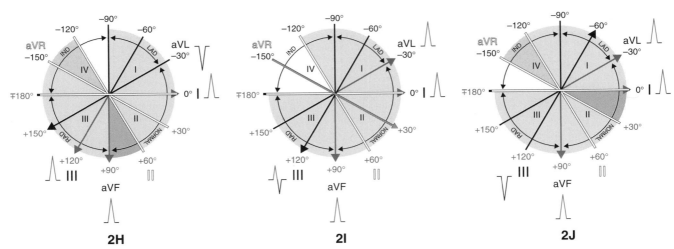

2H

2I

2J

If the QRS axis lies in quadrant III (+90° to +180°):

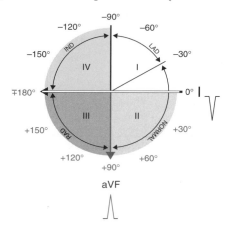

Figure	Leads				Location of QRS Axis
	I	aVF	II	aVR	
2K	−	+	+	−	+90° to +120°
2L	−	+	+	±	+120°
2M	−	+	+	+	+120° to +150°
2N	−	+	±		+150°
2O	−	+	−	+	+150° to +180°

+, Predominantly positive; −, predominantly negative; ±, equiphasic.

Determine the net positivity or negativity of the QRS complexes in leads II and aVR.
If lead II is *positive* and:

   2K. Lead aVR is predominantly negative, the QRS axis is between +90° and +120°.
   2L. Lead aVR is equiphasic, the QRS axis is exactly +120°.

   2M. Lead aVR is predominantly positive, the QRS axis is between +120° and +150°.
If lead II is *equiphasic:*
   2N. The QRS axis is exactly +150°.
If lead II is *negative* and:
   2O. Lead aVR is predominantly positive, the QRS axis is between +150° and +180°.

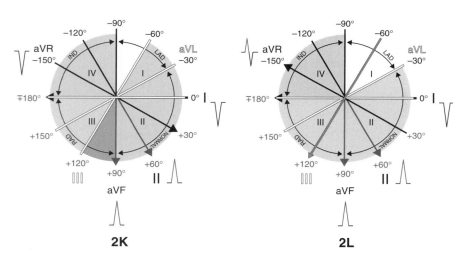

2K   **2L**

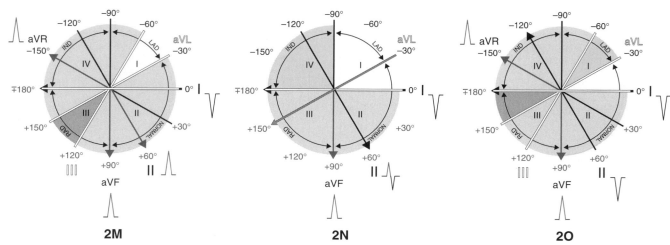

2M   **2N**   **2O**

If the QRS axis lies in quadrant IV (−90° to −180°):

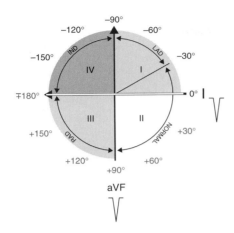

Determine the net positivity or negativity of the QRS complexes in leads III and aVL.

If lead III is *positive* and:

2P. Lead aVL is predominantly negative, the QRS axis is between −150° and −180°.

Method D: Step 2, P-T

Figure	Leads				Location of QRS Axis
	I	aVF	III	aVL	
2P	−	−	+	−	−150° to −180°
2Q	−	−	±		−150°
2R	−	−	−	−	−120° to −150°
2S	−	−	−	±	−120°
2T	−	−	−	+	−90° to −120°

+, Predominantly positive; −, predominantly negative; ±, equiphasic.

If lead III is *equiphasic:*

2Q. The QRS axis is exactly −150°.

If lead III is *negative* and:

2R. Lead aVL is predominantly negative, the QRS axis is between −120° and −150°.

2S. Lead aVL is equiphasic, the QRS axis is exactly −120°.

2T. Lead aVL is predominantly positive, the QRS axis is between −90° and −120°.

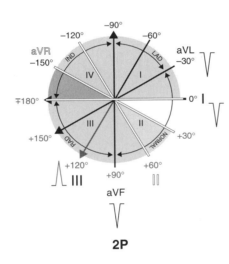

2P

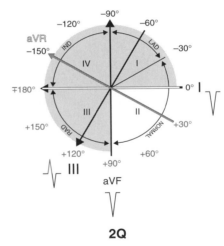

2Q

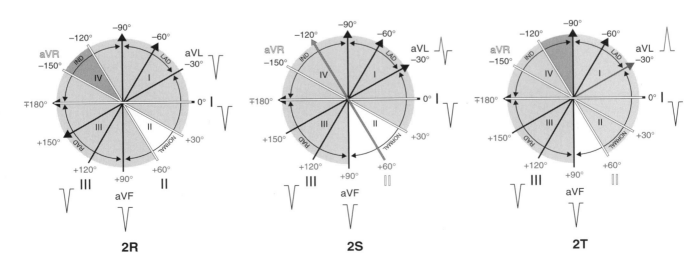

2R   **2S**   **2T**

Method E: The "Perpendicular" Method

The "perpendicular" method uses the perpendicular of a lead with equiphasic or almost equiphasic QRS complexes to determine the position of the QRS axis.

Step 1. Identify the lead with equiphasic (or almost equiphasic) QRS complexes, and label it "**A**" on the hexaxial reference figure.

          AND

Determine the perpendicular to this lead, and label it "**B.**"

Step 2. Identify the lead axis that lies parallel to the perpendicular "**B**," and label it "**C.**"

          AND

Determine whether the QRS complexes in the lead represented by the lead axis "**C**" are predominantly positive or negative.

Step 3. If the QRS complexes are predominantly positive in the lead represented by lead axis

Method E

Lead "A"	Lead Axis "C"	Poles of Lead Axis "C"	
		+	−
I	aVF	+90°	−90°
II	aVL	−30°	+150°
III	aVR	−150°	+30°
aVR	III	+120°	−60°
aVL	II	+60°	−120°
aVF	I	0°	±180°

+, Predominantly positive; −, predominantly negative; ±, equiphasic.

"**C**," the QRS axis lies in the direction of the positive pole of lead axis "**C.**"

Step 4. If the QRS complexes are predominantly negative in the lead represented by lead axis "**C**," the QRS axis lies in the direction of the negative pole of lead axis "**C.**"

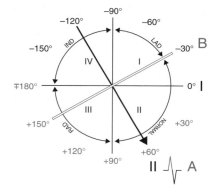

Step 1

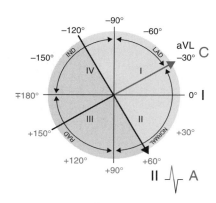

Step 2

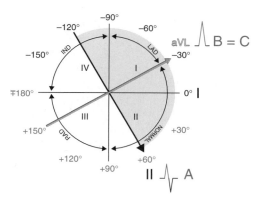

Step 3

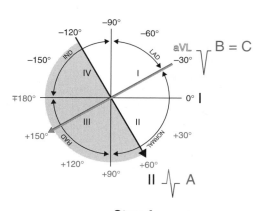

Step 4

Chapter Review Questions Answer Keys

CHAPTER 1

1. (B) The inner layer of the serous pericardium is called the *visceral pericardium* or **epicardium.**

2. (C) The **right** heart pumps blood into the **pulmonary** circulation (the blood vessels within the lungs and those carrying blood to and from the lungs). The **left** heart pumps blood into the **systemic** circulation (the blood vessels in the rest of the body and those carrying blood to and from the body).

3. (A) The right ventricle pumps unoxygenated blood through the **pulmonic** valve and into the lungs through the **pulmonary** artery. In the lungs, the blood picks up oxygen and releases excess carbon dioxide.

4. (C) The period of relaxation and filling of the ventricles with blood is called **ventricular diastole.**

5. (B) The electrical conduction system of the heart is composed of the following structures: the SA node, internodal atrial conduction tracts, AV junction, bundle branches, and the Purkinje network. The **coronary sinus** is not a component of the electrical conduction system.

6. (C) The **bundle of His** is part of the electrical conduction system lying between the AV node and the bundle branches. It is not an accessory conduction pathway.

7. (A) **Conductivity** is the ability of cardiac cells to conduct electrical impulses.

8. (D) When a myocardial cell is in the resting state, a high concentration of **positively** charged **sodium** ions ($Na+$) (cations) is present outside the cell.

9. (B) Cardiac cells cannot be stimulated to depolarize during the **absolute refractory period** because they have not sufficiently repolarized.

10. (C) The **SA node** is normally the dominant and primary pacemaker of the heart because it possesses the highest level of automaticity.

11. (B) **Reentry** is a condition in which the progression of an electrical impulse is delayed or blocked in one or more segments of the electrical conduction system while being conducted normally through the rest of the electrical conduction system. The delayed or blocked electrical impulse is then conducted into the adjacent electrical conduction system.

CHAPTER 2

1. (C) The ECG is a record of the electrical activity (electric current) generated by the **depolarization and repolarization of the atria and ventricles.** The electrical impulses responsible for initiating depolarization of the atria and ventricles are too small to be detected by the ECG electrodes; and the mechanical contraction and relaxation of the atria and ventricles do not generate electrical activity.

2. (D) Dark vertical lines are **0.20 second** (5 mm) apart, whereas light vertical lines are **0.04 second** (1 mm) apart.

3. (B) The sensitivity of the ECG machine is calibrated so that a **1-millivolt** electrical signal produces a **10-mm** deflection on the ECG, equivalent to two large squares on the ECG paper.

4. (B) Atrial depolarization is recorded as the P wave, **ventricular depolarization as the QRS complex,** atrial repolarization as the atrial T wave, and ventricular repolarization as the T wave.

5. (D) Atrial depolarization is recorded as the P wave, ventricular depolarization as the QRS complex, atrial repolarization as the atrial T wave, **and ventricular repolarization as the T wave.**

6. (D) When electrical activity of the heart is not being detected, the ECG is a **straight, flat line,** referred to as the **baseline** or **isoelectric line.**

7. (D) **Muscle tremors, poor electrode contact, and external chest compressions** can all cause artifacts on an ECG tracing.

8. (A) An ECG lead composed of a single positive electrode and a zero reference point (the central terminal) is called a **unipolar lead.**

9. (C) A lead obtained using a positive electrode and a central terminal is called a *unipolar lead.* Unipolar leads include the three augmented leads (aVR, **aVL,** aVF) and the six precordial leads (V_1, V_2, **V_3**, V_4, **V_5**, V_6).

10. (B) Monitoring lead II is obtained by attaching the negative electrode to **the right arm** and the positive electrode to the **left leg.**

11. (C) If the positive ECG electrode is attached to the left leg or lower left anterior chest, all of the electric currents generated in the heart that flow toward the positive electrode will be recorded as **positive (upright)** deflections. The electric currents flowing away from the positive electrode will be recorded as negative (inverted) deflections.

12. (A) Monitoring lead MCL_1 is obtained by attaching the positive **electrode to the right side of the anterior chest in the fourth intercostal space just right of the sternum.**

CHAPTER 3

1. (D) Increased left atrial pressure and left atrial dilatation and hypertrophy as found in **hypertension, mitral and aortic valvular disease, acute MI,** and pulmonary edema secondary to left heart failure may cause wide, notched P waves.

2. (C) The normal PR interval is between **0.12 and 0.20 second.**

3. (C) An ectopic P wave represents atrial depolarization occurring in an **abnormal direction** or **sequence** or both.

4. (B) A normal QRS complex represents normal **depolarization of the ventricles.**

5. (A) The time from the onset of the QRS complex to the peak of the R wave is the **ven-**

tricular activation time (VAT). The VAT represents the time taken for depolarization of the interventricular septum plus depolarization of the ventricle from the endocardium to the epicardium under the facing lead.

6. (B) Aberrant ventricular conduction may occur in the following supraventricular arrhythmias:
   —Premature atrial contractions (PACs)
   —Premature junctional contractions (PJCs)
   —**Atrial tachycardia**
   —Atrial flutter
   —Atrial fibrillation
   —Junctional tachycardia
   —Paroxysmal supraventricular tachycardia

7. (C) The **atrio-His fibers** is an accessory conduction pathway that connects the atria with the lowest part of the AV node near the bundle of His and not with the ventricles directly as do the other accessory conduction pathways. For this reason it does not cause ventricular preexcitation but preexcitation of the bundle of His (i.e., atrio-His preexcitation). Delta waves are absent.

8. (C) Abnormal ventricular repolarization (the **T wave**) may result from myocardial ischemia, acute MI, myocarditis, pericarditis, ventricular enlargement (hypertrophy), electrolyte imbalance (e.g., excess serum potassium), or administration of certain cardiac drugs (e.g., quinidine, procainamide).

9. (B) An abnormally tall U wave may be present in **hypokalemia, cardiomyopathy,** and left ventricular hypertrophy and may follow administration of digitalis, quinidine, and procainamide.

10. (D) A **prolonged PR interval** (one that is greater in duration than 0.20 second) indicates that a delay of progression of the electrical impulse through the AV node, bundle of His, or, rarely, the bundle branches is present.

11. (A) An abnormal ST segment indicates **abnormal ventricular repolarization,** a common consequence of myocardial ischemia and acute MI. It is also present in ventricular fibrosis or aneurysm, pericarditis, left ventricular enlargement (hypertrophy), and administration of digitalis.

CHAPTER 4

1. (D) The heart rate can be determined by the **6-second count method,** a **heart rate calculator ruler,** the **R-R interval method,** or the triplicate method.

2. (C) In adults, a heart rate less than **60** beats per minute indicates a **bradycardia;** a heart rate greater than **100** beats per minute, a **tachycardia.**

3. (C) When using both the **triplicate** method and the **R-R interval** method of determining the heart rate, the rhythm must be regular or else the calculated rate could be inaccurate.

4. (B) The heart rate is **75** beats per minute. Provided the ECG has a regular rate, one method to determine the rate is to count the large squares (0.20 second squares) between the peaks of two consecutive **R** waves and divide this number into 300.

5. (D) The rate of the P waves is usually **the same as that of the QRS complexes,** but sometimes it may be **less:** if an AV block is present, it may be **greater.**

6. (A) If QRS complexes are present but do not regularly precede or follow the P waves, **a complete AV block (third-degree AV block) is present.** Another term used to describe the condition when QRS complexes occur totally unrelated to the P, P′, or F waves is *atrioventricular (AV) dissociation.*

7. (B) If atrial flutter or fibrillation waves are present, the electrical impulses responsible for them have originated in the **atria.**

8. (D) If the P waves are inverted in lead II, the electrical impulses responsible for the P waves most likely have originated in the **lower atria,** the **AV junction,** or the **ventricles.**

9. (D) A PR interval of less than 0.12 second is usually present in an atrial arrhythmia arising in the atria near the AV junction and in a junctional arrhythmia. It is also present in ventricular preexcitation and atrio-His preexcitation.

10. (A) If the QRS complexes are 0.10 second or less in duration, the electrical impulses responsible for the QRS complexes most likely have originated in the **SA node,** atria, or AV junction.

11. (D) Bizarre-appearing QRS complexes with a duration greater than 0.12 second most likely have a pacemaker site in the distal part of a bundle branch, the **Purkinje network,** or the **ventricular myocardium.** The pacemaker site of such abnormal QRS complexes may also be in the SA node, atria, **AV junction,** or the upper part of a bundle branch **in the presence of a bundle branch block or aberrant ventricular conduction.**

12. (C) The AV conduction ratio is **3:2** when there are two QRS complexes for every three P waves.

CHAPTER 5

1. (B) Typically, the heart rate increases during inspiration and **decreases** during expiration.

2. (C) The most common type of sinus arrhythmia, the one related to respiration, is a normal phenomenon commonly seen in children, young adults, and elderly individuals. It is caused by the inhibitory vagal effect of respiration on the SA node.

3. (D) Another less common type of sinus arrhythmia is not related to respiration. It may occur in healthy individuals but is more commonly found in adult patients **with heart disease** or **acute MI** and in those **on digitalis** or morphine.

4. (A) An arrhythmia originating in the SA node with a regular rate of less than 60 beats per minute is called **sinus bradycardia.**

5. (D) Sinus bradycardia may be caused by **excessive inhibitory vagal tone on the SA node, decrease in sympathetic tone on the SA node,** and **hypothermia,** among other things.

6. (C) A mild sinus bradycardia has a heart beat of **50** to **59** beats per minute.

7. (B) A patient with marked sinus bradycardia who is symptomatic will likely have **hypotension and decreased cerebral perfusion.**

8. (B) Symptomatic sinus bradycardia must be promptly treated with **atropine and transcutaneous pacing.**

9. (C) **Sinus arrest** is an arrhythmia caused by episodes of failure in the automaticity of the SA node resulting in bradycardia or asystole.

10. (D) Sinoatrial (SA) exit block may result from toxicity of such medication as **quinidine, digitalis,** and **atenolol.**

CHAPTER 6

1. (B) An arrhythmia originating in pacemakers that shift back and forth between the SA node and an ectopic pacemaker in the atria or AV junction is called a **wandering atrial pacemaker.** It is characterized by P waves of varying size, shape, and direction in any given lead.

2. (D) The arrhythmia described in question number 1 may normally be seen in **the very young, the elderly,** and **athletes.**

3. (C) An extra atrial contraction consisting of a positive P wave in lead II followed by a normal or abnormal QRS complex, occurring earlier than the next beat of the underlying rhythm, is called **a premature atrial contraction.** It is usually followed by a noncompensatory pause.

4. (B) A nonconducted or blocked PAC is **a P′ wave that is not followed by a QRS complex.**

5. (A) The QRS complex of a PAC usually resembles that of **the underlying rhythm.**

6. (B) Two PACs in a row are called **a couplet.**

7. (D) An arrhythmia originating in an ectopic pacemaker in the atria node with an atrial rate between 160 and 240 beats per minute is called **atrial tachycardia.**

8. (D) The reduction in cardiac output accompanying atrial tachycardia can cause **syncope, lightheadedness,** and **dizziness.** In patients with coronary artery disease, it can also cause angina, congestive heart failure, or an acute MI.

9. (B) Atrial flutter is characterized by **flutter waves with a sawtooth appearance** occurring at a rate of 240 to 360 per minute.

10. (C) **Atrial fibrillation** is characterized by multiple dissimilar, small atrial f waves occurring at a rate of 350 to 600 per minute.

CHAPTER 7

1. (C) Absent P′ waves in junctional arrhythmias indicate that **either** retrograde atrial depolarizations occurred during the QRS complexes or atrial depolarizations have not occurred because of a retrograde AV block between the ectopic pacemaker site in the AV junction and the atria.

2. (C) If the ectopic pacemaker in the AV junction discharges too soon after the preceding QRS complex, **the premature P′ wave may not be followed by a QRS complex.**

3. (B) An extra contraction that originates in an ectopic pacemaker in the AV junction, occurring before the next expected beat of the underlying rhythm, is called a **premature junctional contraction,** or **PJC.**

4. (D) The QRS complex of a PJC usually resembles that of the underlying rhythm, being 0.10 second or less in duration. The QRS complex, however, may be 0.12 second or greater in duration and resemble that of a premature ventricular contraction if aberrant ventricular conduction is present. The QRS complex may precede or follow the P′ wave with which it is associated.

5. (D) PJCs are caused by **increased parasympathetic tone on the SA node,** congestive heart failure, damage to the AV junction, **sympathomimetic drugs, digitalis toxicity,** and an excessive dose of certain cardiac drugs such as quinidine or procainamide, among other causes.

6. (D) More than four to six PJCs per minute may indicate an **enhanced automaticity** or a **reentry mechanism** in the AV junction and **that more serious junctional arrhythmias may occur.**

7. (C) An arrhythmia originating in an escape pacemaker in the AV junction with a rate of 40 to 60 beats per minute is called a **junctional escape rhythm.**

8. (D) An arrhythmia consisting of narrow QRS complexes occurring at a rate of 55 beats per minute and P waves occurring independently at a slower rate is a **junctional escape rhythm—a supraventricular arrhythmia.** The presence of P waves occurring independently of the QRS complexes indicates the presence of **atrioventricular (AV) dissociation.**

9. (B) A common cause of nonparoxysmal junctional tachycardia is **digitalis toxicity.** It can also result from damage to the AV junction secondary to an acute inferior MI.

10. (C) Paroxysmal supraventricular tachycardia is characterized by a heart rate between 160 and 240 beats per minute and **an abrupt onset and termination.** The electrophysiological mechanism responsible for PSVT is a reentry mechanism involving the AV node.

CHAPTER 8

1. (C) An extra contraction consisting of an abnormally wide and bizarre QRS complex originating in an ectopic pacemaker in the ventricles is called a **PVC.**

2. (B) Premature ventricular contractions that originate from a single ectopic pacemaker site are called **unifocal.**

3. (C) A PVC may **trigger ventricular fibrillation if it occurs on the T wave** or **depolarize the SA node,** momentarily suppressing it, so that the next P wave of the underlying rhythm appears later than expected.

4. (A) A PVC that appears relatively normal usually originates **near the bifurcation of the bundle of His.**

5. (C) A QRS that has characteristics of both the PVC and a QRS complex of the underlying rhythm is called a **ventricular fusion beat.**

6. (D) Groups of two or more PVCs are called **ventricular group beats, bursts,** and **salvos.**

7. (D) A reentry mechanism in the ventricles may be responsible for **repetitive ventricular contractions, ventricular tachycardia,** or **ventricular fibrillation.**

8. (B) A form of ventricular tachycardia characterized by QRS complexes that gradually change back and forth from one shape, size, and direction to another over a series of beats is called **torsade de pointes.**

9. (D) **Ventricular fibrillation is a life-threatening arrhythmia** requiring **immediate defibrillation.**

10. (B) Asymptomatic accelerated idioventricular rhythm is characterized by a ventricular rate between 40 and 100 beats per minute. It can occur in the presence of a third-degree AV block and is **usually benign,** requiring no treatment.

11. (B) A ventricular rhythm with a ventricular rate and pulse of less than 40 per minute is a **ventricular escape rhythm.**

CHAPTER 9

1. (C) An arrhythmia that occurs commonly in acute inferior myocardial infarction because of the effect of an increase in vagal tone and ischemia on the AV node is called a **first-degree AV block.**

2. (B) An arrhythmia in which there is a progressive delay following each P wave in the conduction of electrical impulses through the AV node until the conduction of the electrical impulses is completely blocked is called a **second-degree, type I AV block** or Wenckebach block.

3. (A) Second-degree, type I AV block is usually transient and reversible and asymptomatic, yet the patient should be monitored and observed because **it can progress to a higher degree AV block.**

4. (C) An arrhythmia in which a complete block of conduction of electrical impulses occurs in one bundle branch and an intermittent block in the other is called a **second-degree, type II AV block.**

5. (A) **Temporary cardiac pacing** is indicated immediately in a symptomatic second-degree, type II AV block that occurs following an acute anteroseptal MI.

6. (D) A second-degree, advanced AV block has an AV conduction ratio **of 3:1 or greater** (i.e., 3:1, 4:1, 6:1, 8:1, or greater).

7. (C) The absence of conduction of electrical impulses through the AV node, bundle of His, or bundle branches, characterized by independent beating of the atria and ventricles, is called a **third-degree AV block.**

8. (D) An escape pacemaker in the AV junction has an inherent firing rate of **40 to 60** beats per minute.

9. (B) If an AV junctional or ventricular escape pacemaker does not take over following a sudden onset of third-degree AV block, ventricular asystole will occur. This is called an **Adams-Stokes syndrome.**

10. (A) A pacemaker that senses spontaneous occurring P waves and QRS complexes, and (1) paces the atria when P waves fail to appear and (2) paces the ventricles when QRS complexes fail to appear after spontaneously occurring or paced P waves, is called an **optimal sequential pacemaker.**

CHAPTER 10

1. (C) In a patient with symptomatic bradycardia and an ECG showing a second-degree, type II AV block, you should administer oxygen, start an IV line, and begin **transcutaneous pacing.**

2. (D) Patients with symptomatic sinus tachycardia should be treated with the **appropriate treatment for the underlying cause of the tachycardia** (i.e., anxiety, exercise, pain, fever, congestive heart failure, hypoxemia, hypovolemia, hypotension, or shock).

3. (A) If a patient is stable with an ECG showing PSVT after administering oxygen and starting an IV line, you should **attempt vagal maneuvers.** Make sure to verify the absence of known carotid artery disease or carotid bruits before attempting carotid sinus massage.

4. (B) Your patient presents with chest pain and signs and symptoms of an acute MI. His ECG shows atrial tachycardia without a block. After administering oxygen and starting an IV line, you should immediately **consider a loading dose of amiodarone.**

5. (A) A patient with atrial fibrillation of less than 48 hours in duration, who is hemodynamically unstable and hypotensive, should be **immediately cardioverted or receive a loading dose of amiodarone.**

6. (D) Your patient is conscious and hemodynamically stable, with a pulse and an ECG showing monomorphic ventricular tachycardia. After administering oxygen and starting an IV, you should perform **any one of the following: start an infusion of procainamide, administer a 150-mg loading dose of amiodarone IV, or deliver a synchronized shock of 100 J.**

7. (A) If your patient in question number 6 begins to complain of chest pain and then becomes pulseless, you should immediately deliver **an unsynchronized shock of 200 joules.**

8. (D) Pulseless electrical activity is the absence of a detectable pulse and blood pressure in the presence of electrical activity of the heart on the ECG. It may result from a complete absence of ventricular contractions **(electromechanical dissociation [EMD])** or marked decrease in cardiac output because of a variety of causes, such as hypovolemia, cardiac rupture, pericardial tamponade, hypothermia, and so forth.

9. (C) In a cardiac arrest, when you are having difficulty starting a peripheral IV and your patient has just been defibrillated three times, you should **administer 2.0 to 2.5 mg of epinephrine via the tracheal tube.**

10. (D) If you suspect asystole, you should **confirm the arrhythmia in two ECG leads, consider delivering three defibrillation shocks if asystole cannot be definitely confirmed, consider transcutaneous pacing after confirming the presence of asystole and the cardiac arrest was witnessed and of short duration,** and continue CPR as necessary, all in this order.

CHAPTER 11

1. (D) The electrode attached to the right leg is a **ground** electrode to provide a path of least resistance for electrical interference in the body.

2. (B) A **bipolar** lead represents the difference in electrical potential between two electrodes.

3. (B) The 'a' in aVR, aVL, and aVF stands for **augmented.**

4. (B) The electrical currents of **Lead I + Lead III = Lead II** is called *Einthoven's law.*

5. (A) Lead aVL is obtained by measuring the electric current between the positive electrode attached to the **left arm** and the central terminal formed by the electrodes attached to the **right arm and left leg.**

6. (B) A **precordial** lead measures the difference in electrical potential between a chest electrode and the central terminal.

7. (B) The placement of the positive chest electrode is as follows:
V_1–right side of the sternum in the fourth intercostal space
V_2–left side of the sternum in the fourth intercostal space
V_3–midway between V_2 and V_4
V_4–**left midclavicular line in the fifth intercostal space**
V_5–left anterior axillary line at the same level as V_4
V_6–left midaxillary line at the same level as V_4

8. (D) See answer 7 above.

9. (C) For V_{6R}, the positive chest electrode is **placed at the right midaxillary line at the same level as V_{4R}.** The location of V_{4R} is in the midclavicular line in the right fifth intercostal space.

10. (C) Leads II, III, and aVF face the **inferior** or diaphragmatic surface of the heart.

CHAPTER 12

1. (A) The mean of all vectors generated during the depolarization of the atria is the **P axis.**

2. (C) An electric current flowing toward the positive pole produces **a positive deflection** on the ECG.

3. (B) The more parallel the electric current is to the axis of the lead, the **larger** the deflection. The more perpendicular, the smaller the deflection.

4. (A) A predominantly positive QRS complex indicates that the **positive** pole of the vector of the QRS axis lies somewhere on the **positive** side of the perpendicular axis.

5. (C) A QRS complex with right axis deviation is **greater than +90°.**

6. (D) Left axis deviation with a QRS axis greater than −30° occurs in adults in the following cardiac disorders:
—left ventricular enlargement and hypertrophy caused by:
—**hypertension**
—**aortic stenosis**
—**ischemic heart disease**
—left bundle branch block and left anterior fascicular block

7. (C) Right axis deviation occurs in adults with **dextrocardia, right ventricular hypertrophy,** and other disorders.

8. (A) A QRS axis **greater than +90°** (right axis deviation) occurs in adults with the following cardiac and pulmonary disorders:
—COPD
—Pulmonary embolism
—Congenital heart disease
—Cor pulmonale
—Severe pulmonary hypertension

9. (D) Determination of the QRS axis may be useful with an **AMI** to determine if an acute left anterior or posterior fascicular block is present; **in acute pulmonary embolism** to determine if right ventricular stretching and enlargement and subsequent acute right bundle branch block are present; and in **a tachycardia with wide QRS complexes** to differentiate between a tachycardia arising in the ventri

cles and one arising in the SA node, atria, or AV junction with wide QRS complexes from whatever cause.

10. (B)   If the QRS complexes are predominantly positive in Lead aVF, the QRS axis is between **0 and +90°.**

CHAPTER 13

1. (C)   The time from the onset of the QRS complex to the peak of the R wave in the QRS complex is called **the ventricular activation time (VAT)** or the **preintrinsicoid deflection.**

2. (C)   The anterior portion of the septum is supplied with blood from the **left anterior descending coronary artery.**

3. (B)   The main blood supply of the AV node and proximal part of the bundle of His is the AV node artery, which arises from the **right coronary artery** in 85% to 90% of the hearts. In the rest of the hearts, the AV node artery arises from the left circumflex coronary artery.

4. (D)   Common causes of bundle branch and ascicular blocks are cardiomyopathy, **ischemic heart disease, idiopathic de generative disease of the electrical conduction system, severe left ventricular hypertrophy,** and, of course, acute MI.

5. (A)   In the setting of an acute MI, an acute right bundle branch block occurs primarily in an **anteroseptal MI,** and rarely in an inferior MI.

6. (A)   In patients with an acute MI complicated by a bundle branch block, **the incidence of pump failure and ventricular arrhythmias is much higher** than in those not so complicated.

7. (C)   Common causes of chronic right bundle branch blocks include **myocarditis, cardiomyopathy, and cardiac surgery.**

8. (B)   In a right bundle branch block with an intact interventricular septum, the QRS complex in lead V_1 is **wide with a classic triphasic rSR′ pattern.**

9. (A)   When the electrical impulses are prevented from directly entering the anterior and lateral walls of the left ventricle, the condition is called a **left anterior fascicular block.**

10. (C)   The electrical impulses are prevented from entering the interventricular septum and posterior wall of the left ventricle directly when the patient has a **left posterior fascicular block.**

CHAPTER 14

1. (C)   A chronic condition of the heart characterized by an increase in the thickness of a chamber's myocardial wall secondary to the increase in the size of the muscle fibers is called **hypertrophy.**

2. (B)   A patient with mitral valve insufficiency or left heart failure may develop **left atrial and ventricular enlargement.**

3. (D)   Left ventricular hypertrophy, a condition usually caused by increased pressure or volume in the left ventricle, is often found in **systemic hypertension, acute MI, mitral insufficiency, hypertrophic cardiomyopathy, and aortic stenosis or insufficiency.**

4. (A)   The diagnosis of left ventricular hypertrophy is based on the ECG characteristics of increased amplitude or depth of the R and S waves in specific limb and precordial leads, **a QRS axis greater than −15°,** and ST segment depression (not ST segment elevation).

5. (A)   **Pericarditis** is an inflammatory disease directly involving the epicardium, with deposition of inflammatory cells and a variable amount of serous, fibrous, purulent, or hemorrhagic exudate within the sac surrounding the heart.

6. (D)   Signs and symptoms of pericarditis include **chest pain, dyspnea, weakness, malaise, chills, fever,** and tachycardia.

7. (C)   In a diffuse pericarditis, the ST segment is elevated in **all leads except aVR and V_1.**

8. (D)   **Hyperkalemia** is an excess of serum potassium above normal levels of 3.5 to 5.0 milliequivalents per liter (mEq/L).

9. (D)   The ECG changes that occur at various levels of excess serum potassium are: **the QRS complexes widen and the T waves become tall; the ST segments disappear and the T waves become peaked; and the PR intervals become prolonged** and a "sine wave" QRS-ST-T pattern appears.

10. (B)   A medication normally prescribed to heart patients, which when taken in excess causes depression of myocardial contractility, AV block, ventricular asystole, PVCs, and ventricular tachycardia and fibrillation, is **procainamide.**

11. (C)   The ECG changes in acute pulmonary embolism include **a QRS axis of greater than +90°.**

12. (B)   ECG changes indicative of right atrial enlargement and right ventricular hypertrophy and a QRS axis of greater than +90° are characteristic of **chronic cor pulmonale.**

13. (A) ST elevations resembling that of acute MI and pericarditis seen in leads I, II, aVF, and V_2-V_6 are typical of early repolarization. They persist and do not return to the baseline as in a resolving acute MI. Abnormally tall, peaked T waves, abnormal Q waves, and ST elevations in leads III and aVR are absent.

14. (B) The Osborn wave is a sign of **hypothermia.**

15. (D) A delta wave indicates that **a preexcitiation syndrome is present, the QRS complex is greater that 0.10 second in duration, and accessory AV pathway conduction is present.**

16. (D) Abnormal conduction of an electrical impulse through an accessory AV pathway results in **an abnormally short PR interval and a delta wave** in the QRS complex.

CHAPTER 15

1. (B) The artery that arises from the left main coronary artery at an obtuse angle and runs posteriorly along the left atrioventricular groove to end in back of the left ventricle is called the **left circumflex coronary artery.** This is the case in 85% to 90% of hearts. In the remaining percentage, the left circumflex coronary artery continues along the atrioventricular groove to become the posterior descending coronary artery while giving rise to the posterior left ventricular arteries and the AV node artery.

2. (C) The SA node is supplied with blood by the sinoatrial node artery, which arises from either **the left circumflex coronary artery** (in 40% to 50% of hearts) or **the right coronary artery** (in 50% to 60% of hearts).

3. (D) Myocardial ischemia or infarction may be caused by an **occlusion of an atherosclerotic coronary artery, coronary artery spasm, increased myocardial workload,** toxic exposure to cocaine or ethanol, decreased level of oxygen in the blood delivered to the myocardium, and decreased coronary artery blood flow from whatever cause.

4. (D) The increase in existing angina from a CCSC class II to a class III indicates the **onset of unstable angina.**

5. (A) The most common cause of acute MI (occurring in about 90% of acute MIs) is a **coronary thrombosis.**

6. (B) Upon revascularization or reoxygenation, necrotic cells **do not return to normal function.**

7. (C) A myocardial infarction in which the zone of infarction involves the entire full thickness of the ventricular wall, from the endocardium to the epicardial surface, is called a **transmural infarction.**

8. (A) By 6 hours after an acute transmural MI, **only a small percentage of cells remain viable** in the involved myocardium.

9. (C) Inverted or tall peaked T waves in the facing leads during the early phase of an acute MI are an indication of **ischemia.**

10. (B) A Q-wave MI cannot be identified as such **until about 8 to 12 hours after the onset of the MI.** The Q waves reach maximum size in about 24 to 48 hours after onset.

11. (D) The most likely cause of an inferior MI is an occlusion of the **posterior left ventricular arteries.**

12. (B) ST segment elevation in **leads V_1-V_4** is diagnostic of an acute anteroseptal MI during the early phase.

CHAPTER 16

1. (B) A **localized anterior myocardial infarction** presents early with ST segment elevation with tall T waves and taller than normal R waves in the midprecordial leads V_3 and V_4, and late with QS complexes with T wave inversion in leads V_3 and V_4.

2. (D) A **lateral myocardial infarction** presents early with ST segment depression in leads II, III, and aVF and ST segment elevation, tall T waves, and taller than normal R waves in leads I, aVL, and the left precordial lead V_5 or V_6 or both.

3. (A) A **septal myocardial infarction** involves both the anterior wall of the left ventricle overlying the interventricular septum and the anterior two thirds of the interventricular septum.

4. (A) A **septal myocardial infarction** presents late with QS complexes with T wave inversions in leads V_1-V_2 and absent normal "septal" q waves in leads II, III, and aVF.

5. (C) An **anterolateral myocardial infarction** presents early with ST segment elevation, tall T waves, and taller than normal R waves in leads I and aVL and the precordial leads V_3-V_6 and ST segment depression in leads II, III, and aVF.

6. (C) An **extensive anterior myocardial infarction** presents late with abnormal Q waves, small R waves, and T wave inversion in leads I and aVL; and QS waves or complexes with T wave inversion in leads V_1-V_6.

7. (C) An **inferior myocardial infarction** involves the posterior left ventricular arteries arising from the right coronary artery or the left circumflex coronary artery of the left coronary artery.

8. (B) An **inferior myocardial infarction** presents early with ST segment elevation, tall T waves, and taller than normal R waves in leads II, III, and aVF and ST segment depression in leads I and aVL.

9. (A) A **posterior myocardial infarction** presents late with large R waves and tall T waves in leads V_1-V_4, an R wave ≥0.04 second in width with slurring and notching in V_1, and an R/S ratio of ≥1 in V_1.

10. (D) A **right ventricular myocardial infarction** presents early with ST segment elevation, tall T waves, and taller than normal R waves in leads II, III, and aVF; ST segment elevation in V_{4R}; and ST segment depression in leads I and aVL.

CHAPTER 17

1. (D) Initial symptoms of cerebral anoxia include **marked anxiety, agitation, a sense of impending doom,** and **extreme fatigue and weakness.**

2. (C) **Dyspnea on exertion** is usually the first noticeable symptom of left heart failure and first appears after an exercise or effort that previously did not produce shortness of breath.

3. (D) A patient with acute myocardial infarction usually presents with a **rapid** pulse rate. However, it may be **normal** or even **slow** if parasympathetic nervous system activity predominates or a slow arrhythmia is present.

4. (B) A patient suffering from an acute myocardial infarction usually presents with **pale, cold,** and **clammy** skin.

5. (A) Pupils start to dilate within **30 seconds** after cessation of blood flow to the brain, becoming fully dilated within **1.5 to 2 minutes** without oxygen.

6. (B) In left heart failure secondary to an acute myocardial infarction, a third heart sound, S_3, **appears after the second heart sound early in diastole,** resulting from rapid filling of the weakened left ventricle during early diastole.

7. (D) Pretibial edema is pitting edema over the tibia, whereas presacral edema is pitting edema over the lower part of the back over the spine. Generalized edema is called **anasarca.**

8. (B) This patient is most likely suffering from **left heart failure.**

9. (B) This patient is most likely suffering from **right heart failure.**

10. (D) This patient is most likely suffering from **compensated cardiogenic shock** as evidenced by the patient's symptoms, general appearance, and vital signs, which show a tachycardia, rapid and labored respirations, and a systolic blood pressure above 90 mm Hg. Uncompensated cardiogenic shock is considered to be present when the systolic blood pressure is 90 mm Hg or less.

CHAPTER 18

1. (D) **Adenosine diphosphate, serotonin, and thromboxane A_2** are all substances that enhance thrombus formation by stimulating platelet aggregation.

2. (B) **Prothrombin** is a plasma protein that, when activated by tissue factor released from damaged arterial wall tissue, converts to thrombin. Thrombin in turn converts fibrinogen to fibrin

3. (C) **Tissue plasminogen activator** (tPA) is a glycoprotein that initiates the process of dissolving fibrinogen and fibrin.

4. (D) The fourth phase in the formation of a coronary artery thrombus is the conversion of fibrinogen into fibrin, which firms up the thrombus and not **fibrinolysis.**

5. (C) There are only three phases to thrombolysis, which includes the release of tPA, plasmin formation, and fibrinolysis, but not **platelet aggregation.**

6. (C) **Promethazine** hydrochloride is a drug used to relieve nausea or vomiting.

7. (A) **Percutaneous transluminal coronary angioplasty** (PTCA) is a procedure in which a balloon-tipped catheter is inserted into an occluded artery and then the balloon is inflated, thereby fracturing the atherosclerotic plaque and dilating the arterial lumen. This procedure is also referred to as *balloon angioplasty.*

8. (B) The correct dosage of reteplase for thrombolytic therapy is **10-U IV bolus in 2 minutes, repeated in 30 minutes.** When reteplase is given in conjunction with antithrombin therapy, such as the administration of a GP IIb/IIIa receptor inhibitor, the correct dosage is 5-U IV bolus of reteplase in 2 minutes, repeated in 30 minutes.

9. (D) The correct dosage of tenecteplase for thrombolytic therapy is **a 30- to 50-mg IV**

bolus in 5 seconds based on the patient's weight. When tenecteplase is given in conjunction with GP IIb/IIIa receptor inhibitor, the correct dosage is half of the above calculated dosage.

10. (A) Morphine sulfate, nitroglycerin, and diuretics should be avoided in patients with possible acute right ventricular myocardial infarction. Normal saline should help restore cardiac output and elevate the systolic blood pressure to 90 to 100 mm Hg. If normal saline is ineffective, dobutamine is indicated **at a dosage of 2 to 20 µg/kg/min.**

11. (B) **Morphine sulfate 1 to 3 mg IV.** The correct dosage for digoxin is 0.5 mg IV; for aminophylline it is 250 to 500 mg IV; and for furosemide it is 40 to 80 mg IV.

Arrhythmia Interpretation: Self-Assessment

I. Arrhythmias

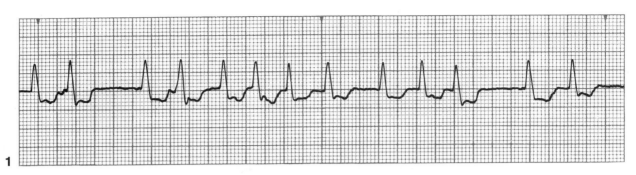

1

Rate: _____

Rhythm: _____

P Waves: _____

PR Int: _____

QRS: _____

Intrp: _____

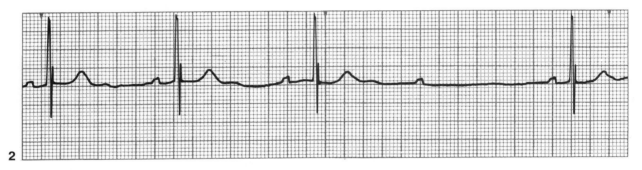

2

Rate: _____

Rhythm: _____

P Waves: _____

PR Int: _____

QRS: _____

Intrp: _____

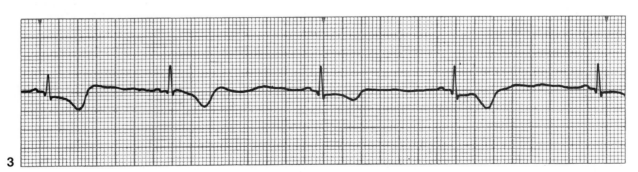

3

Rate: _____

Rhythm: _____

P Waves: _____

PR Int: _____

QRS: _____

Intrp: _____

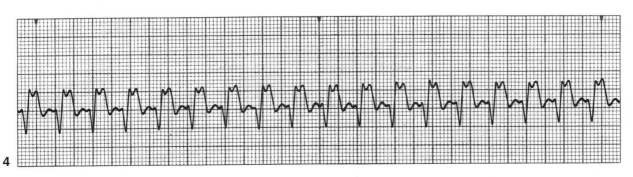

4

Rate: _____

Rhythm: _____

P Waves: _____

PR Int: _____

QRS: _____

Intrp: _____

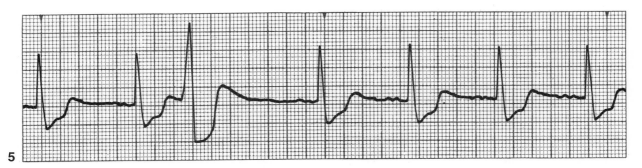

5

Rate: _____

Rhythm: _____

P Waves: _____

PR Int: _____

QRS: _____

Intrp: _____

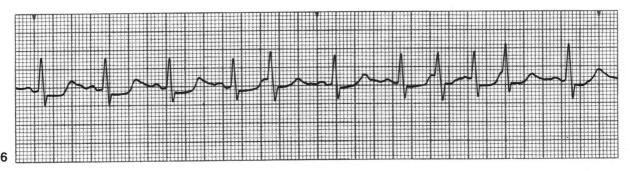

6

Rate: _____

Rhythm: _____

P Waves: _____

PR Int: _____

QRS: _____

Intrp: _____

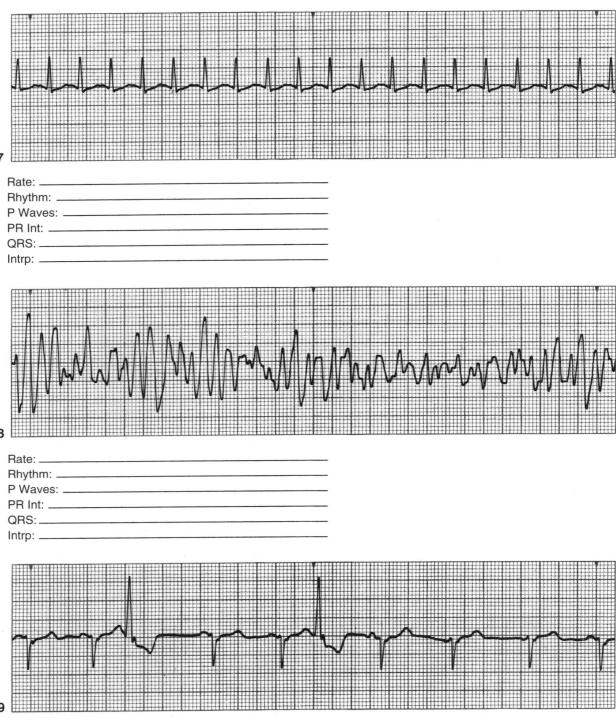

7

Rate: _____

Rhythm: _____

P Waves: _____

PR Int: _____

QRS: _____

Intrp: _____

8

Rate: _____

Rhythm: _____

P Waves: _____

PR Int: _____

QRS: _____

Intrp: _____

9

Rate: _____

Rhythm: _____

P Waves: _____

PR Int: _____

QRS: _____

Intrp: _____

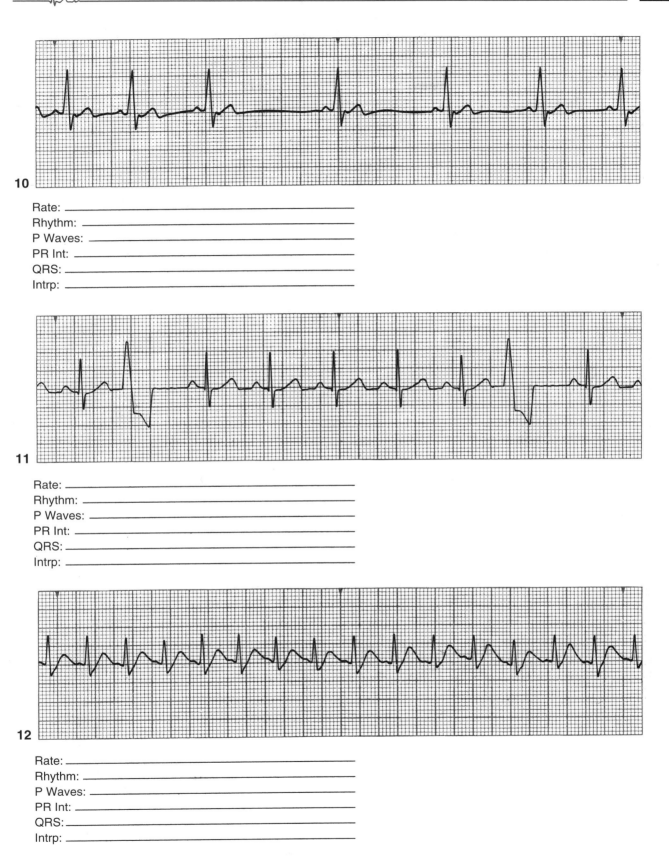

10

Rate: _____

Rhythm: _____

P Waves: _____

PR Int: _____

QRS: _____

Intrp: _____

11

Rate: _____

Rhythm: _____

P Waves: _____

PR Int: _____

QRS: _____

Intrp: _____

12

Rate: _____

Rhythm: _____

P Waves: _____

PR Int: _____

QRS: _____

Intrp: _____

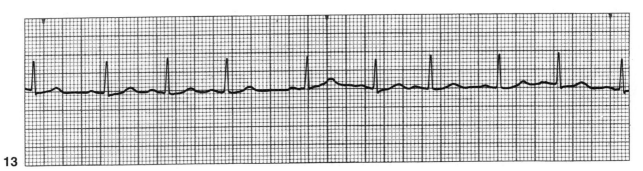

13

Rate: _____

Rhythm: _____

P Waves: _____

PR Int: _____

QRS: _____

Intrp: _____

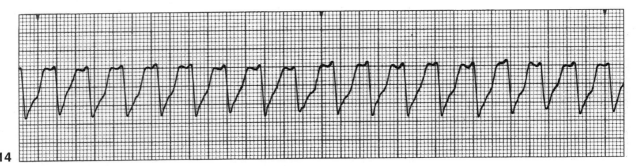

14

Rate: _____

Rhythm: _____

P Waves: _____

PR Int: _____

QRS: _____

Intrp: _____

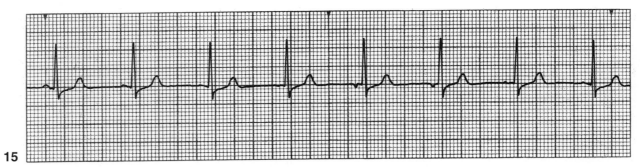

15

Rate: _____

Rhythm: _____

P Waves: _____

PR Int: _____

QRS: _____

Intrp: _____

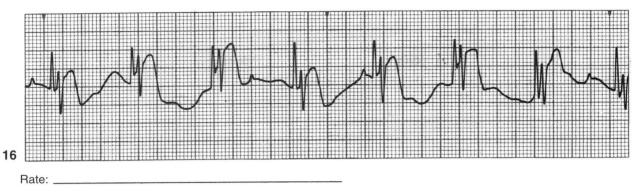

16

Rate: _____

Rhythm: _____

P Waves: _____

PR Int: _____

QRS: _____

Intrp: _____

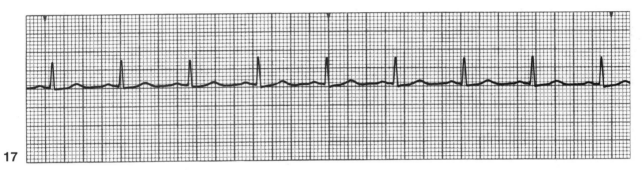

17

Rate: _____

Rhythm: _____

P Waves: _____

PR Int: _____

QRS: _____

Intrp: _____

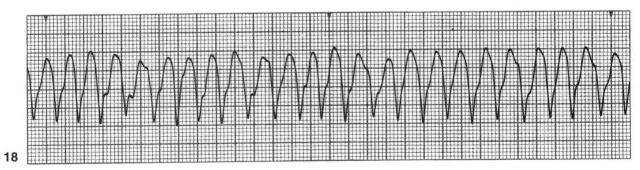

18

Rate: _____

Rhythm: _____

P Waves: _____

PR Int: _____

QRS: _____

Intrp: _____

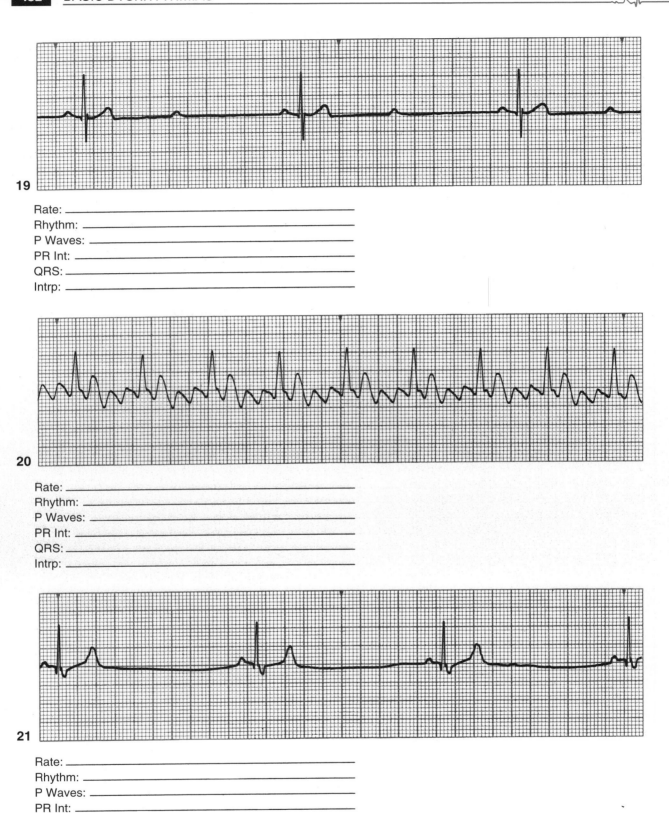

19

Rate: _____

Rhythm: _____

P Waves: _____

PR Int: _____

QRS: _____

Intrp: _____

20

Rate: _____

Rhythm: _____

P Waves: _____

PR Int: _____

QRS: _____

Intrp: _____

21

Rate: _____

Rhythm: _____

P Waves: _____

PR Int: _____

QRS: _____

Intrp: _____

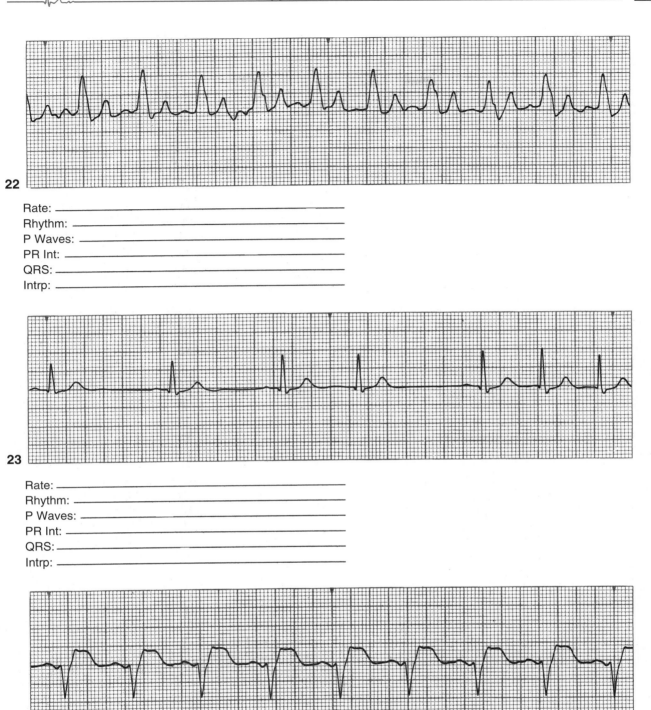

22

Rate: _____

Rhythm: _____

P Waves: _____

PR Int: _____

QRS: _____

Intrp: _____

23

Rate: _____

Rhythm: _____

P Waves: _____

PR Int: _____

QRS: _____

Intrp: _____

24

Rate: _____

Rhythm: _____

P Waves: _____

PR Int: _____

QRS: _____

Intrp: _____

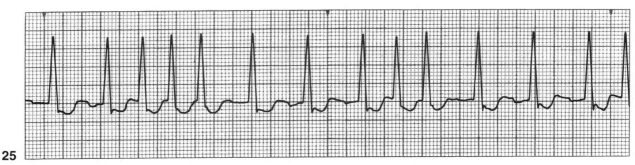

25

Rate: _____

Rhythm: _____

P Waves: _____

PR Int: _____

QRS: _____

Intrp: _____

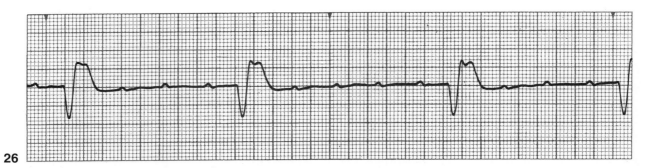

26

Rate: _____

Rhythm: _____

P Waves: _____

PR Int: _____

QRS: _____

Intrp: _____

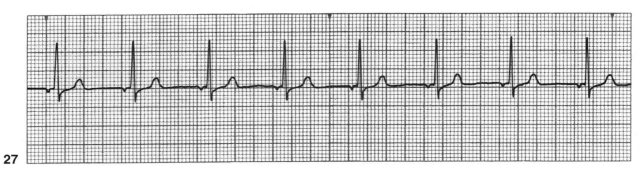

27

Rate: _____

Rhythm: _____

P Waves: _____

PR Int: _____

QRS: _____

Intrp: _____

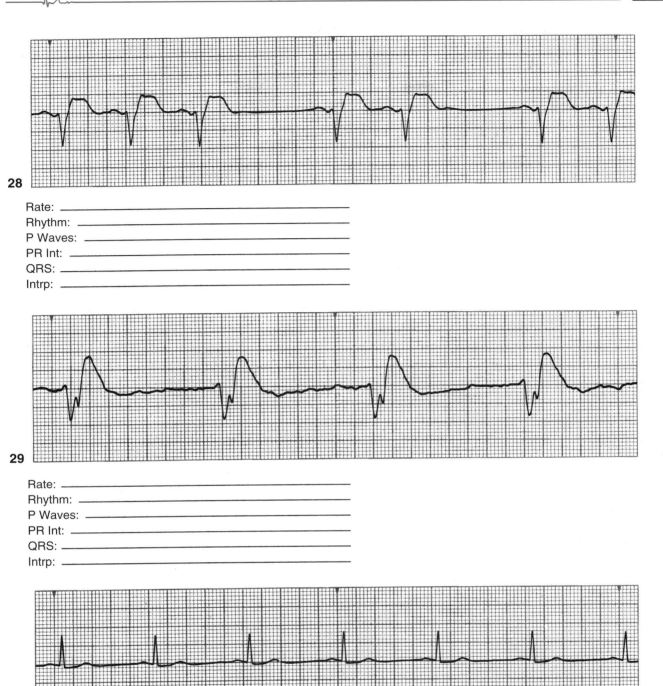

28

Rate: _____

Rhythm: _____

P Waves: _____

PR Int: _____

QRS: _____

Intrp: _____

29

Rate: _____

Rhythm: _____

P Waves: _____

PR Int: _____

QRS: _____

Intrp: _____

30

Rate: _____

Rhythm: _____

P Waves: _____

PR Int: _____

QRS: _____

Intrp: _____

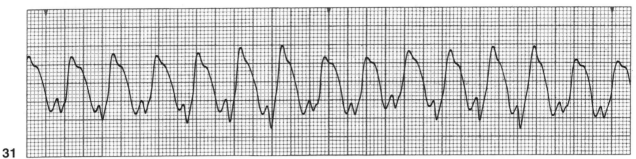

31

Rate: _____

Rhythm: _____

P Waves: _____

PR Int: _____

QRS: _____

Intrp: _____

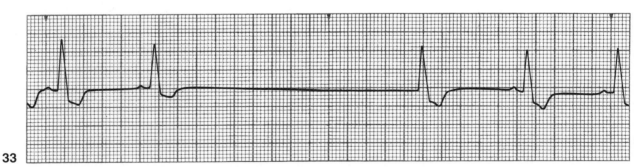

32

Rate: _____

Rhythm: _____

P Waves: _____

PR Int: _____

QRS: _____

Intrp: _____

33

Rate: _____

Rhythm: _____

P Waves: _____

PR Int: _____

QRS: _____

Intrp: _____

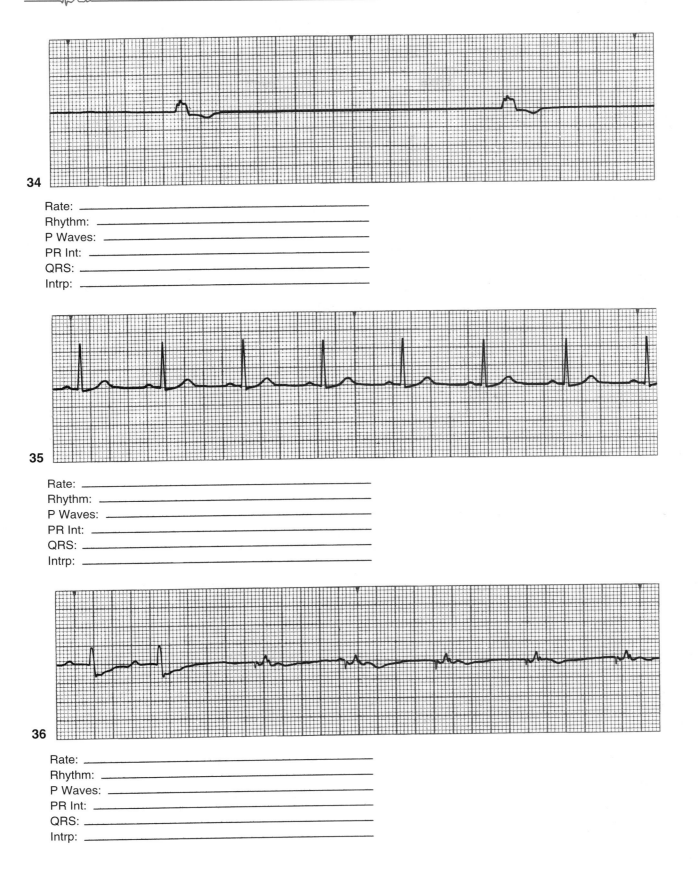

34

Rate: _____

Rhythm: _____

P Waves: _____

PR Int: _____

QRS: _____

Intrp: _____

35

Rate: _____

Rhythm: _____

P Waves: _____

PR Int: _____

QRS: _____

Intrp: _____

36

Rate: _____

Rhythm: _____

P Waves: _____

PR Int: _____

QRS: _____

Intrp: _____

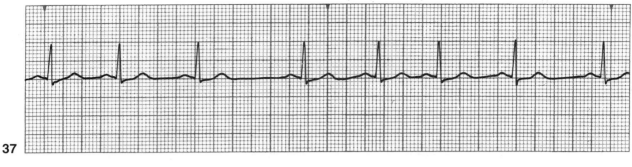

37

Rate: _____

Rhythm: _____

P Waves: _____

PR Int: _____

QRS: _____

Intrp: _____

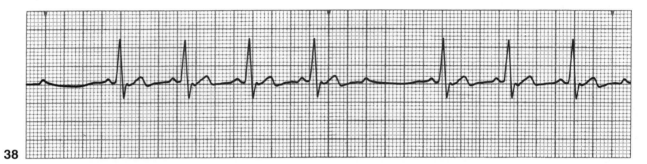

38

Rate: _____

Rhythm: _____

P Waves: _____

PR Int: _____

QRS: _____

Intrp: _____

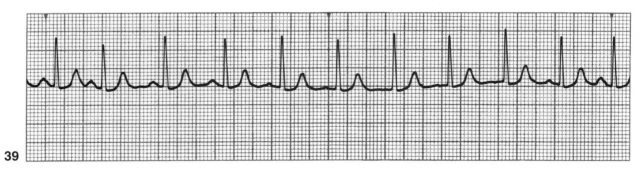

39

Rate: _____

Rhythm: _____

P Waves: _____

PR Int: _____

QRS: _____

Intrp: _____

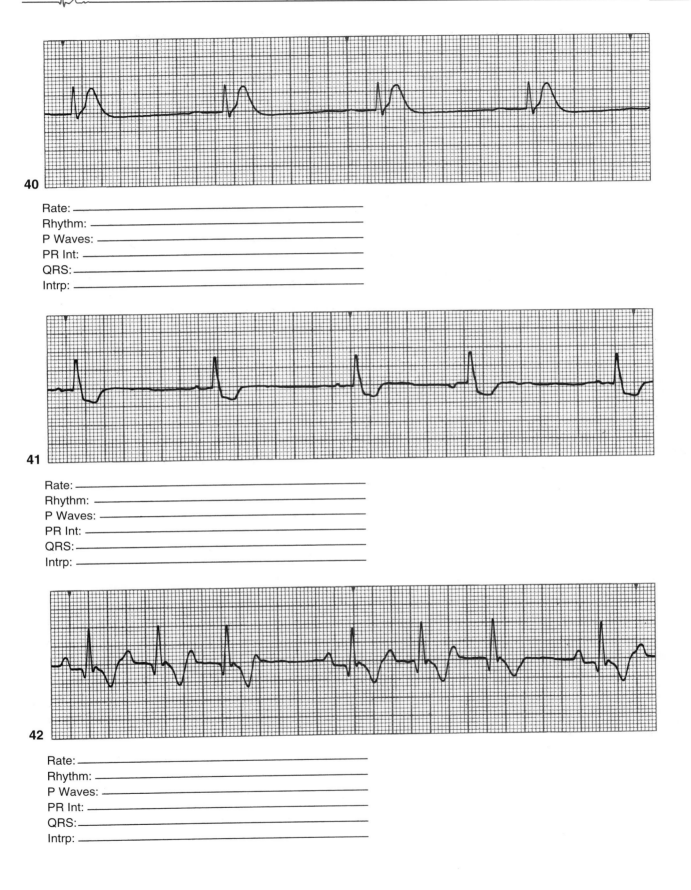

40

Rate: _____

Rhythm: _____

P Waves: _____

PR Int: _____

QRS: _____

Intrp: _____

41

Rate: _____

Rhythm: _____

P Waves: _____

PR Int: _____

QRS: _____

Intrp: _____

42

Rate: _____

Rhythm: _____

P Waves: _____

PR Int: _____

QRS: _____

Intrp: _____

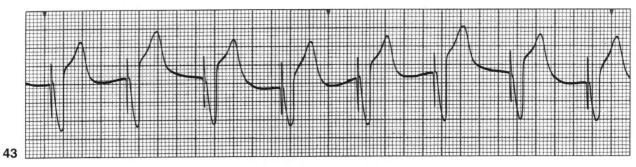

43

Rate: _____

Rhythm: _____

P Waves: _____

PR Int: _____

QRS: _____

Intrp: _____

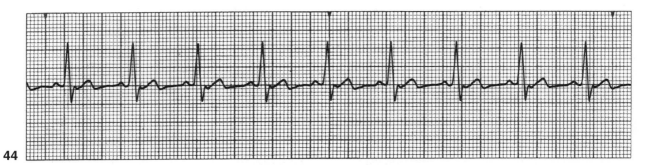

44

Rate: _____

Rhythm: _____

P Waves: _____

PR Int: _____

QRS: _____

Intrp: _____

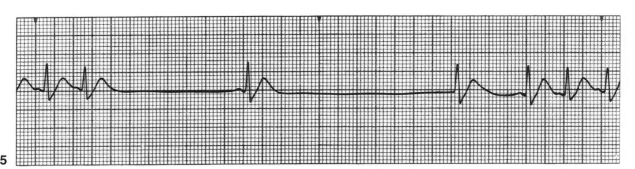

45

Rate: _____

Rhythm: _____

P Waves: _____

PR Int: _____

QRS: _____

Intrp: _____

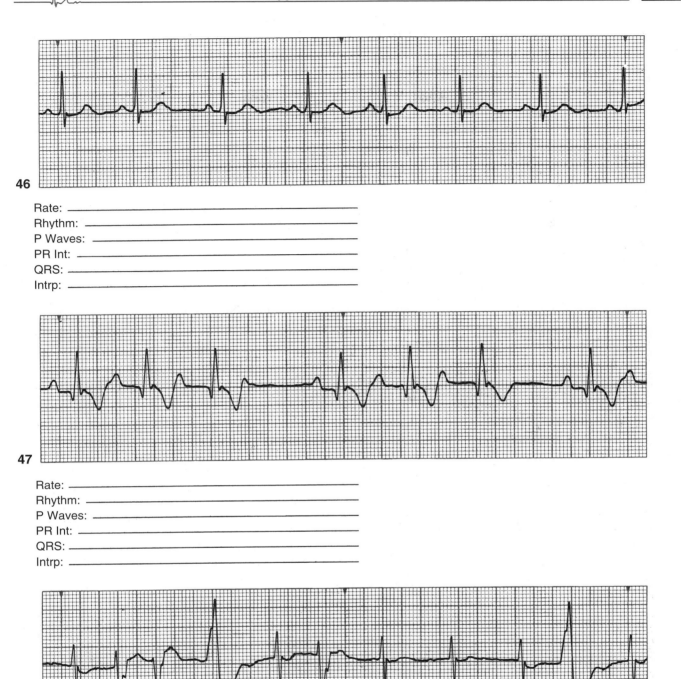

46

Rate: _____

Rhythm: _____

P Waves: _____

PR Int: _____

QRS: _____

Intrp: _____

47

Rate: _____

Rhythm: _____

P Waves: _____

PR Int: _____

QRS: _____

Intrp: _____

48

Rate: _____

Rhythm: _____

P Waves: _____

PR Int: _____

QRS: _____

Intrp: _____

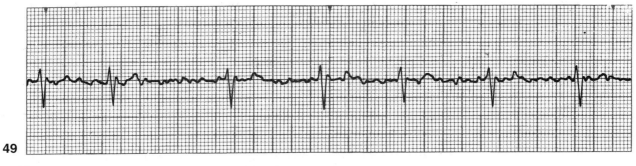

49

Rate: _____

Rhythm: _____

P Waves: _____

PR Int: _____

QRS: _____

Intrp: _____

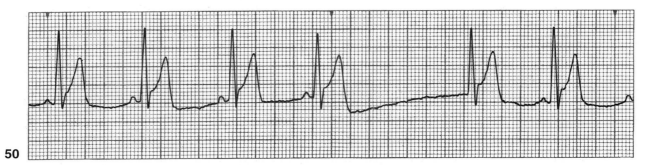

50

Rate: _____

Rhythm: _____

P Waves: _____

PR Int: _____

QRS: _____

Intrp: _____

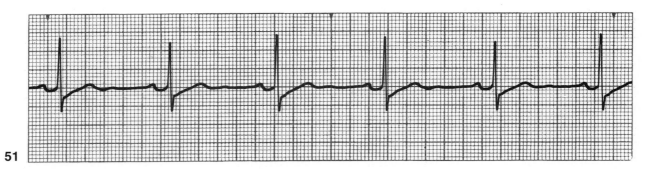

51

Rate: _____

Rhythm: _____

P Waves: _____

PR Int: _____

QRS: _____

Intrp: _____

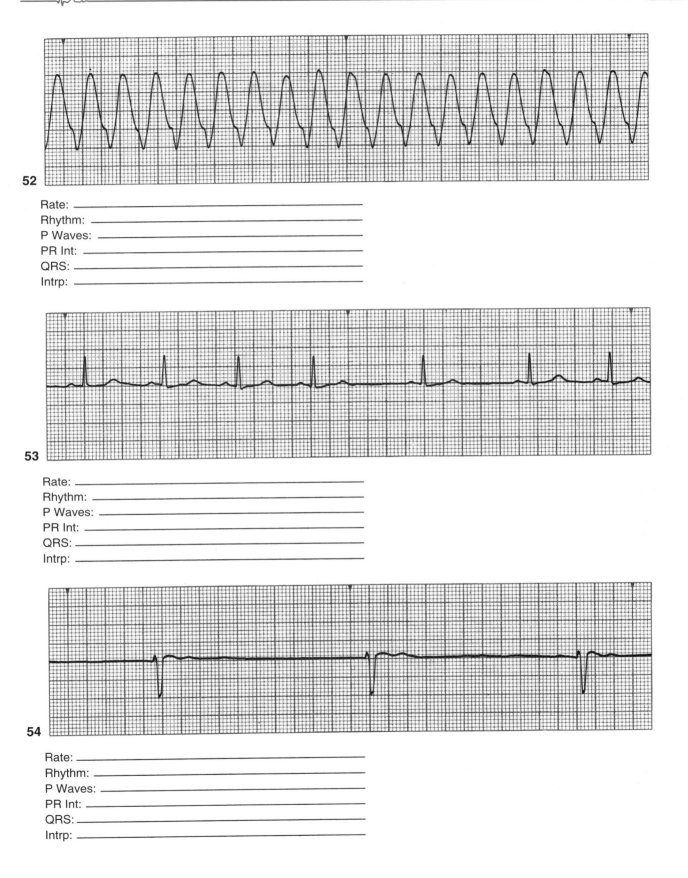

52

Rate: —————————————————————————

Rhythm: ———————————————————————

P Waves: ——————————————————————

PR Int: —————————————————————————

QRS: —————————————————————————

Intrp: —————————————————————————

53

Rate: —————————————————————————

Rhythm: ———————————————————————

P Waves: ——————————————————————

PR Int: —————————————————————————

QRS: —————————————————————————

Intrp: —————————————————————————

54

Rate: —————————————————————————

Rhythm: ———————————————————————

P Waves: ——————————————————————

PR Int: —————————————————————————

QRS: —————————————————————————

Intrp: —————————————————————————

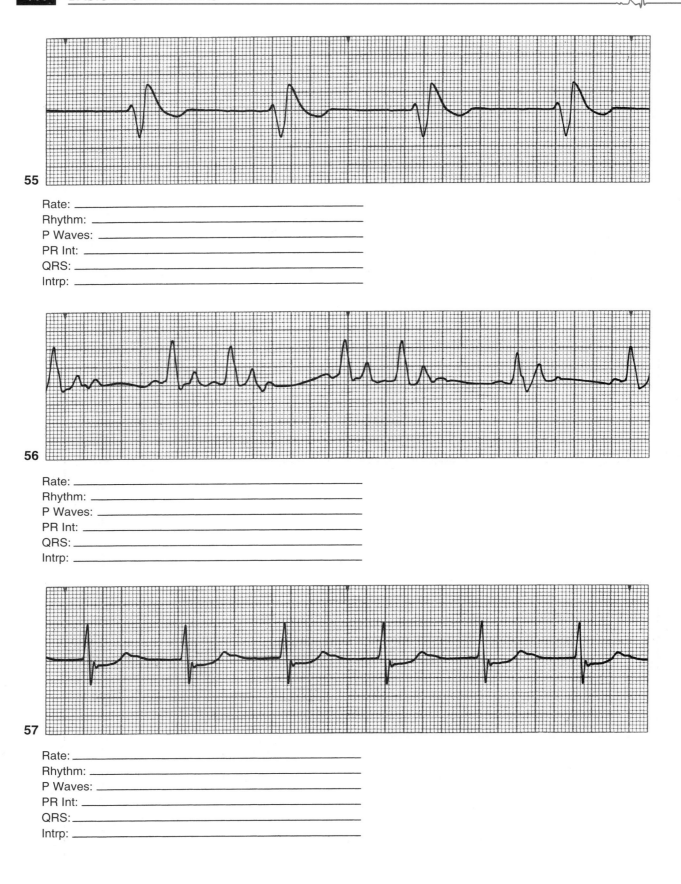

55

Rate: _____

Rhythm: _____

P Waves: _____

PR Int: _____

QRS: _____

Intrp: _____

56

Rate: _____

Rhythm: _____

P Waves: _____

PR Int: _____

QRS: _____

Intrp: _____

57

Rate: _____

Rhythm: _____

P Waves: _____

PR Int: _____

QRS: _____

Intrp: _____

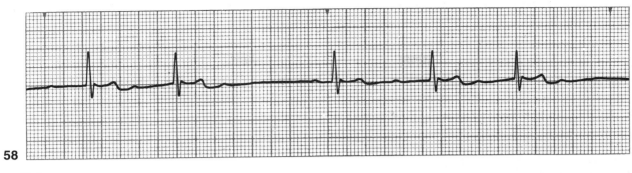

58

Rate: _____
Rhythm: _____
P Waves: _____
PR Int: _____
QRS: _____
Intrp: _____

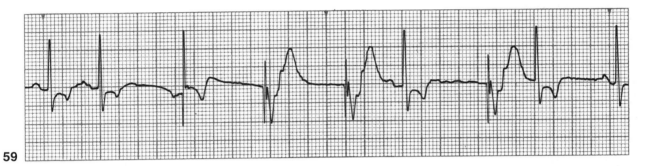

59

Rate: _____
Rhythm: _____
P Waves: _____
PR Int: _____
QRS: _____
Intrp: _____

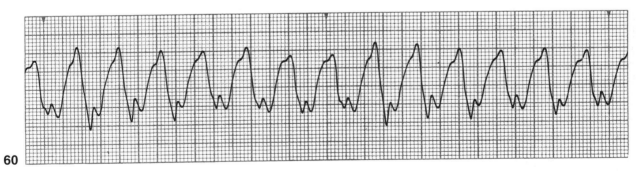

60

Rate: _____
Rhythm: _____
P Waves: _____
PR Int: _____
QRS: _____
Intrp: _____

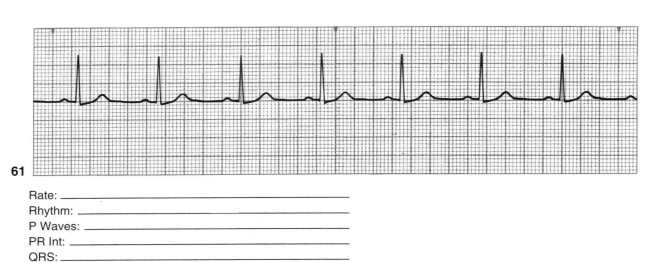

61

Rate: _____

Rhythm: _____

P Waves: _____

PR Int: _____

QRS: _____

Intrp: _____

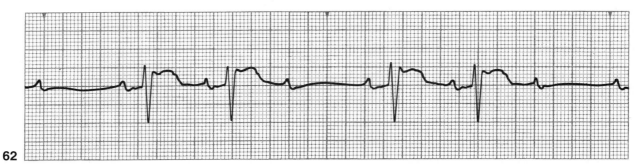

62

Rate: _____

Rhythm: _____

P Waves: _____

PR Int: _____

QRS: _____

Intrp: _____

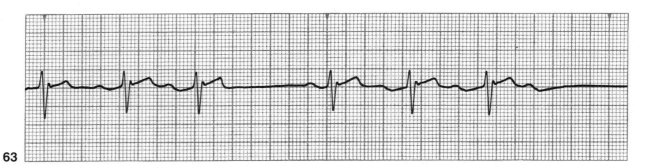

63

Rate: _____

Rhythm: _____

P Waves: _____

PR Int: _____

QRS: _____

Intrp: _____

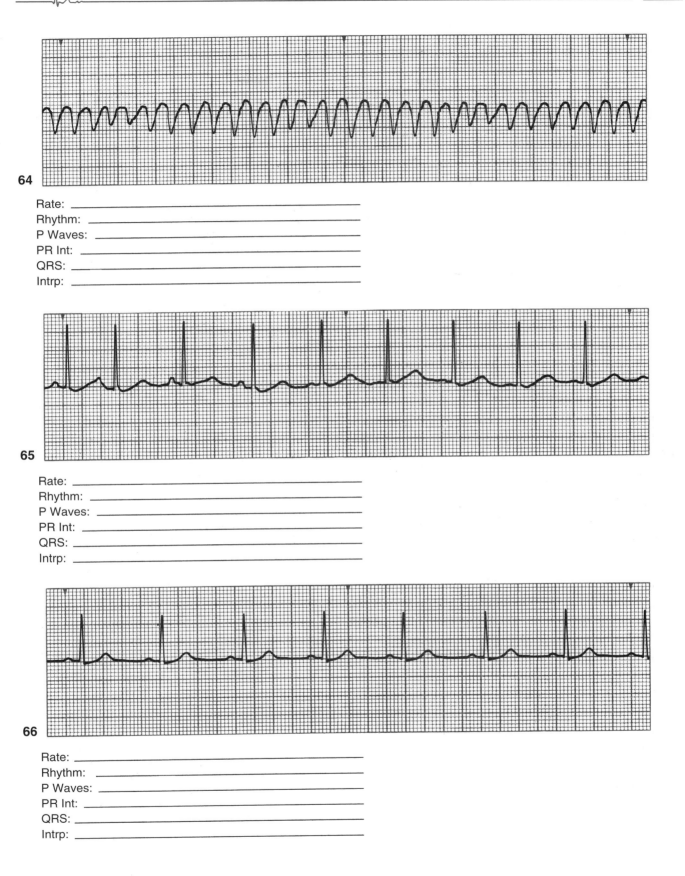

64

Rate: _____

Rhythm: _____

P Waves: _____

PR Int: _____

QRS: _____

Intrp: _____

65

Rate: _____

Rhythm: _____

P Waves: _____

PR Int: _____

QRS: _____

Intrp: _____

66

Rate: _____

Rhythm: _____

P Waves: _____

PR Int: _____

QRS: _____

Intrp: _____

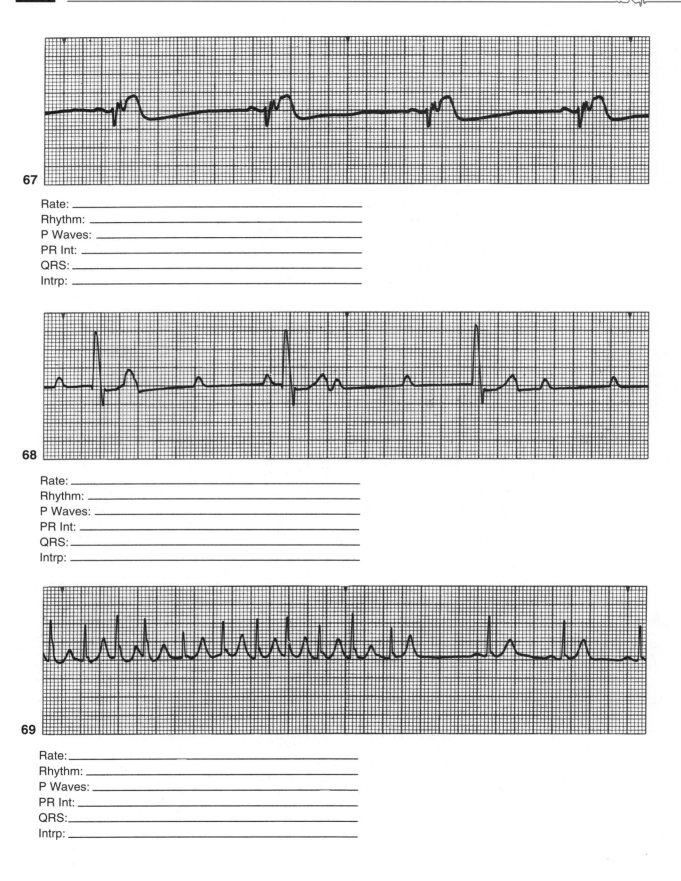

67

Rate: _____

Rhythm: _____

P Waves: _____

PR Int: _____

QRS: _____

Intrp: _____

68

Rate: _____

Rhythm: _____

P Waves: _____

PR Int: _____

QRS: _____

Intrp: _____

69

Rate: _____

Rhythm: _____

P Waves: _____

PR Int: _____

QRS: _____

Intrp: _____

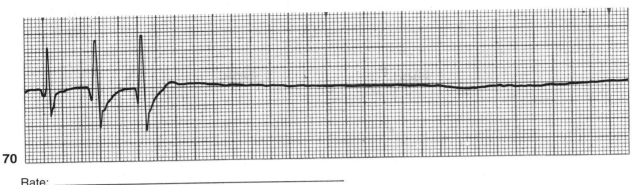

70

Rate: _____

Rhythm: _____

P Waves: _____

PR Int: _____

QRS: _____

Intrp: _____

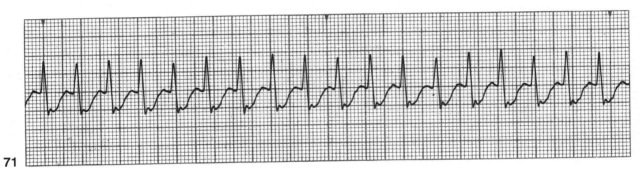

71

Rate: _____

Rhythm: _____

P Waves: _____

PR Int: _____

QRS: _____

Intrp: _____

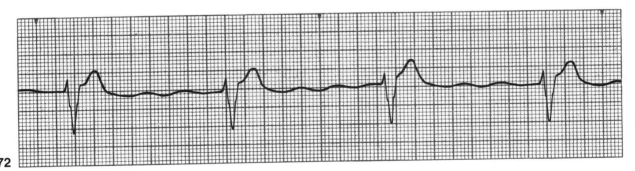

72

Rate: _____

Rhythm: _____

P Waves: _____

PR Int: _____

QRS: _____

Intrp: _____

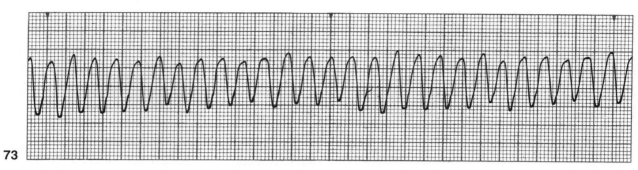

73

Rate: _____

Rhythm: _____

P Waves: _____

PR Int: _____

QRS: _____

Intrp: _____

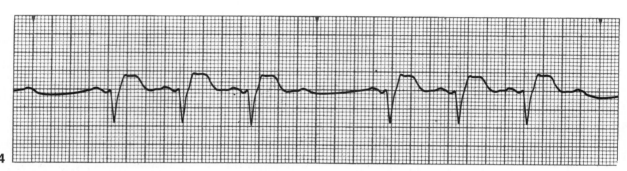

74

Rate: _____

Rhythm: _____

P Waves: _____

PR Int: _____

QRS: _____

Intrp: _____

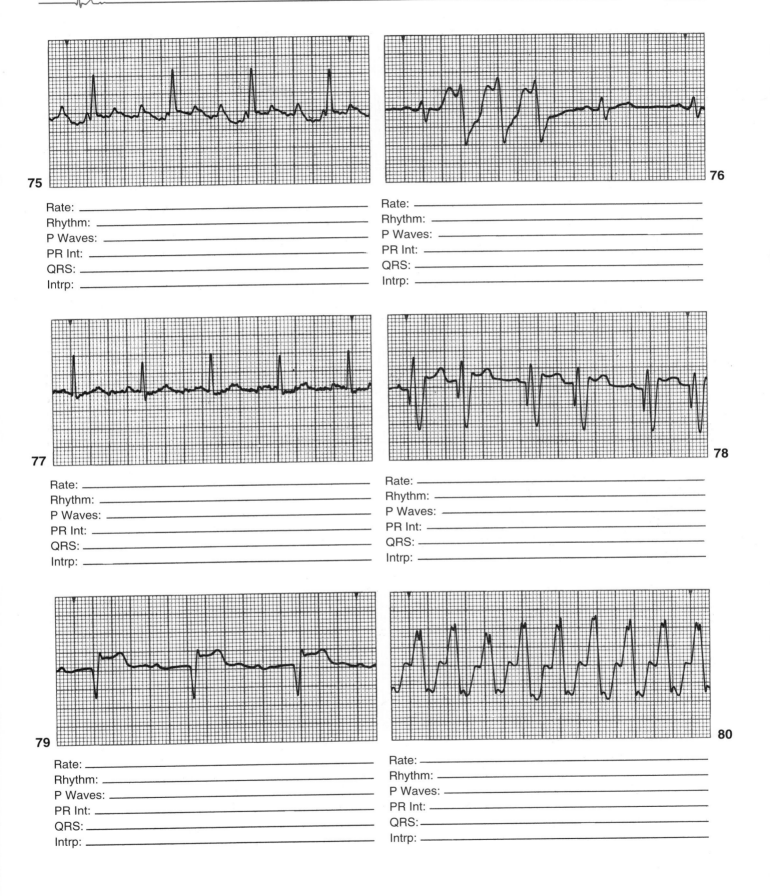

75

Rate: _____
Rhythm: _____
P Waves: _____
PR Int: _____
QRS: _____
Intrp: _____

76

Rate: _____
Rhythm: _____
P Waves: _____
PR Int: _____
QRS: _____
Intrp: _____

77

Rate: _____
Rhythm: _____
P Waves: _____
PR Int: _____
QRS: _____
Intrp: _____

78

Rate: _____
Rhythm: _____
P Waves: _____
PR Int: _____
QRS: _____
Intrp: _____

79

Rate: _____
Rhythm: _____
P Waves: _____
PR Int: _____
QRS: _____
Intrp: _____

80

Rate: _____
Rhythm: _____
P Waves: _____
PR Int: _____
QRS: _____
Intrp: _____

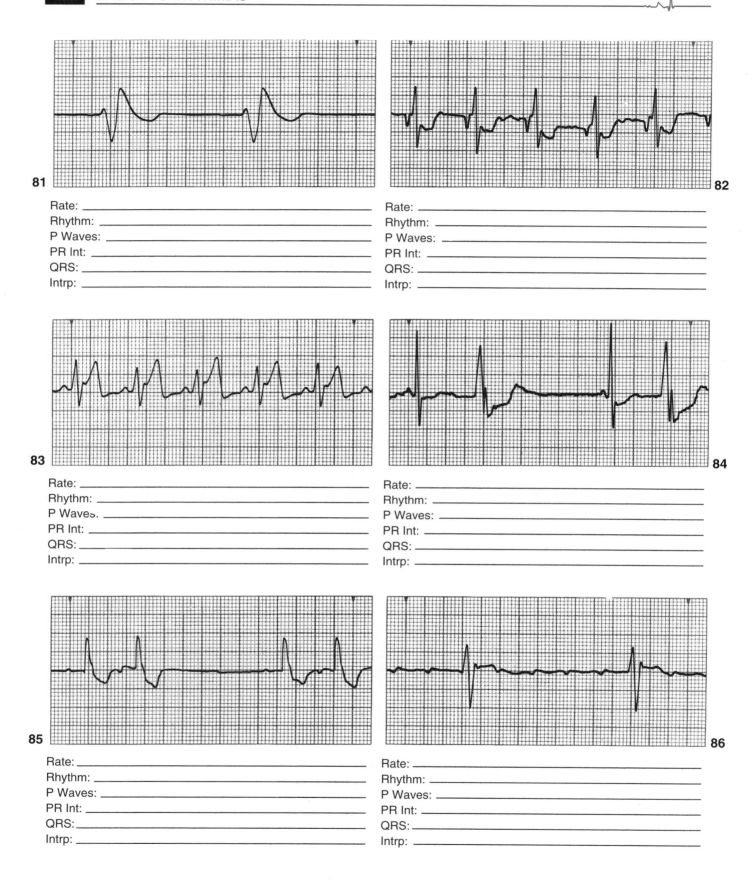

81

Rate: _____

Rhythm: _____

P Waves: _____

PR Int: _____

QRS: _____

Intrp: _____

82

Rate: _____

Rhythm: _____

P Waves: _____

PR Int: _____

QRS: _____

Intrp: _____

83

Rate: _____

Rhythm: _____

P Waves. _____

PR Int: _____

QRS: _____

Intrp: _____

84

Rate: _____

Rhythm: _____

P Waves: _____

PR Int: _____

QRS: _____

Intrp: _____

85

Rate: _____

Rhythm: _____

P Waves: _____

PR Int: _____

QRS: _____

Intrp: _____

86

Rate: _____

Rhythm: _____

P Waves: _____

PR Int: _____

QRS: _____

Intrp: _____

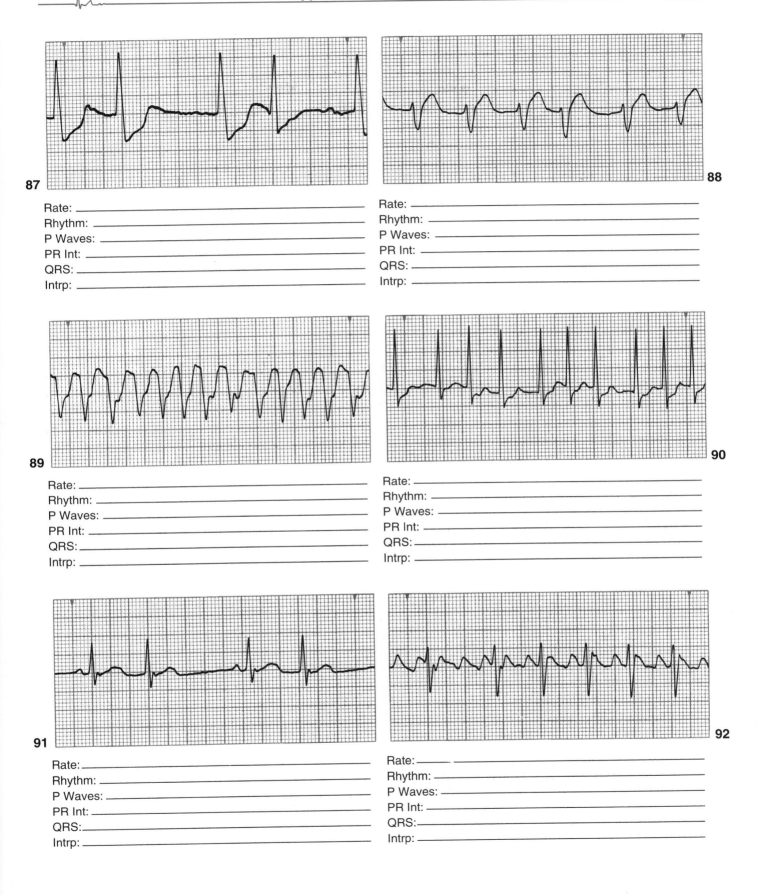

87

Rate: _____
Rhythm: _____
P Waves: _____
PR Int: _____
QRS: _____
Intrp: _____

88

Rate: _____
Rhythm: _____
P Waves: _____
PR Int: _____
QRS: _____
Intrp: _____

89

Rate: _____
Rhythm: _____
P Waves: _____
PR Int: _____
QRS: _____
Intrp: _____

90

Rate: _____
Rhythm: _____
P Waves: _____
PR Int: _____
QRS: _____
Intrp: _____

91

Rate: _____
Rhythm: _____
P Waves: _____
PR Int: _____
QRS: _____
Intrp: _____

92

Rate: _____
Rhythm: _____
P Waves: _____
PR Int: _____
QRS: _____
Intrp: _____

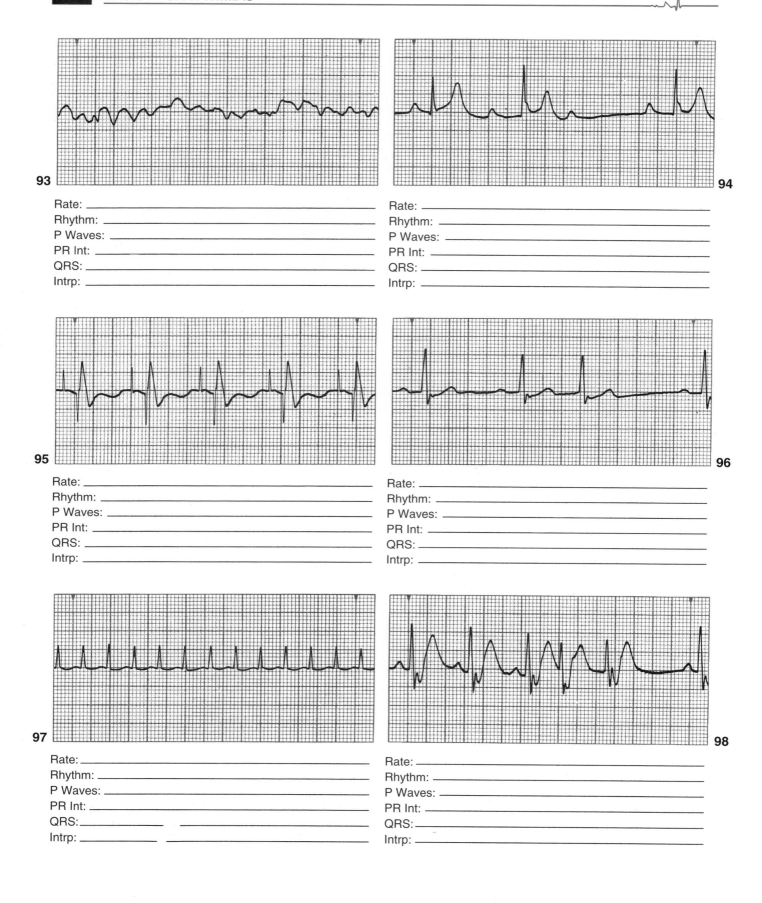

93

Rate: _____
Rhythm: _____
P Waves: _____
PR Int: _____
QRS: _____
Intrp: _____

94

Rate: _____
Rhythm: _____
P Waves: _____
PR Int: _____
QRS: _____
Intrp: _____

95

Rate: _____
Rhythm: _____
P Waves: _____
PR Int: _____
QRS: _____
Intrp: _____

96

Rate: _____
Rhythm: _____
P Waves: _____
PR Int: _____
QRS: _____
Intrp: _____

97

Rate: _____
Rhythm: _____
P Waves: _____
PR Int: _____
QRS: _____   _____
Intrp: _____   _____

98

Rate: _____
Rhythm: _____
P Waves: _____
PR Int: _____
QRS: _____
Intrp: _____

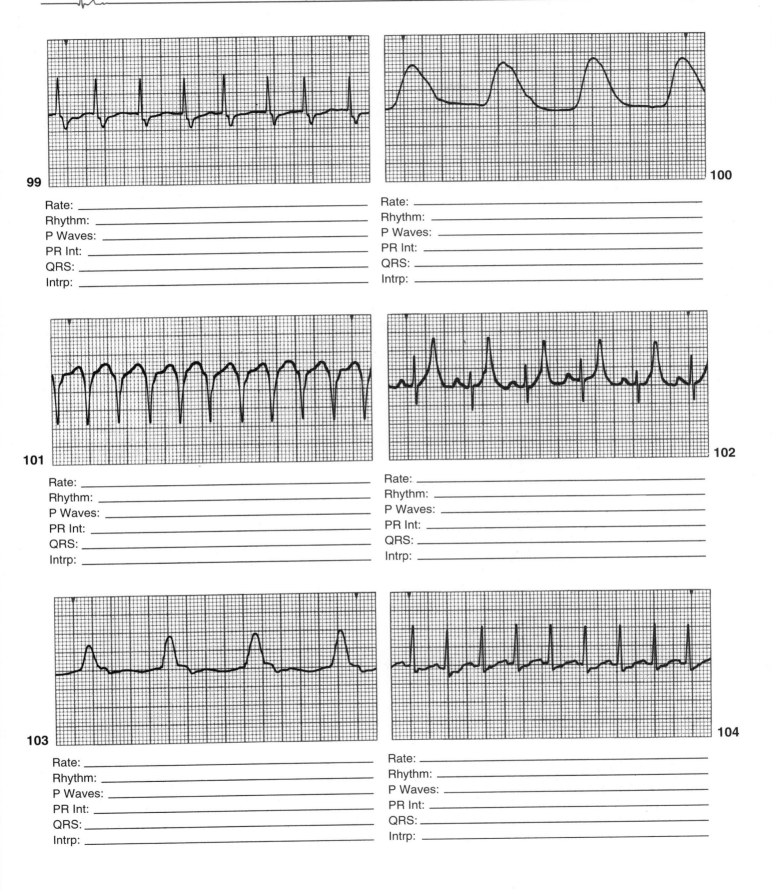

99

Rate: _____
Rhythm: _____
P Waves: _____
PR Int: _____
QRS: _____
Intrp: _____

100

Rate: _____
Rhythm: _____
P Waves: _____
PR Int: _____
QRS: _____
Intrp: _____

101

Rate: _____
Rhythm: _____
P Waves: _____
PR Int: _____
QRS: _____
Intrp: _____

102

Rate: _____
Rhythm: _____
P Waves: _____
PR Int: _____
QRS: _____
Intrp: _____

103

Rate: _____
Rhythm: _____
P Waves: _____
PR Int: _____
QRS: _____
Intrp: _____

104

Rate: _____
Rhythm: _____
P Waves: _____
PR Int: _____
QRS: _____
Intrp: _____

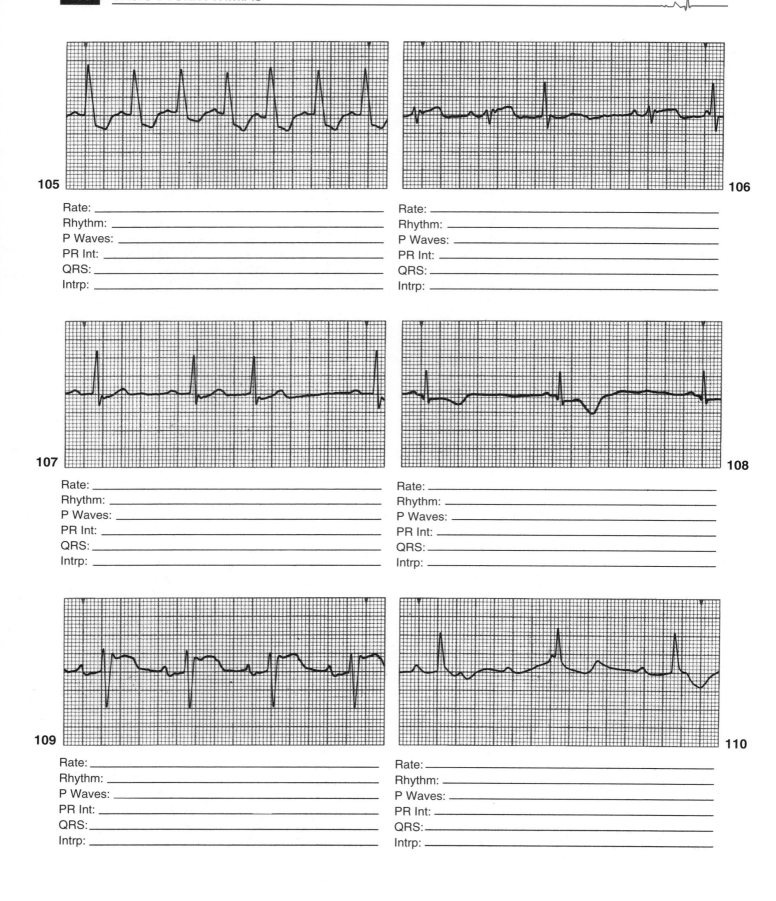

105

Rate: _____
Rhythm: _____
P Waves: _____
PR Int: _____
QRS: _____
Intrp: _____

106

Rate: _____
Rhythm: _____
P Waves: _____
PR Int: _____
QRS: _____
Intrp: _____

107

Rate: _____
Rhythm: _____
P Waves: _____
PR Int: _____
QRS: _____
Intrp: _____

108

Rate: _____
Rhythm: _____
P Waves: _____
PR Int: _____
QRS: _____
Intrp: _____

109

Rate: _____
Rhythm: _____
P Waves: _____
PR Int: _____
QRS: _____
Intrp: _____

110

Rate: _____
Rhythm: _____
P Waves: _____
PR Int: _____
QRS: _____
Intrp: _____

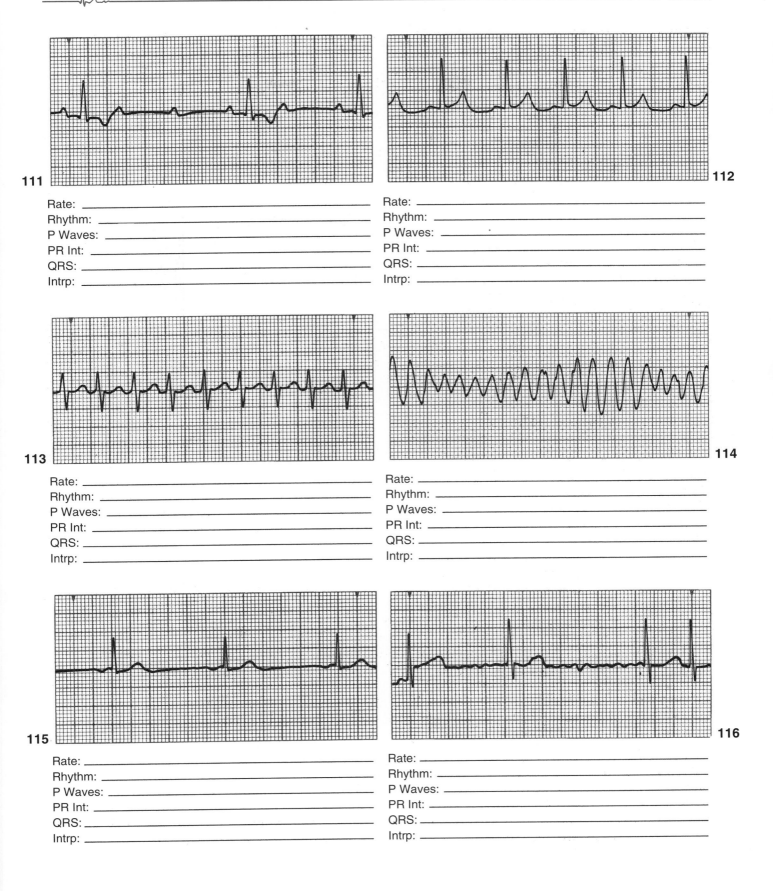

111

Rate: _____
Rhythm: _____
P Waves: _____
PR Int: _____
QRS: _____
Intrp: _____

112

Rate: _____
Rhythm: _____
P Waves: _____
PR Int: _____
QRS: _____
Intrp: _____

113

Rate: _____
Rhythm: _____
P Waves: _____
PR Int: _____
QRS: _____
Intrp: _____

114

Rate: _____
Rhythm: _____
P Waves: _____
PR Int: _____
QRS: _____
Intrp: _____

115

Rate: _____
Rhythm: _____
P Waves: _____
PR Int: _____
QRS: _____
Intrp: _____

116

Rate: _____
Rhythm: _____
P Waves: _____
PR Int: _____
QRS: _____
Intrp: _____

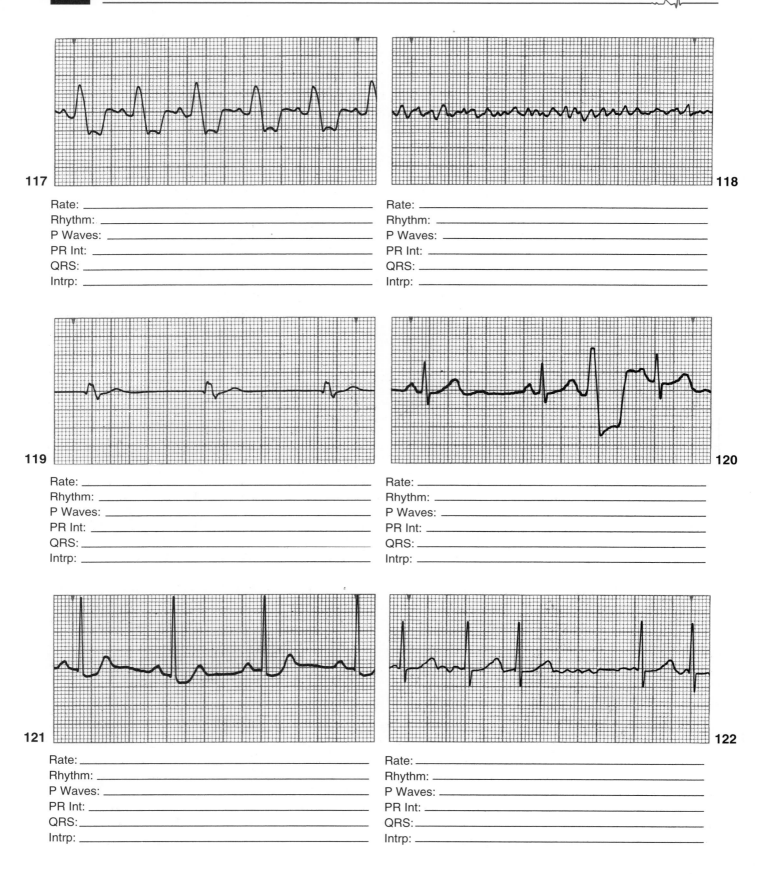

117

Rate: _____

Rhythm: _____

P Waves: _____

PR Int: _____

QRS: _____

Intrp: _____

118

Rate: _____

Rhythm: _____

P Waves: _____

PR Int: _____

QRS: _____

Intrp: _____

119

Rate: _____

Rhythm: _____

P Waves: _____

PR Int: _____

QRS: _____

Intrp: _____

120

Rate: _____

Rhythm: _____

P Waves: _____

PR Int: _____

QRS: _____

Intrp: _____

121

Rate: _____

Rhythm: _____

P Waves: _____

PR Int: _____

QRS: _____

Intrp: _____

122

Rate: _____

Rhythm: _____

P Waves: _____

PR Int: _____

QRS: _____

Intrp: _____

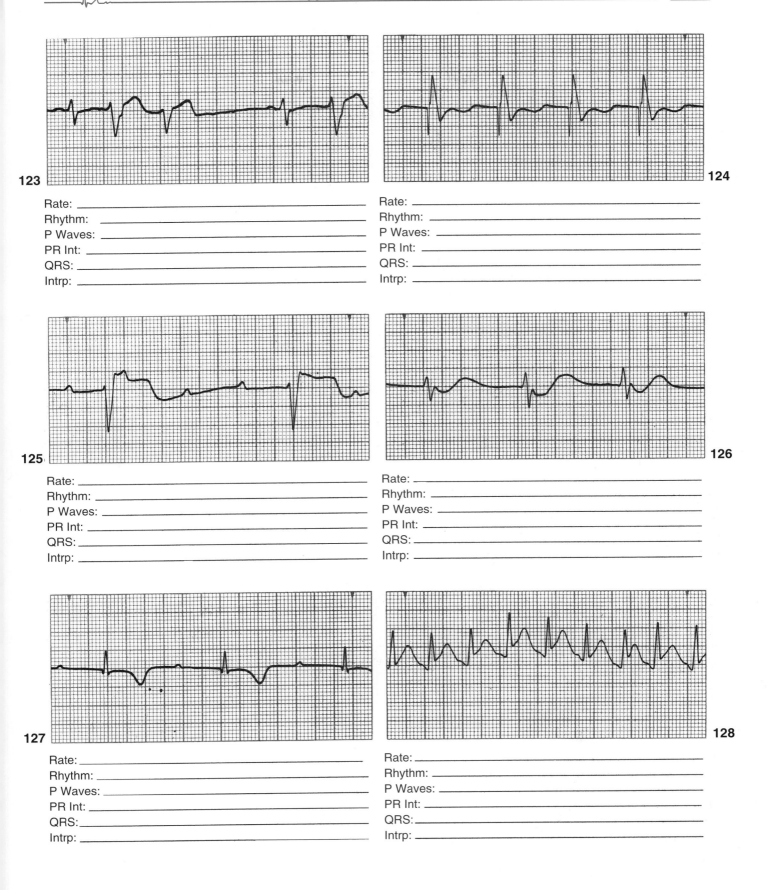

123

Rate: _____
Rhythm: _____
P Waves: _____
PR Int: _____
QRS: _____
Intrp: _____

124

Rate: _____
Rhythm: _____
P Waves: _____
PR Int: _____
QRS: _____
Intrp: _____

125

Rate: _____
Rhythm: _____
P Waves: _____
PR Int: _____
QRS: _____
Intrp: _____

126

Rate: _____
Rhythm: _____
P Waves: _____
PR Int: _____
QRS: _____
Intrp: _____

127

Rate: _____
Rhythm: _____
P Waves: _____
PR Int: _____
QRS: _____
Intrp: _____

128

Rate: _____
Rhythm: _____
P Waves: _____
PR Int: _____
QRS: _____
Intrp: _____

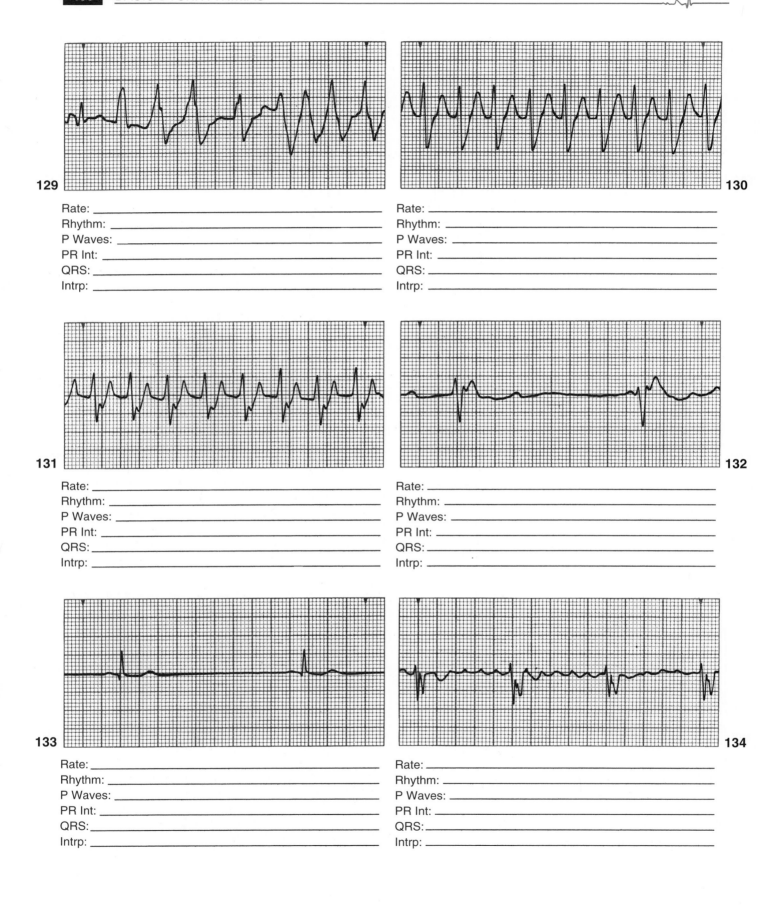

129

Rate: _____

Rhythm: _____

P Waves: _____

PR Int: _____

QRS: _____

Intrp: _____

130

Rate: _____

Rhythm: _____

P Waves: _____

PR Int: _____

QRS: _____

Intrp: _____

131

Rate: _____

Rhythm: _____

P Waves: _____

PR Int: _____

QRS: _____

Intrp: _____

132

Rate: _____

Rhythm: _____

P Waves: _____

PR Int: _____

QRS: _____

Intrp: _____

133

Rate: _____

Rhythm: _____

P Waves: _____

PR Int: _____

QRS: _____

Intrp: _____

134

Rate: _____

Rhythm: _____

P Waves: _____

PR Int: _____

QRS: _____

Intrp: _____

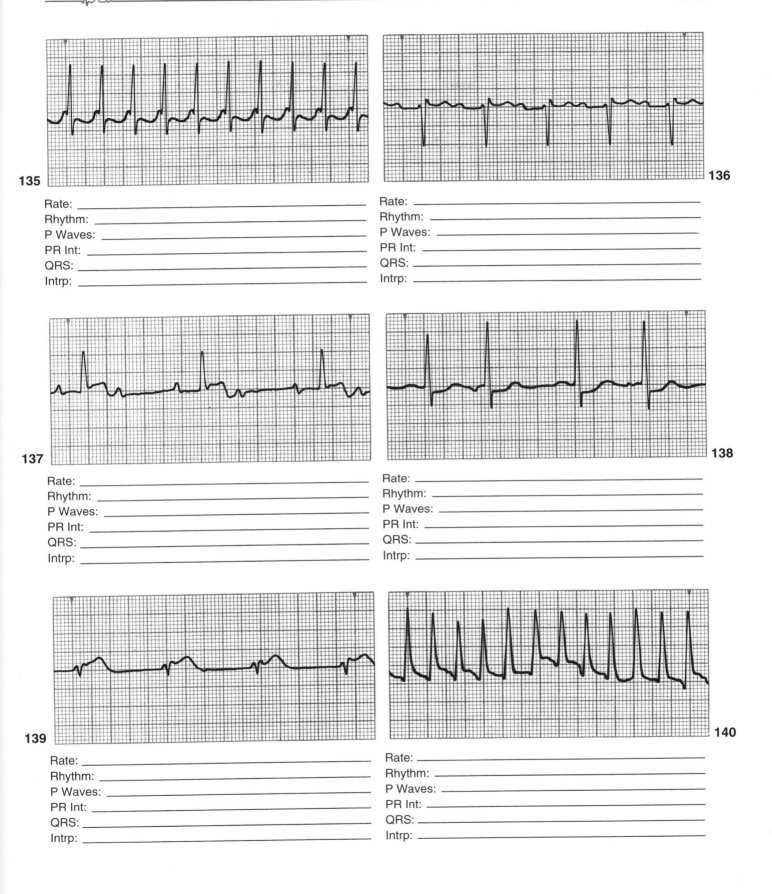

135

Rate: _____
Rhythm: _____
P Waves: _____
PR Int: _____
QRS: _____
Intrp: _____

136

Rate: _____
Rhythm: _____
P Waves: _____
PR Int: _____
QRS: _____
Intrp: _____

137

Rate: _____
Rhythm: _____
P Waves: _____
PR Int: _____
QRS: _____
Intrp: _____

138

Rate: _____
Rhythm: _____
P Waves: _____
PR Int: _____
QRS: _____
Intrp: _____

139

Rate: _____
Rhythm: _____
P Waves: _____
PR Int: _____
QRS: _____
Intrp: _____

140

Rate: _____
Rhythm: _____
P Waves: _____
PR Int: _____
QRS: _____
Intrp: _____

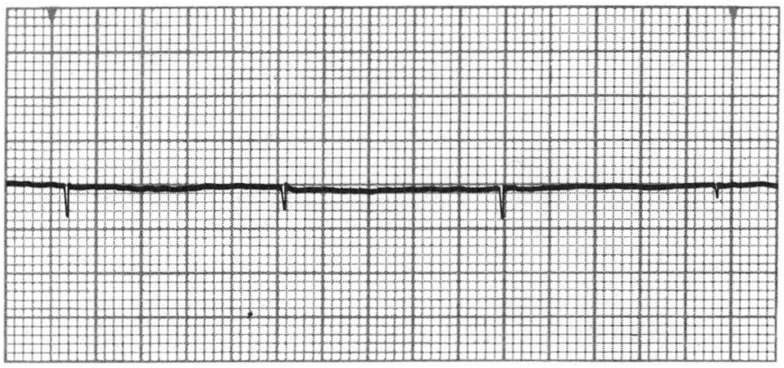

141

Rate: _____
Rhythm: _____
P Waves: _____
PR Int: _____
QRS: _____
Intrp: _____

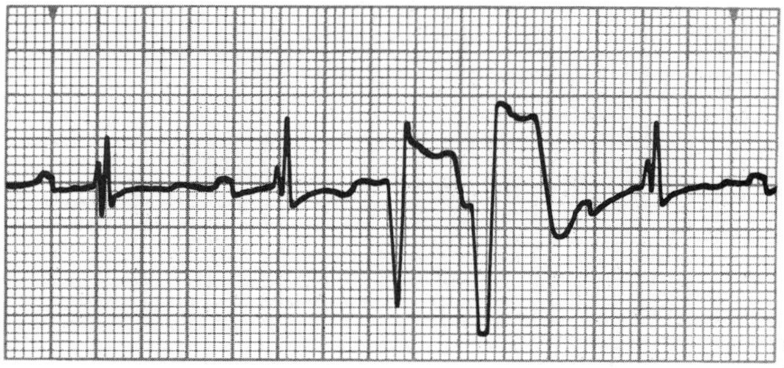

142

Rate: _____
Rhythm: _____
P Waves: _____
PR Int: _____
QRS: _____
Intrp: _____

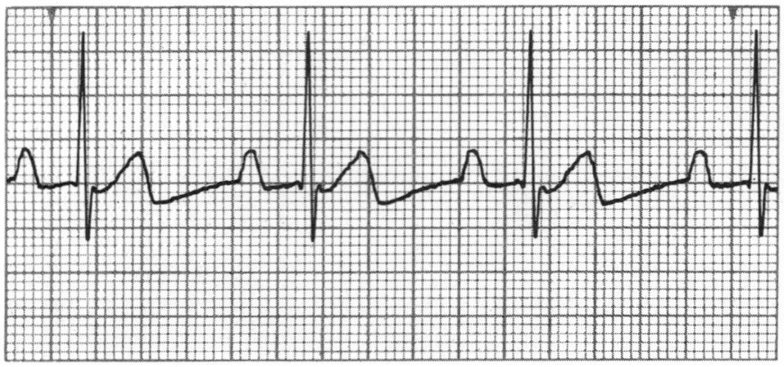

143

Rate: _____
Rhythm: _____
P Waves: _____
PR Int: _____
QRS: _____
Intrp: _____

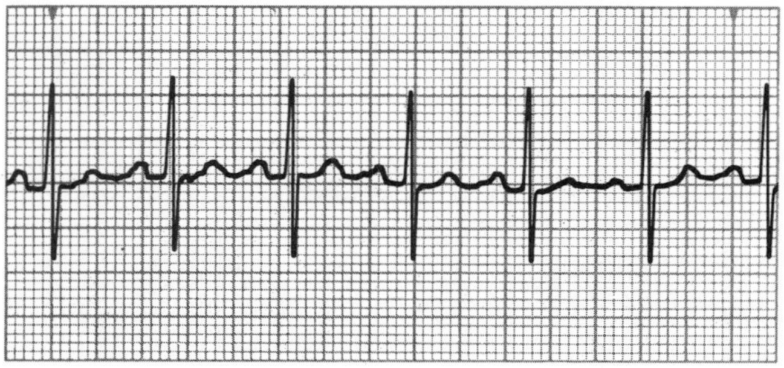

144

Rate: _____
Rhythm: _____
P Waves: _____
PR Int: _____
QRS: _____
Intrp: _____

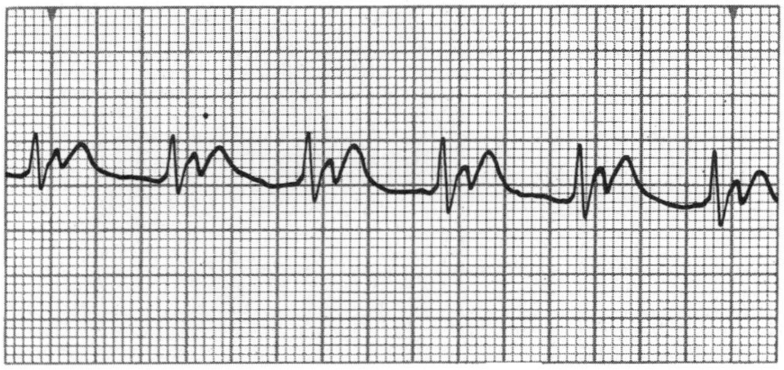

145

Rate: _____
Rhythm: _____
P Waves: _____
PR Int: _____
QRS: _____
Intrp: _____

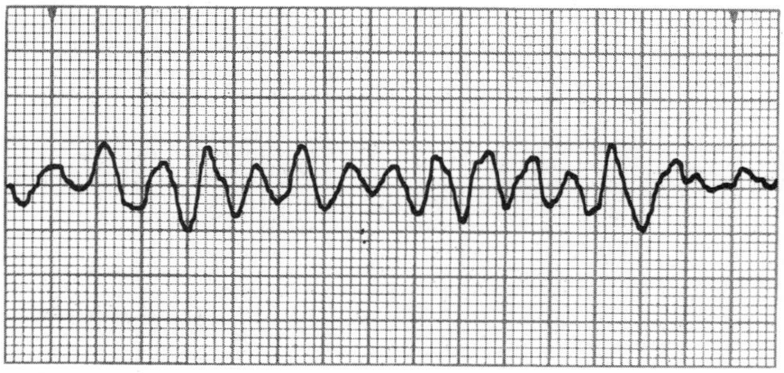

146

Rate: _____
Rhythm: _____
P Waves: _____
PR Int: _____
QRS: _____
Intrp: _____

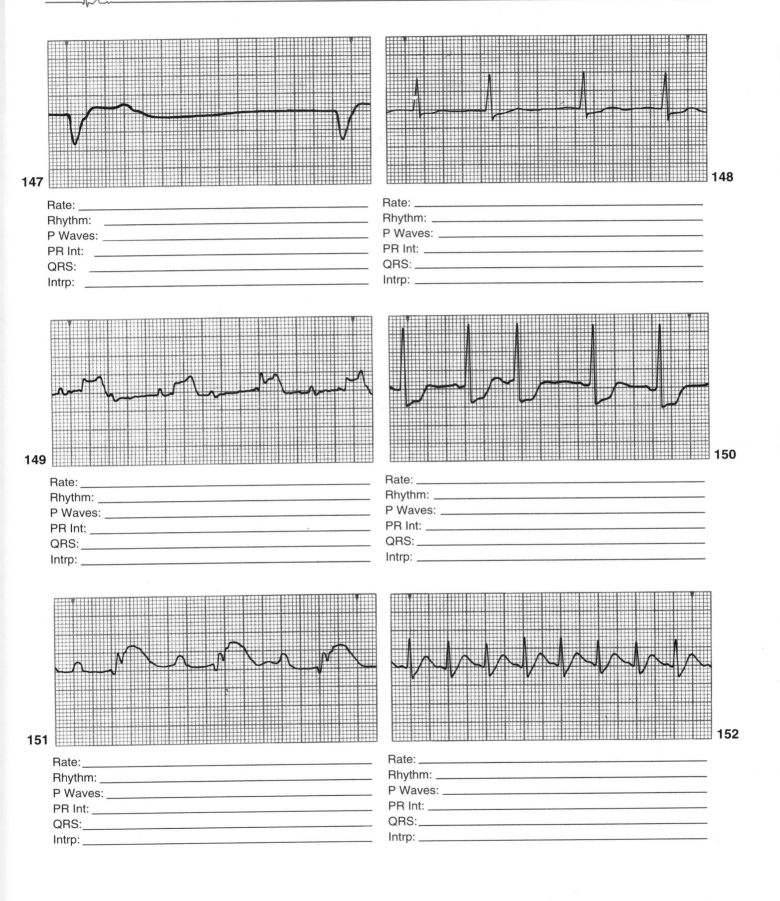

147

Rate: _____
Rhythm: _____
P Waves: _____
PR Int: _____
QRS: _____
Intrp: _____

148

Rate: _____
Rhythm: _____
P Waves: _____
PR Int: _____
QRS: _____
Intrp: _____

149

Rate: _____
Rhythm: _____
P Waves: _____
PR Int: _____
QRS: _____
Intrp: _____

150

Rate: _____
Rhythm: _____
P Waves: _____
PR Int: _____
QRS: _____
Intrp: _____

151

Rate: _____
Rhythm: _____
P Waves: _____
PR Int: _____
QRS: _____
Intrp: _____

152

Rate: _____
Rhythm: _____
P Waves: _____
PR Int: _____
QRS: _____
Intrp: _____

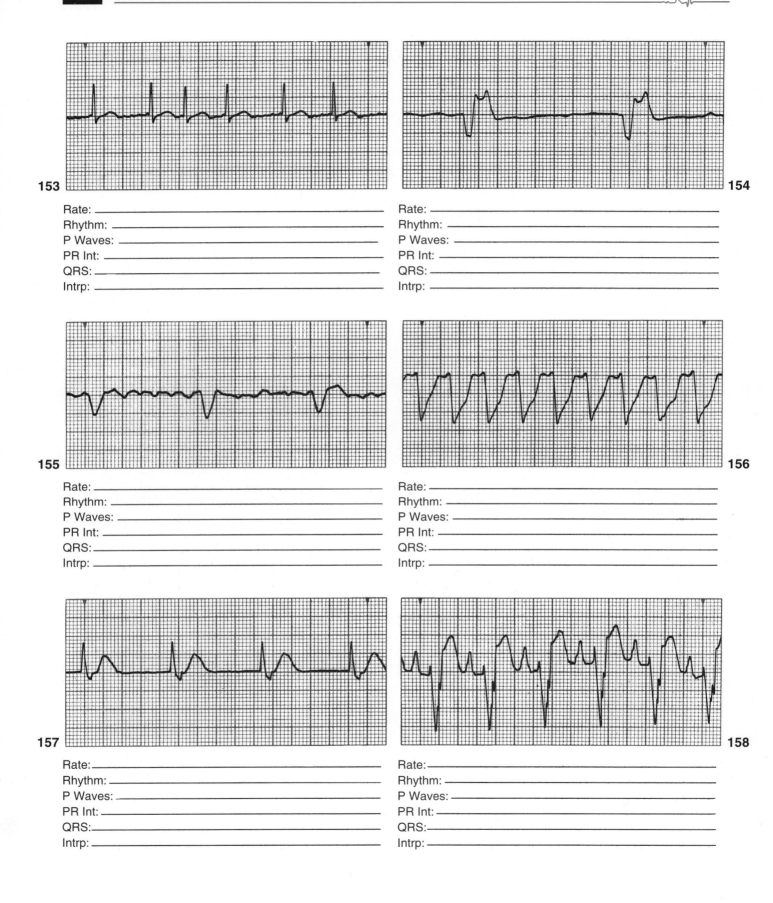

153

Rate: _____
Rhythm: _____
P Waves: _____
PR Int: _____
QRS: _____
Intrp: _____

154

Rate: _____
Rhythm: _____
P Waves: _____
PR Int: _____
QRS: _____
Intrp: _____

155

Rate: _____
Rhythm: _____
P Waves: _____
PR Int: _____
QRS: _____
Intrp: _____

156

Rate: _____
Rhythm: _____
P Waves: _____
PR Int: _____
QRS: _____
Intrp: _____

157

Rate: _____
Rhythm: _____
P Waves: _____
PR Int: _____
QRS: _____
Intrp: _____

158

Rate: _____
Rhythm: _____
P Waves: _____
PR Int: _____
QRS: _____
Intrp: _____

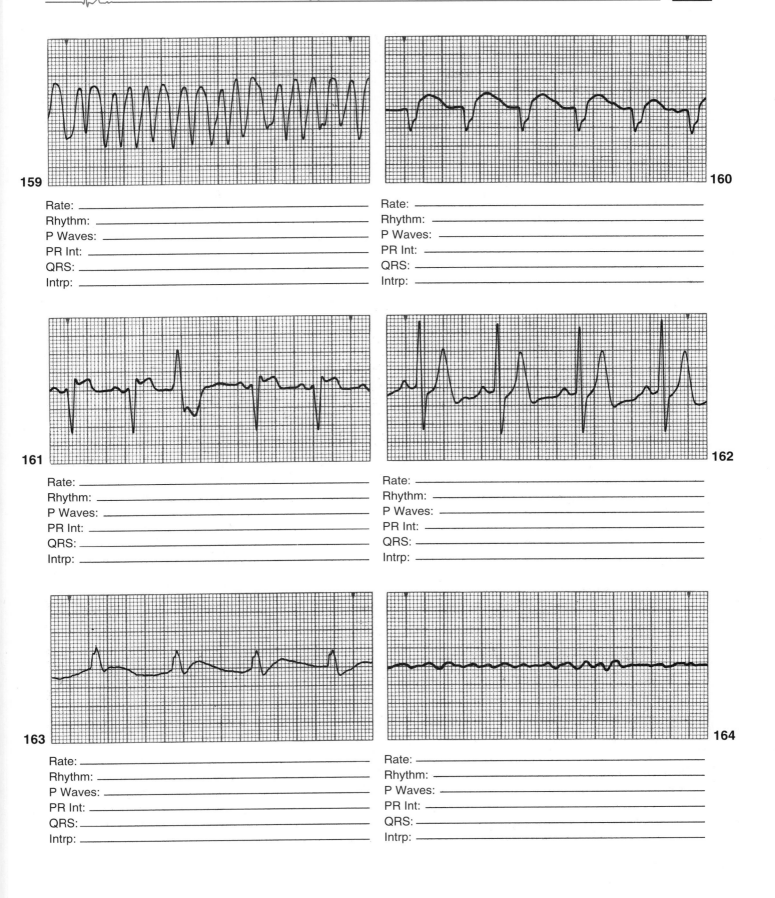

159

Rate: _____
Rhythm: _____
P Waves: _____
PR Int: _____
QRS: _____
Intrp: _____

160

Rate: _____
Rhythm: _____
P Waves: _____
PR Int: _____
QRS: _____
Intrp: _____

161

Rate: _____
Rhythm: _____
P Waves: _____
PR Int: _____
QRS: _____
Intrp: _____

162

Rate: _____
Rhythm: _____
P Waves: _____
PR Int: _____
QRS: _____
Intrp: _____

163

Rate: _____
Rhythm: _____
P Waves: _____
PR Int: _____
QRS: _____
Intrp: _____

164

Rate: _____
Rhythm: _____
P Waves: _____
PR Int: _____
QRS: _____
Intrp: _____

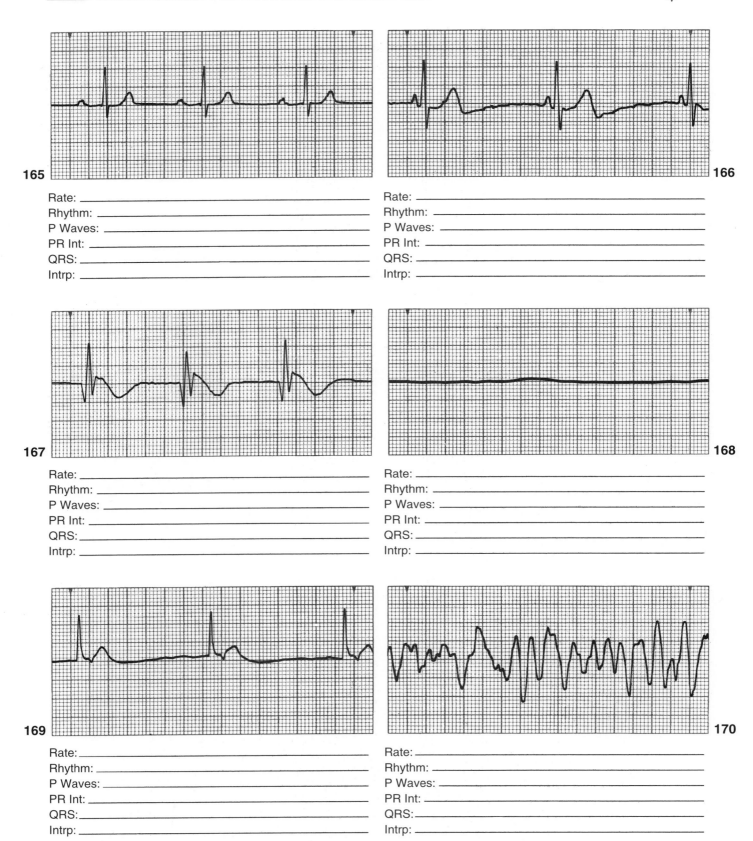

165

Rate: _____
Rhythm: _____
P Waves: _____
PR Int: _____
QRS: _____
Intrp: _____

166

Rate: _____
Rhythm: _____
P Waves: _____
PR Int: _____
QRS: _____
Intrp: _____

167

Rate: _____
Rhythm: _____
P Waves: _____
PR Int: _____
QRS: _____
Intrp: _____

168

Rate: _____
Rhythm: _____
P Waves: _____
PR Int: _____
QRS: _____
Intrp: _____

169

Rate: _____
Rhythm: _____
P Waves: _____
PR Int: _____
QRS: _____
Intrp: _____

170

Rate: _____
Rhythm: _____
P Waves: _____
PR Int: _____
QRS: _____
Intrp: _____

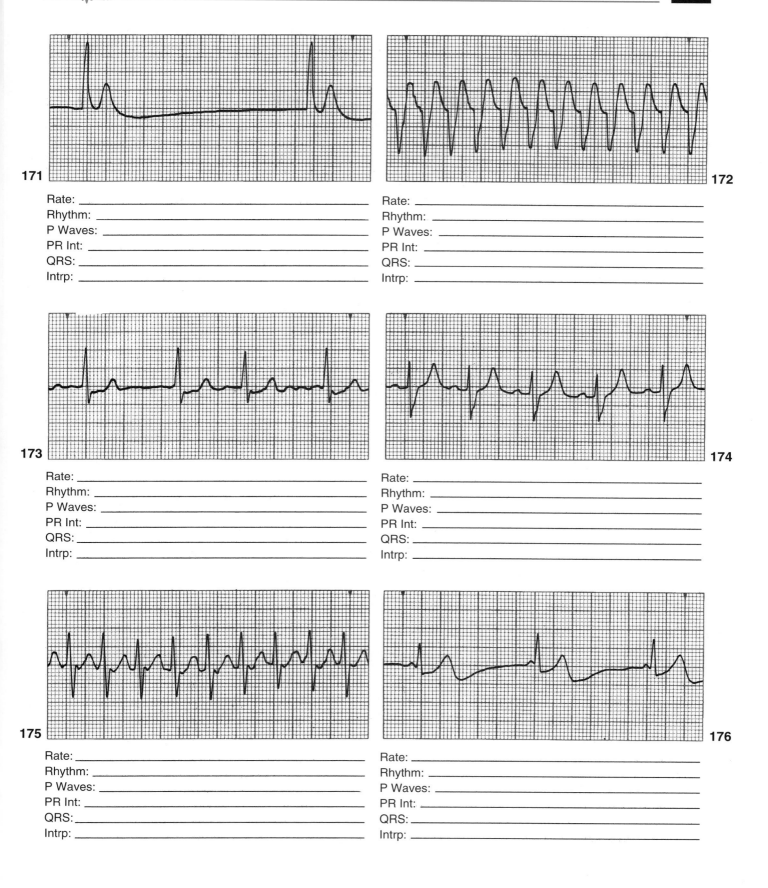

171

Rate: _____
Rhythm: _____
P Waves: _____
PR Int: _____
QRS: _____
Intrp: _____

172

Rate: _____
Rhythm: _____
P Waves: _____
PR Int: _____
QRS: _____
Intrp: _____

173

Rate: _____
Rhythm: _____
P Waves: _____
PR Int: _____
QRS: _____
Intrp: _____

174

Rate: _____
Rhythm: _____
P Waves: _____
PR Int: _____
QRS: _____
Intrp: _____

175

Rate: _____
Rhythm: _____
P Waves: _____
PR Int: _____
QRS: _____
Intrp: _____

176

Rate: _____
Rhythm: _____
P Waves: _____
PR Int: _____
QRS: _____
Intrp: _____

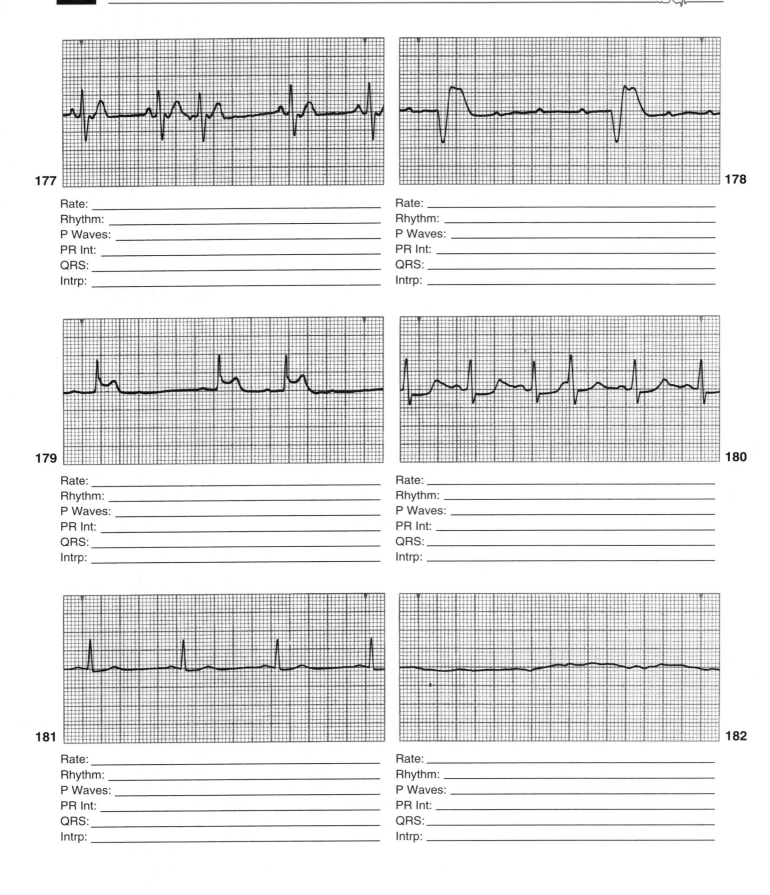

177

Rate: _____
Rhythm: _____
P Waves: _____
PR Int: _____
QRS: _____
Intrp: _____

178

Rate: _____
Rhythm: _____
P Waves: _____
PR Int: _____
QRS: _____
Intrp: _____

179

Rate: _____
Rhythm: _____
P Waves: _____
PR Int: _____
QRS: _____
Intrp: _____

180

Rate: _____
Rhythm: _____
P Waves: _____
PR Int: _____
QRS: _____
Intrp: _____

181

Rate: _____
Rhythm: _____
P Waves: _____
PR Int: _____
QRS: _____
Intrp: _____

182

Rate: _____
Rhythm: _____
P Waves: _____
PR Int: _____
QRS: _____
Intrp: _____

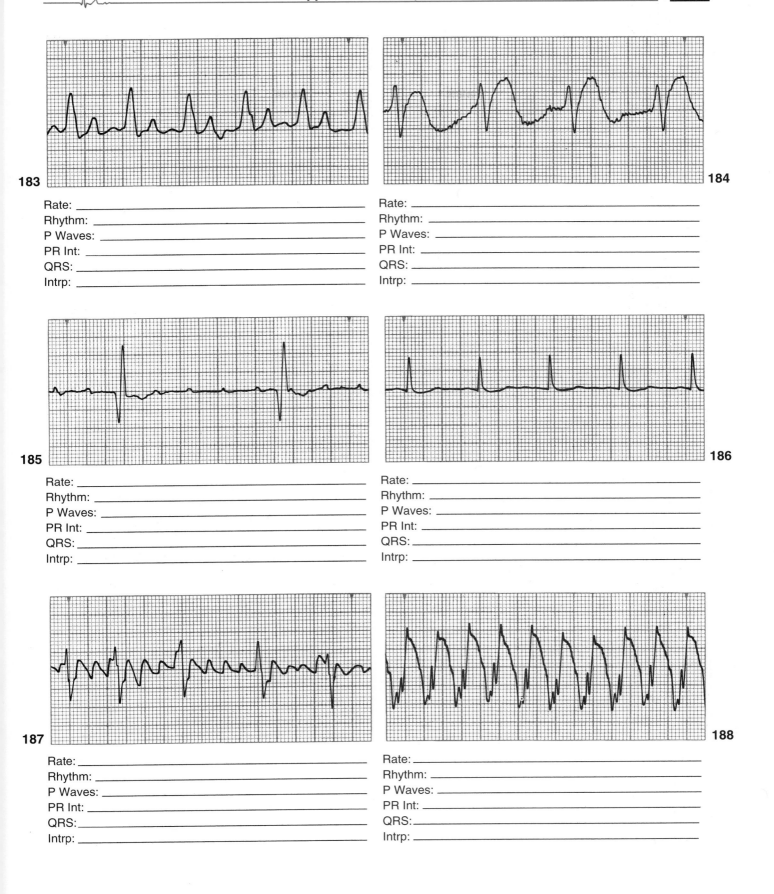

183

Rate: _____
Rhythm: _____
P Waves: _____
PR Int: _____
QRS: _____
Intrp: _____

184

Rate: _____
Rhythm: _____
P Waves: _____
PR Int: _____
QRS: _____
Intrp: _____

185

Rate: _____
Rhythm: _____
P Waves: _____
PR Int: _____
QRS: _____
Intrp: _____

186

Rate: _____
Rhythm: _____
P Waves: _____
PR Int: _____
QRS: _____
Intrp: _____

187

Rate: _____
Rhythm: _____
P Waves: _____
PR Int: _____
QRS: _____
Intrp: _____

188

Rate: _____
Rhythm: _____
P Waves: _____
PR Int: _____
QRS: _____
Intrp: _____

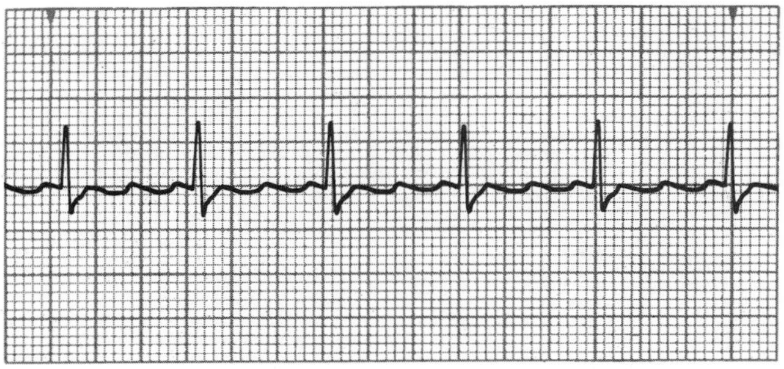

189

Rate: _____
Rhythm: _____
P Waves: _____
PR Int: _____
QRS: _____
Intrp: _____

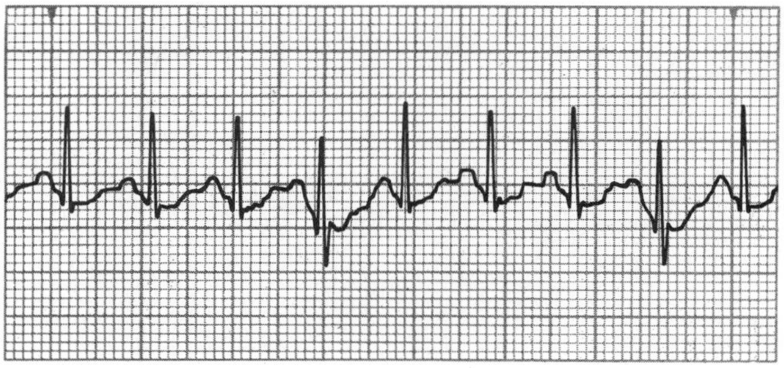

190

Rate: _____
Rhythm: _____
P Waves: _____
PR Int: _____
QRS: _____
Intrp: _____

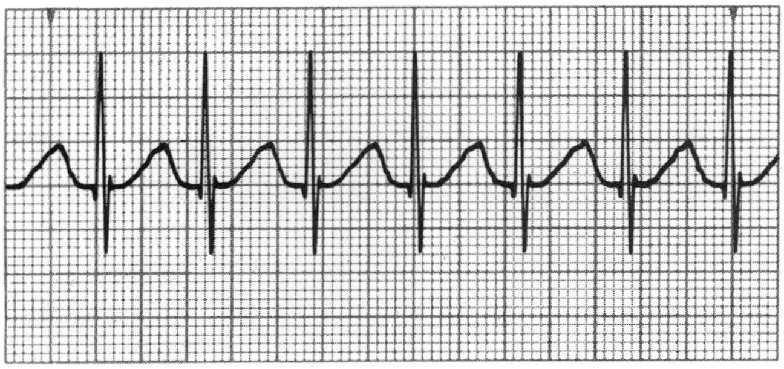

191

Rate: _____
Rhythm: _____
P Waves: _____
PR Int: _____
QRS: _____
Intrp: _____

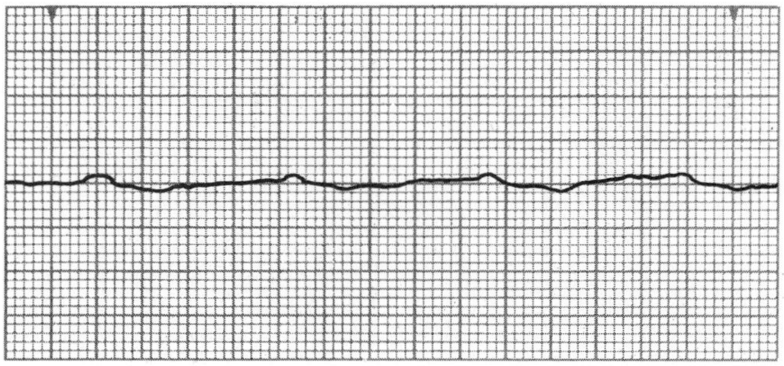

192

Rate: _____
Rhythm: _____
P Waves: _____
PR Int: _____
QRS: _____
Intrp: _____

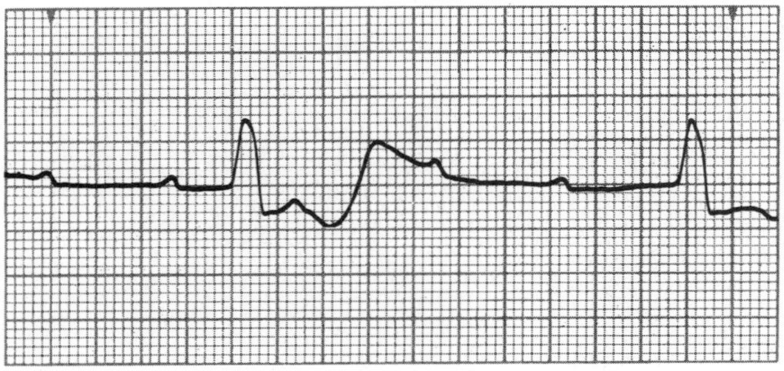

193

Rate: _____
Rhythm: _____
P Waves: _____
PR Int: _____
QRS: _____
Intrp: _____

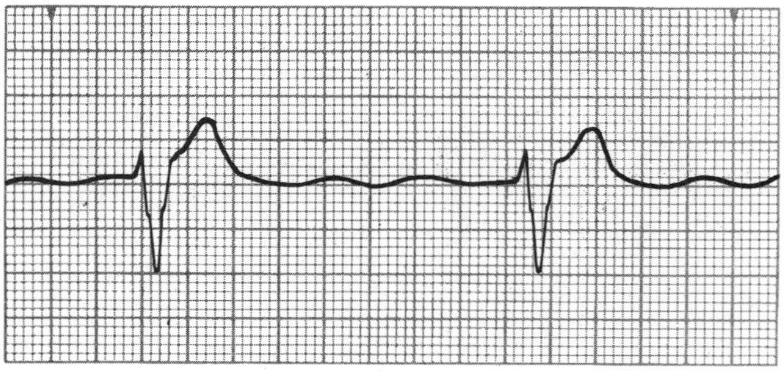

194

Rate: _____
Rhythm: _____
P Waves: _____
PR Int: _____
QRS: _____
Intrp: _____

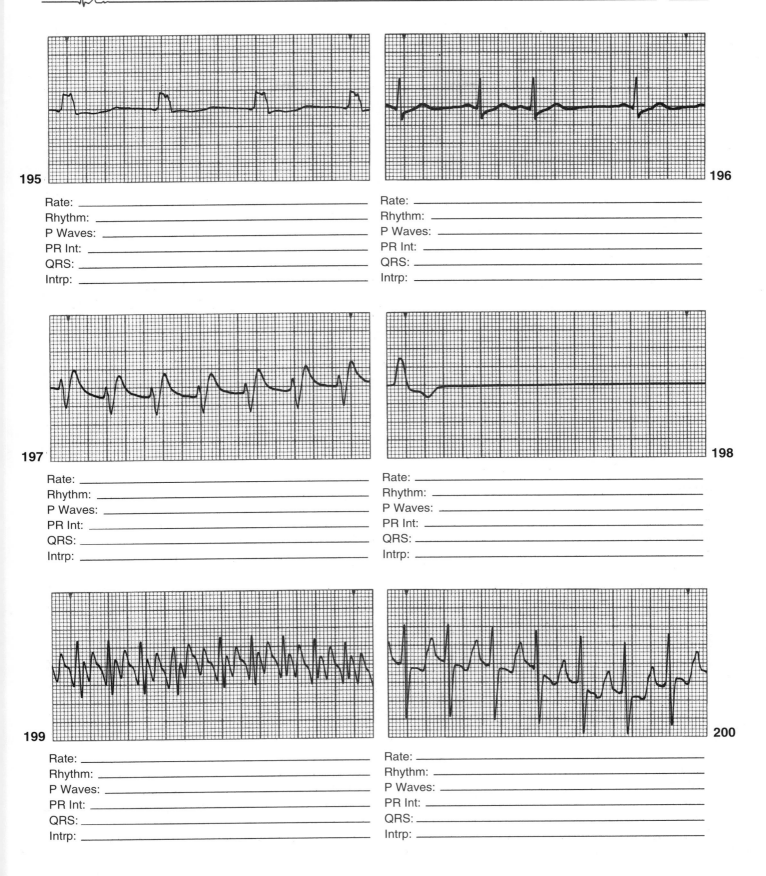

195

Rate: _____
Rhythm: _____
P Waves: _____
PR Int: _____
QRS: _____
Intrp: _____

196

Rate: _____
Rhythm: _____
P Waves: _____
PR Int: _____
QRS: _____
Intrp: _____

197

Rate: _____
Rhythm: _____
P Waves: _____
PR Int: _____
QRS: _____
Intrp: _____

198

Rate: _____
Rhythm: _____
P Waves: _____
PR Int: _____
QRS: _____
Intrp: _____

199

Rate: _____
Rhythm: _____
P Waves: _____
PR Int: _____
QRS: _____
Intrp: _____

200

Rate: _____
Rhythm: _____
P Waves: _____
PR Int: _____
QRS: _____
Intrp: _____

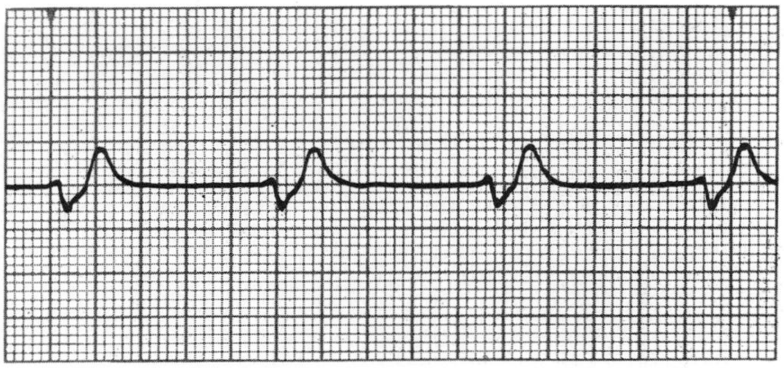

201

Rate: _____

Rhythm: _____

P Waves: _____

PR Int: _____

QRS: _____

Intrp: _____

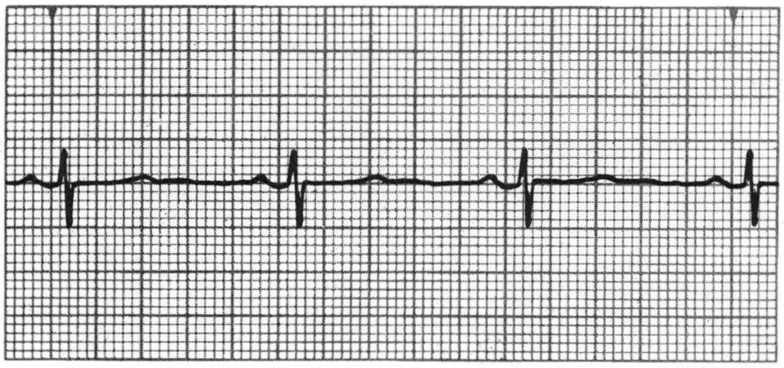

202

Rate: _____

Rhythm: _____

P Waves: _____

PR Int: _____

QRS: _____

Intrp: _____

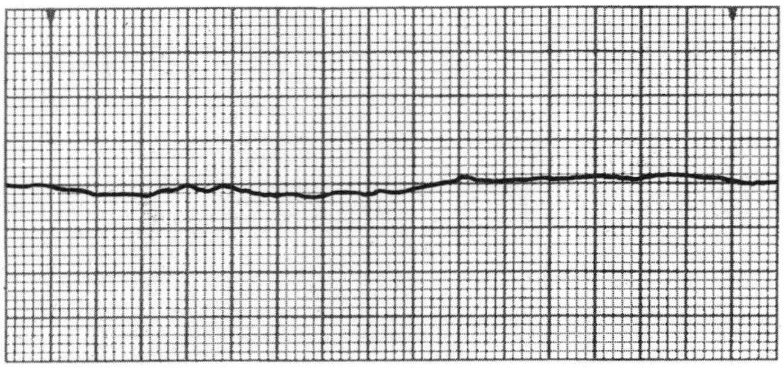

203

Rate: _____

Rhythm: _____

P Waves: _____

PR Int: _____

QRS: _____

Intrp: _____

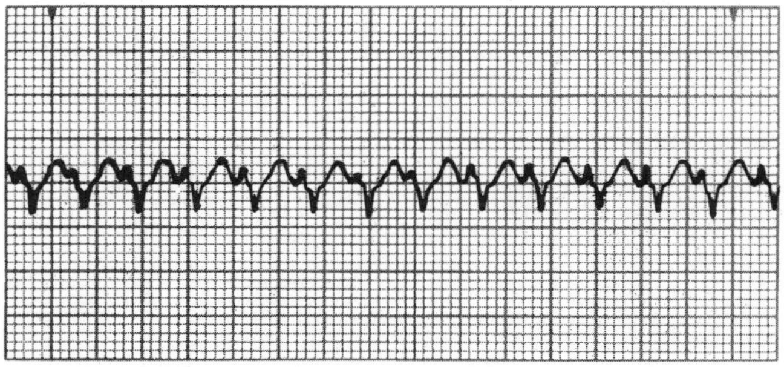

204

Rate: _____

Rhythm: _____

P Waves: _____

PR Int: _____

QRS: _____

Intrp: _____

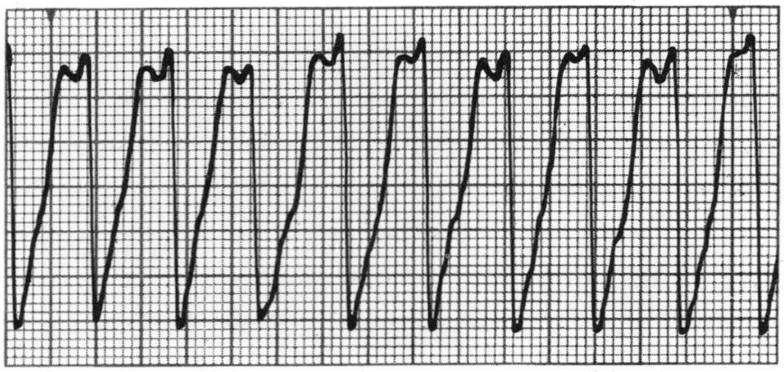

205

Rate: _____

Rhythm: _____

P Waves: _____

PR Int: _____

QRS: _____

Intrp: _____

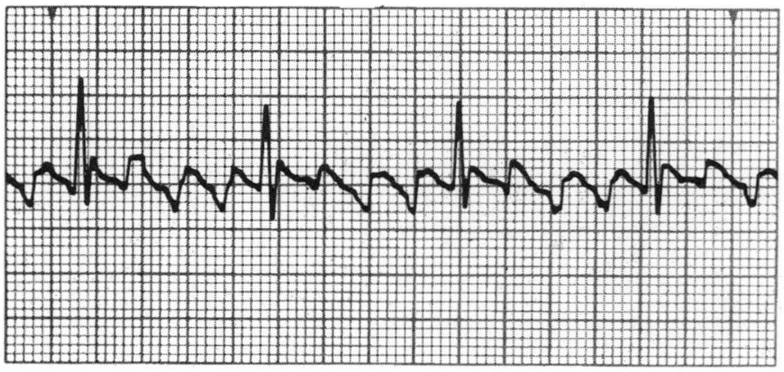

206

Rate: _____

Rhythm: _____

P Waves: _____

PR Int: _____

QRS: _____

Intrp: _____

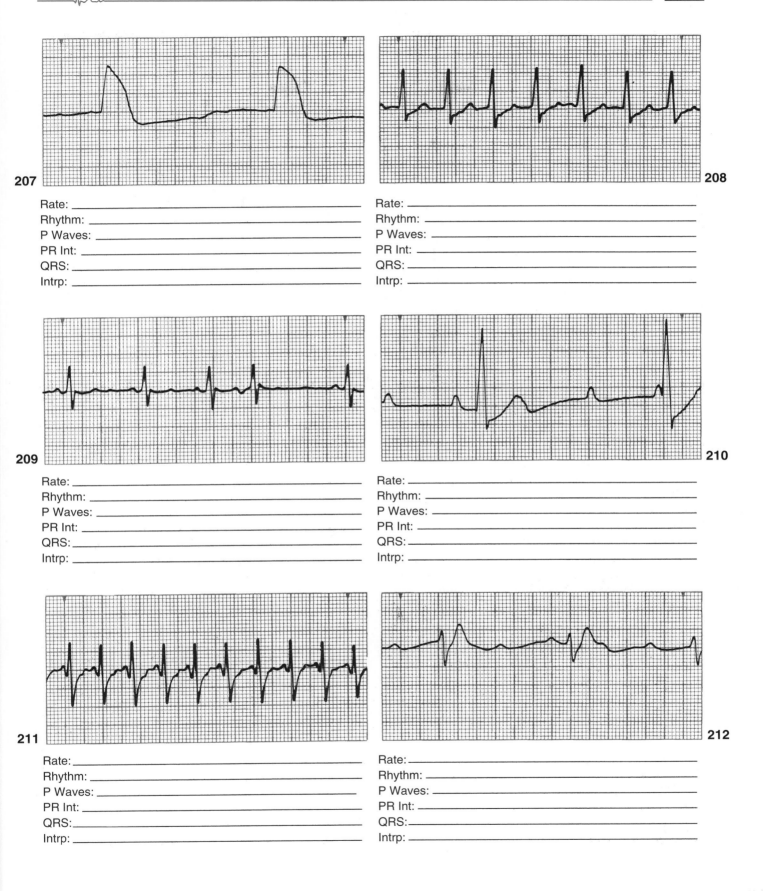

207

Rate: _____
Rhythm: _____
P Waves: _____
PR Int: _____
QRS: _____
Intrp: _____

208

Rate: _____
Rhythm: _____
P Waves: _____
PR Int: _____
QRS: _____
Intrp: _____

209

Rate: _____
Rhythm: _____
P Waves: _____
PR Int: _____
QRS: _____
Intrp: _____

210

Rate: _____
Rhythm: _____
P Waves: _____
PR Int: _____
QRS: _____
Intrp: _____

211

Rate: _____
Rhythm: _____
P Waves: _____
PR Int: _____
QRS: _____
Intrp: _____

212

Rate: _____
Rhythm: _____
P Waves: _____
PR Int: _____
QRS: _____
Intrp: _____

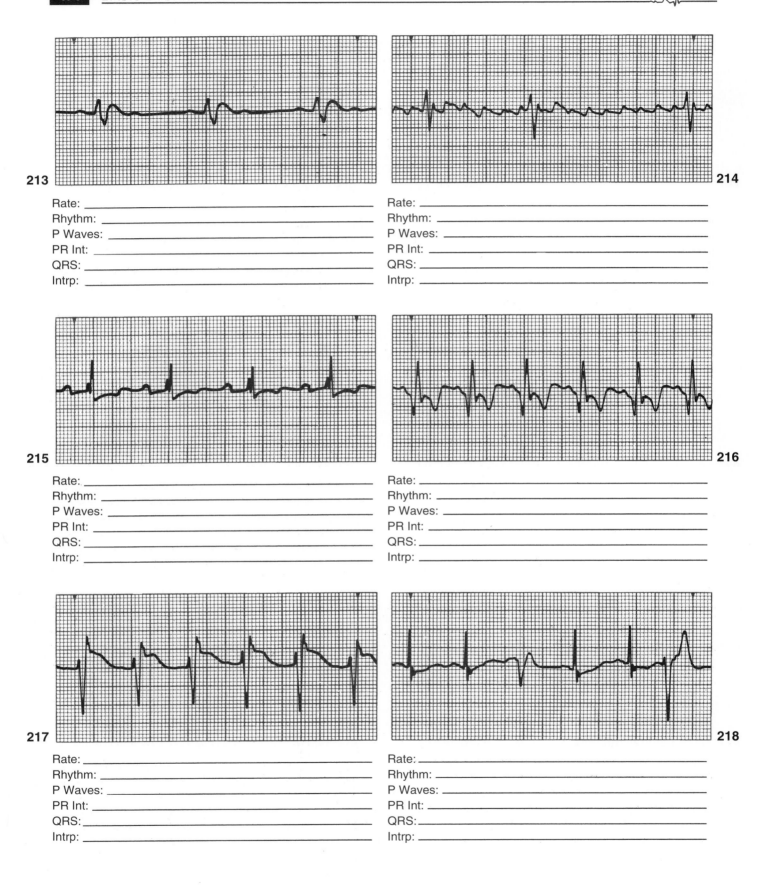

213

Rate: _____
Rhythm: _____
P Waves: _____
PR Int: _____
QRS: _____
Intrp: _____

214

Rate: _____
Rhythm: _____
P Waves: _____
PR Int: _____
QRS: _____
Intrp: _____

215

Rate: _____
Rhythm: _____
P Waves: _____
PR Int: _____
QRS: _____
Intrp: _____

216

Rate: _____
Rhythm: _____
P Waves: _____
PR Int: _____
QRS: _____
Intrp: _____

217

Rate: _____
Rhythm: _____
P Waves: _____
PR Int: _____
QRS: _____
Intrp: _____

218

Rate: _____
Rhythm: _____
P Waves: _____
PR Int: _____
QRS: _____
Intrp: _____

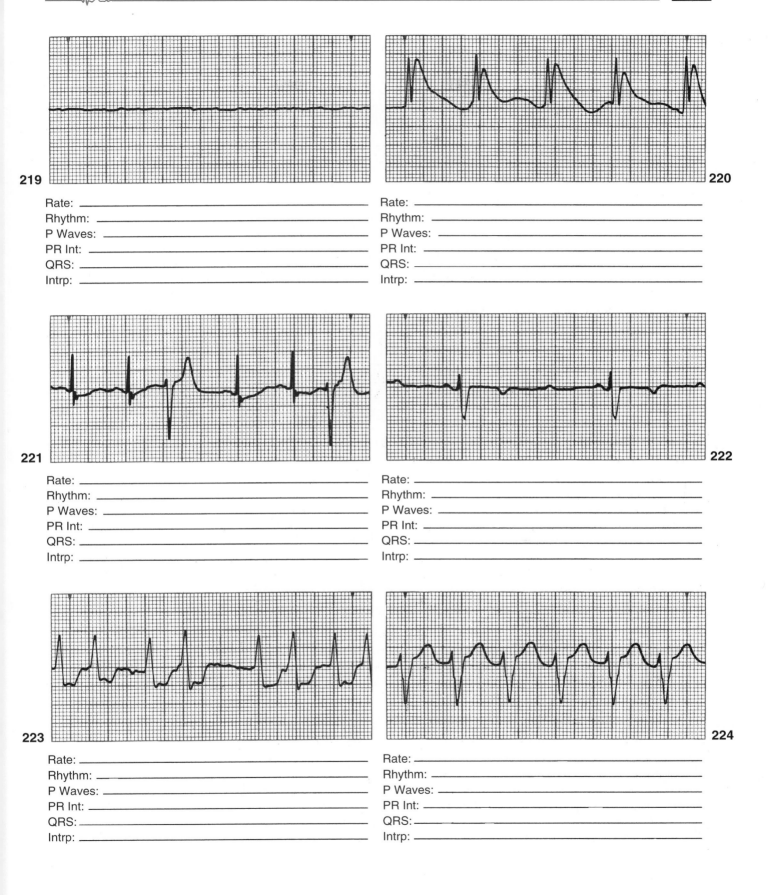

219

Rate: _____
Rhythm: _____
P Waves: _____
PR Int: _____
QRS: _____
Intrp: _____

220

Rate: _____
Rhythm: _____
P Waves: _____
PR Int: _____
QRS: _____
Intrp: _____

221

Rate: _____
Rhythm: _____
P Waves: _____
PR Int: _____
QRS: _____
Intrp: _____

222

Rate: _____
Rhythm: _____
P Waves: _____
PR Int: _____
QRS: _____
Intrp: _____

223

Rate: _____
Rhythm: _____
P Waves: _____
PR Int: _____
QRS: _____
Intrp: _____

224

Rate: _____
Rhythm: _____
P Waves: _____
PR Int: _____
QRS: _____
Intrp: _____

II. Bundle Branch and Fascicular Blocks

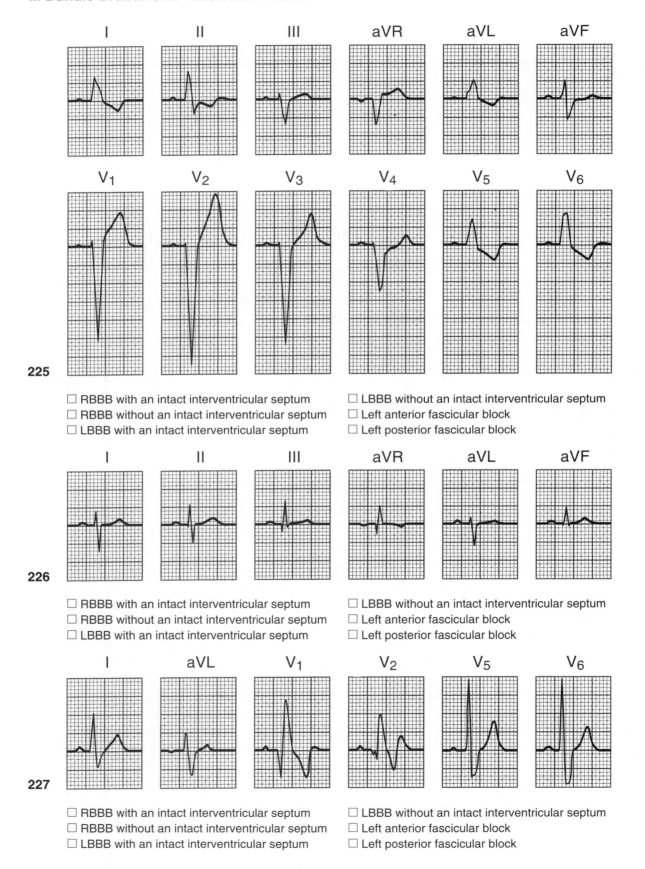

225

- ☐ RBBB with an intact interventricular septum
- ☐ RBBB without an intact interventricular septum
- ☐ LBBB with an intact interventricular septum
- ☐ LBBB without an intact interventricular septum
- ☐ Left anterior fascicular block
- ☐ Left posterior fascicular block

226

- ☐ RBBB with an intact interventricular septum
- ☐ RBBB without an intact interventricular septum
- ☐ LBBB with an intact interventricular septum
- ☐ LBBB without an intact interventricular septum
- ☐ Left anterior fascicular block
- ☐ Left posterior fascicular block

227

- ☐ RBBB with an intact interventricular septum
- ☐ RBBB without an intact interventricular septum
- ☐ LBBB with an intact interventricular septum
- ☐ LBBB without an intact interventricular septum
- ☐ Left anterior fascicular block
- ☐ Left posterior fascicular block

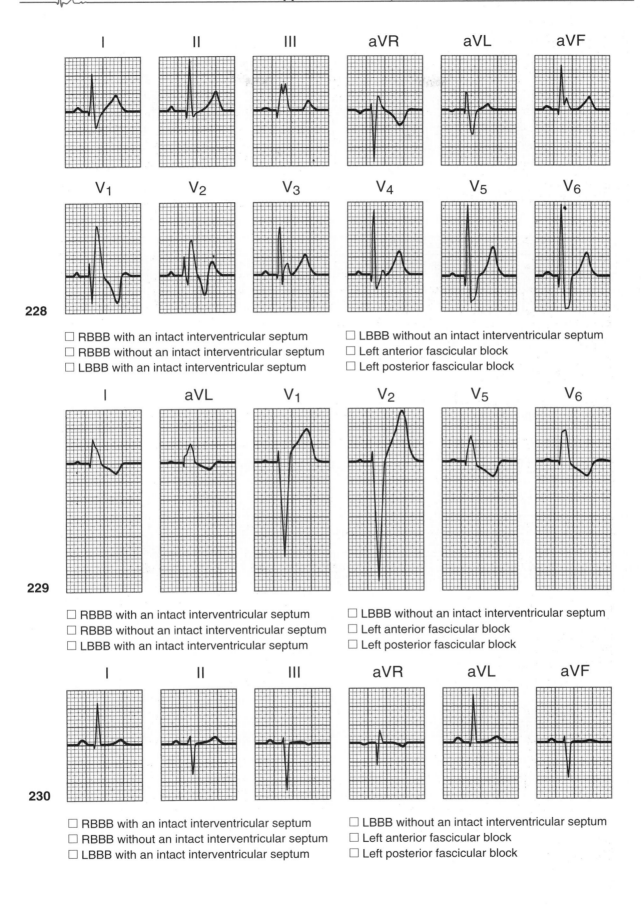

I   II   III   aVR   aVL   aVF

V₁   V₂   V₃   V₄   V₅   V₆

228

☐ RBBB with an intact interventricular septum
☐ RBBB without an intact interventricular septum
☐ LBBB with an intact interventricular septum

☐ LBBB without an intact interventricular septum
☐ Left anterior fascicular block
☐ Left posterior fascicular block

I   aVL   V₁   V₂   V₅   V₆

229

☐ RBBB with an intact interventricular septum
☐ RBBB without an intact interventricular septum
☐ LBBB with an intact interventricular septum

☐ LBBB without an intact interventricular septum
☐ Left anterior fascicular block
☐ Left posterior fascicular block

I   II   III   aVR   aVL   aVF

230

☐ RBBB with an intact interventricular septum
☐ RBBB without an intact interventricular septum
☐ LBBB with an intact interventricular septum

☐ LBBB without an intact interventricular septum
☐ Left anterior fascicular block
☐ Left posterior fascicular block

III. Myocardial Infarctions

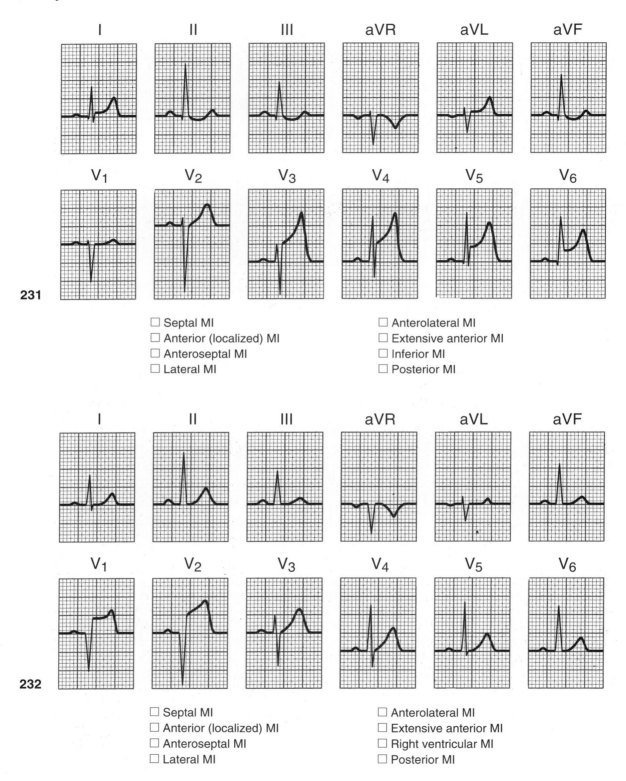

231

- ☐ Septal MI
- ☐ Anterior (localized) MI
- ☐ Anteroseptal MI
- ☐ Lateral MI

- ☐ Anterolateral MI
- ☐ Extensive anterior MI
- ☐ Inferior MI
- ☐ Posterior MI

232

- ☐ Septal MI
- ☐ Anterior (localized) MI
- ☐ Anteroseptal MI
- ☐ Lateral MI

- ☐ Anterolateral MI
- ☐ Extensive anterior MI
- ☐ Right ventricular MI
- ☐ Posterior MI

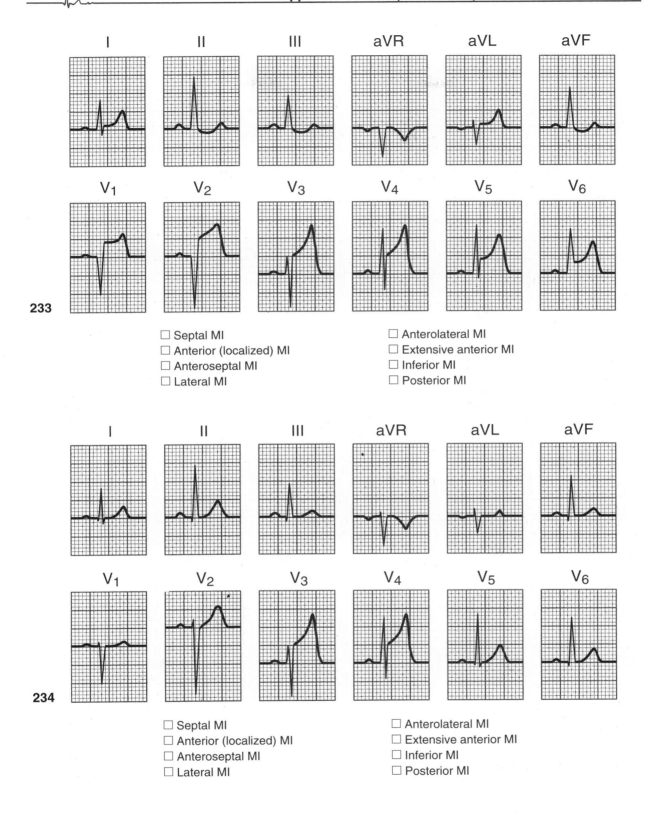

233

- ☐ Septal MI
- ☐ Anterior (localized) MI
- ☐ Anteroseptal MI
- ☐ Lateral MI

- ☐ Anterolateral MI
- ☐ Extensive anterior MI
- ☐ Inferior MI
- ☐ Posterior MI

234

- ☐ Septal MI
- ☐ Anterior (localized) MI
- ☐ Anteroseptal MI
- ☐ Lateral MI

- ☐ Anterolateral MI
- ☐ Extensive anterior MI
- ☐ Inferior MI
- ☐ Posterior MI

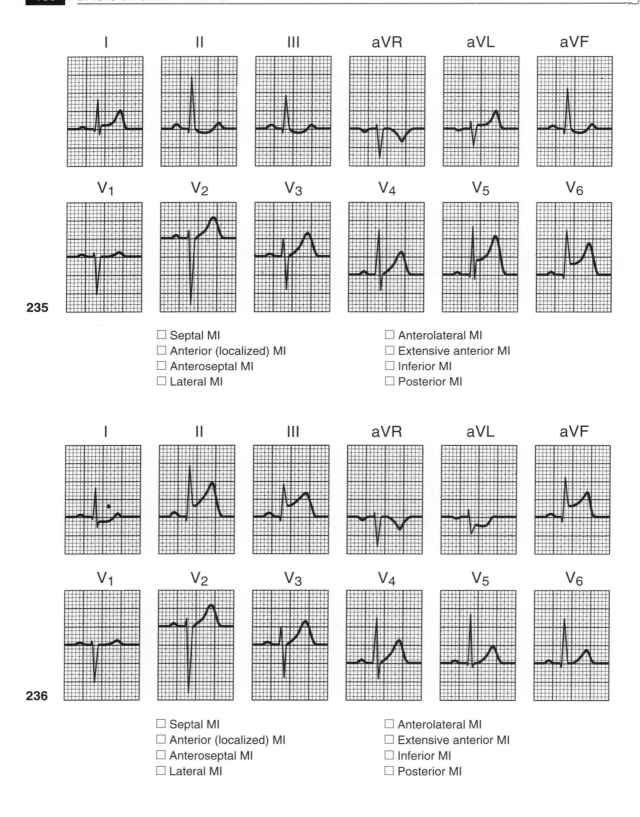

235

☐ Septal MI

☐ Anterior (localized) MI

☐ Anteroseptal MI

☐ Lateral MI

☐ Anterolateral MI

☐ Extensive anterior MI

☐ Inferior MI

☐ Posterior MI

236

☐ Septal MI

☐ Anterior (localized) MI

☐ Anteroseptal MI

☐ Lateral MI

☐ Anterolateral MI

☐ Extensive anterior MI

☐ Inferior MI

☐ Posterior MI

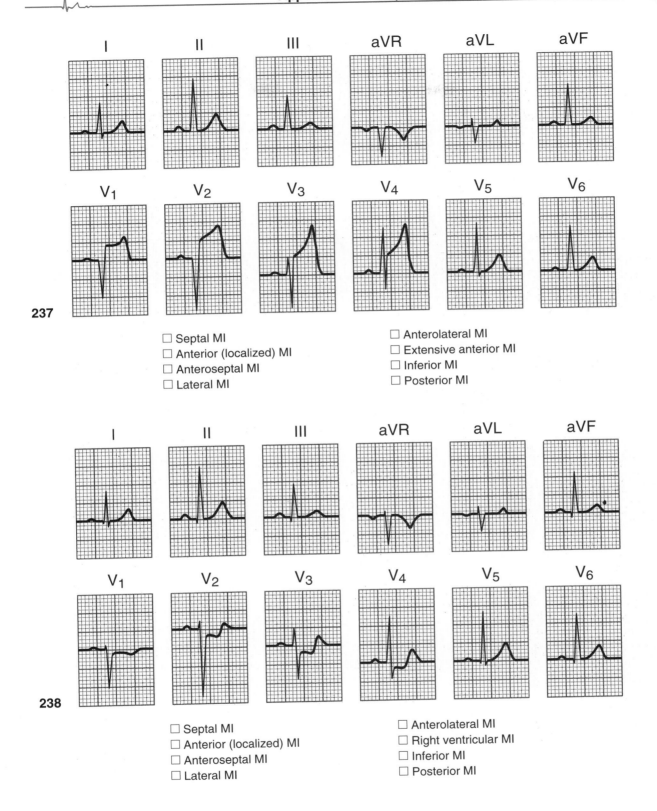

237

□ Septal MI
□ Anterior (localized) MI
□ Anteroseptal MI
□ Lateral MI

□ Anterolateral MI
□ Extensive anterior MI
□ Inferior MI
□ Posterior MI

238

□ Septal MI
□ Anterior (localized) MI
□ Anteroseptal MI
□ Lateral MI

□ Anterolateral MI
□ Right ventricular MI
□ Inferior MI
□ Posterior MI

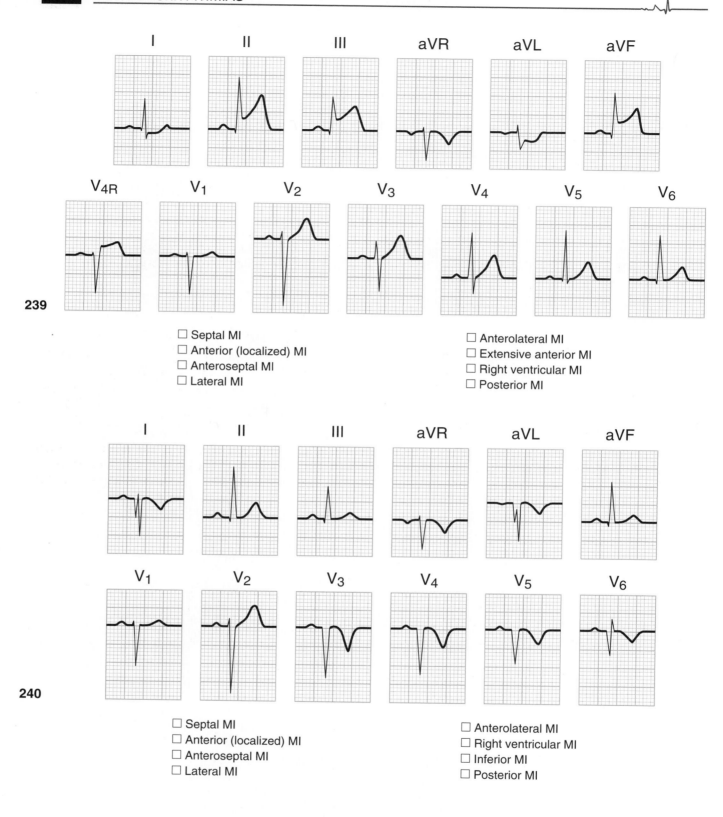

I   II   III   aVR   aVL   aVF

V₄R   V₁   V₂   V₃   V₄   V₅   V₆

239

☐ Septal MI
☐ Anterior (localized) MI
☐ Anteroseptal MI
☐ Lateral MI

☐ Anterolateral MI
☐ Extensive anterior MI
☐ Right ventricular MI
☐ Posterior MI

I   II   III   aVR   aVL   aVF

V₁   V₂   V₃   V₄   V₅   V₆

240

☐ Septal MI
☐ Anterior (localized) MI
☐ Anteroseptal MI
☐ Lateral MI

☐ Anterolateral MI
☐ Right ventricular MI
☐ Inferior MI
☐ Posterior MI

IV. QRS Axes

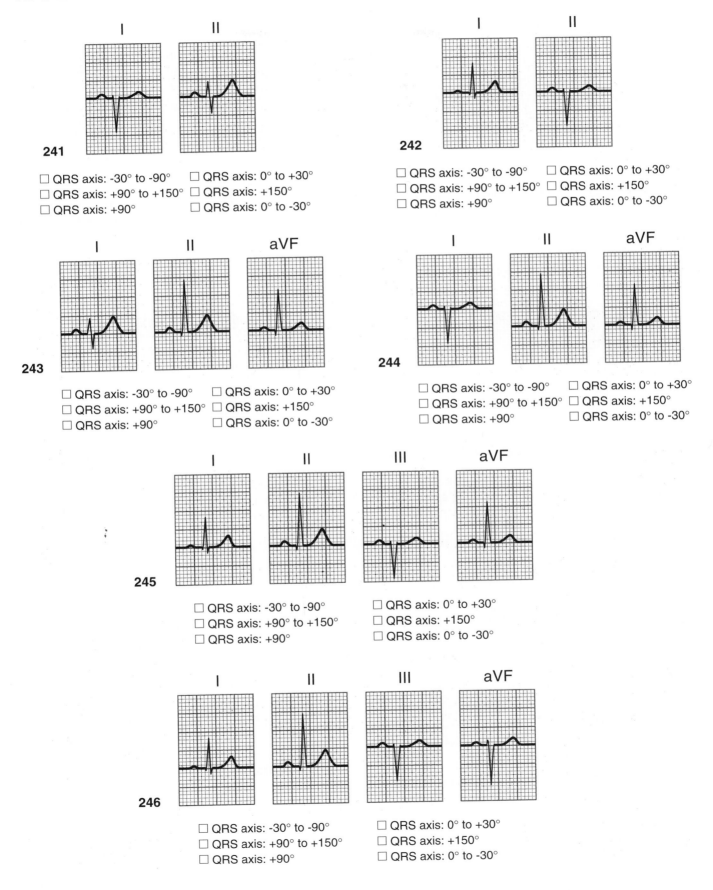

241

☐ QRS axis: -30° to -90°   ☐ QRS axis: 0° to +30°
☐ QRS axis: +90° to +150°   ☐ QRS axis: +150°
☐ QRS axis: +90°   ☐ QRS axis: 0° to -30°

242

☐ QRS axis: -30° to -90°   ☐ QRS axis: 0° to +30°
☐ QRS axis: +90° to +150°   ☐ QRS axis: +150°
☐ QRS axis: +90°   ☐ QRS axis: 0° to -30°

243

☐ QRS axis: -30° to -90°   ☐ QRS axis: 0° to +30°
☐ QRS axis: +90° to +150°   ☐ QRS axis: +150°
☐ QRS axis: +90°   ☐ QRS axis: 0° to -30°

244

☐ QRS axis: -30° to -90°   ☐ QRS axis: 0° to +30°
☐ QRS axis: +90° to +150°   ☐ QRS axis: +150°
☐ QRS axis: +90°   ☐ QRS axis: 0° to -30°

245

☐ QRS axis: -30° to -90°   ☐ QRS axis: 0° to +30°
☐ QRS axis: +90° to +150°   ☐ QRS axis: +150°
☐ QRS axis: +90°   ☐ QRS axis: 0° to -30°

246

☐ QRS axis: -30° to -90°   ☐ QRS axis: 0° to +30°
☐ QRS axis: +90° to +150°   ☐ QRS axis: +150°
☐ QRS axis: +90°   ☐ QRS axis: 0° to -30°

V. ECG Changes: Drug and Electrolyte

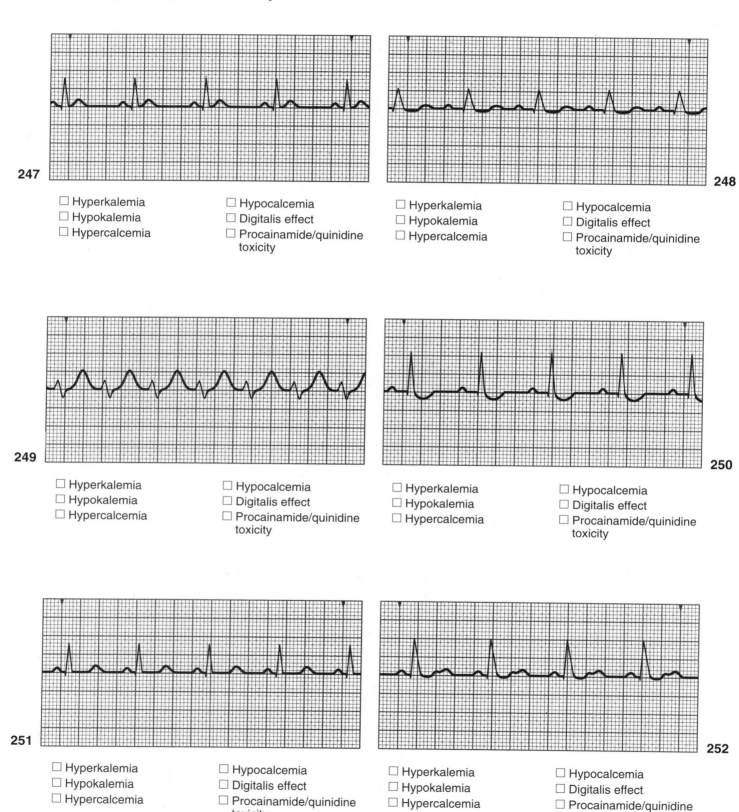

247

☐ Hyperkalemia   ☐ Hypocalcemia
☐ Hypokalemia   ☐ Digitalis effect
☐ Hypercalcemia   ☐ Procainamide/quinidine
                       toxicity

248

☐ Hyperkalemia   ☐ Hypocalcemia
☐ Hypokalemia   ☐ Digitalis effect
☐ Hypercalcemia   ☐ Procainamide/quinidine
                       toxicity

249

☐ Hyperkalemia   ☐ Hypocalcemia
☐ Hypokalemia   ☐ Digitalis effect
☐ Hypercalcemia   ☐ Procainamide/quinidine
                       toxicity

250

☐ Hyperkalemia   ☐ Hypocalcemia
☐ Hypokalemia   ☐ Digitalis effect
☐ Hypercalcemia   ☐ Procainamide/quinidine
                       toxicity

251

☐ Hyperkalemia   ☐ Hypocalcemia
☐ Hypokalemia   ☐ Digitalis effect
☐ Hypercalcemia   ☐ Procainamide/quinidine
                       toxicity

252

☐ Hyperkalemia   ☐ Hypocalcemia
☐ Hypokalemia   ☐ Digitalis effect
☐ Hypercalcemia   ☐ Procainamide/quinidine
                       toxicity

VI. ECG Changes: Miscellaneous

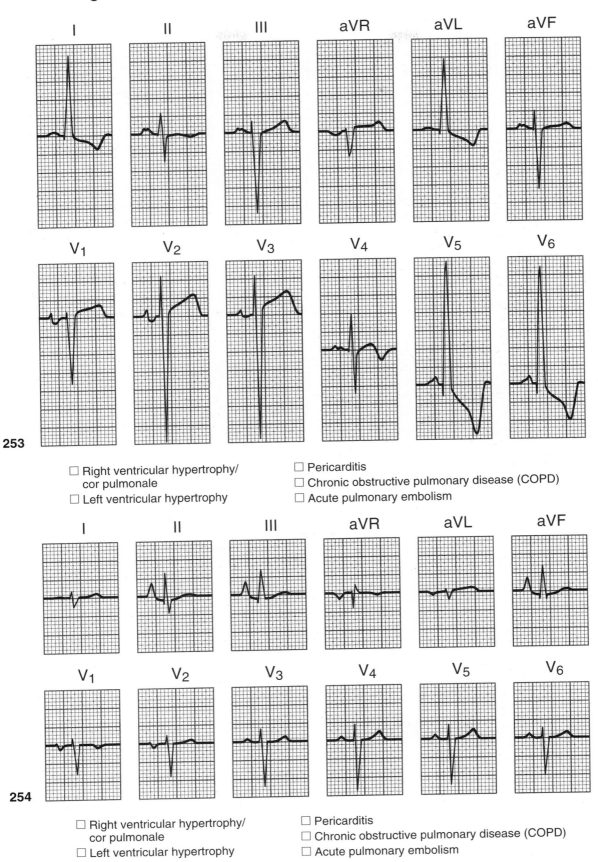

253

☐ Right ventricular hypertrophy/
   cor pulmonale
☐ Left ventricular hypertrophy

☐ Pericarditis
☐ Chronic obstructive pulmonary disease (COPD)
☐ Acute pulmonary embolism

254

☐ Right ventricular hypertrophy/
   cor pulmonale
☐ Left ventricular hypertrophy

☐ Pericarditis
☐ Chronic obstructive pulmonary disease (COPD)
☐ Acute pulmonary embolism

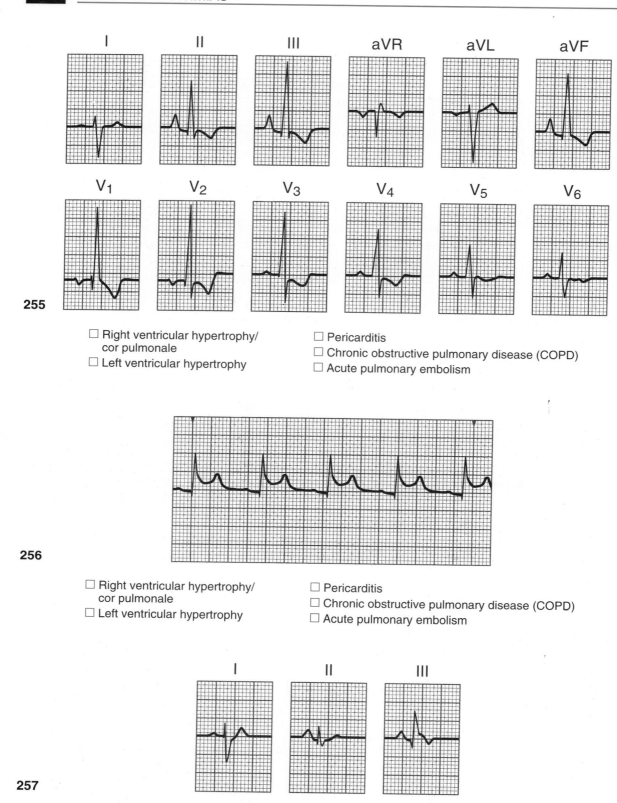

255

- ☐ Right ventricular hypertrophy/ cor pulmonale
- ☐ Left ventricular hypertrophy

- ☐ Pericarditis
- ☐ Chronic obstructive pulmonary disease (COPD)
- ☐ Acute pulmonary embolism

256

- ☐ Right ventricular hypertrophy/ cor pulmonale
- ☐ Left ventricular hypertrophy

- ☐ Pericarditis
- ☐ Chronic obstructive pulmonary disease (COPD)
- ☐ Acute pulmonary embolism

257

- ☐ Right ventricular hypertrophy/ cor pulmonale
- ☐ Left ventricular hypertrophy

- ☐ Pericarditis
- ☐ Chronic obstructive pulmonary disease (COPD)
- ☐ Acute pulmonary embolism

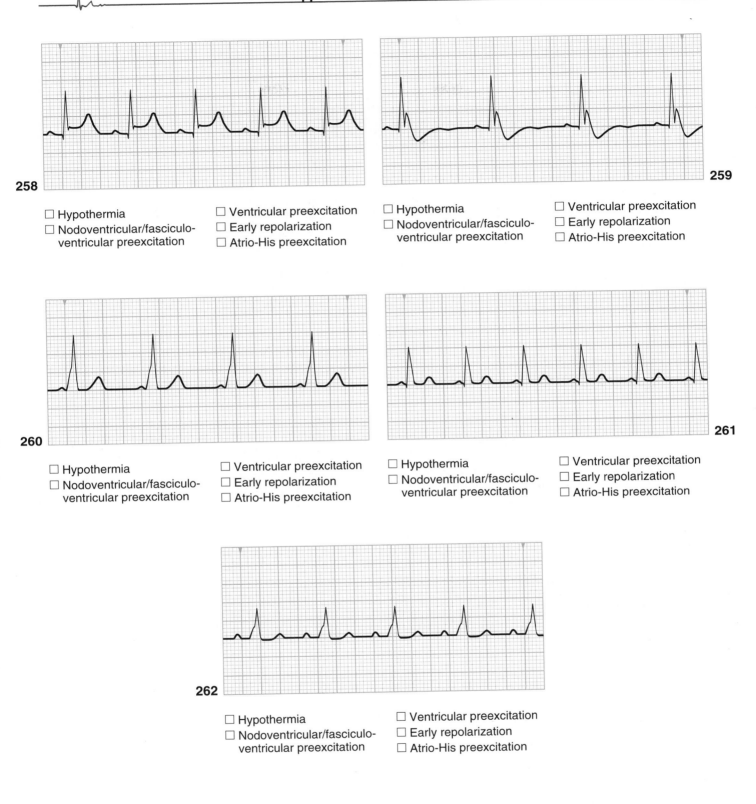

258

☐ Hypothermia
☐ Nodoventricular/fasciculo-
   ventricular preexcitation

☐ Ventricular preexcitation
☐ Early repolarization
☐ Atrio-His preexcitation

259

☐ Hypothermia
☐ Nodoventricular/fasciculo-
   ventricular preexcitation

☐ Ventricular preexcitation
☐ Early repolarization
☐ Atrio-His preexcitation

260

☐ Hypothermia
☐ Nodoventricular/fasciculo-
   ventricular preexcitation

☐ Ventricular preexcitation
☐ Early repolarization
☐ Atrio-His preexcitation

261

☐ Hypothermia
☐ Nodoventricular/fasciculo-
   ventricular preexcitation

☐ Ventricular preexcitation
☐ Early repolarization
☐ Atrio-His preexcitation

262

☐ Hypothermia
☐ Nodoventricular/fasciculo-
   ventricular preexcitation

☐ Ventricular preexcitation
☐ Early repolarization
☐ Atrio-His preexcitation

I. Arrhythmias

1. **Rate:** 126 beats/minute.†
   Rhythm: Irregular.
   P Waves: None; fine atrial fibrillation waves are present.
   PR Int: None.
   QRS: 0.10 second.
   Intrp: Atrial fibrillation (fine).

2. **Rate:** 33 beats/minute.
   Rhythm: Irregular.
   P Waves: Present; the first, second, third, and fifth P waves are followed by QRS complexes.
   PR Int: 0.22 to 0.36 second. The PR intervals progressively increase until a QRS complex fails to follow the P wave.
   QRS: 0.10 second.
   Intrp: Sinus rhythm with second-degree, Type I AV block (Wenckebach).

3. **Rate:** 41 beats/minute.
   Rhythm: Irregular.
   P Waves: Present; precede each QRS complex.
   PR Int: 0.16 second.
   QRS: 0.08 second.
   Intrp: Sinus bradycardia with sinus arrhythmia.

4. **Rate:** 170 beats/minute.
   Rhythm: Regular.
   P Waves: Present; precede each QRS complex.
   PR Int: 0.12 second.
   QRS: About 0.12 second.
   Intrp: Atrial tachycardia with wide QRS complexes.

5. **Rate:** 62 beats/minute.
   Rhythm: Irregular.
   P Waves: Present; precede the second, fourth, fifth, sixth, and seventh QRS complexes. The P waves are abnormal (0.16 second in duration and notched).
   PR Int: 0.26 second.
   QRS: 0.12 second (all QRS complexes except the third QRS complex); 0.14 second (third QRS complex).
   Intrp: Sinus rhythm with first-degree AV block, bundle branch block, and an isolated premature ventricular contraction.

6. **Rate:** 107 beats/minute.
   Rhythm: Irregular.
   P Waves: Present; precede all QRS complexes except the fifth, eighth, ninth, and tenth QRS complexes.
   PR Int: 0.16 second.
   QRS: 0.09 to 0.10 second.
   Intrp: Normal sinus rhythm with premature junctional contractions (fifth, eighth, ninth, and tenth QRS complexes) occurring singly and in group beats; the latter may be considered a short episode of junctional tachycardia.

7. **Rate:** 182 beats/minute.
   Rhythm: Regular.
   P Waves: Present; precede each QRS complex.
   PR Int: 0.08 second.
   QRS: 0.09 second.
   Intrp: Atrial tachycardia.

*Because of the possible distortion of the ECGs during printing, the measurement of the ECG components may vary slightly.
†The heart rates were calculated using R-R interval method 3.

8. **Rate:** Unmeasurable.
   Rhythm: Irregular.
   P Waves: None; coarse ventricular fibrillation waves are present.
   PR Int: None.
   QRS: None.
   Intrp: Ventricular fibrillation (coarse).
9. **Rate:** 89 beats/minute.
   Rhythm: Irregular.
   P Waves: Present; precede all except the third and sixth QRS complexes. The shape and direction of the P waves vary from positive to negative.
   PR Int: 0.6 to 0.12 second.
   QRS: 0.10 second (all QRS complexes except the third and sixth QRS complexes); 0.12 second (third and sixth QRS complexes).
   Intrp: Wandering atrial pacemaker with unifocal (uniform) premature ventricular contractions. Trigeminy is present in the first part of the tracing.
10. **Rate:** 61 beats/minute.
    Rhythm: Irregular.
    P Waves: Present; precede each QRS complex.
    PR Int: 0.12 second.
    QRS: 0.14 second.
    Intrp: Sinus arrhythmia with bundle branch block.
11. **Rate:** 89 beats/minute.
    Rhythm: Irregular.
    P Waves: Present; precede all QRS complexes except the second and eighth QRS complexes.
    PR Int: About 0.16 second.
    QRS: 0.08 second (all QRS complexes except the second and eighth QRS complexes); 0.12 second (second and eighth QRS complexes).
    Intrp: Normal sinus rhythm with isolated unifocal (uniform) premature ventricular contractions.
12. **Rate:** 145 beats/minute.
    Rhythm: Regular.
    P Waves: Present; precede each QRS complex.
    PR Int: About 0.10 second.
    QRS: 0.08 second.
    Intrp: Sinus tachycardia.

13. **Rate:** 87 beats/minute.
    Rhythm: Irregular.
    P Waves: Present; precede each QRS complex.
    PR Int: 0.18 second.
    QRS: 0.06 second.
    Intrp: Sinus arrhythmia.
14. **Rate:** 164 beats/minute.
    Rhythm: Regular.
    P Waves: None.
    PR Int: None.
    QRS: 0.12 second.
    Intrp: Ventricular tachycardia.
15. **Rate:** 74 beats/minute.
    Rhythm: Regular.
    P Waves: Present; precede each QRS complex; shape and direction vary from positive to negative.
    PR Int: 0.08 to 0.12 second.
    QRS: 0.08 second.
    Intrp: Wandering atrial pacemaker.
16. **Rate:** 70 beats/minute (atrial rate: 52 beats/minute).
    Rhythm: Regular.
    P Waves: Present, but have no set relation to the QRS complexes.
    PR Int: None.
    QRS: 0.14 second.
    Intrp: Accelerated idioventricular rhythm with AV dissociation.
17. **Rate:** 83 beats/minute.
    Rhythm: Regular.
    P Waves: Present; precede each QRS complex.
    PR Int: 0.16 second.
    QRS: 0.06 second.
    Intrp: Normal sinus rhythm.
18. **Rate:** 229 beats/minute.
    Rhythm: Regular.
    P Waves: None.
    PR Int: None.
    QRS: 0.12 second.
    Intrp: Ventricular tachycardia.
19. **Rate:** 26 beats/minute.
    Rhythm: Regular.
    P Waves: Present; the first, third, and fifth P waves are followed by QRS complexes. AV conduction ratio is 2:1.
    PR Int: 0.19 second.
    QRS: 0.10 second.
    Intrp: Sinus rhythm with second-shape, 2:1 AV block.

20. **Rate:** 84 beats/minute.
    Rhythm: Regular.
    P Waves: None; atrial flutter waves are present.
    PR Int: None.
    QRS: 0.10 second.
    Intrp: Atrial flutter.
21. **Rate:** 30 beats/minute.
    Rhythm: Regular.
    P Waves: Present; precede each QRS complex.
    PR Int: 0.17 to 0.18 second.
    QRS: 0.12 second.
    Intrp: Sinus bradycardia with bundle branch block.
22. **Rate:** 98 beats/minute.
    Rhythm: Regular.
    P Waves: Present; precede each QRS complex.
    PR Int: About 0.16 second.
    QRS: About 0.19 second.
    Intrp: Normal sinus rhythm with bundle branch block.
23. **Rate:** 62 beats/minute.
    Rhythm: Irregular.
    P Waves: Present; precede the first, second, third, and fifth QRS complexes.
    PR Int: 0.18 second.
    QRS: 0.12 second.
    Intrp: Normal sinus rhythm with bundle branch block and premature junctional contractions.
24. **Rate:** 82 beats/minute.
    Rhythm: Regular.
    P Waves: Present; precede each QRS complex. The P waves are abnormally wide.
    PR Int: 0.16 second.
    QRS: 0.16 second.
    Intrp: Normal sinus rhythm with bundle branch block.
25. **Rate:** 129 beats/minute.
    Rhythm: Irregular.
    P Waves: None; fine atrial fibrillation waves are present.
    PR Int: None.
    QRS: About 0.10 second.
    Intrp: Atrial fibrillation (fine).

26. **Rate:** 31 beats/minute.
    Rhythm: Irregular.
    P Waves: Present; a QRS complex follows the first, fifth, and tenth P waves. AV conduction ratios are 4:1 and 5:1.
    PR Int: 0.34 second.
    QRS: 0.16 second.
    Intrp: Sinus rhythm with second-degree, advanced AV block and bundle branch block.
27. **Rate:** 75 beats/minute.
    Rhythm: Regular.
    P Waves: Present; negative P waves precede each QRS complex.
    PR Int: 0.08 second.
    QRS: 0.08 second.
    Intrp: Accelerated junctional rhythm.
28. **Rate:** 62 beats/minute.
    Rhythm: Irregular. The R-R intervals between the third and fourth QRS complexes and the fifth and sixth QRS complexes are twice the R-R interval of the underlying sinus rhythm.
    P Waves: Present; precede each QRS complex.
    PR Int: 0.18 second.
    QRS: 0.18 second.
    Intrp: Sinus rhythm with sinoatrial (SA) exit block and bundle branch block.
29. **Rate:** 37 beats/minute.
    Rhythm: Regular.
    P Waves: None; atrial fibrillation waves are present.
    PR Int: None,
    QRS: About 0.24 second.
    Intrp: Atrial fibrillation (fine) with third-degree AV block, bundle branch block, and ventricular escape rhythm. AV dissociation is present.
30. **Rate:** 60 beats/minute.
    Rhythm: Regular.
    P Waves: Present; precede each QRS complex.
    PR Int: 0.16 second.
    QRS: 0.06 second.
    Intrp: Normal sinus rhythm.
31. **Rate:** 135 beats/minute.
    Rhythm: Regular.
    P Waves: None.
    PR Int: None.
    QRS: 0.26 second.
    Intrp: Ventricular tachycardia.

32. **Rate:** 163 beats/minute.
    Rhythm: Regular.
    P Waves: None.
    PR Int: None.
    QRS: 0.10 second.
    Intrp: Junctional tachycardia.
33. **Rate:** 41 beats/minute.
    Rhythm: Irregular.
    P Waves: Present; precede the first, second, fourth, and fifth QRS complexes. The R-R interval between the second and fourth QRS complexes is four times the R-R interval of the underlying sinus rhythm.
    PR Int: 0.14 second.
    QRS: 0.12 second.
    Intrp: Sinus rhythm with sinoatrial (SA) exit block, bundle branch block, and an isolated junctional escape beat (third QRS complex).
34. **Rate:** 17 beats/minute.
    Rhythm: Undeterminable.
    P Waves: None.
    PR Int: None.
    QRS: 0.16 second.
    Intrp: Ventricular escape rhythm.
35. **Rate:** 70 beats/minute.
    Rhythm: Regular.
    P Waves: Present; precede each QRS complex.
    PR Int: 0.16 second.
    QRS: 0.06 second.
    Intrp: Normal sinus rhythm.
36. **Rate:** 64 beats/minute.
    Rhythm: Irregular.
    P Waves: Present; precede the first and second QRS complexes. Pacemaker spikes precede the rest of the QRS complexes.
    PR Int: 0.26 second.
    QRS: 0.08 second (first and second QRS complexes); 0.12 second (third, fourth, fifth, sixth, and seventh QRS complexes).
    Intrp: Sinus rhythm with first-degree AV block followed by ventricular asystole and a ventricular demand pacemaker rhythm.
37. **Rate:** 72 beats/minute.
    Rhythm: Irregular.
    P Waves: Present; precede each QRS complex.
    PR Int: 0.16 second.
    QRS: 0.08 second.
    Intrp: Sinus arrhythmia.

38. **Rate:** 75 beats/minute.
    Rhythm: Irregular.
    P Waves: Present; all but the first and sixth P waves are followed by QRS complexes. AV conduction ratio is 5:4.
    PR Int: 0.12 to 0.14 second.
    QRS: 0.14 second.
    Intrp: Sinus rhythm with second-degree, type II AV block and bundle branch block.
39. **Rate:** 101 beats/minute.
    Rhythm: Irregular.
    P Waves: Present; precede each QRS complex. The shape and direction of the P waves vary from positive to negative.
    PR Int: 0.12 to 0.18 second.
    QRS: 0.06 second.
    Intrp: Wandering atrial pacemaker.
40. **Rate:** 37 beats/minute.
    Rhythm: Regular.
    P Waves: Present; precede each QRS complex.
    PR Int: 0.34 second.
    QRS: 0.08 second.
    Intrp: Sinus bradycardia with first-degree AV block.
41. **Rate:** 42 beats/minute.
    Rhythm: Irregular.
    P Waves: Present; precede each QRS complex. The fourth P wave is negative; the rest are positive.
    PR Int: 0.18 to 0.20 second.
    QRS: 0.12 second.
    Intrp: Sinus bradycardia with bundle branch block and an isolated premature atrial contraction.
42. **Rate:** 66 beats/minute.
    Rhythm: Irregular.
    P Waves: Present; all the P waves except the fourth and eighth P waves are followed by QRS complexes.
    PR Int: 0.22 to 0.40 second. The PR intervals progressively increase until a QRS complex fails to follow the P wave.
    QRS: 0.14 second.
    Intrp: Sinus rhythm with second-degree, type I AV block (Wenckebach) and bundle branch block.
43. **Rate:** 74 beats/minute.
    Rhythm: Regular.
    P Waves: None.
    PR Int: None.
    QRS: 0.12 second.
    Intrp: Pacemaker rhythm (ventricular pacemaker).

44. **Rate:** 88 beats/minute.
Rhythm: Regular.
P Waves: Present; precede each QRS complex.
PR Int: 0.12 second.
QRS: 0.14 second.
Intrp: Normal sinus rhythm with bundle branch block.

45. **Rate:** 61 beats/minute.
Rhythm: Irregular.
P Waves: Present; precede all but the fourth QRS complex.
PR Int: 0.12 second.
QRS: 0.08 second.
Intrp: Sinus rhythm with sinus arrest and a premature junctional contraction.

46. **Rate:** 71 beats/minute.
Rhythm: Regular.
P Waves: Present; precede each QRS complex.
PR Int: 0.18 second.
QRS: About 0.10 second.
Intrp: Normal sinus rhythm.

47. **Rate:** 66 beats/minute.
Rhythm: Irregular.
P Waves: Present; all but the fourth and eighth P waves are followed by QRS complexes.
PR Int: 0.22 to 0.40 second. The PR intervals progressively increase until a QRS complex fails to follow the P wave.
QRS: About 0.15 second.
Intrp: Sinus rhythm with second-degree, type I AV block (Wenckebach) and bundle branch block.

48. **Rate:** 102 beats/minute.
Rhythm: Irregular.
P Waves: None; fine atrial fibrillation waves are present.
PR Int: None.
QRS: About to 0.10 second (first, fifth, seventh, eighth, ninth, and tenth QRS complexes); 0.12 to 0.16 second (second, third, fourth, sixth, and tenth QRS complexes). The shape and direction of the second, third, and fourth QRS complexes differ from each other. The second QRS complex is similar to the sixth QRS complex; the fourth QRS complex is similar to the tenth QRS complex.
Intrp: Atrial fibrillation (fine) with third-degree AV block, accelerated junctional rhythm, multifocal (multiform) PVCs (group beats), and a short burst of ventricular tachycardia. AV dissociation is present.

49. **Rate:** 63 beats/minute.
Rhythm: Irregular.
P Waves: None; coarse atrial fibrillation waves are present.
PR Int: None.
QRS: 0.13 second.
Intrp: Atrial fibrillation (coarse) with bundle branch block.

50. **Rate:** 57 beats/minute.
Rhythm: Irregular. The R-R interval between the fourth and fifth QRS complexes is less than twice the R-R interval of the underlying sinus rhythm.
P Waves: Present; precede all but the fifth QRS complex.
PR Int: 0.12 second.
QRS: About 0.12 second.
Intrp: Sinus rhythm with sinus arrest and incomplete bundle branch block, and an isolated junctional escape beat.

51. **Rate:** 52 beats/minute.
Rhythm: Regular.
P Waves: Present; precede each QRS complex.
PR Int: 0.20 second.
QRS: 0.08 second.
Intrp: Normal sinus rhythm.

52. **Rate:** 183 beats/minute.
    Rhythm: Regular.
    P Waves: None.
    PR Int: None.
    QRS: 0.16 second.
    Intrp: Ventricular tachycardia.

53. **Rate:** 65 beats/minute.
    Rhythm: Irregular.
    P Waves: Present; precede each QRS complex.
    PR Int: 0.16 second.
    QRS: 0.08 second.
    Intrp: Sinus arrhythmia.

54. **Rate:** 27 beats/minute.
    Rhythm: Regular.
    P Waves: None.
    PR Int: None.
    QRS: 0.12 second.
    Intrp: Junctional escape rhythm with bundle branch block.

55. **Rate:** 40 beats/minute.
    Rhythm: Regular.
    P Waves: None.
    PR Int: None.
    QRS: 0.16 second.
    Intrp: Ventricular escape rhythm.

56. **Rate:** 59 beats/minute.
    Rhythm: Irregular.
    P Waves: Present; the second, third, fifth, sixth, eighth, and tenth P waves are followed by QRS complexes. AV conduction ratios are 3:2 and 2:1.
    PR Int: About 0.16 second.
    QRS: About 0.16 second.
    Intrp: Sinus rhythm with second-degree, type II 3:2 AV block and 2:1 AV block and bundle branch block.

57. **Rate:** 58 beats/minute.
    Rhythm: Regular.
    P Waves: Present; negative P waves follow each QRS complex.
    PR Int: None.
    QRS: 0.12 second.
    Intrp: Junctional escape rhythm with incomplete bundle branch block.

58. **Rate:** 53 beats/minute.
    Rhythm: Irregular.
    P Waves: Present; the first, second, fourth, fifth, and sixth P waves are followed by QRS complexes.
    PR Int: 0.22 to 0.46 second. The PR intervals progressively increase until a QRS complex fails to follow the P wave.
    QRS: 0.08 second.
    Intrp: Sinus rhythm with second-degree, type I AV block (Wenckebach).

59. **Rate:** 80 beats/minute.
    Rhythm: Irregular.
    P Waves: Present; precede the first, second, third, sixth, eighth, and ninth QRS complexes. The third P wave is negative; the fifth wave is buried in the preceding T wave. Pacemaker spikes precede the third, fourth, fifth, and seventh QRS complexes.
    PR Int: 0.12 to 0.18 second.
    QRS: 0.07 second (first, second, sixth, eighth, and ninth QRS complexes); 0.16 second (fourth, fifth, and seventh QRS complexes). The third QRS complex is a fusion beat—a combination of the normally conducted QRS complex and the pacemaker induced ventricular QRS complex.
    Intrp: Sinus rhythm with episodes of ventricular demand pacemaker rhythm.

60. **Rate:** 135 beats/minute.
    Rhythm: Regular.
    P Waves: None.
    PR Int: None.
    QRS: About 0.32 to 0.36 second.
    Intrp: Ventricular tachycardia.

61. **Rate:** 70 beats/minute.
    Rhythm: Regular.
    P Waves: Present; precede each QRS complex.
    PR Int: 0.16 second.
    QRS: 0.06 second.
    Intrp: Normal sinus rhythm.

62. **Rate:** 52 beats/minute.
Rhythm: Irregular.
P Waves: Present; the second, third, fifth, and sixth P waves are followed by QRS complexes. The AV conduction ratio is 3:2.
PR Int: 0.24 to 0.26 second.
QRS: 0.16 second.
Intrp: Sinus rhythm with second-degree, type II AV block and bundle branch block.

63. **Rate:** 64 beats/minute.
Rhythm: Irregular.
P Waves: Present; the first, second, fourth, fifth, and sixth P waves are followed by QRS complexes.
PR Int: 0.24 to 0.36 second. The PR intervals progressively increase until a QRS complex fails to follow the P wave.
QRS: 0.12 second.
Intrp: Sinus rhythm with second-degree, type I AV block (Wenckebach) and bundle branch block.

64. **Rate:** 284 beats/minute.
Rhythm: Regular.
P Waves: None.
PR Int: None.
QRS: About 0.12 second.
Intrp: Ventricular tachycardia.

65. **Rate:** 87 beats/minute.
Rhythm: Irregular.
P Waves: Present; precede each QRS complex.
PR Int: 0.12 to 0.16 second.
QRS: 0.04 second.
Intrp: Wandering atrial pacemaker.

66. **Rate:** 70 beats/minute.
Rhythm: Regular.
P Waves: Present; precede each QRS complex.
PR Int: 0.16 second.
QRS: 0.07 second.
Intrp: Normal sinus rhythm.

67. **Rate:** 37 beats/minute.
Rhythm: Regular.
P Waves: Present; precede each QRS complex.
PR Int: 0.18 second.
QRS: 0.12 second.
Intrp: Sinus bradycardia with bundle branch block.

68. **Rate:** 30 beats/minute (atrial rate: 82 beats/minute).
Rhythm: Regular.
P Waves: Present, but have no set relation to the QRS complexes.
PR Int: None.
QRS: 0.14 second.
Intrp: Third-degree AV block with wide QRS complexes.

69. **Rate:** 125 beats/minute (average); 165 beats/minute (first part); 79 beats/minute (second part).
Rhythm: Irregular.
P Waves: Present; precede each QRS complex. In the first part, the P waves are superimposed on the preceding T waves.
PR Int: 0.16 second.
QRS: About 0.04 second.
Intrp: Paroxysmal supraventricular tachycardia with reversion to normal sinus rhythm.

70. **Rate:** 120 beats minute (three beats).
Rhythm: Regular (three beats).
P Waves: None.
PR Int: None.
QRS: 0.14 second.
Intrp: Supraventricular tachycardia with wide QRS complexes or ventricular tachycardia followed by ventricular asystole.

71. **Rate:** 174 beats/minute.
Rhythm: Regular.
P Waves: None.
PR Int: None.
QRS: 0.10 second.
Intrp: Supraventricular tachycardia.

72. **Rate:** 36 beats/minute.
Rhythm: Regular.
P Waves: None.
PR Int: None.
QRS: 0.18 second.
Intrp: Junctional escape rhythm with bundle branch block or ventricular escape rhythm.

73. **Rate:** 263 beats/minute.
Rhythm: Regular.
P Waves: None.
PR Int: None.
QRS: About 0.12 second.
Intrp: Ventricular tachycardia.

74. **Rate:** 69 beats/minute.
    Rhythm: Irregular.
    P Waves: Present; the second, third, fourth, sixth, seventh, and eighth P waves are followed by QRS complexes. AV conduction ratio is 4:3.
    PR Int: 0.16 second.
    QRS: 0.20 second.
    Intrp: Sinus rhythm with second-degree, type II AV block and bundle branch block.

75. **Rate:** 72 beats/minute.
    Rhythm: Regular.
    P Waves: P waves are present. A QRS complex follows every third P wave.
    PR Int: 0.32 second.
    QRS: 0.08 second.
    Intrp: Supraventricular tachycardia with 3:1 AV block.

76. **Rate:** 104 beats/minute.
    Rhythm: Irregular.
    P Waves: Present; precede the first, fifth, and sixth QRS complex.
    PR Int: 0.18 second.
    QRS: 0.12 second (first, fifth, and sixth complexes); about 0.16 second (second, third, and fourth QRS complex).
    Intrp: Sinus rhythm with bundle branch block and unifocal (uniform) premature ventricular contractions occurring in a burst of three (ventricular tachycardia); R-on-T phenomenon.

77. **Rate:** 82 beats/minute.
    Rhythm: Regular.
    P Waves: Present; precede each QRS complex.
    PR Int: About 0.16 second.
    QRS: 0.08 second.
    Intrp: Normal sinus rhythm.

78. **Rate:** 100 beats/minute.
    Rhythm: Irregular.
    P Waves: Present; precede each QRS complex.
    PR Int: 0.12 to 0.14 second.
    QRS: About 0.18 second.
    Intrp: Sinus rhythm with bundle branch block and premature atrial contractions (atrial bigeminy).

79. **Rate:** 56 beats/minute.
    Rhythm: Regular.
    P Waves: Present; precede each QRS complex.
    PR Int: 0.36 to 0.42 second. The PR intervals progressively increase.
    QRS: About 0.12 second.
    Intrp: Sinus rhythm with second-degree AV block (type undeterminable, probably type I AV block [Wenckebach]) and bundle branch block.

80. **Rate:** 181 beats/minute.
    Rhythm: Regular.
    P Waves: None.
    PR Int: None.
    QRS: About 0.18 second.
    Intrp: Supraventricular tachycardia with wide QRS complexes or ventricular tachycardia.

81. **Rate:** 40 beats/minute.
    Rhythm: Undeterminable.
    P Waves: None.
    PR Int: None.
    QRS: About 0.20 second.
    Intrp: Ventricular escape rhythm.

82. **Rate:** 94 beats/minute.
    Rhythm: Regular.
    P Waves: Present; negative P waves precede each QRS complex.
    PR Int: 0.08 second.
    QRS: 0.10 second.
    Intrp: Accelerated junctional rhythm.

83. **Rate:** 94 beats/minute.
    Rhythm: Regular.
    P Waves: Present; precede each QRS complex.
    PR Int: 0.12 second.
    QRS: 0.12 second.
    Intrp: Normal sinus rhythm with bundle branch block.

84. **Rate:** 68 beats/minute.
    Rhythm: Irregular.
    P Waves: Present; precede the first and third QRS complexes.
    PR Int: About 0.08 second.
    QRS: 0.08 second (first and third QS complex); 0.18 second (second and fourth QRS complex).
    Intrp: Atrial rhythm with premature ventricular contractions (ventricular bigeminy).

85. **Rate:** 68 beats/minute.
    Rhythm: Irregular.
    P Waves: Present; precede each QRS complex. The first and third P waves are positive; the second and fourth P waves are negative.
    PR Int: 0.20 second.
    QRS: 0.12 second.
    Intrp: Sinus rhythm with first-degree AV block, bundle branch block, and premature atrial contractions (atrial bigeminy).

86. **Rate:** 34 beats/minute (atrial rate: 163 beats/minute).
    Rhythm: Undeterminable.
    P Waves: Present, but the negative P waves have no set relation to the QRS complexes.
    PR Int: None.
    QRS: 0.16 second.
    Intrp: Third-degree AV block with wide QRS complexes.

87. **Rate:** 75 beats/minute.
    Rhythm: Irregular.
    P Waves: None; fine atrial fibrillation waves are present.
    PR Int: None.
    QRS: 0.16 second.
    Intrp: Atrial fibrillation (fine).

88. **Rate:** 107 beats/minute.
    Rhythm: Irregular.
    P Waves: Present; precede each QRS complex.
    PR Int: 0.14 second.
    QRS: 0.12 second.
    Intrp: Sinus tachycardia with first-degree AV block, bundle branch block, and an isolated premature junctional contraction (fourth QRS complex).

89. **Rate:** 230 beats/minute.
    Rhythm: Slightly irregular.
    P Waves: None.
    PR Int: None.
    QRS: 0.12 second.
    Intrp: Ventricular tachycardia.

90. **Rate:** 170 beats/minute.
    Rhythm: Irregular.
    P Waves: None; fine atrial fibrillation waves are present.
    PR Int: None.
    QRS: 0.08 second.
    Intrp: Atrial fibrillation (fine).

91. **Rate:** 80 second beats/minute.
    Rhythm: Irregular.
    P Waves: Present; precede the first and third QRS complexes.
    PR Int: 0.14 second.
    QRS: 0.12 second.
    Intrp: Sinus rhythm with bundle branch block and premature junctional contractions (bigeminy).

92. **Rate:** 115 beats/minute.
    Rhythm: Irregular.
    P Waves: None; atrial flutter waves are present.
    PR Int: None.
    QRS: 0.12 second.
    Intrp: Atrial flutter with wide QRS complexes.

93. **Rate:** Unmeasurable.
    Rhythm: Irregular.
    P Waves: None; coarse ventricular fibrillation waves are present.
    PR Int: None.
    QRS: None.
    Intrp: Ventricular fibrillation (coarse).

94. **Rate:** 46 beats/minute.
    Rhythm: Irregular.
    P Waves: Present; the first, second, and fourth P waves are followed by QRS complexes.
    PR Int: 0.20 to 0.32 second. The PR intervals progressively increase until a QRS complex fails to follow the P wave.
    QRS: 0.10 second.
    Intrp: Sinus rhythm with second-degree, type I AV block (Wenckebach).

95. **Rate:** 82 beats/minute.
    Rhythm: Regular.
    P Waves: None; atrial and ventricular pacemaker spikes are present.
    PR Int: None.
    QRS: 0.16 second.
    Intrp: Pacemaker rhythm (AV or optimal sequential pacemaker).

96. **Rate:** 61 beats/minute.
    Rhythm: Irregular.
    P Waves: Present; precede the first, second, and fourth QRS complexes.
    PR Int: 0.22 second.
    QRS: 0.11 second.
    Intrp: Normal sinus rhythm with incomplete bundle branch block and an isolated premature junctional contraction (third QRS complex).

97. **Rate:** 224 beats/minute.
    Rhythm: Regular.
    P Waves: None.
    PR Int: None.
    QRS: 0.06 second.
    Intrp: Supraventricular tachycardia.
98. **Rate:** 98 beats/minute.
    Rhythm: Irregular.
    P Waves: Present; precede the first, second, third, and sixth QRS complexes.
    PR Int: 0.16 second.
    QRS: 0.16 to 0.18 second.
    Intrp: Normal sinus rhythm with bundle branch block and premature junctional contractions (group beats).
99. **Rate:** 136 beats/minute.
    Rhythm: Regular.
    P Waves: Present; negative P waves follow each QRS complex.
    PR Int: None.
    QRS: 0.06 second.
    Intrp: Junctional tachycardia.
100. **Rate:** 63 beats/minute.
    Rhythm: None.
    P Waves: None; positive wide artifacts are present.
    PR Int: None.
    QRS: None.
    Intrp: Ventricular asystole with artifacts (chest compressions).
101. **Rate:** 184 beats/minute.
    Rhythm: Regular.
    P Waves: None.
    PR Int: None.
    QRS: 0.10 second.
    Intrp: Supraventricular tachycardia.
102. **Rate:** 102 beats/minute.
    Rhythm: Regular.
    P Waves: Present; precede each QRS complex.
    PR Int: 0.16 second.
    QRS: 0.06 second.
    Intrp: Sinus tachycardia. Abnormally tall T waves characteristic of hyperkalemia are present.
103. **Rate:** 68 beats/minute.
    Rhythm: Regular.
    P Waves: None.
    PR Int: None.
    QRS: About 0.22 second.
    Intrp: Accelerated idioventricular rhythm.

104. **Rate:** 164 beats/minute.
    Rhythm: Regular.
    P Waves: Present; precede each QRS complex.
    PR Int: 0.12 second.
    QRS: 0.08 second.
    Intrp: Atrial tachycardia.
105. **Rate:** 123 beats/minute.
    Rhythm: Regular.
    P Waves: Present; precede each QRS complex.
    PR Int: 0.14 second.
    QRS: 0.12 second.
    Intrp: Sinus tachycardia with bundle branch block.
106. **Rate:** 76 beats/minute.
    Rhythm: Irregular.
    P Waves: Present; precede the second and fourth QRS complex. The fifth QRS complex is superimposed on a P wave.
    PR Int: 0.16 second.
    QRS: 0.08 second (third and fifth QRS complexes); 0.12 second (first, second, and fourth QRS complexes).
    Intrp: Normal sinus rhythm with bundle branch block and premature junctional contractions.
107. **Rate:** 61 beats/minute.
    Rhythm: Irregular.
    P Waves: Present; precede the first, second, and fourth QRS complexes.
    PR Int: 0.24 second.
    QRS: 0.10 second.
    Intrp: Sinus rhythm with first-degree AV block and an isolated premature junctional contraction.
108. **Rate:** 41 beats/minute.
    Rhythm: Regular.
    P Waves: Present; precede each QRS complex.
    PR Int: About 0.14 second.
    QRS: 0.08 second.
    Intrp: Sinus bradycardia.
109. **Rate:** 69 beats/minute.
    Rhythm: Regular.
    P Waves: Present; precede each QRS complex.
    PR Int: About 0.24 second.
    QRS: 0.14 second.
    Intrp: Sinus rhythm with first-degree AV block and bundle branch block.

110. **Rate:** 48 beats/minute (atrial rate: 125 beats/minute).
    Rhythm: Regular.
    P Waves: Present, but have no set relation to the QRS complexes.
    PR Int: None.
    QRS: 0.10 second.
    Intrp: Third-degree AV block.

111. **Rate:** 41 beats/minute.
    Rhythm: Irregular.
    P Waves: Present; the first, fourth, and sixth P waves are followed by QRS complexes. AV conduction ratios are 2:1 and 3:1.
    PR Int: 0.20 second.
    QRS: 0.12 second.
    Intrp: Sinus rhythm with second-degree, 2:1 and advanced AV block.

112. **Rate:** 92 beats/minute.
    Rhythm: Regular.
    P Waves: Present; precede each QRS complex.
    PR Int: 0.14 second.
    QRS: About 0.06 second.
    Intrp: Normal sinus rhythm.

113. **Rate:** 161 beats/minute.
    Rhythm: Regular.
    P Waves: None.
    PR Int: None.
    QRS: 0.09 second.
    Intrp: Supraventricular tachycardia.

114. **Rate:** 320 beats/minute.
    Rhythm: Slightly irregular.
    P Waves: None.
    PR Int: None.
    QRS: 0.14 to 0.20 second.
    Intrp: Torsade de pointes.

115. **Rate:** 50 beats/minute.
    Rhythm: Regular.
    P Waves: Present; precede each QRS complex.
    PR Int: 0.16 second.
    QRS: 0.08 second.
    Intrp: Junctional escape rhythm with first-degree AV block.

116. **Rate:** 60 beats/minute.
    Rhythm: Irregular.
    P Waves: None; fine atrial fibrillation waves are present.
    PR Int: None.
    QRS: 0.08 second.
    Intrp: Atrial fibrillation (fine).

117. **Rate:** 97 beats/minute.
    Rhythm: Regular.
    P Waves: Present; precede each QRS complex.
    PR Int: 0.16 second.
    QRS: 0.16 second.
    Intrp: Normal sinus rhythm with bundle branch block.

118. **Rate:** Unmeasurable.
    Rhythm: Irregular.
    P Waves: None; coarse ventricular fibrillation waves present.
    PR Int: None.
    QRS: None.
    Intrp: Ventricular fibrillation (coarse).

119. **Rate:** 48 beats/minute.
    Rhythm: Regular.
    P Waves: Present; follow each QRS complex.
    PR Int: None.
    QRS: About 0.16 second.
    Intrp: Junctional escape rhythm with bundle branch block or acclerated idioventricular rhythm.

120. **Rate:** 73 beats/minute.
    Rhythm: Irregular.
    P Waves: Present; precede the first, second, and fourth QRS complexes.
    PR Int: 0.18 second.
    QRS: 0.08 second (first, second, and fourth QRS complexes); 0.16 second (third QRS complex).
    Intrp: Normal sinus rhythm with an isolated premature ventricular contraction (interpolated).

121. **Rate:** 62 beats/minute.
    Rhythm: Regular.
    P Waves: Present; precede each QRS complex.
    PR Int: 0.20 second.
    QRS: About 0.08 second.
    Intrp: Normal sinus rhythm.

122. **Rate:** 78 beats/minute.
    Rhythm: Irregular.
    P Waves: None; fine atrial fibrillation waves are present.
    PR Int: None.
    QRS: 0.08 second.
    Intrp: Atrial fibrillation (fine).

123. **Rate:** 87 beats/minute.
Rhythm: Irregular.
P Waves: Present; precede the first and fourth QRS complexes.
PR Int: 0.16 second.
QRS: 0.10 second (first and fourth QRS complexes); about 0.16 to 0.18 second (second, third, and fifth QRS complexes).
Intrp: Normal sinus rhythm with multiform premature ventricular contractions (group beats).

124. **Rate:** 80 beats/minute.
Rhythm: Regular.
P Waves: None; ventricular pacemaker spikes are present.
PR Int: None.
QRS: 0.16 second.
Intrp: Pacemaker rhythm (ventricular pacemaker).

125. **Rate:** 31 beats/minute (atrial rate: 97 beats/minute).
Rhythm: Undeterminable.
P Waves: Present, but have no set relation to the QRS complexes.
PR Int: None.
QRS: 0.12 to 0.14 second.
Intrp: Third-degree AV block with wide QRS complexes.

126. **Rate:** 57 beats/minute.
Rhythm: Regular.
P Waves: None.
PR Int: None.
QRS: About 0.12 second.
Intrp: Junctional escape rhythm with bundle branch block.

127. **Rate:** 47 beats/minute.
Rhythm: Regular.
P Waves: Present; precede each QRS complex.
PR Int: 0.48 second.
QRS: 0.08 second.
Intrp: Sinus bradycardia with first-degree AV block.

128. **Rate:** 149 beats/minute.
Rhythm: Regular.
P Waves: Present; precede each QRS complex.
PR Int: Unmeasurable.
QRS: 0.08 second.
Intrp: Atrial tachycardia.

129. **Rate:** 160 beats/minute.
Rhythm: Irregular.
P Waves: Undeterminable.
PR Int: Undeterminable.
QRS: 0.12 second (first QRS complex); ≥0.16 second (rest of the QRS complexes).
Intrp: A wide QRS complex followed by multiform ventricular tachycardia.

130. **Rate:** 160 beats/minute.
Rhythm: Regular.
P Waves: None.
PR Int: None.
QRS: 0.14 second.
Intrp: Supraventricular tachycardia with wide QRS complexes or ventricular tachycardia.

131. **Rate:** 150 beats/minute.
Rhythm: Regular.
P Waves: Present; follow each QRS complex.
PR Int: None.
QRS: 0.10 second.
Intrp: Junctional tachycardia.

132. **Rate:** 31 beats/minute (atrial rate: unmeasurable).
Rhythm: Undeterminable.
P Waves: Present, but have no set relation to the QRS complexes.
PR Int: None.
QRS: About 0.15 second.
Intrp: Third-degree AV block with wide QRS complexes.

133. **Rate:** 31 beats/minute.
Rhythm: Undeterminable.
P Waves: Present; precede each QRS complex.
PR Int: 0.14 second.
QRS: 0.08 second.
Intrp: Sinus bradycardia.

134. **Rate:** 59 beats/minute.
Rhythm: Regular.
P Waves: None; atrial flutter waves are present.
PR Int: None.
QRS: 0.12 to 0.16 second.
Intrp: Atrial flutter with bundle branch block.

135. **Rate:** 178 beats/minute.
Rhythm: Regular.
P Waves: None.
PR Int: None.
QRS: 0.08 second.
Intrp: Supraventricular tachycardia.

136. **Rate:** 91 beats/minute.
     Rhythm: Regular.
     P Waves: Present; precede each QRS complex.
     PR Int: 0.28 second.
     QRS: 0.12 second.
     Intrp: Sinus rhythm with first-degree AV block and bundle branch block.

137. **Rate:** 47 beats/minute.
     Rhythm: Regular.
     P Waves: Present; the first, third, and fifth P waves are followed by QRS complexes.
     PR Int: 0.28 second.
     QRS: 0.12 second.
     Intrp: Sinus rhythm with second-degree, 2:1 AV block and bundle branch block.

138. **Rate:** 78 beats/minute.
     Rhythm: Irregular.
     P Waves: Present; precede each QRS complex. The second and fourth P waves are abnormal, each in a different way.
     PR Int: About 0.22 second (first and third PR intervals); about 0.16 second (second and fourth PR intervals).
     QRS: About 0.10 second.
     Intrp: Sinus rhythm with multifocal premature atrial contractions.

139. **Rate:** 64 beats/minute.
     Rhythm: Regular.
     P Waves: None.
     PR Int: None.
     QRS: About 0.10 second.
     Intrp: Accelerated junctional rhythm.

140. **Rate:** 222 beats/minute.
     Rhythm: Regular.
     P Waves: None.
     PR Int: None.
     QRS: 0.12 second.
     Intrp: Supraventricular tachycardia with wide QRS complexes or ventricular tachycardia.

141. **Rate:** None (pacemaker spikes: 63 beats/minute).
     Rhythm: Regular.
     P Waves: None; pacemaker spikes are present.
     PR Int: None.
     QRS: None.
     Intrp: Ventricular asystole with pacemaker spikes without capture.

142. **Rate:** 99 beats/minute.
     Rhythm: Irregular.
     P Waves: Present; precede the first, second, and fifth QRS complexes.
     PR Int: 0.28 second.
     QRS: 0.10 second (first, second, and fifth QRS complexes); 0.12 to 0.16 second (third and fourth QRS complexes).
     Intrp: Sinus rhythm with first-degree AV block and multiform premature ventricular contractions (group beats).

143. **Rate:** 61 beats/minute.
     Rhythm: Regular.
     P Waves: Present: precede each QRS complex. P waves are abnormally tall (P pulmonale).
     PR Int: 0.26 second.
     QRS: 0.10 second.
     Intrp: Sinus rhythm with first-degree AV block.

144. **Rate:** 114 beats/minute.
     Rhythm: Regular.
     P Waves: Present; precede each QRS complex.
     PR Int: 0.16 second.
     QRS: 0.08 second.
     Intrp: Sinus tachycardia.

145. **Rate:** 100 beats/minute.
     Rhythm: Regular.
     P Waves: Present; negative P waves follow each QRS complex.
     PR Int: None.
     QRS: 0.10 second.
     Intrp: Junctional tachycardia.

146. **Rate:** Unmeasurable.
     Rhythm: Irregular.
     P Waves: None; coarse ventricular fibrillation waves are present.
     PR Int: None.
     QRS: None.
     Intrp: Ventricular fibrillation (coarse).

147. **Rate:** 21 beats/minute.
     Rhythm: Undeterminable.
     P Waves: None.
     PR Int: None.
     QRS: 0.16 second.
     Intrp: Ventricular escape rhythm.

148. **Rate:** 68 beats/minute.
     Rhythm: Irregular.
     P Waves: None; fine atrial fibrillation waves are present.
     PR Int: None.
     QRS: 0.10 second.
     Intrp: Atrial fibrillation (fine).

149. **Rate:** 65 beats/minute (atrial rate: 113 beats/minute).
     Rhythm: Regular.
     P Waves: Present, but have no set relation to the QRS complexes.
     PR Int: None.
     QRS: Undeterminable.
     Intrp: Third-degree AV block.
150. **Rate:** 88 beats/minute.
     Rhythm: Irregular.
     P Waves: Present; precede each QRS complex. Third wave negative.
     PR Int: About 0.14 second.
     QRS: About 0.08 second.
     Intrp: Normal sinus rhythm with an isolated premature junctional contraction.
151. **Rate:** 55 beats/minute.
     Rhythm: Regular.
     P Waves: Present; abnormally wide, positive P waves precede each QRS complex.
     PR Int: About 0.40 second.
     QRS: About 0.10 second.
     Intrp: Sinus rhythm with first-degree AV block. Possible 2:1 AV block.
152. **Rate:** 148 beats/minute.
     Rhythm: Regular.
     P Waves: Present; precede each QRS complex.
     PR Int: Undeterminable; P waves are buried in the preceding QRS complexes.
     QRS: 0.10 second.
     Intrp: Sinus tachycardia.
153. **Rate:** 118 beats/minute.
     Rhythm: Irregular.
     P Waves: None; fine atrial fibrillation waves are present.
     PR Int: None.
     QRS: 0.08 second.
     Intrp: Atrial fibrillation (fine).
154. **Rate:** 36 beats/minute.
     Rhythm: Undeterminable.
     P Waves: None.
     PR Int: None.
     QRS: About 0.16 second.
     Intrp: Ventricular escape rhythm.
155. **Rate:** 50 beats/minute.
     Rhythm: Regular.
     P Waves: None; atrial flutter waves are present.
     PR Int: None.
     QRS: 0.16 second.
     Intrp: Atrial flutter with bundle branch block.

156. **Rate:** 163 beats/minute.
     Rhythm: Regular.
     P Waves: None.
     PR Int: None.
     QRS: 0.16 second.
     Intrp: Ventricular tachycardia.
157. **Rate:** 63 beats/minute.
     Rhythm: Regular.
     P Waves: Present; negative P waves follow each QRS complex.
     PR Int: None.
     QRS: About 0.08 second.
     Intrp: Accelerated junctional rhythm.
158. **Rate:** 103 beats/minute.
     Rhythm: Regular.
     P Waves: Present: P waves precede each QRS complex. The P waves are abnormally tall (P pulmonale).
     PR Int: 0.19 second.
     QRS: About 0.15 second.
     Intrp: Sinus tachycardia with bundle branch block.
159. **Rate:** 312 beats/minute.
     Rhythm: Slightly irregular.
     P Waves: None.
     PR Int: None.
     QRS: 0.12 to 0.14 second.
     Intrp: Ventricular tachycardia (multiform).
160. **Rate:** 101 beats/minute.
     Rhythm: Regular.
     P Waves: None.
     PR Int: None.
     QRS: 0.14 second.
     Intrp: Junctional tachycardia with wide QRS complexes or ventricular tachycardia.
161. **Rate:** 92 beats/minute.
     Rhythm: Irregular.
     P Waves: Present; precede the first, second fourth, and fifth QRS complexes.
     PR Int: 0.14 second.
     QRS: 0.16 second.
     Intrp: Normal sinus rhythm with bundle branch block and an isolated premature ventricular contraction (interpolated).
162. **Rate:** 70 beats/minute.
     Rhythm: Regular.
     P Waves: Present; precede each QRS complex.
     PR Int: About 0.18 second.
     QRS: 0.12 second.
     Intrp: Normal sinus rhythm with bundle branch block.

163. **Rate:** 72 beats/minute.
  Rhythm: Regular.
  P Waves: None.
  PR Int: None.
  QRS: 0.12 to 0.16 second.
  Intrp: Accelerated idioventricular rhythm.
164. **Rate:** Unmeasurable.
  Rhythm: Irregular.
  P Waves: None; fine ventricular waves are present.
  PR Int: None.
  QRS: None.
  Intrp: Ventricular fibrillation (fine).
165. **Rate:** 57 beats/minute.
  Rhythm: Regular.
  P Waves: Present; precede each QRS complex.
  PR Int: 0.24 second.
  QRS: About 0.10 second.
  Intrp: Sinus bradycardia with first-degree AV block.
166. **Rate:** 43 beats/minute.
  Rhythm: Regular.
  P Waves: Present; positive P waves precede each QRS complex.
  PR Int: 0.10 second.
  QRS: About 0.10 second.
  Intrp: Sinus bradycardia with atrio-His preexcitation.
167. **Rate:** 57 beats/minute.
  Rhythm: Regular.
  P Waves: None.
  PR Int: None.
  QRS: About 0.16 second.
  Intrp: Accelerated idioventricular rhythm.
168. **Rate:** None.
  Rhythm: None.
  P Waves: None.
  PR Int: None.
  QRS: None.
  Intrp: Ventricular asystole.
169. **Rate:** 43 beats/minute.
  Rhythm: Regular.
  P Waves: Present; negative P waves follow each QRS complex.
  PR Int: None.
  QRS: About 0.10 second.
  Intrp: Junctional escape rhythm.
170. **Rate:** Unmeasurable.
  Rhythm: Irregular.
  P Waves: None; coarse ventricular fibrillation waves are present.
  PR Int: None.
  QRS: None.
  Intrp: Ventricular fibrillation (coarse).

171. **Rate:** 25 beats/minute.
  Rhythm: Undeterminable.
  P Waves: None.
  PR Int: None.
  QRS: 0.10 to 0.12 second.
  Intrp: Junctional escape rhythm with wide QRS complexes.
172. **Rate:** 213 beats/minute.
  Rhythm: Regular.
  P Waves: None.
  PR Int: None.
  QRS: 0.12 second.
  Intrp: Supraventricular tachycardia with wide QRS complexes or ventricular tachycardia.
173. **Rate:** 70 beats/minute.
  Rhythm: Irregular.
  P Waves: None; fine atrial fibrillation waves are present.
  PR Int: None.
  QRS: 0.10 second.
  Intrp: Atrial fibrillation (fine).
174. **Rate:** 89 beats/minute.
  Rhythm: Regular.
  P Waves: Present; precede each QRS complex.
  PR Int: About 0.18 second.
  QRS: 0.12 second.
  Intrp: Normal sinus rhythm with bundle branch block.
175. **Rate:** 165 beats/minute.
  Rhythm: Regular.
  P Waves: None.
  PR Int: None.
  QRS: 0.10 second.
  Intrp: Supraventricular tachycardia.
176. **Rate:** 48 beats/minute.
  Rhythm: Regular.
  P Waves: Present; appear to precede each QRS complex.
  PR Int: 0.08 second.
  QRS: 0.08 second.
  Intrp: Sinus bradycardia with atrio-His preexcitation.

177. **Rate:** 79 beats/minute.
Rhythm: Irregular.
P Waves: Present; positive P waves precede the first, second, fourth, and fifth QRS complexes. A negative P wave precedes the third QRS complex.
PR Int: 0.12 second (first, second, fourth, and fifth QRS complexes); 0.09 second (third QRS complex).
QRS: 0.10 second.
Intrp: Normal sinus rhythm with an isolated premature junctional contraction.

178. **Rate:** 33 beats/minute (atrial rate: 39 beats/minute).
Rhythm: Undeterminable.
P Waves: Present; the first and fifth P waves are followed by QRS complexes. AV conduction ratio is 4:1.
PR Int: 0.34 second.
QRS: 0.14 second.
Intrp: Sinus rhythm with second-degree advanced AV block and wide QRS complexes.

179. **Rate:** 59 beats/minute.
Rhythm: Irregular.
P Waves: Present; the first, third, and fourth P waves are followed by QRS complexes.
PR Int: 0.20 to 0.28 second.
QRS: About 0.05 second.
Intrp: Sinus rhythm with second-degree AV block (probably Type I [Wenckebach]).

180. **Rate:** 96 beats/minute.
Rhythm: Irregular. An incomplete compensatory pause follows the fourth QRS complex.
P Waves: Present; precede the second, third, fifth, and sixth QRS complexes.
PR Int: 0.18 second.
QRS: 0.10 second.
Intrp: Normal sinus rhythm with an isolated premature junctional contraction.

181. **Rate:** 60 beats/minute.
Rhythm: Regular.
P Waves: Present; precede each QRS complex.
PR Int: 0.15 second.
QRS: 0.07 second.
Intrp: Normal sinus rhythm.

182. **Rate:** Unmeasurable.
Rhythm: Irregular.
P Waves: None; fine ventricular fibrillation waves are present.
PR Int: None.
QRS: None.
Intrp: Ventricular fibrillation (fine).

183. **Rate:** 98 beats/minute.
Rhythm: Regular.
P Waves: Present; precede each QRS complex.
PR Int: About 0.20 second.
QRS: About 0.16 second.
Intrp: Normal sinus rhythm with bundle branch block.

184. **Rate:** 64 beats/minute.
Rhythm: Regular.
P Waves: None.
PR Int: None.
QRS: About 0.16 second.
Intrp: Accelerated idioventricular rhythm.

185. **Rate:** 35 beats/minute (atrial rate: 167 beats/minute).
Rhythm: Undeterminable.
P Waves: Present, but have no set relation to the QRS complexes.
PR Int: None.
QRS: 0.12 second.
Intrp: Third-degree AV block with wide QRS complexes.

186. **Rate:** 79 beats/minute.
Rhythm: Regular.
P Waves: Present; precede each QRS complex.
PR Int: 0.15 second.
QRS: 0.08 second.
Intrp: Normal sinus rhythm.

187. **Rate:** 87 beats/minute.
Rhythm: Irregular.
P Waves: None; atrial flutter waves are present. The AV conduction ratios vary.
PR Int: None.
QRS: 0.10 second.
Intrp: Atrial flutter.

188. **Rate:** 181 beats/minute.
Rhythm: Regular.
P Waves: None.
PR Int: None.
QRS: About 0.22 second.
Intrp: Supraventricular tachycardia with wide QRS complexes or ventricular tachycardia.

189. **Rate:** 103 beats/minute.
Rhythm: Regular.
P Waves: None; atrial flutter waves are present.
PR Int: None.
QRS: 0.06 second.
Intrp: Atrial flutter.

190. **Rate:** 161 beats/minute.
Rhythm: Regular.
P Waves: Present; precede each QRS complex.
PR Int: 0.12 second.
QRS: 0.08 second.
Intrp: Atrial tachycardia.

191. **Rate:** 130 beats/minute.
Rhythm: Regular.
P Waves: None.
PR Int: None.
QRS: About 0.10 second.
Intrp: Supraventricular tachycardia.

192. **Rate:** Ventricular rate: none (atrial rate: 70 beats/minute).
Rhythm: Regular.
P Waves: Present.
PR Int: None.
QRS: None.
Intrp: Ventricular asystole.

193. **Rate:** 31 beats/minute (atrial rate 106 beats/minute).
Rhythm: Undeterminable.
P Waves: Present, but have no set relation to the QRS complexes.
PR Int: None.
QRS: About 0.14 second.
Intrp: Third-degree AV block with wide QRS complexes.

194. **Rate:** 36 beats/minute.
Rhythm: Undeterminable.
P Waves: None.
PR Int: None.
QRS: 0.16 second.
Intrp: Junctional escape rhythm with wide QRS complexes or ventricular escape rhythm.

195. **Rate:** 59 beats/minute.
Rhythm: Regular.
P Waves: Present; negative P waves precede each QRS complex.
PR Int: 0.05 to 0.06 second.
QRS: About 0.14 second.
Intrp: Junctional escape rhythm with bundle branch block.

196. **Rate:** 71 beats/minute.
Rhythm: Irregular. A complete compensatory pause follows the third QRS complex.
P Waves: Present; precede each QRS complex.
PR Int: 0.16 second.
QRS: 0.08 second.
Intrp: Normal sinus rhythm with an isolated premature atrial contraction.

197. **Rate:** 122 beats/minute.
Rhythm: Regular.
P Waves: None.
PR Int: None.
QRS: 0.12 second.
Intrp: Junctional tachycardia with wide QRS complexes or ventricular tachycardia.

198. **Rate:** None.
Rhythm: None.
P Waves: None.
PR Int: None.
QRS: 0.16 second.
Intrp: A single wide QRS complex, probably ventricular in origin, followed by ventricular asystole.

199. **Rate:** 169 beats/minute.
Rhythm: Irregular.
P Waves: None; atrial flutter waves are present. The AV conduction ratios vary.
PR Int: None.
QRS: 0.08 second.
Intrp: Atrial flutter.

200. **Rate:** 128 beats/minute.
Rhythm: Regular.
P Waves: Present; precede each QRS complex. The P waves are abnormally tall (P pulmonale).
PR Int: 0.24 second.
QRS: About 0.12 second.
Intrp: Sinus tachycardia with first-degree AV block and bundle branch block.

201. **Rate:** 63 beats/minute.
Rhythm: Regular.
P Waves: None.
PR Int: None.
QRS: About 0.16 second.
Intrp: Accelerated junctional rhythm with wide QRS complexes or accelerated idioventricular rhythm.

202. **Rate:** 60 beats/minute.
  Rhythm: Regular.
  P Waves: Present; precede each QRS complex.
  PR Int: 0.16 second.
  QRS: 0.07 second.
  Intrp: Normal sinus rhythm.
203. **Rate:** Unmeasurable.
  Rhythm: None.
  P Waves: None; fine ventricular fibrillation waves are present.
  PR Int: None.
  QRS: None.
  Intrp: Ventricular fibrillation (fine).
204. **Rate:** 238 beats/minute.
  Rhythm: Regular.
  P Waves: None.
  PR Int: None.
  QRS: About 0.10 second.
  Intrp: Supraventricular tachycardia.
205. **Rate:** 165 beats/minute.
  Rhythm: Regular.
  P Waves: None.
  PR Int: None.
  QRS: About 0.24 second.
  Intrp: Ventricular tachycardia.
206. **Rate:** 72 beats/minute.
  Rhythm: Regular.
  P Waves: None; atrial flutter waves are present.
  PR Int: None.
  QRS: 0.08 second.
  Intrp: Atrial flutter.
207. **Rate:** 33 beats/minute.
  Rhythm: Undeterminable.
  P Waves: None.
  PR Int: None.
  QRS: Unmeasurable; greater than 0.12 second.
  Intrp: Ventricular escape rhythm.
208. **Rate:** 126 beats/minute.
  Rhythm: Regular.
  P Waves: None.
  PR Int: None.
  QRS: 0.11 second.
  Intrp: Junctional tachycardia with incomplete bundle branch block.

209. **Rate:** 81 beats/minute.
  Rhythm: Irregular.
  P Waves: Present; precede each QRS complex. The shape and direction of the fourth P wave differs from the others.
  PR Int: 0.13 second (first, second, third, and fifth PR intervals); 0.18 second (fourth PR interval).
  QRS: 0.10 second (first, second, third, and fifth QRS complex).
  Intrp: Normal sinus rhythm with an isolated premature atrial contraction.
210. **Rate:** 31 beats/minute (atrial rate: 83 beats/minute).
  Rhythm: Undeterminable.
  P Waves: Present, but have no set relation to the QRS complexes.
  PR Int: None.
  QRS: About 0.14 second.
  Intrp: Third-degree AV block with wide QRS complexes.
211. **Rate:** 180 beats/minute.
  Rhythm: Regular.
  P Waves: Present: precede each QRS complex.
  PR Int: 0.08 second.
  QRS: 0.12 second.
  Intrp: Atrial tachycardia with atrio-His preexcitation and bundle branch block.
212. **Rate:** 45 beats/minute (atrial rate 111 beats/minute).
  Rhythm: Regular.
  P Waves: Present, but have no set relation to the QRS complexes.
  PR Int: None.
  QRS: 0.12 second.
  Intrp: Third-degree AV block.
213. **Rate:** 52 beats/minute.
  Rhythm: Regular.
  P Waves: Present; the first, third, and fifth P waves are followed by QRS complexes. The AV conduction ratio is 2:1.
  PR Int: 0.20 second.
  QRS: 0.14 second.
  Intrp: Sinus rhythm with second-degree, 2:1 AV block and bundle branch block.

214. Rate: 44 beats/minute.
Rhythm: Irregular.
P Waves: None; atrial flutter waves are present. The AV conduction ratios vary.
PR Int: None.
QRS: About 0.14 second.
Intrp: Atrial flutter with wide QRS complexes.

215. Rate: 71 beats/minute.
Rhythm: Regular.
P Waves: Present; precede each QRS complex.
PR Int: 0.26 second.
QRS: 0.10 second.
Intrp: Sinus rhythm with first-degree AV block.

216. Rate: 103 beats/minute.
Rhythm: Regular.
P Waves: Present; precede each QRS complex.
PR Int: 0.12 second.
QRS: 0.14 second.
Intrp: Sinus tachycardia with bundle branch block.

217. Rate: 104 beats/minute.
Rhythm: Regular.
P Waves: None.
PR Int: None.
QRS: 0.14 second.
Intrp: Junctional tachycardia with wide QRS complexes or ventricular tachycardia.

218. Rate: 109 beats/minute.
Rhythm: Irregular.
P Waves: Present: precede the first, second, third, fourth, and fifth QRS complexes.
PR Int: 0.14 second.
QRS: 0.09 second (first, second, third, fourth, and fifth QRS complexes); 0.11 second (sixth QRS complex).
Intrp: Normal sinus rhythm with premature ventricular contractions and a fusion beat (third QRS complex).

219. Rate: None.
Rhythm: None.
P Waves: None.
PR Int: None.
QRS: None.
Intrp: Ventricular asystole.

220. Rate: 81 beats/minute.
Rhythm: Regular.
P Waves: None.
PR Int: None.
QRS: 0.10 second.
Intrp: Accelerated junctional rhythm with possible Osborn waves.

221. Rate: 109 beats/minute.
Rhythm: Irregular.
P Waves: Present; precede the first, second, fourth, and fifth QRS complexes.
PR Int: About 0.14 second.
QRS: 0.09 second (first, second, fourth, and fifth QRS complexes); 0.11 second (third and sixth QRS complexes).
Intrp: Normal sinus rhythm with unifocal (uniform) premature ventricular contractions (trigeminy).

222. Rate: 37 beats/minute.
Rhythm: Undeterminable.
P Waves: Present; the second and fifth P waves are followed by QRS complexes. The third and sixth P waves are buried in the preceding T waves. The AV conduction ratio is 3:1.
PR Int: 0.16 second.
QRS: 0.14 second.
Intrp: Sinus rhythm with second-degree, advanced AV block and bundle branch block.

223. Rate: 128 beats/minute.
Rhythm: Irregular.
P Waves: None; final atrial fibrillation waves are present.
PR Int: None.
QRS: 0.12 to 0.16 second.
Intrp: Atrial fibrillation (fine) with bundle branch block.

224. Rate: 108 beats/minute.
Rhythm: Regular.
P Waves: None.
PR Int: None.
QRS: 0.16 second.
Intrp: Ventricular tachycardia.

II. Bundle Branch and Fascicular Blocks
225. Left bundle branch block with an intact interventricular septum.
226. Left posterior fascicular block.
227. Right bundle branch block without an intact interventricular septum.
228. Right bundle branch block with an intact interventricular septum.

229. Left bundle branch block without an intact interventricular septum.
230. Left anterior fascicular block.

III. Myocardial Infarctions
231. Anterolateral myocardial infarction.
232. Septal myocardial infarction.
233. Extensive anterior myocardial infarction.
234. Anterior (localized) myocardial infarction.
235. Lateral myocardial infarction.
236. Inferior myocardial infarction.
237. Anteroseptal myocardial infarction.
238. Posterior myocardial infarction.
239. Right ventricular MI.
240. Anterolateral MI.

IV. QRS Axes
241. QRS axis: $+150°$.
242. QRS axis: $-30°$ to $-90°$.
243. QRS axis: $+90°$.
244. QRS axis: $+90°$ to $+150°$.
245. QRS axis: $0°$ to $+30°$.
246. QRS axis: $0°$ to $-30°$.

V. ECG Changes: Drug and Electrolyte
247. Hypercalcemia.
248. Procainamide/quinidine toxicity.
249. Hyperkalemia.
250. Digitalis effect.
251. Hypocalcemia.
252. Hypokalemia.

VI. ECG Changes: Miscellaneous
253. Left ventricular hypertrophy.
254. Chronic obstructive pulmonary disease (COPD).
255. Right ventricular hypertrophy/cor pulmonale.
256. Pericarditis.
257. Acute pulmonary embolism.
258. Early repolarization.
259. Hypothermia.
260. Ventricular preexcitation.
261. Atrio-His preexcitation.
262. Nodoventricular/fasciculoventricular preexcitation.

Glossary

Abciximab A platelet GP IIb/IIIa receptor inhibitor that blocks the GP IIb/IIIa receptors on activated platelets from binding to vWF and fibrinogen, thus inhibiting platelet adhesion and aggregation and further thrombus formation.

ABCs Airway, breathing, and circulation. The determination of unresponsiveness, breathlessness, and pulselessness and their management.

Aberrancy See *Aberrant ventricular conduction (aberrancy)*.

Aberrant ventricular conduction (aberrancy) An electrical impulse originating in the SA node, atria, or AV junction that is temporarily conducted abnormally through the bundle branches, resulting in a bundle branch block. This is usually caused by the appearance of the electrical impulse at the bundle branches prematurely, before the bundle branches have been sufficiently repolarized. Aberrancy may occur with atrial fibrillation, atrial flutter, premature atrial and junctional contractions, and sinus, atrial, and junctional tachycardias. Also referred to simply as *ventricular aberrancy*.

Absolute refractory period (ARP) of the ventricles The period of ventricular depolarization and most of ventricular repolarization during which the ventricles cannot be stimulated to depolarize. It begins with the onset of the QRS complex and ends at about the peak of the T wave.

Accelerated idioventricular rhythm (AIVR) An arrhythmia originating in an ectopic pacemaker in the ventricles with a rate between 40 and 100 beats per minute. Also referred to as *accelerated ventricular rhythm*, *idioventricular tachycardia*, and *slow ventricular tachycardia*.

Accelerated junctional rhythm An arrhythmia originating in an ectopic pacemaker in the AV junction, with a rate between 60 and 100 beats per minute.

Accelerated rhythm Three or more consecutive beats originating in an ectopic pacemaker with a rate faster than the inherent rate of the escape pacemaker but less than 100 beats per minute. Examples are accelerated junctional rhythm and accelerated idioventricular rhythm (AIVR).

Accelerated ventricular rhythm See *Accelerated idioventricular rhythm (AIVR)*.

Accessory conduction pathways Several distinct abnormal electrical conduction pathways within the heart that bypass the AV node, the bundle of His, or both, thus allowing the electrical impulses to travel from the atria to the ventricles more rapidly than usual. They include the accessory atrioventricular (AV) pathways (the bundles of Kent), the atrio-His fibers, and the nodoventricular/fasciculoventricular fibers.

Accessory atrioventricular (AV) pathways (bundles of Kent) Abnormal accessory conduction pathways located between the atria and the ventricles that bypass the AV junction, resulting in the so-called *Wolff-Parkinson-White (WPW) conduction*. The result is an abnormally wide QRS complex with a delta wave and an abnormally short PR interval, the classic form of *ventricular preexcitation*. When this type of AV conduction is associated with a paroxysmal supraventricular tachycardia with normal QRS complexes, it is known as the *Wolff-Parkinson-White (WPW) syndrome*. Three separate accessory AV pathways have been found: type A WPW conduction pathway, type B WPW conduction pathway, and posteroseptal WPW conduction pathway.

Accessory AV pathway conduction See *Accessory atrioventricular (AV) pathways (bundles of Kent)*.

Acidosis A disturbance in the acid-base balance of the body caused by excessive amounts of carbon dioxide (respiratory acidosis), lactic acid (metabolic acidosis), or both.

Actin One of the contractile protein filaments in myofibrils that give the myocardial cells the property of contractility. The other is myosin.

Action potential See *Cardiac action potential*.

Activase Trade name for alteplase (t-PA), a thrombolytic agent.

Acute coronary syndromes Include silent ischemia, stable and unstable angina, acute MI, and sudden cardiac death.

Acute myocardial infarction (acute MI, AMI) A condition that is present when necrosis of the myocardium occurs because of prolonged and complete interruption of blood flow to the area. The area of the myocardium involved identifies the acute myocardial infarction:

Anterior MI

Septal MI	Lateral MI
Anterior (localized) MI	Anterolateral MI
Anteroseptal MI	Extensive anterior MI

Inferior (diaphragmatic) MI

Inferolateral MI

Posterior MI
Right ventricular MI

Adams-Stokes syndrome Sudden attacks of unconsciousness, with or without convulsions, caused by a sudden slowing or stopping of the heart beat.

Adenosine An antiarrhythmic used to convert paroxysmal supraventricular tachycardia (PSVT) with narrow QRS complexes and narrow-QRS-complex tachycardia of unknown origin (with pulse).

Adenosine diphosphate (ADP) A substance released from platelets after the platelets are activated following damage to the blood vessel walls. Adenosine diphosphate promotes thrombus formation by stimulating platelet aggregation. Other substances released on platelet activation are serotonin and thromboxane A_2.

ADP See *Adenosine diphosphate (ADP)*.

Adrenalin Trade name for epinephrine. See *epinephrine*.

Adrenergic Having the characteristics of the sympathetic nervous system; sympathomimetic.

Advanced life support Emergency medical care beyond basic life support, including one or more of the following: starting an intravenous (IV) line, administering IV fluids, administering drugs, defibrillating, inserting an esophageal obturator airway or endotracheal tube, and monitoring and interpreting the ECG.

Afterdepolarization An abnormal condition of latent pacemaker and myocardial cells (nonpacemaker cells) in which spontaneous depolarization occurs because of a spontaneous and rhythmic increase in the level of phase 4 membrane action potential following a normal depolarization. If afterdepolarization occurs early in phase 4, it is called *early afterdepolarization;* if late in phase 4, it is called *delayed afterdepolarization.* This abnormal condition is also referred to as *triggered activity.*

Agonal Occurring at the moment of or just before death.

Agonal rhythm Cardiac arrhythmia present in a dying heart. Ventricular escape rhythm.

Alteplase (t-PA) A thrombolytic agent that converts plasminogen, a plasma protein, to plasmin, which in turn dissolves the fibrin binding the platelets together within a thrombus (fibrinolysis), causing the thrombus to break apart (thrombolysis). Trade name: Activase.

Amplitude (voltage) With respect to ECGs, the height or depth of a wave or complex measured in millimeters (mm).

Aneurysm Dilation of an artery (such as the aorta) or a chamber of the heart (such as the ventricle).

Anion An ion with a negative charge (e.g., Cl^-, PO_4^{---}, SO_4^{--}).

Anoxia Absence or lack of oxygen.

Antegrade (or anterograde) conduction Conduction of the electrical impulse in a forward direction, that is, from the SA node or atria to the ventricles or from the AV junction to the ventricles.

Anterior leads Leads I, aVL, and V_1-V_6.

Anterior (localized) MI A myocardial infarction commonly caused by occlusion of the diagonal arteries of the left anterior descending (LAD) coronary artery and characterized by early changes in the ST segments and T waves (i.e., ST elevation and tall, peaked T waves) and the appearance later of abnormal Q waves in leads V_3-V_4.

Anterior MI A myocardial infarction caused by the occlusion of the left anterior descending (LAD) coronary artery or the left circumflex coronary artery or any of their branches, singly or in combination. Anterior MI includes septal, anterior (localized), anteroseptal, lateral, anterolateral, and extensive anterior myocardial infarctions and is characterized by early changes in the ST segments and T waves (i.e., ST elevation and tall, peaked T waves) and the appearance early or later of abnormal Q waves in two or all of leads I, aVL, and V_1-V_6, depending on the site of the infarction.

Anterolateral MI A myocardial infarction commonly caused by occlusion of the diagonal arteries of the left anterior descending (LAD) coronary artery alone or in conjunction with the anterolateral marginal artery of the left circumflex coronary artery and characterized by early changes in the ST segments and T waves (i.e., ST elevation and tall, peaked T waves) and the appearance later of abnormal Q waves in leads I, aVL, and V_3-V_6.

Anteroseptal MI A myocardial infarction commonly caused by occlusion of the left anterior descending (LAD) coronary artery involving both the septal perforator and diagonal arteries and characterized by early changes in the ST segments and T waves (i.e., ST elevation and tall, peaked T waves) in leads V_1-V_4 and the appearance early of abnormal Q waves in leads V_1-V_2 and then later in leads V_3-V_4.

Anticoagulant A substance that blocks the conversion of prothrombin to thrombin and inhibits the action of thrombin on fibrinogen, thus preventing the conversion of fibrinogen to fibrin threads. Low-molecular-weight (LMW) heparin, unfractionated heparin.

Antiplatelet agent Any compound or drug that inhibits platelet adhesion and aggregation and further thrombus formation. Includes aspirin and platelet GP IIb/IIIa receptor inhibitors such as abciximab and eptifibatide.

Aorta The main trunk of the arterial system of the body consisting of the ascending aorta, the aortic arch, and the descending aorta. The descending aorta is further divided into the thoracic and abdominal aorta.

Aortic dissection Splitting of the media layer of the aorta, leading to the formation of a dissecting aneurysm.

Aortic valve The one-way valve located between the left ventricle and the ascending aorta.

Apex of the heart The pointed lower end of the heart formed by the pointed lower ends of the right and left ventricles.

Arrhythmia A rhythm other than a normal sinus rhythm when (1) the heart rate is less than 60 or greater than 100 beats per minute, (2) the rhythm is irregular, (3) premature contractions occur, or (4) the normal progression of the electrical impulse through the electrical conduction system is blocked. Also known as *dysrhythmia*, a more appropriate term but one not used as frequently.

Artifacts Mechanically or electrically produced extraneous spikes and waves recorded on an ECG record. Common causes of artifacts are muscle tremor, alternating current (AC) interference, loose electrodes, interference related to biotelemetry, and external chest compression. Artifacts are also referred to as *electrical interference* or *noise.*

Artificial pacemaker An electronic device used to stimulate the heart to beat when the electrical conduction system of the heart malfunctions, causing bradycardia or ventricular asystole. An artificial pacemaker consists of an electronic pulse generator, a battery, and a wire lead that senses the electrical activity of the heart and delivers electrical impulses to the atria or ventricles or both when the pacemaker senses an absence of electrical activity.

Aspirin An antiplatelet agent.

Asymptomatic bradycardia A bradycardia with a systolic blood pressure greater than 90 to 100 mm Hg and stable and the absence of congestive heart failure, chest pain, dyspnea, signs and symptoms of decreased cardiac output, and premature ventricular contractions. Treatment may not be indicated even if the heart rate falls below 50 beats per minute.

Asystole Absence of contractions of the ventricles or the entire heart.

Atenolol A β-adrenergic blocking agent used primarily in the treatment of tachyarrhythmias, hypertension, angina pectoris, and acute MI.

Atherosclerotic plaque A lesion in the arterial wall that varies in size and composition from a well-demarcated, yellowish, raised area or swelling on the intimal surface of an artery produced by subintimal fatty deposits (atheroma) to a large, protruding, dull, white, fibrous plaque filled with pools of gruel-like lipid and foam cells filled with lipid, surrounded by fibrous tissue, necrotic debris, various amounts of blood, and calcium, all covered by a fibrous cap.

Atrial and ventricular demand pacemaker An artificial pacemaker that paces either the atria or ventricles when there is no appropriate spontaneous underlying atrial or ventricular rhythm.

Atrial arrhythmias Arrhythmias originating in the atria, such as wandering atrial pacemaker (WAP), premature atrial contractions (PACs), atrial tachycardia (ectopic atrial tachycardia, multifocal atrial tachycardia), atrial flutter, and atrial fibrillation.

Atrial demand pacemaker (AAI) An artificial pacemaker that senses spontaneously occurring P waves and paces the atria when they do not appear.

Atrial depolarization The electrical process of discharging the resting (polarized) myocardial cells producing the P, P′, F, and f waves and causing the atria to contract.

Atrial diastole The interval or period during which the atria are relaxed and filling with blood. The period between atrial contractions.

Atrial dilatation Distension of the atria because of increased pressure and/or volume within the atria; it may be acute or chronic.

Atrial enlargement Includes atrial dilatation and hypertrophy. Common causes include heart failure, ventricular hypertrophy from whatever cause, pulmonary diseases, pulmonary or systemic hypertension, heart valve stenosis or insufficiency, and acute myocardial infarction. See *Left atrial enlargement (left atrial dilatation and hypertrophy), Right atrial enlargement (right atrial dilatation and hypertrophy).*

Atrial fibrillation An arrhythmia arising in numerous ectopic pacemakers in the atria characterized by very rapid atrial fibrillation (f) waves and an irregular, often rapid ventricular response. Atrial fibrillation is "fast" if the ventricular rate is greater than 100 per minute and "slow" if it is less than 60. When fast, atrial fibrillation is considered uncontrolled (untreated) atrial fibrillation; when slow it is controlled (treated) atrial fibrillation.

Atrial fibrillation (f) waves Irregularly shaped, rounded (or pointed), and dissimilar atrial waves originating in multiple ectopic pacemakers in the atria at a rate between 350 and 600 (average, 400) beats per minute. May be "fine" (less than 1 mm in height) or "coarse" (1 mm or greater in height).

Atrial flutter An arrhythmia arising in an ectopic pacemaker in the atria, characterized by abnormal atrial flutter waves with a sawtooth appearance and usually a regular ventricular response after every other or every fourth F wave. If the QRS complexes occur irregularly at varying F wave-to-QRS complex ratios, a variable AV block is present. Atrial flutter may be transient (paroxysmal) or chronic (persistent). When fast, atrial flutter is considered uncontrolled (untreated) atrial flutter; when slow it is controlled (treated) atrial flutter.

Atrial flutter-fibrillation An arrhythmia arising in the atria alternating between atrial flutter and atrial fibrillation.

Atrial flutter (F) waves Regularly shaped, usually pointed atrial waves with a sawtooth appearance originating in an ectopic pacemaker in the atria at a rate between 240 and 360 (average, 300) beats per minute.

Atrial hypertrophy Increase in the thickness of the atrial wall because of chronic increase in pressure and/or volume within the atria.

"Atrial kick" Refers to the complete filling of the ventricles brought on by the contraction of the atria during the last part of ventricular diastole just before the ventricles contract.

Atrial overload Refers to increased pressure and/or volume within the atria.

Atrial repolarization The electrical process by which the depolarized atria return to their polarized, resting state. Atrial repolarization produces the atrial T (Ta) wave.

Atrial standstill Absence of electrical activity of the atria.

Atrial synchronous ventricular pacemaker (VDD) An artificial pacemaker that is synchronized with the patient's atrial rhythm and paces the ventricles when an AV block occurs.

Atrial systole The interval or period during which the atria are contracting and emptying of blood.

Atrial tachycardia An arrhythmia originating in an ectopic pacemaker in the atria with a rate between 160 and 240 beats per minute. It includes ectopic atrial tachycardia and multifocal atrial tachycardia (MAT). Atrial tachycardia may occur with or without an AV block, which may be constant or variable. It may occur with narrow QRS complexes or abnormally wide QRS complexes because of preexisting bundle branch block, aberrant ventricular conduction, or ventricular preexcitation. When abnormal QRS complexes occur with the tachycardia because of aberrant ventricular conduction, the tachycardia is called *atrial tachycardia with aberrant ventricular conduction (aberrancy).*

Atrial T wave (Ta) Represents atrial repolarization; often buried in the following QRS complex.

Atrio-His preexcitation Abnormal conduction of the electrical impulses from the atria to the bundle of His via the atrio-His fibers (James fibers) bypassing the AV node, resulting in PR intervals that are usually shortened to less than 0.12 second and normal QRS complexes.

Atrio-His fibers (James fibers) Abnormal accessory conduction pathways connecting the atria with the lower part of the AV node at its junction with the bundle of His. See *Atrio-His preexcitation.*

Atrioventricular (AV) block See *AV block and specific AV blocks.*

Atrioventricular (AV) dissociation Occurs when the atria and ventricles beat independently.

Atrioventricular (AV) junction The part of the electrical conduction system that normally conducts the electrical impulse from the atria to the ventricles. It consists of the AV node and the bundle of His.

Atrioventricular (AV) node The part of the electrical conduction system, located in the posterior floor of the right atrium near the interatrial septum, through which the electrical impulses are normally conducted from the atria to the bundle of His.

Atrium The thin-walled chamber into which venous blood flows before reaching the ventricle. The two atria, the right and left atria, form the upper part of the heart, or the base, and are separated from the ventricles by the mitral and tricuspid valves.

Atropine A drug that counteracts parasympathetic activity in the heart, thereby increasing the heart rate and enhancing the conduction of the electrical impulses through the AV node; used to treat sinus bradycardia, sinus arrest/sinoatrial exit block, second- and third- degree AV blocks with narrow QRS complexes, ventricular asystole, and pulseless electrical activity.

Augmented (unipolar) leads Leads aVR, aVL, and aVF; each obtained using a positive electrode attached to one extremity and a negative electrode to a central terminal.

Lead aVR The positive electrode attached to the right arm and the negative electrode to the central terminal.

Lead aVL The positive electrode attached to the left arm and the negative electrode to the central terminal.

Lead aVF The positive electrode attached to the left leg and the negative electrode to the central terminal.

Automaticity, property of The property of a cell to reach a threshold potential and generate electrical impulses spontaneously. Also referred to as the *property of self-excitation.*

Autonomic nervous system Part of the nervous system that is involved in the constant control of involuntary bodily functions, including the control of cardiac output (by regulating the heart rate and stroke volume) and blood pressure (by regulating blood vessel activity). It includes the sympathetic (adrenergic) and parasympathetic (cholinergic or vagal) nervous systems, each producing opposite effects when stimulated.

AV Abbreviation for atrioventricular.

AV block Delay or failure of conduction of electrical impulses through the AV junction.

AV block, first-degree An arrhythmia in which there is a constant delay in the conduction of electrical impulses through the AV node. It is characterized by abnormally prolonged PR intervals (greater than 0.20 second).

AV block, second-degree, type I (Wenckebach) An arrhythmia in which progressive prolongation of the conduction of electrical impulses through the AV node occurs until conduction is completely blocked. It is characterized by progressive lengthening of the PR interval until a QRS complex fails to appear after a P wave. This phenomenon is cyclical.

AV block, second-degree, type II An arrhythmia in which a complete block of conduction of the electrical impulses occurs in one bundle branch and an intermittent block in the other. It is characterized by regularly or irregularly absent QRS complexes (producing, commonly, an AV conduction ratio of 4:3 or 3:2) and a bundle branch block.

AV block, second-degree, 2:1 and advanced An arrhythmia caused by defective conduction of electrical impulses through the AV node or bundle branches or both. It is characterized by regularly or irregularly absent QRS complexes (producing, commonly, an AV conduction ratio of 2:1 or greater) with or without a bundle branch block.

AV blocks with wide QRS complexes Second-degree AV block, type II and 2:1 and advanced AV block, and third-degree AV block with wide QRS complexes require a temporary transcutaneous pacemaker immediately, whether or not the bradycardia is symptomatic.

AV block, third-degree (complete AV block) An arrhythmia in which there is a complete block of the conduction of electrical impulses through the AV node, bundle of His, or bundle branches. It is characterized by independent beating of the atria and ventricles. Third-degree AV block may be transient and reversible or permanent (chronic).

AV conduction ratio The ratio of P, P′, F, or f waves to QRS complexes. For example, an AV conduction ratio of 4:3 indicates that for every four P waves, three are followed by QRS complexes.

AV dissociation Occurs when the atria and ventricles beat independently.

AV junction See *Atrioventricular (AV) junction.*

AV node See *Atrioventricular (AV) node.*

AV sequential pacemaker (DVI) An artificial pacemaker that paces either the atria or ventricles or both sequentially when spontaneous ventricular activity is absent.

Axis Used alone, usually refers to the QRS axis—the single large vector representing the mean (or average) of all the ventricular vectors. It is usually graphically displayed as an arrow. See *P axis, ST axis,* and *T axis.*

Axis of a lead (lead axis) A hypothetical line joining the poles of a lead. A lead axis has a direction and a polarity.

β-blocker Beta blocker, beta-adrenergic blocking agent, β-adrenergic blocking agent. See *Beta blockers.*

Bachmann's bundle A branch of the internodal atrial conduction tracts that extends across the atria, conducting the electrical impulses from the SA node to the left atrium.

Balloon angioplasty The insertion of a balloon-tipped catheter into the occluded or narrowed coronary artery to reopen the artery by inflating the balloon, fracturing the atheromatous plaque, and dilating the arterial lumen. This procedure, also called *percutaneous transluminal coronary angioplasty (PTCA),* is often followed by insertion of a coronary artery stent.

Baseline The part of the ECG during which electrical activity of the heart is absent. Commonly the interval between the end of the T wave and the onset of the P wave (the TP segment) is considered the baseline and is used as the reference for the measurement of the amplitude of the ECG waves and complexes.

Base of the heart The upper part of the heart formed by the right and left atria.

Beta blockers A group of drugs that block sympathetic activity; used primarily to treat tachyarrhythmias, hypertension, angina, and acute MI. *Atenolol, esmolol,* and *metoprolol.*

Bidirectional ventricular tachycardia Ventricular tachycardia characterized by two distinctly different forms of QRS complexes alternating with each other, indicating the presence of two ventricular ectopic pacemakers.

Bigeminy An arrhythmia in which every other beat is a premature contraction. The premature beat may be atrial, junctional, or ventricular in origin (i.e., atrial bigeminy, junctional bigeminy, ventricular bigeminy).

Biological death Present when irreversible brain damage has occurred, usually within 10 minutes after cardiac arrest, if untreated.

Biphasic deflection A deflection having both a positive and a negative component (e.g., a biphasic P wave, a biphasic T wave).

Bipolar limb leads Leads I, II, and III.

Bleeding diathesis A tendency toward abnormally inadequate blood clotting and an increase in bleeding.

Block Delay or failure of conduction of an electrical impulse through the electrical conduction system because of tissue damage or increased parasympathetic (vagal) tone.

Blocked PAC A P′ wave not followed by a QRS complex.

Blood thinner A term used to indicate an anticoagulant, such as warfarin, used to reduce the prothrombin activity, thus inhibiting clot formation.

Bolus A single large dose of a drug that provides an initial high therapeutic blood level of the drug.

Bradycardia An arrhythmia with a rate of less than 60 per minute.

Bradycardias Arrhythmias with rates of less than 60 per minute (e.g., sinus bradycardia; sinus arrest and sinoatrial [SA] exit block; junctional escape rhythm; ventricular escape rhythm; second-degree, type I AV block [Wenckebach]; second-degree, type II AV block; second-degree, 2:1 and advanced AV block; and third-degree AV block).

Bretylium tosylate An antiarrhythmic once used in the treatment of premature ventricular contractions (PVCs), ventricular fibrillation, and ventricular tachycardia.

Bundle branch block (BBB) Defective conduction of electrical impulses through the right or left bundle branch from the bundle of His to the Purkinje network, causing a right or left bundle branch block. It may be complete or incomplete (partial) or permanent (chronic) or intermittent (transient). It may be present with or without an intact interventricular septum.

Bundle branches The part of the electrical conduction system in the ventricles consisting of the right and left bundle branches that conducts the electrical impulses from the bundle of His to the Purkinje network of the myocardium.

Bundle of His The part of the electrical conduction system located in the upper part of the interventricular septum that conducts the electrical impulses from the AV node to the right and left bundle branches. The bundle of His and the AV node form the AV junction.

Bundles of Kent See *Accessory atrioventricular (AV) pathways.*

Buried P wave Refers to a P wave partially or completely hidden in a preceding T wave. This occurs when a sinus, atrial, or junctional P wave occurs during the repolarization of a previous beat as in a sinus, atrial, or junctional tachycardia or a premature atrial or junctional premature beat.

Bursts (or salvos) Refers to the occurrence of two or more consecutive premature atrial, junctional, or ventricular contractions.

CABG See *Coronary artery bypass grafting (CABG).*

Calcium channel blocker A drug that blocks the entry of calcium ions (Ca⁺⁺) into cells, especially those of cardiac and vascular smooth muscle. Used as an antiarrhythmic, antihypertensive, and antianginal drug. *Diltiazem.*

Calcium chloride A calcium salt (electrolyte) used to replenish blood calcium levels after administration of excessive calcium channel blockers or to reverse the effects of hyperkalemia and hypermagnesemia on the heart.

Calibration (or standardization) Accomplished by inserting a standard 1-millivolt (mV) electrical signal to produce a 10-mm deflection (two large squares) on the ECG.

Camel's hump Descriptive term referring to the distinctive narrow, positive wave—the Osborn wave—that occurs at the junction of the QRS complex and the ST segment in hypothermic patients with a core body temperature of ≤95° F. Also referred to as the "J wave" or the "J deflection."

Capture Refers to the ability of a pacemaker's electrical impulse to depolarize the atria or ventricles or both.

Capture beat A normally conducted QRS complex of the underlying rhythm occurring within a ventricular tachycardia.

Cardiac action potential Refers to the membrane potential of a myocardial cell and the changes it undergoes during depolarization and repolarization. The phases of the cardiac action potential include the following:
Phase 0: depolarization phase
Phase 1: early rapid repolarization phase
Phase 2: plateau phase of slow repolarization
Phase 3: terminal phase of rapid repolarization
Phase 4: period between action potentials

Cardiac arrest The sudden and unexpected cessation of an adequate circulation to maintain life in a patient who was not expected to die.

Cardiac cells Cells of the heart, consisting of the myocardial (or "working") cells and the specialized cells of the electrical conduction system of the heart.

Cardiac cycle The interval from the beginning of one heart beat to the beginning of the next one. The cardiac cycle normally consists of a P wave, a QRS complex, and a T wave. It represents a sequence of atrial contraction and relaxation and ventricular contraction and relaxation, in that order.

Cardiac output The amount of blood circulated by the heart in 1 minute, in liters per minute. Obtained by multiplying the amount of blood expelled by the left ventricle with each contraction (stroke volume) by the heart rate per minute.

Cardiac pacemaker An artificial pacemaker. See *Artificial pacemaker.*

Cardiac standstill Absence of atrial and ventricular contractions. This term is used interchangeably with ventricular asystole.

Cardiac tamponade Acute compression of the heart because of effusion of fluid into the pericardial cavity (as occurs in pericarditis) or accumulation of blood in the pericardium from rupture of the heart or penetrating trauma.

Cardiac vector A graphic presentation, using an arrow, representing the moment-to-moment electric current generated by depolarization or repolarization of a small segment of the atrial or ventricular wall.

Cardioaccelerator center One of the nerve centers of the sympathetic nervous system, located in the medulla oblongata, a part of the brainstem. Impulses from the cardioaccelerator center reach the electrical conduction system of the heart and the atria and ventricles by way of the sympathetic nerves.

Cardiogenic Originating in the heart.

Cardiogenic shock A life-threatening complication of acute myocardial infarction caused by the inability of the damaged ventricles to maintain an adequate systemic circulation. One of the consequences of pump failure.

Cardioinhibitor center One of the nerve centers of the parasympathetic nervous system, located in the medulla oblongata, a part of the brain512stem. Impulses from the cardioinhibitor center by way of the right and left vagus nerves innervate the atria, SA node, and AV junction, and to a small extent the ventricles.

Cardiomyopathy A primary disease of the myocardium affecting the bundle branches, causing bundle branch and fascicular blocks, often of unknown etiology.

Cardioversion Application of a synchronized countershock to convert certain arrhythmias—atrial flutter, atrial fibrillation, paroxysmal supraventricular tachycardia (PSVT), wide-QRS-complex tachycardia of unknown origin with pulse, and ventricular tachycardia with pulse—to an organized supraventricular rhythm.

Carotid artery disease Primarily atherosclerotic in nature, with progressive formation of lumen-narrowing (stenotic) atheromatous plaques. A carotid occlusive disease.

Carotid bruit An abnormal sound or murmur heard by auscultation over a stenotic (narrowed) carotid artery, usually a sign of an atheromatous plaque.

Carotid sinus A slightly dilated section of the common carotid artery at the point where it bifurcates, containing sensory nerve endings involved in the nervous reflexes regulating blood pressure and heart rate.

Carotid sinus massage Application of pressure to one of the carotid sinuses with the fingertips to convert paroxysmal supraventricular tachycardia (PSVT) and narrow-QRS-complex tachycardia of unknown origin (with pulse).

Catecholamines Hormone-like substances, such as epinephrine and norepinephrine, that have a strong sympathetic action on the heart and peripheral blood vessels, increasing the cardiac output and blood pressure.

Cation An ion with a positive charge (e.g., K^+, Na^+).

cc Abbreviation for cubic centimeter. It is often substituted for ml.

Cell membrane potential The difference in electrical potential across the cell membrane (i.e., the difference between the electrical potential within the cell and a reference potential in the extracellular fluid surrounding the cell).

Central terminal The central terminal, in the case of the augmented ECG leads, consists of connecting together two of the three electrodes used (the right and left arm electrodes and the left leg electrode) other than the positive electrode. In the case of the precordial leads, the central terminal consists of connecting all three extremity electrodes—the right and left arm electrodes and the left leg electrode. The central terminal is considered to be an *indifferent, zero reference point.*

Cerebrovascular disease General term for a brain dysfunction caused by an inadequacy of the cerebral blood supply.

Cerebrovascular accident (CVA) Cerebral ischemia caused by a decrease in blood flow resulting from obstruction of a blood vessel by an embolus or a thrombus, or from cerebrovascular hemorrhage. Cerebral stroke.

Chambers of the heart Consists of the two thin-walled atria (the right and left atrium) and the two thick-walled ventricles (the right and left ventricle).

Chronic obstructive pulmonary disease (COPD) A chronic disease of the lungs characterized by a chronic productive cough and dyspnea. Typical ECG pattern: poor R-wave progression in the precordial leads V_1 through V_5 or V_6.

Circulatory system The blood vessels in the body, including the systemic and pulmonary circulatory systems.

Clinical death Present the moment the patient's cardiac output ceases, as evidenced by the absence of a pulse and blood pressure; occurs immediately after the onset of cardiac arrest. Common causes are ventricular fibrillation, pulseless ventricular tachycardia, ventricular asystole, and pulseless electrical activity.

Coagulation Clotting. The process of changing from a liquid to a solid (i.e., changing from liquid blood to a solid blood clot or thrombus).

Coarse atrial fibrillation Atrial fibrillation with large fibrillatory waves—1 mm or greater in height.

Coarse ventricular fibrillation Ventricular fibrillation with large fibrillatory waves—greater than 3 mm in height.

Collagen fibers The white protein fibers present in the connective tissue within the intima of the arterial wall that, when exposed to blood after an injury, immediately bind to the platelets directly (via GP Ia receptors) and indirectly through vWF (via GP Ib and GP IIb/IIIa receptors). This action adheres the platelets to the arterial wall and activates them.

Compensatory pause The R-R interval following a premature contraction. It may be full or incomplete, depending on whether the SA node, for example, is depolarized by the premature contraction. If the SA node is not depolarized by the premature contraction, the compensatory pause is called "full" (or "fully"); the sum of a "full" compensatory pause and the preceding R-R interval is equal to the sum of two R-R intervals of the underlying rhythm. If the SA node is depolarized by the premature contraction, resetting the timing of the SA node, the compensatory pause is called "incomplete"; the sum of an "incomplete" compensatory pause and the preceding R-R interval is less than the sum of two R-R intervals of the underlying rhythm.

Complete atrioventricular (AV) block See *AV block, third-degree.*

Complete bundle branch block (right, left) Complete disruption of the conduction of electrical impulses through the right or left bundle branch. The duration of the QRS complex is 0.12 second or greater.

Components of the electrocardiogram Includes the P wave, PR interval, PR segment, QRS complex, ST segment, T wave, U wave, QT interval, TP segment, and R-R interval.

Conducted PAC A positive P' wave (in Lead II) followed by a QRS complex.

Conducted PJC A negative P' wave (in Lead II) followed by a QRS complex.

Conductivity, property of The property of cardiac cells to conduct electrical impulses.

Congestive heart failure (CHF) Excessive blood or tissue fluid in the lungs or body or both caused by the inefficient pumping of the ventricles. One of the consequences of pump failure. May be of recent origin (acute) or of prolonged duration (chronic).

Contractile filament See *Myofibril.*

Contractility, property of The property of cardiac cells to contract when they are depolarized by an electrical impulse.

Controlled atrial flutter A "treated" atrial flutter with a slow ventricular rate of about 60 to 75 beats per minute.

COPD See *Chronic obstructive pulmonary disease (COPD).*

Coronary artery circulation The coronary artery circulation consists of the left coronary artery (LCA) and the right coronary artery (RCA). The left coronary artery has a short main stem, the left main coronary artery, which branches into the left anterior descending (LAD) coronary artery and the left circumflex coronary artery. The arteries that commonly arise from the left anterior descending (LAD) coronary artery, the left circumflex coronary artery, and the right coronary artery are listed below.

Left anterior descending coronary artery
Diagonal arteries
Septal perforator arteries
Right ventricular arteries

Left circumflex coronary artery
Left atrial circumflex arteries
Anterolateral marginal artery
Posterolateral marginal arteries
Distal left circumflex artery

Right coronary artery
Conus artery
Sinoatrial node artery
Anterior right ventricular artery
Right atrial artery
Acute marginal artery
Posterior descending coronary artery
AV node artery
Posterior left ventricular arteries

Coronary artery disease Progressive narrowing and eventual obstruction of the coronary arteries by atherosclerosis.

Coronary artery stenting The procedure of inserting a cylindrical coil or wire mesh into an obstructed coronary artery and expanding it (usually by balloon inflation) to compress the surrounding atherosclerotic tissue and dilate the obstructed lumen.

Coronary artery bypass grafting (CABG) The surgical procedure of bypassing a critically narrowed or obstructed coronary artery using an internal mammary (thoracic) artery or a saphenous vein. Other arteries used for grafting include the radial artery, the inferior gastroepiploic artery, and the inferior epigastric artery.

Coronary artery angioplasty See *Percutaneous transluminal coronary angioplasty (PTCA).*

Coronary artery stent A cylindrical coil or wire mesh. See *Coronary artery stenting.*

Coronary circulation Passage of blood through the coronary arteries and their branches and the capillaries in the heart and then back to the right atrium via the coronary venules and veins and the coronary sinus.

Coronary occlusion (or obstruction) Obstruction of a coronary artery, usually by a blood clot (coronary thrombus); the major cause of acute myocardial infarction.

Coronary sinus The outlet in the right atrium draining the coronary venous system.

Coronary thrombosis The formation of a blood clot (thrombus) within a coronary artery, resulting in coronary artery obstruction; the major cause of acute myocardial infarction.

Coronary vasospasm Coronary artery spasm. One of the causes of coronary artery obstruction.

Cor pulmonale Right heart disease with right ventricular hypertrophy and right atrial dilatation caused by pulmonary hypertension secondary to chronic lung disease.

Corrected QT interval (QTc) The average duration of the QT interval normally expected at a given heart rate.

Coumadin Trade name for warfarin, an anticoagulant. See *Warfarin.*

Countershock See *Synchronized countershock.*

Coupled beats Atrial or ventricular ectopic beats occurring in groups of two. Also called *paired beats, couplet.*

Couplet Two consecutive premature contractions. Also referred to as *coupled beats, paired beats.*

Coupling Ventricular bigeminy with the premature ventricular contractions following the QRS complexes of the underlying rhythm at equal coupling intervals.

Coupling interval The R-R interval between a premature contraction and the preceding QRS complex of the underlying rhythm.

C-reactive protein A plasma protein that becomes abnormally elevated in many acute inflammatory conditions and in tissue necrosis as occurs in acute MI. It becomes elevated in about 24 hours after acute MI.

Current of injury The theoretical cause of ST segment elevation in acute myocardial infarction; an electrical manifestation of the inability of cardiac cells "injured" by severe ischemia to maintain a normal resting membrane potential during diastole.

CVA See *Cerebrovascular accident (CVA).*

Cyanosis Slightly bluish, grayish, slatelike, or purplish discoloration of the skin caused by the presence of unoxygenated blood.

Defibrillation shock An unsynchronized direct-current (DC) shock used to terminate pulseless ventricular tachycardia and ventricular fibrillation.

Deflection Refers to the waves in the ECG. A deflection may be positive (upright), negative (inverted), biphasic (both positive and negative), or equiphasic (equally positive and negative). When a series of waves, such as a QRS complex, is composed of positive and negative deflections, it may be (1) predominantly positive (the sum total of the positive and negative deflections is positive, no matter by how much), (2) predominantly negative (the sum total of the positive and negative deflections is negative, no matter by how much), or (3) equiphasic (the positive deflections are equal to the negative deflections).

Delayed afterdepolarization See *Afterdepolarization.*

Delta wave The slurring of the onset of the QRS complex—the fusion of the depolarization wave of a prematurely activated ventricle, the result of premature ventricular excitation, and the depolarization wave of the other, normally activated ventricle. Present in ventricular preexcitation and nodoventricular/fasciculoventricular preexcitation.

Demand pacemakers Artificial pacemakers that have a sensing device that senses the heart's electrical activity and fires at a preset rate when the heart's electrical activity drops below a predetermined rate level.

Demand pacing Refers to a mode of pacing by an artificial pacemaker in which the pacemaker is turned on when an appropriate underlying spontaneous atrial or ventricular rhythm fails to occur.

Depolarization The electrical process by which the resting potential of a polarized, resting cell of the atria, ventricles, or electrical conduction system is reduced to a less negative value.

Depolarization waves The parts of the ECG representing the depolarization of the atria and ventricles—the P wave (atrial depolarization) and the QRS complex (ventricular depolarization).

Depolarized state The condition of the cell when it has been completely depolarized.

Diabetic hemorrhagic retinopathy A disorder of the retinal blood vessels characterized by degeneration of the blood vessels and hemorrhage within the eye, the result of long-standing, poorly controlled diabetes.

Diastole (electrical) Phase 4 of the action potential.

Diastole (mechanical) The period of atrial or ventricular relaxation.

Diazepam An antianxiety agent used to produce amnesia in conscious patients before cardioversion of certain arrhythmias. A drug that relieves apprehension and anxiety. Trade name: Valium.

Digitalis A cardiac glycoside obtained from the leaves of *Digitalis lanata*, used to decrease rapid ventricular rate in atrial flutter, atrial fibrillation, and paroxysmal supraventricular tachycardia (PSVT) and to improve ventricular contraction in congestive heart failure.

Digitalis effect The changes in the ECG caused by the administration of digitalis. They include prolongation of the PR interval over 0.2 second; depression of the ST segment by 1 mm or more in many of the leads, with a characteristic "scooped-out" appearance; alteration of the T waves so that they appear flattened, inverted, or biphasic; and shortening of the QT interval to less than normal for the heart rate.

Digitalis overdose Excessive administration of digitalis, often accompanied by signs and symptoms of digitalis toxicity, which includes the appearance of arrhythmias, such as sinus arrhythmia and bradycardia; premature atrial, junctional, and ventricular contractions; atrial, junctional, and ventricular tachycardias; accelerated idioventricular rhythm (AIVR); ventricular fibrillation; and AV blocks. In fact, almost any arrhythmia may be caused by excess digitalis.

Digitalis toxicity Digitalis overdose.

Digitalization The process of administering an adequate amount of digitalis over a period of time in the treatment of certain arrhythmias. See *Digoxin*.

Digoxin A cardiac glycoside obtained from the leaves of *Digitalis lanata*, used in the treatment of atrial flutter, atrial fibrillation, and paroxysmal supraventricular tachycardia (PSVT) and to improve ventricular contraction in congestive heart failure.

Dilatation and hypertrophy Refers to the two kinds of enlargement of the atria and ventricles.

Diltiazem hydrochloride A calcium channel blocker drug used to treat atrial tachycardia without block, atrial flutter, atrial fibrillation, and paroxysmal supraventricular tachycardia (PSVT).

Direct-current (DC) shock Used as defibrillation shock, synchronized countershock, and unsynchronized shock to terminate various arrhythmias. See *Defibrillation shock, Synchronized countershock,* and *Unsynchronized shock.*

Directional coronary atherectomy (DCA) The mechanical removal of a noncalcified thrombus through a catheter inserted in the occluded or narrowed coronary artery.

Diuretic A drug used in congestive heart failure to decrease excess body fluid by increasing the secretion of urine by the kidney.

Diving reflex The technique of immersing the patient's face in ice water to elicit the parasympathetic reflex in an attempt to terminate paroxysmal supraventricular tachycardia (PSVT) and narrow-QRS-complex tachycardia of unknown origin (with pulse). It should only be tried if other vagal maneuvers are not effective and ischemic heart disease is not present or suspected.

Dobutamine (Dobutrex) Adrenergic agent used to increase cardiac output and elevate the blood pressure.

Dominant coronary artery (right, left) Refers to the coronary artery, right or left, that gives rise to both the posterior left ventricular arteries and the posterior descending coronary artery.

Dominant (or primary) pacemaker of the heart The SA node.

Dopamine hydrochloride A sympathomimetic that increases blood pressure; used in the treatment of hypotension and shock.

Downsloping ST segment depression A type of ST segment depression that is most specific for myocardial ischemia, including that present in acute subendocardial non-Q-wave MI.

Dropped beats Nonconducted P waves in AV blocks.

Dropped P waves Absent P waves in sinus arrest and sinoatrial (SA) exit block.

Dual-chamber pacemaker An artificial pacemaker that paces the atria, ventricles, or both when appropriate.

Dying heart A heart with feeble, ineffectual ventricular contractions and an ECG showing markedly abnormal QRS complexes, usually a ventricular escape rhythm.

Dysrhythmia A rhythm other than a normal sinus rhythm. A term more correct than "arrhythmia" but less frequently used.

Early afterdepolarization See *Afterdepolarization.*

Early repolarization A normal variant of myocardial repolarization in which the ST segment is elevated or depressed 1 to 3 mm above or below the baseline, respectively. Most commonly elevated in leads I, II, and aVF and the precordial leads V_2-V_6.

ECG Abbreviation for electrocardiogram.

ECG artifacts See *Artifacts.*

ECG calipers A device used in determining the heart rate and rhythm and measuring the various intervals and segments in an ECG tracing.

ECG grid The grid on the ECG paper is formed by dark and light horizontal and vertical lines. It is used to measure the time in seconds (sec) and distance in millimeters (mm) along the horizontal lines and voltage (amplitude) in millimeters (mm) along the vertical lines. The dark vertical lines are 0.20 second (5 mm) apart; the light vertical lines, 0.04 second (1 mm) apart. The dark horizontal lines are 5 mm apart; the light horizontal lines, 1 mm apart. A large square is 5 × 5 mm; a small square, 1 × 1 mm.

ECG lead One of twelve ECG leads that measure the difference in electrical potential generated by the heart, obtained by using a positive and a negative electrode—the positive electrode attached to an extremity or the anterior chest wall and the negative electrode to an extremity or a central terminal. Includes leads I, II, III, aVR, aVL, aVF, and V_1 through V_6.

ECG lead V_{4R} A precordial lead obtained by placing the positive electrode in the right midclavicular line in the right fifth intercostal space. Used primarily to rule out a right ventricular myocardial infarction after the initial finding of an inferior myocardial infarction.

ECG monitor The screen of an oscilloscope used in viewing the ECG.

Ectopic atrial tachycardia An atrial tachycardia that originates in a single atrial ectopic pacemaker site, characterized by P′ waves that are usually identical.

Ectopic beats Premature beats originating in ectopic pacemakers in the atria, AV junction, and ventricles (e.g., premature atrial contractions [PACs], premature junctional contractions [PJCs], and premature ventricular contractions [PVCs]).

Ectopic focus A pacemaker other than the SA node.

Ectopic pacemakers Abnormal pacemakers in the atria, AV junction, bundle branches, Purkinje network, and ventricular myocardium.

Ectopic P wave (P′ wave) A P wave produced by the depolarization of the atria in an abnormal direction, initiated by an electrical impulse arising in an ectopic pacemaker in the atria, AV junction, or ventricles. The ectopic P wave may be either positive (upright) or negative (inverted) in lead II and may precede or follow the QRS complex.

Ectopic rhythms Arrhythmias originating in ectopic pacemakers in the atria, AV junction, and ventricles.

Atrial. Wandering atrial pacemaker (WAP), premature atrial contractions (PACs), atrial tachycardia (ectopic atrial tachycardia, multifocal atrial tachycardia), atrial flutter, atrial fibrillation

Junctional. Premature junctional contractions (PJCs), non paroxysmal junctional tachycardia (accelerated junc tional rhythm, junctional tachycardia), paroxysmal supraventricular tachycardia (PSVT)

Ventricular. Accelerated idioventricular rhythm (AIVR), pre mature ventricular contractions (PVCs), ventricular tachycardia (VT), ventricular fibrillation (VF)

Ectopic tachycardias Abnormal rhythms originating in ectopic pacemakers having a rate of over 100 beats per minute, such as atrial tachycardia (ectopic atrial tachycardia, multifocal atrial tachycardia), atrial flutter, atrial fibrillation, junctional tachycardia, paroxysmal supraventricular tachycardia (PSVT), and ventricular tachycardia (VT).

Ectopic ventricular arrhythmias Abnormal rhythms originating in ectopic pacemakers in the ventricles, such as accelerated idioventricular rhythm (AIVR), premature ventricular contractions (PVCs), ventricular tachycardia, and

ventricular fibrillation.

Ectopy A condition signifying the presence of ectopic beats and rhythms (e.g., ventricular ectopy).

Edema A condition in which the body tissues have accumulated excessive tissue fluid or exudate (as in congestive heart failure).

Einthoven's equilateral triangle An equilateral triangle depicted in the frontal plane using the lead axes of the three limb leads as the sides with the heart and its zero reference point in the center.

Einthoven's law The sum of the electrical currents recorded in leads I and III equals the sum of the electrical currents recorded in lead II.

Electric current The flow of electricity along a conductor in a closed circuit.

Electrical activity of the heart The electric current generated by the depolarization and repolarization of the atria and ventricles, which can be graphically displayed on the ECG.

Electrical alternans Periodic alternation in the size of the QRS complexes between normal and small, coincident with respiration; typically present in cardiac tamponade.

Electrical axis and vector A graphic presentation, using an arrow, of the electric current generated by the depolarization and repolarization of the atria and ventricles.

Electrical conduction system of the heart Includes the sinoatrial (SA) node, internodal atrial conduction tracts, interatrial conduction tract (Bachmann's bundle), atrioventricular (AV) node, bundle of His, right and left bundle branches, and Purkinje network.

Electrical conduction system of the ventricles The His-Purkinje system, which includes the bundle of His, the right and left bundle branches, and the Purkinje network.

Electrical impulse The tiny electric current that normally originates in the SA node automatically and is conducted through the electrical conduction system to the atria and ventricles, causing them to depolarize and contract.

Electrical nonuniformity A condition of the ventricles during the vulnerable period of ventricular repolarization (i.e., the relative refractory period of the ventricles coincident with the peak of the T wave) when the ventricular muscle fibers may be completely repolarized, partially repolarized, or completely refractory. Stimulation of the ventricles at this point by an intrinsic electrical impulse, such as that generated by a PVC or by an extrinsic impulse from a cardiac pacemaker or an electrical countershock, may result in nonuniform conduction of the electrical impulse through the muscle fibers, setting up a reentry mechanism that may precipitate repetitive ventricular contractions and result in ventricular tachycardia or fibrillation. Responsible for the "R-on-T phenomenon."

Electrical potential Refers to the amount of electric current generated by the depolarization and repolarization of the heart and expressed as millivolts (mV). It ranges between 0 to ±20 mV or more.

Electrocardiogram (ECG) The graphic display of the electrical activity of the heart generated by the depolarization and repolarization of the atria and ventricles. The ECG includes the QRS complex; the P, T, and U waves; the PR, ST, and TP segments; and the PR, QT, and R-R intervals.

Electrode A sensing device that detects electrical activity, such as that of the heart. May be positive or negative.

Electrolyte A substance that when in solution dissociates into cations and anions, thus becoming capable of conducting electricity.

Electrolyte imbalance Abnormal concentrations of serum electrolytes within the body caused by excessive intake or loss of such electrolytes as calcium, carbonate, chloride, potassium, and sodium.

Electromechanical dissociation (EMD) A condition of the heart in which the electrical activity of the heart is present and can be recorded on the ECG, but effective ventricular contractions, blood pressure, and pulse are absent.

Embolism Obstruction of a blood vessel by an embolus that reduces or stops blood flow, resulting in ischemia or necrosis of the tissue supplied by the blood vessel.

Embolus A mass of solid, liquid, or gaseous material carried from one part of the circulatory system to another.

End-diastolic PVC A PVC occurring at about the same time that a QRS complex of the underlying rhythm is expected to occur.

Endocardium The thin membrane lining the inside of the heart.

Enhanced automaticity An abnormal condition of latent pacemaker cells in which their firing rate is increased beyond their inherent rate because of a spontaneous increase in the slope of phase-4 depolarization. See *Slope of phase-4 depolarization.*

Enoxaparin A low-molecular-weight (LMW) heparin used as an anticoagulant. See *Anticoagulant.*

Epicardial surface The outside surface of the heart.

Epicardium The thin membrane lining the outside of the heart.

Epinephrine (Adrenalin) A hormone and drug produced by the adrenal gland and other tissues of the body. It is an alpha- and beta-stimulator causing an increase in blood pressure by means of peripheral artery vasoconstriction and an increase in cardiac output by increasing heart rate and force of ventricular contraction. Used in the treatment of bronchial asthma, acute allergic disorders, bradycardia from whatever cause, ventricular fibrillation/pulseless ventricular tachycardia, ventricular asystole, and pulseless electrical activity.

Eptifibatide A platelet GP IIb/IIIa receptor inhibitor that blocks the GP IIb/IIIa receptors on activated platelets from binding to vWF and fibrinogen, thus inhibiting platelet adhesion and aggregation and further thrombus formation.

Equiphasic deflection A biphasic deflection in which the sum of the positive (upright) deflection or deflections in an ECG are equal to that of the negative (inverted) deflection or deflections.

Escape beat or complex A QRS complex arising in an escape (or secondary pacemaker) in the AV junction or ventricles when the underlying rhythm slows to less than the escape or secondary pacemaker's inherent firing rate. Such rhythms are called *junctional* or *ventricular escape beats* or *complexes.*

Escape (or secondary) pacemaker A latent pacemaker in the AV junction or ventricles that takes over pacing the heart when the pacemaker of the underlying rhythm slows to less than the latent pacemaker's inherent firing rate or stops functioning altogether.

Escape rhythm Three or more consecutive QRS complexes that result when the underlying rhythm slows to less than the escape or secondary pacemaker's inherent firing rate, or stops altogether and the escape pacemaker takes over. Examples of escape rhythms are junctional escape rhythm and ventricular escape rhythm.

Esmolol A beta-adrenergic blocking agent used primarily in the treatment of tachyarrhythmias, hypertension, angina pectoris, and acute MI.

Essentially regular rhythm A rhythm in which the shortest and longest R-R interval varies by less than 0.16 second (four small squares) in an ECG tracing.

Excitability, property of The ability of a cell to respond to stimulation.

Extensive anterior MI A myocardial infarction commonly caused by occlusion of the left anterior descending (LAD) coronary artery alone or in conjunction with the anterolateral marginal artery of the left circumflex coronary artery and characterized by early changes in the ST segments and T waves (i.e., ST elevation and tall, peaked T waves) in leads I, aVL, and V_1-V_6 and the appearance early of abnormal Q waves in leads V_1-V_2 and then later in leads I, aVL, and V_3-V_6.

External cardiac pacing Transcutaneous pacing (TCP, TC pacing). A technique to treat bradycardias from whatever cause, ventricular asystole, and pulseless electrical activity using an external artificial pacemaker.

Extrasystole A premature beat or contraction independent of the underlying rhythm caused by an electrical impulse originating in an ectopic focus in the atria, AV junction, or ventricles. Examples of extrasystoles are premature atrial contractions (PACs), premature junctional contractions (PJCs), and premature ventricular contractions (PVCs).

Facing ECG leads Leads that view specific surfaces of the heart (e.g., leads V_1-V_4 are facing leads viewing the anterior of the heart).

Fascicle A band or bundle of muscle or nerve fibers. The left anterior fascicle and the left posterior fascicle form the two major divisions of the left bundle branch before it divides into the Purkinje fibers, forming the Purkinje network. See *Left bundle branch (LBB).*

Fascicular block Absent conduction of electrical impulses through one of the fascicles of the left bundle branch (i.e., left anterior fascicular block, left posterior fascicular block).

Fascicular premature ventricular contraction (PVC) A PVC with an almost normal QRS complex originating in the ventricles near the bifurcation of the bundle of His.

Fasciculoventricular fibers (Mahaim fibers) An accessory conduction pathway located between the bundle of His and the ventricles, resulting in fasciculoventricular preexcitation.

Fasciculoventricular preexcitation Abnormal conduction of the electrical impulses through the fasciculoventricular fibers, resulting in abnormally wide QRS complexes of greater than 0.10 second in duration and of abnormal shape, with a delta wave. PR intervals are normal.

Fast sodium channels Structures in the cell membrane called "pores" that facilitate the rapid flow of sodium ions into the cell during depolarization, rapidly changing the electrical potential within the cell from negative to positive. Fast sodium channels are typically found in the myocardial cells and the cells of the electrical conduction system other than those of the SA and AV nodes.

Fibrillation Chaotic, disorganized beating of the myocardium in which each myofibril contracts and relaxes independently, producing rapid, tremulous, and ineffectual contractions. Fibrillation may occur in both the atria and ventricles.

Fibrillation (f) waves On the ECG, these waves appear as numerous irregularly shaped, rounded (or pointed), and dissimilar waves originating in multiple ectopic foci in the atria or ventricles.

Fibrin An elastic threadlike filament that binds the platelets firmly together to form the thrombus after being converted from fibrinogen.

Fibrinogen A plasma protein that converts to fibrin, an elastic threadlike filament, when exposed to thrombin.

Fibrinolysis The process of dissolving the fibrin strands binding the platelets together within a thrombus, initiating the breakup of the thrombus (thrombolysis).

Fine atrial fibrillation Atrial fibrillation with fine fibrillatory waves—less than 1 mm in height.

Fine ventricular fibrillation Ventricular fibrillation with small fibrillatory waves—less than 3 mm in height.

Firing rate The rate at which electrical impulses are generated in a pacemaker, whether it is the SA node or an ectopic or escape pacemaker.

First-degree AV block An arrhythmia in which there is a constant delay in the conduction of electrical impulses through the AV node. It is characterized by abnormally prolonged PR intervals (greater than 0.20 second).

Fixed coupling Equal intervals of time between each premature beat and the preceding QRS complex of the underlying rhythm (i.e., equal [constant] coupling intervals).

Fixed-rate pacemakers Artificial pacemakers designed to fire constantly at a preset rate without regard to the patient's own heart's electrical activity.

Fluid bolus A rapidly administered predetermined volume of IV fluid, such as 0.9% saline or Ringer's lactate solution, to reverse hypotension and shock.

Flutter Rapid, regular, repetitive beating of the atria or ventricles.

Flutter-fibrillation Refers to the simultaneous occurrence of flutter and fibrillation as in atrial flutter-fibrillation.

Flutter (F) waves On the ECG, these waves appear as numerous repetitive, similar, usually pointed waves originating in an ectopic pacemaker in the atria or ventricles.

Frequent PVCs Five or more PVCs per minute.

Frontal plane A flat surface passing through the body at right angles to a plane passing through the body from front to back in the midline (sagittal plane), as viewed from the front of the body.

Full (fully) compensatory pause See *Compensatory pause*.

Furosemide A rapid-acting diuretic used to treat congestive heart failure by promoting the excretion of urine to reduce pulmonary congestion and edema. Trade name: Lasix.

Fusion beat, ventricular A ventricular complex unlike the QRS complexes of the underlying rhythm and those of the ventricular arrhythmia in a given ECG lead, having features of both. This results from the stimulation of the ventricles by two electrical impulses, one originating in the SA node or an ectopic focus in the atria or AV junction and the other in an ectopic focus in the ventricles. A fusion beat can occur in accelerated idioventricular rhythm (AIVR), pacemaker rhythm, premature ventricular contractions (PVCs), and ventricular tachycardia.

f waves See *Atrial fibrillation (f) waves*.

F waves See *Atrial flutter (F) waves*.

Gap junction A structure within the intercalated disks located at the junctions of the branches of myocardial cells, permitting very rapid conduction of electrical impulses from one cell to another.

Glycoprotein (GP) receptors Adhesive glycoproteins located on platelet surface that bind with various components of connective tissue and blood to form thrombi. The major receptors and their function include the following:
GP Ia binds the platelets directly to collagen fibers present in connective tissue.
GP Ib binds the platelets to von Willebrand factor (vWF).
GP IIb/IIIa binds the platelets to vWF and, after the platelets are activated, to fibrinogen.

Goals in the management of an acute MI The three major goals in the management of acute MI are:
• Prevent the further expansion of the original thrombus and/or prevent the formation of a new thrombus
• Dissolve or lyse the existing thrombus (thrombolysis)
• Enlarge the lumen of the occluded section of the affected coronary artery

GP Ia receptor The platelet receptor that binds the platelets directly to collagen fibers present in connective tissue.

GP Ib receptor The platelet receptor that binds the platelets to von Willebrand factor (vWF).

GP IIb/IIIa receptor The platelet receptor that binds the platelets to vWF and, after the platelets are activated, to fibrinogen.

GP IIb/IIIa receptor inhibitor Inhibits platelet adhesion and aggregation by blocking the platelets' GP IIb/IIIa receptors. Abciximab, eptifibatide.

Gram (g) Measurement of metric weight equal to about 1 cubic centimeter (cc) or 1 milliliter (ml) of water. 1000 g is equal to 1 kilogram (kg).

Grid, ECG See *ECG grid*.

Ground electrode The ECG lead other than the positive and negative leads that grounds the input to prevent extraneous noise from entering the amplifier circuit.

Group beating Repetitive sequence of two or more consecutive beats followed by a dropped beat as seen in second-degree AV block.

Group beats Occurrence of two or more consecutive atrial, junctional, or ventricular premature contractions preceded and followed by the underlying rhythm.

Gruel The semiliquid, lipid-rich mixture often seen within the atherosclerotic plaque.

Heart rate The number of heart beats, QRS complexes, or R-R intervals per minute.

Heart rate calculator ruler A rulerlike device used to calculate the heart rate.

Hemiblock Blockage to the conduction of electrical impulses in one of the fascicles (anterior or posterior) of the left bundle branch. See *left anterior fascicular block (LAFB), left posterior fascicular block (LPFB)*.

Hemodynamically stable (or unstable) Refers to a patient who is normotensive, without chest pain or congestive heart failure, and not having an acute myocardial infarction or ischemic episode. A patient who is *hemodynamically unstable*, on the other hand, is hypotensive with evidence of poor peripheral perfusion, has chest pain or congestive heart failure, or is having an acute myocardial infarction or ischemic episode.

Hemorrhagic diathesis Any tendency to spontaneous bleeding or bleeding from minor trauma caused by a defect in clotting or a defect in the structure of blood vessels.

Hemostatic defects Abnormal conditions that stop the flow of blood within the vessels.

Heparin An anticoagulant. Types of heparin include low-molecular-weight (LMW) heparin and unfractionated heparin. See *Anticoagulant*.

Hexaxial reference figure A guide for determining the direction of the QRS axis in the frontal plane, formed by the lead axes of the three limb leads and three augmented leads, spaced 30° apart around a zero reference point.

His-Purkinje system (of the ventricles) The part of the electrical system consisting of the bundle of His, bundle branches, and Purkinje network.

"Hockey stick" pattern The ventricular "strain" pattern in the QRS-ST-T complex produced by a downsloping ST segment depression and T wave inversion; characteristic of long-standing right or left ventricular hypertrophy. Synonymous with *left* or *right ventricular strain pattern*.

Horizontal plane A flat surface passing through the body at right angles to the sagittal and frontal planes and, in the case of electrocardiography, dividing the chest into an upper and a lower half at the level of the heart.

Hypercalcemia Elevated levels of calcium in the blood.

Hypercapnia Excessive amount of carbon dioxide in the blood.

Hypercarbia Hypercapnia.

Hyperkalemia Excessive amount of potassium in the blood.

Hypertension Blood pressure over 140/90 mm Hg.

Hypertrophy See *Ventricular hypertrophy*.

Hyperventilation Increased ventilation of the alveoli caused by abnormally rapid, deep, and prolonged respirations; the result is a loss of carbon dioxide from the body and eventually alkalosis.

Hypocalcemia Low amount of calcium in the blood.

Hypocapnia Low amount of carbon dioxide in the blood.

Hypocarbia Hypocapnia. Low amount of carbon dioxide in the blood.

Hypokalemia Low amount of potassium in the blood.

Hypotension Low blood pressure; generally considered to be a systolic blood pressure of 80 to 90 mm Hg or less.

Hypothermia A state of low body temperature. When the core body temperature drops to ≤95° F, a distinctive narrow, positive wave—the Osborn wave—appears in the ECG. See *Osborn wave*.

Hypoventilation Decreased ventilation of the alveoli.

Hypovolemia Decreased amount of blood in the body's cardiovascular system.

Hypoxemia Reduced oxygenation of the blood.

Hypoxia Reduced amount of oxygen. Hypoxia is used interchangeably with the term *anoxia*.

ICHD code See *Intersociety Commission for Heart Disease Resources (ICHD) Code*.

Idioventricular Pertaining to the ventricles.

Idioventricular rhythm See *Ventricular escape rhythm*.

Idioventricular tachycardia See *Accelerated idioventricular rhythm (AIVR)*.

IM Abbreviation for intramuscular.

Incomplete AV block (second-degree AV block) An arrhythmia in which one or more P waves are not conducted to the ventricles. See *Second-degree, type I AV block (Wenckebach); Second-degree, type II AV block; Second-degree, 2:1 and advanced AV block*.

Incomplete bundle branch block (right, left) Defective conduction of electrical impulses through the right or left bundle branch from the bundle of His to the Purkinje network in the myocardium, resulting in a slightly widened QRS complex (i.e., greater than 0.10 second but less than 0.12 second).

Incomplete compensatory pause The R-R interval following a premature contraction that if added to the R-R interval preceding the premature complex would result in a sum less than the sum of two R-R intervals of the underlying rhythm. See *Compensatory pause*.

Indeterminate axis A QRS axis between −90° and ±180° (i.e., *extreme right axis deviation*).

Indifferent, zero reference point See *Central terminal*.

Infarction Death (necrosis) of tissue caused by interruption of the blood supply to the affected tissue.

Inferior (diaphragmatic) MI A myocardial infarction commonly caused by occlusion of the posterior left ventricular arteries of the right coronary artery or, less commonly, of the left circumflex coronary artery of the left coronary artery and characterized by early changes in the ST segments and T waves (i.e., ST elevation and tall, peaked T waves) and the appearance later of abnormal Q waves in leads II, III, and aVF.

Inferior vena cava One of the two largest veins in the body that empty venous blood into the right atrium.

Inferolateral MI A myocardial infarction that may be caused (1) by occlusion of (a) the laterally located diagonal arteries of the left anterior descending (LAD) coronary artery and/or the anterolateral marginal artery of the left circumflex coronary artery and (b) the posterior left ventricular arteries of the right coronary artery or, less commonly, of the left circumflex coronary artery of the left coronary artery or (2) by occlusion of the left circumflex artery of a dominant left coronary artery. The infarct is characterized by early changes in the ST segments and T waves (i.e., ST elevation and tall, peaked T waves) and the appearance later of abnormal Q waves in leads I, II, III, aVL, aVF, and V_5 or V_6.

Infranodal Below the AV node.

Infrequent PVCs Less than five PVCs per minute.

Infusion Administration of a fluid other than blood into a vein.

Inherent firing rate The rate at which a given pacemaker of the heart normally generates electrical impulses.

INR International Normalized Ratio, the standard measure of the degree of anticoagulation attained by the administration of an anticoagulant such as warfarin. Based on the prothrombin time (PT), the optimal degree of anticoagulation is present when the INR is within the range of 2.0 to 3.0.

Instantaneous electrical axis or vector A graphic presentation, using an arrow, of the electric current generated by the depolarization or repolarization of the atria and ventricles at any given moment.

Integrilin Trade name for eptifibatide, a GP IIb/IIIa receptor inhibitor.

Interatrial conduction tract See *Bachmann's bundle*.

Interatrial septum The membranous wall separating the right and left atria.

Intercalated disks Specialized structures located at the junctions of the branches of myocardial cells that permit very rapid conduction of electrical impulses from one cell to another.

Internodal atrial conduction tracts Part of the electrical conduction system of the heart consisting of three pathways of specialized conducting tissue located in the walls of the right atrium between the SA node and AV node.

Interpolated PVC A PVC that occurs between two normally conducted QRS complexes without greatly disturbing the underlying rhythm. A full compensatory pause, commonly present with PVCs, is absent.

Intersociety Commission for Heart Disease Resources (ICHD) Code A three-letter code specifying the capabilities of an artificial pacemaker. The first letter of the code indicates which chamber is paced (A, atria; V, ventricles; D, both atria and ventricles); the second letter indicates which chamber is sensed (A, atria; V, ventricles; D, both atria and ventricles); the third letter indicates the response of the pacemaker to a P wave or QRS complex (I, pacemaker output inhibited by a P wave or QRS complex; D, pacemaker output inhibited by a QRS complex and triggered by a P wave).

Intervals The sections of the ECG between waves and complexes of the ECG. Includes waves, complexes, and segments. See *P-P interval, PR interval, QT interval,* and *R-R interval.*

Interventricular septum The membranous, muscular wall separating the right and left ventricles. The anterior portion of the interventricular septum is supplied by the left anterior descending (LAD) coronary artery; the posterior portion is supplied by the posterior descending coronary artery.

Intima The innermost layer lining a blood vessel.

Intracardiac Within the heart.

Intravenous (IV) drip The very slow administration of fluid into a vein.

Intraventricular conduction disturbance Defective conduction of electrical impulses from the AV junction to the myocardium via the bundle branches and Purkinje fibers, resulting in an abnormally wide QRS complex. It occurs most commonly as a right or left bundle branch block and to a lesser extent as a nonspecific, diffuse intraventricular conduction defect (IVCD) seen in myocardial infarction, fibrosis, and hypertrophy; electrolyte imbalance; and excessive administration of certain cardiac drugs.

Intrinsicoid deflection The downstroke of the R wave; the part of the QRS complex that begins at the peak of the last R wave and ends at the J point or tip of the following S wave. Follows the ventricular activation time (VAT) (or preintrinsicoid deflection).

Intrinsicoid deflection time (IDT) See *Ventricular activation time (VAT).*

Ion An atom or group of atoms having a positive charge (cation) or a negative one (anion).

Ischemia Reduced blood flow to tissue caused by narrowing or occlusion of the artery supplying blood to it. Ischemia results in tissue anoxia. Ischemia may be localized under the endocardium (subendocardial ischemia) or under the epicardium (subepicardial ischemia).

Ischemic heart disease Heart disease caused by a deficiency of the blood supply to the heart (the myocardium, the electrical conduction system, and other structures), caused by obstruction or constriction of the coronary arteries. Manifestations of ischemic heart disease include acute MI, angina pectoris, bundle branch and fascicular blocks, right and left heart failure, and arrythmias.

Ischemic T waves Symmetrically positive and abnormally tall, peaked T waves, or symmetrically and deeply inverted T waves that appear over an ischemic myocardium. Generally, the ischemic T waves are upright over subendocardial ischemia and inverted over subepicardial ischemia.

Isoelectric line The flat (sometimes wavy) line in an ECG during which electrical activity is absent. Synonymous with *baseline.*

Isolated beat A premature contraction occurring singly.

IV Abbreviation for intravenous.

IV bolus A single, relatively large dose of a drug given intravenously.

IV fluids Sterile fluids such as 0.9% saline or Ringer's lactate solution administered intravenously.

IV line A catheter or needle, a solution administration set, and an intravenous solution used to administer drugs and fluids intravenously.

James fibers The other name for atrio-His fibers, the abnormal accessory conduction pathway connecting the atria with the lower part of the AV node at its junction with the bundle of His.

J deflection See *Osborn wave.*

Joules Unit of electrical energy delivered for 1 second by an electrical source, such as a defibrillator. Used interchangeably with the term *Watt-seconds.*

J point See *Junction (or "J") point.*

Junction (AV) See *Atrioventricular (AV) junction.*

Junctional arrhythmia An arrhythmia arising in an ectopic or escape pacemaker in the AV junction, such as premature junctional contractions, junctional escape rhythm, non-paroxysmal junctional tachycardia (accelerated junctional rhythm, junctional tachycardia), and paroxysmal supraventricular tachycardia (PSVT).

Junctional escape beats (complexes) and rhythms Beats (or complexes) and rhythms originating in an escape pacemaker in the AV junction that occur when the rate of the underlying supraventricular rhythm drops to less than 40 to 60 beats per minute.

Junctional escape rhythm An arrhythmia originating in an escape pacemaker in the AV junction with a rate of 40 to 60 beats per minute.

Junctional tachycardia An arrhythmia originating in an ectopic pacemaker in the AV junction with a rate greater than 100 beats per minute. When abnormal QRS complexes occur with the tachycardia because of aberrant ventricular conduction, the tachycardia is called *junctional tachycardia with aberrant ventricular conduction (aberrancy).*

Junction (or "J") point The point where the QRS complex becomes the ST segment or the ST-T wave.

J wave See *Osborn wave.*

K⁺ Symbol for potassium.

kg Abbreviation for kilogram.

Kilogram A unit of metric weight measurement. One kilogram (kg) is equal to 1000 grams, or 2.2 pounds.

KVO Abbreviation for "keep the vein open."

L Abbreviation for liter.

LAD Left anterior descending coronary artery. See *Coronary circulation*.

Large squares The areas on ECG paper enclosed by the dark horizontal and vertical lines of the grid.

Latent (or subsidiary) pacemaker cells Cells in the electrical conduction system with the property of automaticity, located below the SA node. These cells hold the property of automaticity in reserve should the SA node fail to function properly or electrical impulses fail to reach them for any reason, such as a disruption in the electrical conduction system.

Lateral leads Leads V_5 and V_6. The *left precordial leads*.

Lateral MI A myocardial infarction commonly caused by occlusion of the laterally located diagonal arteries of the left anterior descending (LAD) coronary artery and/or the anterolateral marginal artery of the left circumflex coronary artery and characterized by early changes in the ST segments and T waves (i.e., ST elevation and tall, peaked T waves) and the appearance later of abnormal Q waves in leads I, aVL, and V_5 or V_6.

LBB See *Left bundle branch (LBB)*.

LBBB See *Left bundle branch block (LBBB)*.

Lead A lead of the ECG. See *ECG lead*.

Lead axis See *Axis of a lead (lead axis)*.

Lead I, monitoring lead See *Monitoring lead I*.

Lead II, monitoring lead See *Monitoring lead II*.

Lead III, monitoring lead See *Monitoring lead III*.

Lead MCL₁, monitoring lead See *Monitoring lead MCL₁*.

Lead MCL₆, monitoring lead See *Monitoring lead MCL₆*.

Left anterior fascicular block (LAFB) Absent conduction of electrical impulses through the left anterior fascicle of the left bundle branch. Typical ECG pattern: q_1r_3 pattern. Also referred to as *left anterior hemiblock*.

Left atrial enlargement (left atrial dilatation and hypertrophy) Usually caused by increased pressure and/or volume in the left atrium. It is found in mitral valve stenosis and insufficiency, acute myocardial infarction, left heart failure, and left ventricular hypertrophy from various causes, such as aortic stenosis or insufficiency, systemic hypertension, and hypertrophic cardiomyopathy.

Left axis deviation (LAD) A QRS axis greater than $-30°$ ($-30°$ to $-90°$).

Left bundle branch block (LBBB) Defective conduction of electrical impulses through the left bundle branch. Left bundle branch block may be complete or incomplete and be present with or without an intact interventricular septum.

Left bundle branch (LBB) Part of the electrical conduction system of the heart that conducts electrical impulses into the left ventricle. It consists of the left common bundle branch (or main stem), which divides into two bundles of fibers, the left anterior fascicle (LAF) and the left posterior fascicle (LPF).

Left posterior fascicular block (LPFB) Absent conduction of electrical impulses through the left posterior fascicle of the left bundle branch. Typical ECG pattern: q_3r_1 pattern. Also referred to as *left posterior hemiblock*.

Left precordial (or lateral) leads Leads V_5 and V_6.

Left ventricular failure Inadequacy of the left ventricle to maintain normal circulation of blood. This results in pulmonary congestion and edema.

Left ventricular hypertrophy (LVH) Increase in the thickness of the left ventricular wall because of chronic increase in pressure and/or volume within the ventricle. Common causes include mitral insufficiency, aortic stenosis or insufficiency, and systemic hypertension.

Lenegre's disease/Lev's disease Idiopathic degenerative disease of the electrical conduction system with fibrosis and/or sclerosis and disruption of the conduction fibers. A cause of bundle branch and fascicular blocks.

Leukocytes White blood cells.

Lidocaine An antiarrhythmic used to treat premature ventricular contractions (PVCs) and monomorphic and polymorphic ventricular tachycardia with a pulse.

Life-threatening arrhythmias Include ventricular fibrillation, pulseless ventricular tachycardia, ventricular asystole, and pulseless electrical activity.

Limb or extremity leads The three standard (bipolar) limb leads (leads I, II, and III) and the three augmented (unipolar) leads (leads aVR, aVL, and aVF).

Lingual aerosol Pertains to a method of delivering a drug by spraying it under the tongue.

Liter (L) A metric measurement of volume. One liter is equal to 1000 milliliters (ml), or 1.1 quarts.

LMW heparin Low-molecular-weight (LMW) heparin, an anticoagulant.

Loading dose A single large dose of a drug that produces an initial high therapeutic blood level necessary to treat certain conditions.

Lovenox Trade name for enoxaparin, a low-molecular-weight (LMW) heparin used as an anticoagulant. See *Anticoagulant*.

Lower case letters Lower case letters, such as q, r, s, are used to designate small deflections of the ECG.

Low-molecular-weight (LMW) heparin An anticoagulant.

LPF See *Left posterior fascicle (LPF)*.

LVH See *Left ventricular hypertrophy (LVH)*.

Lyse To break up, to disintegrate (e.g., to lyse a thrombus).

Lysis The process of breaking up or disintegrating (e.g., thrombolysis).

Magnesium sulfate An electrolyte solution used to treat polymorphic ventricular tachycardia (with pulse), torsade de pointes (with pulse), and ventricular fibrillation/pulseless ventricular tachycardia if indicated.

Mahaim fibers See *Nodoventricular/fasciculoventricular fibers (Mahaim fibers)*.

Marked bradycardia A bradycardia with a heart rate between 30 and 45 beats per minute or less accompanied by hypotension and signs and symptoms of decreased perfusion of the brain and other organs.

Marked sinus bradycardia See *Marked bradycardia*.

MAT See *Multifocal atrial tachycardia (MAT)*.

MCL₁ See *Monitoring ECG lead MCL₁*.

Mean QRS axis The average of all the ventricular vectors; the QRS axis, or simply, the axis.

Mean vector An average of one or more vectors.

Medulla oblongata Part of the brainstem connecting the cerebral hemispheres with the spinal cord; it contains specialized nerve centers for special senses, respiration, and circulation, including the sympathetic and parasympathetic nervous systems with their respective cardioaccelerator and cardioinhibitor centers.

Membrane potential The electrical potential measuring the difference between the interior of a cell and the surrounding extracellular fluid.

mEq Abbreviation for milliequivalents.

Meter A metric unit of linear measurement. One meter is equal to 1000 millimeters, or 39.37 inches.

Metoprolol A beta blocker. See *Beta blockers.*

mg Abbreviation for milligrams.

μg Abbreviation for microgram.

microgram (μg) A metric unit of measurement of weight. One thousand micrograms are equal to 1 milligram.

Midclavicular line An imaginary line beginning in the middle of the left clavicle and running parallel to the sternum slightly inside the left nipple.

Midprecordial (or anterior) leads Leads V_3 and V_4.

Mild bradycardia A bradycardia with a heart rate between 50 and 59 beats per minute and absence of hypotension and signs and symptoms of decreased perfusion of the brain or other organs.

Mild sinus bradycardia See *Mild bradycardia.*

Milliequivalents (mEq) The weight of a substance dissolved in 1 milliliter of solution.

Milligram (mg) A metric unit of weight. One thousand milligrams are equal to 1 kilogram, or 2.2 pounds.

Milliliter (ml) A metric unit of measurement of volume. One thousand milliliters are equal to 1 liter, or 1.1 quarts.

Millimeter (mm) A metric unit of linear measurement. One thousand millimeters are equal to 1 meter, or 39.37 inches.

Millimeter of mercury (mm Hg) A metric unit of weight used in the determination of blood pressure.

Millivolt (mV) A unit of electrical energy. One thousand millivolts are equal to 1 volt.

Mitral stenosis Pathologic narrowing of the orifice of the mitral valve, commonly the result of rheumatic fever or age-related calcification of the valve leaflets. One of the causes of left atrial enlargement.

Mitral valve The one-way valve located between the left atrium and the left ventricle.

ml Abbreviation for milliliter.

mm Abbreviation for millimeter.

mm Hg Abbreviation for millimeters of mercury.

Monitored cardiac arrest Cardiac arrest in a patient who is being monitored.

Monitoring lead I The single ECG lead used for monitoring the heart for arrhythmias. Lead I is obtained by attaching the negative electrode to the right arm or the upper right anterior chest wall and the positive electrode to the left arm or the upper left anterior chest wall.

Monitoring lead II The single ECG lead commonly used for monitoring the heart solely for arrhythmias. Lead II is obtained by attaching the negative electrode to the right arm or the upper right anterior chest wall and the positive electrode to the left leg or the lower left anterior chest wall at the intersection of the left fifth intercostal space and the midclavicular line.

Monitoring lead III The single ECG lead used for monitoring the heart for arrhythmias. Lead III is obtained by attaching the negative electrode to the left arm or the upper left anterior chest wall and the positive electrode to the left leg or the lower left anterior chest wall at the intersection of the fifth intercostal space and the midclavicular line.

Monitoring lead MCL$_1$ An ECG lead commonly used in the monitoring of arrhythmias in the hospital, particularly in differentiating supraventricular arrhythmias with aberrant ventricular conduction (aberrancy) from ventricular arrhythmias. Lead MCL$_1$ is obtained by attaching the positive electrode to the right side of the anterior chest in the fourth intercostal space just right of the sternum. The negative electrode is attached to left chest in the midclavicular line below the clavicle.

Monitoring lead MCL$_6$ The single ECG lead commonly used for monitoring the heart solely for arrhythmias. Lead MCL$_6$ is obtained by attaching the negative electrode to the upper left anterior chest wall and the positive electrode to the lower left anterior chest wall at the intersection of the sixth intercostal space and the midaxillary line.

Morphine sulfate A narcotic analgesic and sedative used to produce amnesia in conscious patients before cardioversion of certain arrhythmias. Also used as a vasodilator to relieve congestive heart failure secondary to left heart failure.

"M" (or rabbit ears) pattern Refers to the rSR' pattern of the QRS complex in V_1, representative of a right bundle branch block.

Multifocal Indicates an arrhythmia originating in different pacemaker sites (e.g., a ventricular arrhythmia with QRS complexes that differ in size, shape, and direction).

Multifocal atrial tachycardia (MAT) An atrial tachycardia that originates in three or more different ectopic pacemaker sites, characterized by P' waves that usually vary in size, shape, and direction in each given lead.

Multifocal premature ventricular contractions (PVCs) Different-appearing premature ventricular contractions (PVCs) in the same tracing that originate from different ectopic pacemaker sites in the ventricles.

Multiform Applies to a ventricular arrhythmia with QRS complexes that differ in size, shape, and direction, originating in single or multiple pacemaker sites.

Multiform premature ventricular contractions (PVCs) Different-appearing premature ventricular contractions (PVCs) in the same tracing that originate in one or more ectopic pacemaker sites in the ventricles.

Multiform ventricular tachycardia Ventricular tachycardia with QRS complexes that differ markedly from beat to beat.

Muscle tremor The cause of extraneous spikes and waves in the ECG brought on by voluntary or involuntary muscle movement or shivering; often seen in elderly persons or in a cold environment.

mV Abbreviation for millivolt.

Myocardial Pertaining to the muscular part of the heart.

Myocardial infarction (MI) See *Acute myocardial infarction (acute MI, AMI).*

Myocardial injury Reversible changes in the myocardial cells from prolonged lack of oxygen. ECG manifestations include ST elevation or depression over injured myocardial cells.

Myocardial ischemia Reversible changes in myocardial cells from a temporary lack of oxygen. ECG manifestations include symmetrical T wave elevation or inversion over ischemic myocardial cells.

Myocardial necrosis (infarction) Irreversible damage to myocardial cells causing their death, the result of prolonged lack of oxygen. ECG manifestations include abnormal Q waves over necrotic myocardial cells.

Myocardial (or "working") cells Myocardial cells other than those in the electrical conduction system of the ventricles.

Myocardial rupture Rupture of the myocardial wall, usually occurring in the left ventricle in the area of necrosis following an acute transmural myocardial infarction.

Myocardium Cardiac muscle.

Myofibril Tiny structure within a muscle cell that contracts when stimulated. Contains the contractile protein filaments actin and myosin.

Myosin One of the contractile protein filaments in myofibrils that give the myocardial cells the property of contractility. The other is actin.

Na⁺ Symbol for sodium ion.

Necrosis Death of tissue.

Nervous control of the heart Emanates from the autonomic nervous system, which includes the sympathetic (adrenergic) and parasympathetic (cholinergic or vagal) nervous systems, each producing opposite effects when stimulated.

Nitroglycerin An explosive used as a vasodilator to relieve angina pectoris and to relieve severe pulmonary congestion and edema (congestive heart failure) secondary to left heart failure. Also used in acute coronary syndromes to enhance coronary blood flow and to reduce ventricular preload by decreasing venous return through venous dilation.

Nodoventricular fibers (Mahaim fibers) An accessory conduction pathway located between the lower part of the AV node and the ventricles, resulting in nodoventricular preexcitation.

Nodoventricular preexcitation Abnormal conduction of the electrical impulses through the nodoventricular fibers, resulting in abnormally wide QRS complexes of greater than 0.10 second in duration and of abnormal shape, with a delta wave. PR intervals are normal.

Noise Extraneous spikes, waves, and complexes in the ECG signal caused by muscle tremor, 60-cycle AC interference, improperly attached electrodes, and biomedical telemetry-related events, such as out-of-range ECG transmission and weak transmitter batteries.

Noncompensatory pause The R-R interval following a premature contraction that, if added to the R-R interval preceding the premature complex, would result in a sum less than the sum of two R-R intervals of the underlying rhythm. Synonymous with *incomplete compensatory pause*. See *Compensatory pause*.

Nonconducted PAC A positive P′ wave (in Lead II) not followed by a QRS complex. A blocked PAC.

Nonconducted PJC A negative P′ wave (in Lead II) not followed by a QRS complex. A blocked PJC.

Nonconducted P wave A P wave not followed by a QRS complex. A dropped beat.

Nonpacemaker cell A cardiac cell without the property of automaticity.

Nonparoxysmal junctional tachycardia An arrhythmia originating in an ectopic pacemaker in the AV junction with a rate between 60 and 150 beats per minute. It includes accelerated junctional rhythm (60 to 100 beats per minute) and junctional tachycardia (100 to 150 beats per minute). It may occur with narrow QRS complexes or abnormally wide QRS complexes because of preexisting bundle branch block or aberrant ventricular conduction. When abnormal QRS complexes occur with the tachycardia because of aberrant ventricular conduction, the tachycardia is called *junctional tachycardia with aberrant ventricular conduction (aberrancy)*.

Non-Q-wave MI A myocardial infarction where abnormal Q waves are absent in the ECG. In the majority of such MIs, a nontransmural MI is present; in the rest it is transmural.

Nonsustained ventricular tachycardia Paroxysms of three or more PVCs separated by the underlying rhythm. Paroxysmal ventricular tachycardia.

Nontransmural Not extending from the endocardium to the epicardium (i.e., partial involvement of the myocardial wall, either in the subendocardial area or the midportion of the myocardium).

Nontransmural myocardial infarction A myocardial infarction in which the ventricular wall is only partially involved by the infarction.

Norepinephrine (Levarterenol) Adrenergic agent used in the treatment of hypotension and shock. Levophed.

Normal QRS axis A QRS axis between −30° and +90°.

Normal saline Incorrect term for the intravenous saline solution containing 0.9% sodium chloride (0.9% saline).

Normal sinus rhythm (NSR) Normal rhythm of the heart, originating in the SA node with a rate of 60 to 100 beats per minute.

Notch A sharply pointed upright or downward wave in the QRS complex or T wave that does not go below or above the baseline, respectively.

Opposite (or reciprocal) ECG leads See *"Reciprocal" ECG changes*.

Optimal sequential pacemaker (DDD) An artificial pacemaker that paces the atria or ventricles or both when spontaneous atrial or ventricular activity is absent.

Oral anticoagulant See *Warfarin sodium*.

Osborn wave The distinctive narrow, positive wave that occurs at the junction of the QRS complex and the ST segment—the QRS-ST junction—in hypothermic patients with a core body temperature of ≤95° F. Also referred to as the "J wave," the "J deflection," or the "camel's hump." Associated ECG changes include prolonged PR and QT intervals and widening of the QRS complex.

Overdrive suppression The suppression of spontaneous depolarization of the SA node or an escape or ectopic pacemaker by a series of electrical impulses (from whatever source) that depolarize the pacemaker cells prematurely. Following termination of the electrical impulses, there may be a slight delay in the appearance of the next expected spontaneous depolarization of the affected pacemaker cells because of a depressing effect that premature depolarization has on their automaticity.

Overload Refers to increased pressure, volume, or both within a chamber of the heart from various causes, resulting in chamber enlargement from dilatation, hypertrophy, or both. Examples are right atrial enlargement, left atrial enlargement, right ventricular hypertrophy, and left ventricular hypertrophy.

PAC Abbreviation for premature atrial contraction.

Pacemaker, artificial An electronic device used to stimulate the heart to beat when the electrical conduction system of the heart malfunctions, causing bradycardia or ventricular asystole. An artificial pacemaker consists of an electronic pulse generator, a battery, and a wire lead that senses the electrical activity of the heart and delivers electrical impulses to the atria or ventricles or both when the pacemaker senses an absence of electrical activity.

Pacemaker cell A myocardial cell with the property of automaticity.

Pacemaker of the heart The SA node or an escape or ectopic pacemaker in the electrical system of the heart or in the myocardium. May be sinus nodal, atrial, AV junctional, or ventricular.

Pacemaker rhythm An arrhythmia produced by an artificial pacemaker.

Pacemaker site The site of the origin of an electrical impulse. It can be the SA node or an escape or ectopic pacemaker in any part of the electrical system of the heart or in the myocardium.

Pacemaker spike The narrow sharp deflection in the ECG caused by the electrical impulse generated by an artificial pacemaker.

Paired beats Atrial or ventricular ectopic beats occurring in groups of two. Also called *coupled beats, couplet.*

Paired PVCs Two consecutive PVCs.

Parasympathetic (cholinergic or vagal) activity The inhibitory action on the heart, blood vessels, and other organs brought on by the stimulation of the parasympathetic nervous system. The effect on the heart and blood vessels results in a decrease in heart rate, cardiac output, and blood pressure and, sometimes, an AV block.

Parasympathetic (cholinergic or vagal) nervous system Part of the autonomic nervous system involved in the control of involuntary bodily functions, including the control of cardiac and blood vessel activity. Activation of this system depresses cardiac activity and produces effects opposite to those of the sympathetic nervous system. Some effects of parasympathetic stimulation are slowing of the heart rate, decreased cardiac output, drop in blood pressure, nausea, vomiting, bronchial spasm, sweating, faintness, and hypersalivation.

Parasympathetic (cholinergic or vagal) tone Pertains to the degree of parasympathetic activity.

Paroxysm Sudden occurrence; spasm or seizure.

Paroxysmal supraventricular tachycardia (PSVT) An arrhythmia with a rate between 160 and 240 beats per minute and usually an abrupt onset and termination. It originates in the AV junction as a reentry mechanism involving the AV node alone (AV nodal reentry tachycardia—AVNRT) or the AV node and an accessory conduction pathway (AV reentry tachycardia—AVRT). It may occur with narrow QRS complexes or abnormally wide QRS complexes because of preexisting bundle branch block or aberrant ventricular conduction. When abnormal QRS complexes occur only with the paroxysmal supraventricular tachycardia because of aberrant ventricular conduction, the tachycardia is called *paroxysmal supraventricular tachycardia (PSVT) with aberrant ventricular conduction (aberrancy).*

Paroxysmal ventricular tachycardia A short burst of ventricular tachycardia consisting of three or more QRS complexes.

Paroxysms of beats Bursts of three or more beats. Three or more beats are considered to be a tachycardia.

P axis The mean of all the vectors generated during the depolarization of the atria.

PEA See *Pulseless electrical activity.*

PCI See *Percutaneous coronary interventions (PCI).*

Peak of the T wave Coincident with the vulnerable period of ventricular repolarization, during which a premature ventricular contraction (PVC) can initiate ventricular tachycardia or ventricular fibrillation.

Percutaneous coronary interventions (PCI) Catheter-based techniques to enlarge the lumen of the occluded section of the affected coronary artery mechanically by means of one or more of the following:
- Percutaneous transluminal coronary angioplasty (PTCA)
- Coronary artery stenting
- Directional coronary atherectomy (DCA)
- Rotational atherectomy

Percutaneous transluminal coronary angioplasty (PTCA) Inserting a balloon-tipped catheter into the occluded or narrowed coronary artery and then inflating the balloon, thus fracturing the atheromatous plaque and dilating the arterial lumen. This procedure, also referred to as *balloon angioplasty,* is the most commonly performed invasive treatment for coronary artery occlusion. It is often followed by insertion of a coronary artery stent.

Perfusion Passage of a fluid such as blood through the vessels of a tissue or organ.

Pericardial effusion Fluid within the pericardial cavity or sac.

Pericardial tamponade Accumulation of fluid under pressure within the pericardial cavity.

Pericarditis Inflammation of the pericardium accompanied by chest pain somewhat resembling that of acute myocardial infarction. The ECG in acute pericarditis mimics that of acute myocardial infarction because of marked ST segment elevation.

Pericardium The tough fibrous sac containing the heart and origins of the superior vena cava, inferior vena cava, aorta, and pulmonary artery. The pericardium consists of an inner, two-layered, fluid-secreting membrane (serous pericardium) and an outer, tough, fibrous sac (fibrous pericardium). The inner layer of the serous pericardium, the visceral pericardium, or as it is more commonly known, the *epicardium,* covers the heart itself; the outer layer, the parietal pericardium, lines the fibrous pericardium. Between the two layers of the serous pericardium is the pericardial space or cavity (or sac), which contains the pericardial fluid.

Peripheral vascular resistance The resistance to blood flow in the systemic circulation that depends on the degree of constriction or dilation of the small arteries, arterioles, venules, and small veins making up the peripheral vascular system.

Peripheral vasoconstriction Constriction of blood vessels, especially the small arteries, arterioles, venules, and small veins, causing an increase in blood pressure and a decrease in the circulation of blood beyond the point of vasoconstriction.

Peripheral vasodilatation Dilation of blood vessels, especially the small arteries, arterioles, venules, and small veins, causing a decrease in blood pressure.

Perpendicular of a lead axis (perpendicular axis) A line intersecting or connecting with the lead axis at ±90° (or a right angle), at its electrically "zero" point. Also referred to simply as the *perpendicular.*

pH Symbol for the concentration of hydrogen ions (H$^+$) in a solution.

Phases of acute MI
   Phase 1: (0 to 2 hours)
   Phase 2: (2 to 24 hours)
   Phase 3: (24 to 72 hours)
   Phase 4: (2 to 8 weeks)
Phases of depolarization and repolarization See *Cardiac action potential.*
Phases of thrombolysis (1) Release of tPA from the endothelium of the blood vessel wall into the plasma; (2) plasmin formation by conversion of plasminogen attached to the fibrin strands within the thrombus through the action of tPA; (3) fibrinolysis by the breakdown of fibrin through the action of plasmin, causing the platelets to separate from each other and the thrombus to break apart.
Physiological AV block An AV block that occurs only when a rapid atrial arrhythmia, such as atrial fibrillation, atrial flutter, and atrial tachycardia, is present.
PJC Abbreviation for premature junctional contraction.
Plasmin An enzyme that dissolves fibrin within the thrombus, helping to break the thrombus apart (thrombolysis). See *Plasminogen.*
Plasminogen A plasma glycoprotein that converts to an enzyme, plasmin, when activated by tissue-type plasminogen activator (tPA). Plasmin, in turn, dissolves the fibrin strands (fibrinolysis) binding the platelets together within a thrombus, initiating thrombolysis.
Platelet activation The second phase of thrombus formation that occurs after the platelets become bound to the collagen fibers. The platelets become activated and change their shape from smooth ovals to tiny spheres while releasing adenosine diphosphate (ADP), serotonin, and thromboxane A_2 (TxA$_2$), substances that stimulate platelet aggregation. Platelet activation is also stimulated by the lipid-rich gruel within the atherosclerotic plaque. At the same time, the GP IIb/IIIa receptor is turned on to bind with fibrinogen. While this is going on, tissue factor is being released from the tissue and platelets.
Platelet aggregation The third phase of thrombus formation. Once activated, the platelets bind to each other by means of fibrinogen, which binds to the platelets' GP IIb/IIIa receptors. Stimulated by ADP and TxA$_2$, the binding of fibrinogen to the GP IIb/IIIa receptors is greatly enhanced, resulting in a rapid growth of the platelet plug. By this time, the prothrombin has been converted to thrombin by the tissue factor.
Platelet GP IIb/IIIa receptor inhibitor A compound that blocks the GP IIb/IIIa receptors on activated platelets from binding to fibrinogen, thus inhibiting platelet adhesion and aggregation and further thrombus formation. GP IIb/IIIa receptor inhibitors include abciximab and eptifibatide.
Platelet adhesion The first phase of thrombus formation. After the denudation or rupture of an atherosclerotic plaque, the platelets are exposed to collagen fibers and von Willebrand factor (vWF). The platelets' receptors GP Ia binds with the collagen fibers and GP Ib and GP IIb/IIIa with vWF, which in turn also binds with collagen fibers. The result is the adhesion of platelets to the collagen fibers within the plaque, forming a layer of platelets overlying the damaged plaque.
Platelets Small cells present in the blood that are necessary for coagulation of blood and maintenance of hemostasis. Contain adhesive glycoproteins (GP) receptors that bind with various components of connective tissue and blood to form thrombi. The major receptors are GP Ia, GP Ib, and GP IIb/IIIa. Platelets also contain several substances that when released upon platelet activation promote thrombus formation by stimulating platelet aggregation. These include adenosine diphosphate (ADP), serotonin, and thromboxane A_2 (TxA$_2$).
Pleura The serous membrane enveloping the lungs and lining the thoracic cavity, completely enclosing a space filled with fluid, the pleural cavity.
P mitrale A wide notched P wave occurring in the presence of left atrial dilatation and hypertrophy. Typically associated with severe mitral stenosis.
Pneumothorax, tension Accumulation of air under positive pressure within the pleural cavity.
Polarity The condition of being positive or negative.
Polarized (or resting) state of the cell The condition of the cell after repolarization, when the interior of the cell is negative and the outside is positive.
Poor R-wave progression Refers to the presence of small R waves in the precordial leads V_1 through V_5 or V_6 characteristic of chronic obstructive pulmonary disease (COPD).
Postdefibrillation arrhythmia An arrhythmia occurring after defibrillatory shocks (e.g., premature beats, bradycardias, and tachycardias).
Posterior MI A myocardial infarction commonly caused by occlusion of the distal left circumflex artery and/or posterolateral marginal artery of the left circumflex artery and characterized by early changes in the ST segments and T waves (i.e., ST depression in V_1-V_4, inverted T waves in V_1-V_2).
Potential (electrical) The difference in the concentration of ions across a cell membrane, for instance, measured in millivolts.
P-P interval The section of the ECG between the onset of one P wave and the onset of the following P wave.
P prime (P′) wave An abnormal P wave originating in an ectopic pacemaker in the atria or AV junction or, rarely, in the ventricles. Usually negative in lead II.
P pulmonale A wide, tall P wave (greater than 2.5 mm in height) occurring in the presence of right atrial dilatation and hypertrophy. Typically associated with pulmonary disease such as COPD, pulmonary embolism, and cor pulmonale.
Precordial Pertaining to the precordium.
Precordial reference figure An outline of the chest wall in the horizontal plane superimposed by the six precordial lead axes and their angles of reference in degrees, radiating out from the heart's zero reference point.
Precordial thump A sharp, brisk blow delivered to the midportion of the sternum with a clenched fist in an initial attempt to terminate ventricular fibrillation or pulseless ventricular tachycardia.
Precordial (unipolar) leads Leads V_1, V_2, V_3, V_4, V_5, and V_6; each obtained using a positive electrode attached to a specific area of the anterior chest wall and a central terminal. The positive electrode for each precordial lead is attached as follows:
   V_1: Right side of the sternum in the fourth intercostal space.
   V_2: Left side of the sternum in the fourth intercostal space.

V_3: Midway between V_2 and V_4.

V_4: Left midclavicular line in the fifth intercostal space.

V_5: Left anterior axillary line at the same level as V_4.

V_6: Left midaxillary line at the same level as V_4.

V_1 and V_2: The right precordial (or septal) leads overlie the right ventricle.

V_3 and V_4: The midprecordial (or anterior) leads overlie the interventricular septum and part of the left ventricle.

V_5 and V_6: The left precordial (or lateral) leads overlie the left ventricle.

Precordium The region of the thorax over the heart, the midportion of the sternum.

Preexcitation syndrome An abnormal ECG pattern consisting of an abnormally short PR interval or an abnormally wide QRS complex with a delta wave, or both, that results when electrical impulses travel from the atria or AV junction into the ventricles through accessory conduction pathways, causing the ventricles to depolarize earlier than they normally would. Accessory conduction pathways are abnormal strands of myocardial fibers that conduct electrical impulses (1) from the atria to the ventricles (accessory AV pathways), (2) from the atria to the AV junction (atrio-His fibers), or (3) from the AV junction to the ventricles (nodoventricular/fasciculoventricular fibers), bypassing various parts of the normal electrical conduction system. Preexcitation syndromes include *ventricular preexcitation, atrio-His preexcitation*, and *nodoventricular/fasciculoventricular preexcitation*.

Preintrinsicoid deflection The part of the QRS complex measured from its onset to the peak of the R wave, or, if there is more than one R wave, to the peak of the last R wave. See *Ventricular activation time (VAT)*.

Premature atrial contraction (PAC) An extra beat consisting of an abnormal P wave originating in an ectopic pacemaker in the atria followed by a normal or abnormal QRS complex. PACs with abnormal QRS complexes that occur only with the PACs are called *PACs with aberrancy*; such PACs resemble PVCs. Also called *premature atrial beats (PABs) or complexes*.

Premature ectopic beat (contraction) An extra beat or contraction originating in the atria, AV junction or ventricles, such as premature atrial contraction (PAC), premature junctional contraction (PJC), and premature ventricular contraction (PVC).

Premature junctional contraction (PJC) An extra beat that originates in an ectopic pacemaker in the AV junction, consisting of a normal or abnormal QRS complex with or without an abnormal P wave. If a P wave is present, the PR interval is shorter than normal. PJCs with abnormal QRS complexes that occur only with the PJCs are called *PJCs with aberrancy*. Such PJCs resemble PVCs.

Premature ventricular contraction (PVC) An extra beat consisting of an abnormally wide and bizarre QRS complex originating in an ectopic pacemaker in the ventricles.

Prinzmetal's angina A severe form of angina pectoris occurring at rest, caused by coronary artery spasm.

Procainamide hydrochloride An antiarrhythmic used to treat premature ventricular contractions and ventricular tachycardia.

Procainamide toxicity Excessive administration of procainamide, manifested by wide QRS complexes, low and wide T waves, U waves, prolonged PR intervals, depressed ST segments, and prolonged QT intervals.

Promethazine hydrochloride A drug used primarily for the prevention and control of nausea and vomiting.

Prophylaxis Preventive treatment.

Prothrombin A plasma protein that, when activated by exposure of the blood to tissue factor released from damaged arterial wall tissue, converts to thrombin. Thrombin in turn converts fibrinogen to fibrin.

PR (P'R) interval The section of the ECG between the onset of the P (or P') wave and the onset of the QRS complex. Normal PR interval is 0.12 to 2.0 second.

PR segment The section of the ECG between the end of the P wave and the onset of the QRS complex.

Pseudoelectromechanical dissociation A life-threatening condition in which the ventricular contractions are too weak to produce a detectable pulse and blood pressure because of the failure of the myocardium or electrical conduction system or both from a variety of causes. A form of pulseless electrical activity.

PTCA Percutaneous transluminal coronary angioplasty (PTCA).

Pulmonary circulation Passage of blood from the right ventricle through the pulmonary artery, all of its branches, and capillaries in the lungs and then to the left atrium through the pulmonary venules and veins. The blood vessels within the lungs and those carrying blood to and from the lungs.

Pulmonary embolism Obstruction (occlusion) of pulmonary arteries by small amounts of solid, liquid, or gaseous material carried to the lungs through the veins. Typical ECG pattern: $S_1Q_3T_3$ pattern.

Pulmonary infarction Localized necrosis of lung tissue caused by obstruction of the arterial blood supply, commonly caused by pulmonary embolism.

Pulmonic valve The one-way valve located between the right ventricle and the pulmonary artery.

Pulseless electrical activity The absence of a detectable pulse and blood pressure in the presence of electrical activity of the heart as evidenced by some type of an ECG rhythm other than ventricular fibrillation or ventricular tachycardia.

Pulseless ventricular tachycardia A life-threatening arrhythmia equivalent to ventricular fibrillation and treated the same way, by immediate defibrillation.

Pulse oximetry The continuous measurement of the oxygen saturation of hemoglobin and the pulse.

Pump failure Partial or total failure of the heart to pump blood forward effectively, causing congestive heart failure and cardiogenic shock. It is a complication of acute myocardial infarction, occurring more frequently in the presence of a bundle branch block.

Purkinje fibers Tiny, immature muscle fibers forming an intricate web, the Purkinje network, spread widely throughout the subendocardial tissue of the ventricles, whose ends finally terminate at the myocardial cells.

Purkinje network of the ventricles The part of the electrical conduction system between the bundle branches and the ventricular myocardium consisting of the Purkinje fibers and their terminal branches.

PVC Abbreviation for premature ventricular contraction.

P wave Normally, the first wave of the P-QRS-T complex representing the depolarization of the atria. The P wave may be positive (upright), symmetrically tall and peaked, or wide and notched; negative (inverted); biphasic (partially upright, partially inverted); or flat.

q₁r₃ pattern Typical ECG pattern of an initial small q wave in lead I and an initial small r wave in lead III indicative of a left anterior fascicular block.

q₃r₁ pattern Typical ECG pattern of an initial small q wave in lead III and an initial small r wave in lead I indicative of a left posterior fascicular block.

QRS axis The single large vector representing the mean (or average) of all the ventricular vectors.

QRS complex Normally, the wave following the P wave, consisting of the Q, R, and S waves, and representing ventricular depolarization. May be normal (narrow), 0.10 second or less, or abnormal (wide), greater than 0.10 second.

qRS pattern The QRS pattern present in leads V₅-V₆ typical of right bundle branch block with an intact interventricular septum. An example of a QRS complex with a "terminal S" wave.

QRS-ST-T pattern Refers to the abnormally wide, "sine-wave" appearing QRS-ST-T complex that occurs in hyperkalemia.

QSR pattern The QRS pattern present in leads V₁-V₂ typical of right bundle branch block with a damaged interventricular septum.

QS wave A QRS complex that consists entirely of a single, large negative deflection.

QTc See *Corrected QT interval (QTc)*.

QT interval The section of the ECG between the onset of the QRS complex and the end of the T wave, representing ventricular depolarization and repolarization.

Quadrants Refers to the four quadrants of the hexaxial reference figure—quadrants I, II, III, and IV.

Quadrigeminy A series of groups of four beats, usually consisting of three normally conducted QRS complexes followed by a premature contraction that may be atrial, junctional, or ventricular in origin (i.e., atrial quadrigeminy, junctional quadrigeminy, ventricular quadrigeminy).

Quinidine sulfate An antiarrhythmic used to treat premature atrial and junctional contractions.

Quinidine toxicity Excessive administration of quinidine, manifested electrocardiographically by wide, often notched P waves; wide QRS complexes; low, wide T waves; U waves; prolonged PR intervals; depressed ST segments; and prolonged QT intervals.

Q wave The first negative deflection of the QRS complex not preceded by an R wave.

Q wave myocardial infarction (MI) A myocardial infarction in which abnormal Q waves are present in the ECG. In the majority of the Q wave MIs a transmural myocardial infarction is present; in the rest, the infarction involves only the subendocardium or midportion of the myocardium.

Rabbit ears pattern See *rSR' pattern*.

Rate conversion table A table converting the number of small squares between two adjacent R waves into the heart rate per minute.

Rate of impulse formation (the firing rate) See *Slope of phase-4 depolarization*.

R double prime (R") The third R wave in a QRS complex.

"Reciprocal" ECG changes ECG changes of evolving acute myocardial infarction present in opposite ECG leads, being, for the most part, opposite in direction to those in the facing ECG leads (i.e., a mirror image). For example, an elevated ST segment and a symmetrically tall, peaked T wave in a facing ECG lead is mirrored as a depressed ST segment and a deeply inverted T wave in an opposite ECG lead.

Reentry mechanism A mechanism by which an electrical impulse repeatedly exits and reenters an area of the heart causing one or more ectopic beats.

Refractory Inability to respond to a stimulus.

Refractory period The time during which a cell or fiber may or may not be depolarized by an electrical stimulus depending on the strength of the electrical impulse. It extends from phase 0 to the end of phase 3 and is divided into the *absolute refractory period (ARP)* and *relative refractory period (RRP)*. The absolute refractory period extends from phase 0 to about midway through phase 3. The relative refractory period extends from about midway through phase 3 to the end of phase 3.

Relative refractory period (RRP) of the ventricles The period of ventricular repolarization during which the ventricles can be stimulated to depolarize by an electrical impulse stronger than usual. It begins at about the peak of the T wave and ends with the end of the T wave.

ReoPro Trade name for abciximab.

Reperfusion therapy Treatment to reopen an occluded atherosclerotic coronary artery using a thrombolytic agent or a mechanical means such as percutaneous coronary interventions that include percutaneous transluminal coronary angioplasty (PTCA), coronary artery stenting, directional coronary atherectomy (DCA), and rotational atherectomy.

Repolarization The electrical process by which a depolarized cell returns to its polarized, resting state.

Repolarization wave The progression of the repolarization process through the atria and ventricles that appears on the ECG as the atrial and ventricular T waves.

Repolarized state The condition of the cell when it has been completely repolarized.

Resting membrane potential Electrical measurement of the difference between the electrical potential of the interior of a fully repolarized, resting cell and that of the extracellular fluid surrounding it.

Resting state of a cell The condition of a cell when a layer of positive ions surrounds the cell membrane and an equal number of negative ions lines the inside of the cell membrane directly opposite each positive ion. A cell in such a condition is called a *polarized cell*.

Resuscitation The restoration of life by artificial respiration and external chest compression.

Retavase Trade name for reteplase (r-PA), a thrombolytic agent.

Reteplase (r-PA) A thrombolytic agent that converts plasminogen, a plasma protein, to plasmin, which in turn dissolves the fibrin binding the platelets together within a thrombus (fibrinolysis), causing the thrombus to break apart (thrombolysis). Trade name: Retavase.

Retrograde atrial depolarization Abnormal depolarization of the atria that begins near the AV junction, producing a negative P' wave in Lead II. Typically associated with junctional arrhythmias.

Retrograde AV block Delay or failure of backward conduction through the AV junction into the atria of electrical impulses originating in the bundle of His or ventricles.

Retrograde conduction Conduction of an electrical impulse in a direction opposite to normal (i.e., from the AV junction or ventricles [through the AV junction] to the atria or SA node). Same as *retrograde AV conduction.*

Right atrial enlargement (right atrial dilatation and hypertrophy) Usually caused by increased pressure and/or volume in the right atrium. It is found in pulmonary valve stenosis, tricuspid valve stenosis and insufficiency (relatively rare), and pulmonary hypertension and right ventricular hypertrophy from various causes. These include chronic obstructive pulmonary disease (COPD), cor pulmonale, status asthmaticus, pulmonary embolism, pulmonary edema, mitral valve stenosis or insufficiency, and congenital heart disease.

Right axis deviation (RAD) A QRS axis greater than +90°. Extreme right axis deviation—a QRS axis between −90° and ±180° (indeterminate axis).

Right bundle branch (RBB) Part of the electrical conduction system of the heart that conducts electrical impulses into the right ventricle.

Right bundle branch block (RBBB) Defective conduction of electrical impulses through the right bundle branch. It may be complete or incomplete and be present with or without an intact interventricular septum. Typical ECG patterns:

- **rSR′ pattern** in lead V_1, the so-called *"M" (or rabbit ears) pattern*
- **Tall "terminal" R waves** in leads aVR and V_1-V_2
- **Deep and slurred "terminal" S waves** in leads I, aVL, and V_5-V_6
- **qRS pattern** in leads V_5-V_6—typical of right bundle branch block with an intact interventricular septum
- **QSR pattern** in leads V_1-V_2—typical of right bundle branch block without an intact interventricular septum

Right heart failure Inadequacy of the right ventricle to maintain the normal circulation of blood. This results in distended veins of the body, especially the jugular veins; body tissue edema; and congestion and distension of the liver and spleen. The lungs are typically clear.

Right precordial (or septal) leads Leads V_1-V_2.

Right precordial (unipolar) leads Leads V_{2R}, V_{3R}, V_{4R}, V_{5R}, and V_{6R}; each obtained using a positive electrode attached to a specific area of the right anterior chest wall and a central terminal. The right precordial leads overlie the right ventricle. The positive electrode for each right precordial lead is attached as follows:

V_{2R}: Right side of the sternum in the fourth intercostal space
V_{3R}: Midway between V_{2R} and V_{4R}
V_{4R}: Right midclavicular line in the right fifth intercostal space
V_{5R}: Right anterior axillary line at the same level as V_{4R}
V_{6R}: Right midaxillary line at the same level as V_{4R}

Right ventricular hypertrophy (RVH) Increase in the thickness of the right ventricular wall because of chronic increase in pressure and/or volume within the ventricle. It is found in pulmonary valve stenosis and other congenital heart defects (e.g., atrial and ventricular septal defects), tricuspid valve insufficiency (relatively rare), and pulmonary hyper-

tension from various causes. These include chronic obstructive pulmonary disease (COPD), status asthmaticus, pulmonary embolism, pulmonary edema, and mitral valve stenosis or insufficiency.

Right ventricular MI A myocardial infarction caused by the occlusion of the right coronary artery and characterized by early changes in the ST segments and T waves (i.e., ST elevation and tall, peaked T waves) and taller than normal R waves in leads II, III, and aVF and ST segment elevation in V_{4R} and the appearance later of abnormal QS waves or complexes with T wave inversion in leads II, III, and aVF and T wave inversion in V_{4R}.

Ringer's lactate solution Frequently used sterile IV solution containing sodium, potassium, calcium, and chloride ions in about the same concentrations as present in blood, in addition to lactate ions.

R-on-T phenomenon An ominous type of premature ventricular contraction (PVC) that falls on the T wave of the preceding QRS-T complex. This can cause ventricular tachycardia or ventricular fibrillation.

Rotational atherectomy The use of a rotational, drill-like device to remove a calcified thrombus.

r-PA See *Reteplase (r-PA).*

RP′ interval The section of the ECG between the onset of the QRS complex and the onset of the P′ wave following it. This is present in junctional arrhythmias and occasionally in ventricular arrhythmias.

R prime (R′) The second R wave in a QRS complex.

R-R interval The section of the ECG between the onset of one QRS complex and the onset of an adjacent QRS complex or between the peaks of two adjacent R waves.

RS pattern Refers to the appearance of a QRS complex in which there is an initial tall R wave followed by a deep S wave.

rSR′ pattern A typical QRS complex pattern in V_1 present in right bundle branch block. Also referred to as the *"M"* or *rabbit ears pattern.*

R wave The positive wave or deflection in the QRS complex. An upper case "R" indicates a large R wave; a lower case "r," a small R wave. May be tall or small; narrow or wide, slurred, or notched.

Salvos Refers to two or more consecutive premature contractions. Bursts.

SA node The dominant pacemaker of the heart located in the wall of the right atrium near the inlet of the superior vena cava.

Sawtooth appearance Description given atrial flutter waves.

Scooped-out appearance Description given to the depression of the ST segment caused by digitalis. Also referred to as the *"digitalis effect."*

S double prime (S″) The third S wave in the QRS complex.

Secondary pacemaker of the heart A pacemaker in the electrical system of the heart other than the SA node; an escape or ectopic pacemaker.

Second-degree AV block An arrhythmia in which one or more P waves are not conducted to the ventricles. Incomplete AV block. See *AV block, second-degree, type I (Wenckebach); AV block, second-degree, type II;* and *AV block, second-degree, 2:1 and advanced.*

Second-degree, type I AV block (Wenckebach) An arrhythmia in which progressive prolongation of the conduction of electrical impulses through the AV node occurs until conduction is completely blocked. It is characterized by progressive lengthening of the PR interval until a QRS complex fails to appear after a P wave. This phenomenon is cyclical.

Second-degree, type II AV block An arrhythmia in which a complete block of conduction of the electrical impulses occurs in one bundle branch and an intermittent block in the other. It is characterized by regularly or irregularly absent QRS complexes (producing, commonly, an AV conduction ratio of 4:3 or 3:2). The QRS complexes, typically, are abnormally wide (greater than 0.12 second in duration).

Second-degree, 2:1 and advanced AV block An arrhythmia caused by defective conduction of the electrical impulses through the AV node or the bundle branches or both. It is characterized by regularly or irregularly absent QRS complexes (producing, commonly, an AV conduction ratio of 2:1 or greater). The QRS complexes may be narrow (0.10 second or less) or abnormally wide (greater than 0.12 second in duration).

Segment A section of the ECG between two waves (e.g., PR segment, ST segment, and TP segment). A segment does not include waves or intervals.

Self-excitation, property of The property of a cell to reach a threshold potential and generate electrical impulses spontaneously without being externally stimulated. Also referred to as the *property of automaticity.*

Septal depolarization Refers to the depolarization of the interventricular septum early in ventricular depolarization, producing the septal q and r waves.

Septal leads Leads V$_1$-V$_2$. The *right precordial leads.*

Septal MI A myocardial infarction commonly caused by occlusion of the left anterior descending (LAD) coronary artery beyond the first diagonal branch, involving the septal perforator arteries, and characterized by early changes in the ST segments and T waves (i.e., ST elevation and tall, peaked T waves) and the early appearance of abnormal Q waves in leads V$_1$-V$_2$.

Septal q waves The small q waves produced by the normal left-to-right depolarization of the interventricular septum early in ventricular depolarization. Present in one or more of leads I, II, III, aVL, aVF, and V$_5$-V$_6$.

Septal r waves The small r waves produced by the normal left-to-right depolarization of the interventricular septum early in ventricular depolarization. Present in the right precordial leads V$_1$ and V$_2$.

Septum A wall separating two cavities.

Serotonin A substance released from platelets after the platelets are activated after damage to the blood vessel walls. Serotonin is a potent vasoconstrictor and promotes thrombus formation by stimulating platelet aggregation. Other substances released on platelet activation are adenosine diphosphate (ADP) and thromboxane A$_2$ (TxA$_2$).

Serum cardiac markers Proteins and enzymes released from damaged or necrotic myocardial tissue into the blood. These serum markers include myoglobin, CK-MB (creatinine kinase MB isoenzyme), and troponin T and I (cTnT, cTnI).

Shock A state of cardiovascular collapse caused by numerous factors such as severe AMI, hemorrhage, anaphylactic reaction, severe trauma, pain, strong emotions, drug toxicity, or other causes. A patient in decompensated shock typically has dulled senses and staring eyes, a pale and cyanotic color, cold and clammy skin, systolic blood pressure of 80 to 90 mm Hg or less, a feeble rapid pulse (over 110 beats per minute), and a urinary output of less than 20 ml per hour.

Short vertical lines The vertical lines inscribed at every 3-second interval along the top of the ECG paper.

Sick sinus syndrome A clinical entity manifested by syncope or near-syncope, dizziness, increased congestive heart failure, angina, and/or palpitations as a result of a dysfunctioning sinus node, especially in the elderly. The ECG may show marked sinus bradycardia, sinus arrest, sinoatrial (SA) block, chronic atrial fibrillation or flutter, AV junctional escape rhythm, or tachyarrhythmias interspersing with the bradycardias (sinus-tachyarrhythmia syndrome).

Single-chamber pacemaker Artificial pacemaker that paces either the atria or the ventricles when appropriate.

Sinoatrial (SA) exit block An arrhythmia caused by a block in the conduction of the electrical impulse from the SA node to the atria, resulting in bradycardia, episodes of asystole, or both.

Sinoatrial (SA) node See *SA node.*

Sinus arrest An arrhythmia caused by a decrease in the automaticity of the SA node, resulting in bradycardia, episodes of asystole, or both.

Sinus arrhythmia Irregularity of the heart rate caused by fluctuations of parasympathetic activity on the SA node during breathing.

Sinus bradycardia An arrhythmia originating in the SA node with a rate of less than 60 beats per minute.

Sinus node arrhythmias Arrhythmias arising in the sinus (SA) node include sinus arrhythmia, sinus bradycardia, sinus arrest and sinoatrial (SA) exit block, and sinus tachycardia.

Sinus P wave A P wave produced by the depolarization of the atria initiated by an electrical impulse arising in the SA node.

Sinus tachycardia An arrhythmia originating in the SA node with a rate of over 100 beats per minute.

Site of origin Pacemaker site.

6-second count method A method of determining the heart rate by counting the number of QRS complexes within a 6-second interval and multiplying this number by 10 to get the heart rate per minute.

6-second intervals The period between every third 3-second interval mark.

Slope of phase-4 depolarization Refers to the rate at which a cell membrane depolarizes spontaneously, becoming progressively less negative, during phase 4—the period between action potentials. As soon as the threshold potential is reached, rapid depolarization of the cell (phase 0) occurs. The rate of spontaneous depolarization is dependent on the degree of sloping of phase-4 depolarization. The steeper the slope of phase-4 depolarization, the faster is the rate of spontaneous depolarization and the rate of impulse formation (the firing rate). The flatter the slope, the slower is the firing rate.

Slow calcium-sodium channels A mechanism in the membrane of certain cardiac cells, predominantly those of the SA and AV nodes, by which positively charged calcium and sodium ions enter the cells slowly during depolarization, changing the potential within these cells from negative to positive. The result is a slower rate of depolarization as compared with the depolarization of cardiac cells with fast sodium channels.

Slow ventricular tachycardia See *Accelerated idioventricular rhythm (AIVR).*

Slurring of the QRS complex The delta wave.

Small squares The areas on ECG paper enclosed by the light horizontal and vertical lines of the grid.

Sodium bicarbonate Chemical substance with alkaline properties used to increase the pH or alkalinity of the body when acidosis is present; considered in the treatment of ventricular fibrillation, pulseless ventricular tachycardia, ventricular asystole, and pulseless electrical activity if indicated.

Sodium-potassium pump A mechanism in the cell membrane, activated during phase 4—the period between action potentials, that transports excess sodium out of the cell and potassium back in to help maintain a stable membrane potential between action potentials.

Specialized cells of the electrical conduction system of the heart One of two kinds of cardiac cells in the heart, the other being the myocardial (or "working") cells. The specialized cells conduct electrical impulses extremely rapidly (six times faster than do the myocardial cells), but do not contract. Some of these cells, the pacemaker cells, are also capable of generating electrical impulses spontaneously, having the property of automaticity.

Spikes Artifacts in the ECG. If numerous and occurring randomly, they are most likely caused by muscle tremor, AC interference, loose electrodes, or biotelemetry-related interference. If they are regular, occurring at a rate of about 60 to 80/minute, they are most likely caused by an artificial pacemaker.

Spontaneous depolarization Property possessed by pacemaker cells allowing them to achieve threshold potential and depolarize without external stimulation.

S prime (S′) The second S wave in the QRS complex.

S₁Q₃T₃ pattern Typical ECG changes in lead I and lead III that occur in acute pulmonary embolism (i.e., large S wave in lead I and a Q wave and inverted T wave in lead III).

Standard (bipolar) limb leads Standard limb leads I, II, and III; each obtained using a positive electrode attached to one extremity and a negative electrode to another extremity as follows:

Lead I: The positive electrode attached to the left arm and the negative electrode to the right arm.

Lead II: The positive electrode attached to the left leg and the negative electrode to the right arm. Commonly used as a monitoring lead in prehospital emergency cardiac care.

Lead III: The positive electrode attached to the left leg and the negative electrode to the left arm.

Standardization of the ECG tracing A means of standardizing the amplitude of the waves and complexes of the ECG using a 1 millivolt/10 mm standardization impulse.

Standard leads Usually refers to the 12 ECG leads—*leads I, II, III, aVR, aVL, aVF, and V₁ through V₆.*

Standard paper speed A rate of 25 mm per second.

ST axis The mean of all the vectors generated during the ST segment.

Stent A cylindrical coil or wire mesh. See *Coronary artery stenting.*

Strain pattern Refers to the combination of a downsloping ST segment depression and a T wave inversion, characteristic of long-standing right or left ventricular hypertrophy. Along with the R wave, gives the so-called "hockey stick" appearance to the QRS-ST-T complex.

ST segment The section of the ECG between the end of the QRS complex, the "J" point, and onset of the T wave. May be flat (horizontal), downsloping, or upsloping.

ST segment depression An ECG sign of severe myocardial ischemia, appearing in the leads facing the ischemia. An ST segment is considered to be depressed when it is ≥1 mm (≥0.1 mV) below the baseline, measured 0.04 second (1 small square) after the J point of the QRS complex. It may be flat, upsloping, or downsloping. ST depression is also seen in the leads opposite those with ST elevation.

ST segment elevation An ECG sign of severe, extensive, myocardial ischemia and injury in the evolution of an acute Q-wave MI, usually indicating a transmural involvement. Less frequently, it may be seen in an acute non-Q-wave MI. An ST segment is considered to be elevated when it is ≥1 mm (≥0.1 mV) above the baseline, measured 0.04 second (1 small square) after the J point of the QRS complex. ST elevation usually occurs in the leads facing the myocardial ischemia and injury. ST elevation is also present in pericarditis and early repolarization.

ST-T wave The section of the ECG between the end of the QRS complex and the end of the T wave that includes the ST segment and T wave.

Subendocardial Located under the endocardium.

Subendocardial, non-Q-wave MI A myocardial infarction localized in the subendocardial area of the myocardium with absent Q waves in the ECG most of the time. See *Non-Q wave myocardial infarction.*

Subepicardial Located under the epicardium.

Sublingual Under the tongue. Subglossal.

Substernal Under the sternum (retrosternal).

Sudden cardiac death Sudden and unexpected death usually from coronary heart disease in patients with relatively minor or vague premonitory symptoms who appear well. Usual cause: a life- threatening arrhythmia.

Superior vena cava One of the two largest veins in the body that empty venous blood into the right atrium.

Supernormal period The short terminal phase of repolarization (phase 3) of cardiac cells near the end of the T wave, just before the cells return to their resting potential, during which a stimulus weaker than is normally required can depolarize the cardiac cells.

Supernormal period of ventricular repolarization The last phase of repolarization during which the cell can be stimulated to depolarize by an electrical stimulus weaker than usual (i.e., a subthreshold stimulus).

Supraventricular Refers to the part of the heart above the bundle branches; includes the SA node, atria, and AV junction.

Supraventricular arrhythmia An arrhythmia originating above the bifurcation of the bundle of His.

Supraventricular tachycardia An arrhythmia originating above the bifurcation of the bundle of His in the SA node, atria, or AV junction, with a rate of over 100 beats per minute.

Sustained ventricular tachycardia Prolonged ventricular tachycardia.

S wave The first negative or downward wave of deflection of the QRS complex that is preceded by an R wave. An upper case "S" indicates a large S wave; a lower case "s" indicates a small S wave. May be deep and narrow or wide and slurred.

Sympathetic (adrenergic) activity The excitatory action on the heart, blood vessels, and other organs brought on by the stimulation of the sympathetic nervous system. The effect on the heart and blood vessels results in an increase in heart rate, cardiac output, and blood pressure.

Sympathetic (adrenergic) nervous system Part of the autonomic nervous system involved in the control of involuntary bodily functions, including the control of cardiac and blood vessel activity. This system stimulates cardiac activity and produces effects opposite to those of the parasympathetic nervous system, which depresses cardiac activity. Some effects of sympathetic stimulation are an increase in heart rate, cardiac output, and blood pressure.

Sympathetic tone Pertains to the degree of sympathetic activity.

Sympathomimetic drugs Drugs that mimic the effects of stimulation of the sympathetic nervous system (e.g., epinephrine and norepinephrine).

Symptomatic bradycardia A bradycardia with one or more of the following signs or symptoms: (1) hypotension (systolic blood pressure less than 90 mm Hg), (2) congestive heart failure, (3) chest pain, (4) dyspnea, (5) signs and symptoms of decreased cardiac output, or (6) premature ventricular contractions. Requires treatment immediately.

Symptomatic "relative" bradycardia Normal sinus rhythm or an arrhythmia with a heart rate somewhat above 60 beats per minute with signs or symptoms associated with a symptomatic bradycardia because of the heart rate being too slow relative to the existing metabolic needs. Requires treatment immediately.

Synchronized countershock A direct-current (DC) shock synchronized with the QRS complex used to terminate the following:
- Atrial flutter/Atrial fibrillation
- Paroxysmal supraventricular tachycardia (PSVT) with narrow QRS complexes
- Wide-QRS-complex tachycardia of unknown origin (with pulse)
- Ventricular tachycardia, monomorphic (with pulse)
- Ventricular tachycardia, polymorphic, with normal QT interval (with pulse)

Syncytium A branching and anastomosing network of cells, such as that formed by the interconnection of the cardiac cells to form the myocardium.

Systemic circulation Passage of blood from the left ventricle through the aorta, all its branches, and capillaries in the tissue of the body and then to the right atrium through the venules, veins, and vena cavae. The blood vessels in the body (except those in the lungs) and those carrying blood to and from the body.

Systole (electrical) The period of time from phase 0 to the end of phase 3 of the cardiac action potential.

Systole (mechanical) The period of atrial or ventricular contraction.

Tachycardia Considered to be three or more beats occurring at a rate exceeding 100 beats per minute.

Ta wave Atrial T wave; usually buried in the following QRS complex.

T axis The mean of all the vectors generated during the repolarization of the ventricles (i.e., during the T wave).

Temporary transvenous pacemaker Delivery of electrical impulses generated by an external artificial pacemaker through a catheter threaded through a vein and positioned in the right ventricle.

Tenecteplase (TNK-tPA) A thrombolytic agent that converts plasminogen, a plasma protein, to plasmin, which in turn dissolves the fibrin binding the platelets together within a thrombus (fibrinolysis), causing the thrombus to break apart (thrombolysis). Trade name: TNKase.

Terminal The final wave of the QRS complex.

Terminal R and S waves Typical ECG findings in right bundle branch block—tall "terminal" R waves in leads aVR and V_1-V_2; deep and slurred "terminal" S waves in leads I, aVL, and V_5-V_6.

Third-degree AV block (complete AV block) Complete absence of conduction of electrical impulses from the atria to the ventricles through the AV junction. May be transient and reversible or permanent (chronic). Usually associated with abnormally wide QRS complexes, but the QRS complexes may be narrow. See *AV block, third-degree.*

3-second interval The period between two adjacent 3-second interval lines.

Threshold potential The value of intracellular negativity at which point a cardiac cell can be depolarized after being electrically stimulated.

Thrombin An enzyme formed from prothrombin when prothrombin is exposed to tissue factor released from damaged arterial wall tissue. Thrombin in turn converts fibrinogen to fibrin.

Thrombolysis The breakdown (lysis) of a thrombus (blood clot) by thrombolytic agents such as the normally occurring tissue plasminogen activator (tPA), which converts plasminogen attached to the fibrin strands within the thrombus to plasmin (an enzyme). Plasmin in turn breaks down the fibrin into soluble fragments (fibrinolysis) causing the platelets to separate from each other and the thrombus to break apart. Drugs used for thrombolysis include: alteplase (t-PA) (Activase), reteplase (r-PA) (Retavase), and tenecteplase (TNK-tPA) (TNKase).

Thrombolytic agents A tissue plasminogen activator that converts plasminogen, normally present in the blood, to plasmin, an enzyme that dissolves fibrin (fibrinolysis) within the thrombus, helping to break the thrombus apart (thrombolysis). The following are thrombolytic agents: alteplase (t-PA), reteplase (r-PA), and tenecteplase (TNK-tPA).

Thromboxane A₂ (TxA₂) A substance released from platelets after the platelets are activated following damage to the blood vessel walls. Thromboxane A_2 promotes thrombus formation by stimulating platelet aggregation. Other substances released on platelet activation are adenosine diphosphate (ADP) and serotonin. Aspirin inhibits thromboxane A_2 (TxA_2) formation and its release from the platelets, thus partially impeding platelet aggregation.

Thrombus formation The formation of a blood clot (coagulation) involving a complex interaction between certain blood components (i.e., platelets, prothrombin, and fibrinogen) and von Willebrand factor (vWF), collagen fibers, and tissue factor present in the endothelium and intima lining the blood vessel walls. The four phases of thrombus formation are as follows:

Phase I: Platelet adhesion. See *Platelet adhesion.*
Phase II: Platelet activation. See *Platelet activation.*
Phase III: Platelet aggregation. See *Platelet aggregation.*
Phase IV: Thrombus formation.

Also refers to the fourth phase of thrombus formation when the fibrinogen between the platelets is converted into stronger strands of fibrin by the action of thrombin, itself converted from prothrombin by tissue factor. Plasminogen usually becomes attached to the fibrin during its formation. As the thrombus grows, red cells and leukocytes (white cells) become entrapped in the platelet-fibrin mesh.

Thrombus (blood clot) An aggregation of platelets, fibrin, clotting agents, and red and white blood cells attached to a blood vessel wall.

Tissue plasminogen activator (tPA) A clot-dissolving enzyme normally present in the endothelium of the blood vessel wall that activates plasminogen to convert to plasmin, which, in turn, dissolves the fibrin (fibrinolysis), causing the thrombus to break apart (thrombolysis).

Tissue factor A substance present in tissue, platelets, and leukocytes that when released after injury, initiates the conversion of prothrombin to thrombin.

TNK-tPA Tenecteplase (TNK-tPA), a thrombolytic agent.

TNKase Trade name for tenecteplase (TNK-tPA), a thrombolytic agent.

Torsade de pointes A form of ventricular tachycardia characterized by QRS complexes that gradually change back and forth from one shape and direction to another over a series of beats. A French expression meaning "twisting around a point."

tPA Tissue plasminogen activator (tPA). See Alteplase (t-PA).

TP segment The section of the ECG between the end of the T wave and the onset of the P wave. Used as the baseline reference for the measurement of the amplitude of the ECG waves and complexes.

Transcutaneous overdrive pacing The use of a transcutaneous pacemaker to terminate certain arrhythmias such as *polymorphic ventricular tachycardia with a prolonged QT interval (with pulse)* and *torsade de pointes (with pulse)*. This is done by adjusting the pacemaker's rate to one that is greater than that of the arrhythmia.

Transcutaneous pacing (TCP, TC pacing) The delivery of electrical impulses through the skin to treat bradycardias from whatever cause, ventricular asystole, and pulseless electrical activity using an external artificial pacemaker. External cardiac pacing.

Transmural Extending from the endocardium to the epicardium.

Transmural, Q wave MI An infarction in which the zone of infarction involves the entire full thickness of the ventricular wall, from the endocardium to the epicardial surface. Abnormal Q waves are usually present.

Trendelenburg position One in which the patient is supine on the backboard, the head of which is tilted downward 30 to 40 degrees, and the patient's knees are bent.

Triaxial reference figure A guide for determining the direction of the QRS axis in the frontal plane, formed by the lead axes of the three limb leads or the three augmented leads,

spaced 60° apart around a zero reference point. The two tri-axial reference figures, one formed by the standard limb leads and the other by the augmented leads, superimposed, form the hexaxial reference figure.

Tricuspid valve The one-way valve located between the right atrium and the right ventricle.

Trigeminy A series of groups of three beats, usually consisting of two normally conducted QRS complexes followed by a premature contraction. The premature contraction may be atrial, junctional, or ventricular in origin (i.e., atrial trigeminy, junctional trigeminy, ventricular trigeminy).

Triggered activity See *Afterdepolarization.*

Triphasic rSR' pattern of RBBB See *"M" (or rabbit ears) pattern.*

Triplicate method A method used to determine the heart rate.

T wave The part of the ECG representing repolarization of the ventricles that follows the QRS complex from which it is separated by the ST segment if it is present. It may be positive (symmetrically tall and peaked) or negative (deeply inverted).

T wave elevation/inversion See *Ischemic T waves.*

TxA$_2$ Thromboxane A$_2$ (TxA$_2$).

12-lead electrocardiogram (ECG) The routine (or conventional) ECG consisting of three standard (bipolar) limb leads (leads I, II, and III), three augmented (unipolar) leads (leads aVR, aVL, and aVF), and six precordial (unipolar) leads (leads V$_1$, V$_2$, V$_3$, V$_4$, V$_5$, and V$_6$).

Uncontrolled Refers to arrhythmias such as atrial flutter and atrial fibrillation that are untreated and, consequently, have rapid ventricular rates.

Underlying rhythm The basic rhythm upon which certain arrhythmias are superimposed, such as sinus arrest and sinoatrial (SA) exit block, AV blocks, pacemaker rhythm, and premature atrial, junctional, and ventricular contractions.

Unfractionated heparin An anticoagulant.

Unifocal Pertains to a single ectopic pacemaker.

Unifocal PVCs PVCs that originate in the same ventricular ectopic pacemaker site, usually appearing identical (i.e., uniform).

Uniform PVCs PVCs having the same appearance and configuration, presumably arising from the same ventricular ectopic pacemaker site (i.e., unifocal).

Unipolar chest ("V") leads Leads V$_1$ to V$_6$.

Unipolar limb leads Leads aVR, aVL, and aVF.

Unmonitored cardiac arrest Cardiac arrest that is witnessed by the resuscitation team or that has occurred before the arrival of the team and the patient is not being monitored.

Unsynchronized shock A direct-current (DC) shock not synchronized with the QRS complex, used to treat the following:

- Ventricular tachycardia, polymorphic, with prolonged QT interval (with pulse)
- Torsade de pointes (with pulse)
- Pulseless ventricular tachycardia
- Ventricular fibrillation

Upper case letters Upper case letters, such as Q, R, S, are used to designate large deflections of the ECG.

U wave The positive wave superimposed on or following the T wave. Possibly represents the final phase of repolarization of the ventricles.

Vagal maneuvers Methods to increase the vagal (parasympathetic) tone to convert paroxysmal supraventricular tachycardia. See *Valsalva maneuver*.

Vagal (parasympathetic) tone See *Parasympathetic (vagal) tone*.

Vagus nerve The parasympathetic nerve. Consists of the right and left vagus nerves.

Valsalva maneuver Forceful act of expiration with the mouth and nose closed, producing a bearing down on the abdomen. Used to increase the parasympathetic tone to convert paroxysmal supraventricular tachycardia.

Variable AV block Refers to an AV block with varying AV conduction ratios (i.e., the ratio of P, P′, F, or f waves to QRS complexes varies).

Vasoconstriction Narrowing the lumen of blood vessels.

Vasoconstrictor A drug, hormone, or substance that constricts the lumen of blood vessels.

Vasodilatation Vasodilation. Widening the lumen of blood vessels.

Vasodilator A drug, hormone, or substance that dilates or widens the lumen of blood vessels.

Vasopressor A drug that causes vasoconstriction.

Vasovagal Pertaining to a vascular and neurogenic cause.

VAT See *Ventricular activation time (VAT)*.

Vector A graphic presentation, using an arrow, of the electric current generated by the depolarization or repolarization of the atria and ventricles at any one moment of time.

Ventricle The thick-walled muscular chamber that receives blood from the atrium and pumps it into the pulmonary or systemic circulation. The two ventricles form the larger lower part of the heart and the apex. They are separated from the atria by the mitral and tricuspid valves.

Ventricular activation time (VAT) The time it takes for depolarization of the interventricular septum, the right ventricle, and most of the left ventricle, up to and including the endocardial to epicardial depolarization of the left ventricular wall under the facing lead. Also called the *preintrinsicoid deflection* or *intrinsicoid deflection time (IDT)*.

Ventricular arrhythmia An arrhythmia originating in an ectopic pacemaker in the ventricles. Also referred to as *ventricular ectopy*.

Ventricular asystole (cardiac standstill) Cessation of ventricular contractions.

Ventricular demand pacemaker (VVI) A pacemaker that senses spontaneously occurring QRS complexes and paces the ventricles when they do not appear.

Ventricular diastole The interval or period during which the ventricles are relaxed and filling with blood. The period between ventricular contractions.

Ventricular dilatation Distension of the ventricle because of increased pressure and/or volume within the ventricle; it may be acute or chronic.

Ventricular enlargement Ventricular enlargement includes ventricular dilatation and hypertrophy. Common causes include heart failure, pulmonary diseases, pulmonary or systemic hypertension, heart valve stenosis or insufficiency, congenital heart defects, and acute myocardial infarction. See *Left ventricular hypertrophy (LVH)*, *Right ventricular hypertrophy (RVH)*.

Ventricular escape rhythm An arrhythmia arising in an escape pacemaker in the ventricles with a rate of less than 40 beats per minute.

Ventricular fibrillation/pulseless ventricular tachycardia Two life-threatening ventricular arrhythmias that result in cardiac arrest. Treatment is immediate defibrillation.

Ventricular fibrillation (VF, V-FIB) An arrhythmia originating in multiple ectopic pacemakers in the ventricles characterized by numerous ventricular fibrillatory waves and no QRS complexes.

Ventricular fibrillation (VF) waves Bizarre, irregularly shaped, rounded or pointed, and markedly dissimilar waves originating in multiple ectopic pacemakers in the ventricles.

Ventricular fusion beat See *Fusion beat, ventricular*.

Ventricular hypertrophy Enlargement of the ventricular myocardium, the result of an increase in the size of the muscle fibers because of chronic increase in pressure and/or volume within the ventricle. Common causes include heart failure, pulmonary diseases, pulmonary or systemic hypertension, heart valve stenosis or insufficiency, and congenital heart defects. See *Left ventricular hypertrophy (LVH)*, *Right ventricular hypertrophy (RVH)*.

Ventricular overload Refers to increased pressure and/or volume within the ventricles.

Ventricular preexcitation The premature depolarization of the ventricles associated with an abnormal accessory conduction pathway, such as the accessory AV pathways or nodoventricular/fasciculoventricular fibers that bypass the AV junction or bundle of His, respectively, allowing the electrical impulses to initiate depolarization of the ventricles earlier than usual. This results in an abnormally wide QRS complex of greater than 0.10 second that characteristically has an abnormal slurring and sometimes notching at its onset—the delta wave. The PR interval is usually less than 0.12 second when ventricular preexcitation is the result of an accessory AV pathway and usually normal when nodoventricular/fasciculoventricular fibers are the cause. The term *ventricular preexcitation* is most commonly used to indicate ventricular preexcitation associated with accessory AV pathway conduction.

Ventricular repolarization The electrical process by which the depolarized ventricles return to their polarized, resting state. Ventricular depolarization is represented by the T wave on the ECG.

Ventricular "strain" pattern The changes in the QRS-ST-T complex produced by a downsloping ST segment depression and T wave inversion, characteristic of long-standing right or left ventricular hypertrophy. Also known as the *"hockey stick" pattern*.

Ventricular systole The interval or period during which the ventricles are contracting and emptying of blood.

Ventricular tachycardia (VT, V-TACH) An arrhythmia originating in an ectopic pacemaker in the ventricles with a rate between 100 and 250 beats per minute.

Ventricular T wave (T wave) Represents ventricular repolarization.

Verapamil An antiarrhythmic used to treat paroxysmal atrial and junctional tachycardias.

V leads Leads V_1, V_2, V_3, V_4, V_5, and V_6. See *Precordial (unipolar) leads*.

von Willebrand factor (vWF) A protein stored in the endothelium of blood vessels, that when exposed to blood binds to the platelets' GP Ib and GP IIb/GP IIIa receptors, adhering the platelets to the collagen fibers in the blood vessel wall.

Voltage (amplitude) See *Amplitude (voltage)*.

Vulnerable period of ventricular repolarization The part of the last phase of repolarization during which the ventricles can be stimulated to depolarize prematurely by a greater than normal electrical stimulus. This corresponds to the downslope of the T wave.

vWF See *von Willebrand factor (vWF)*.

Wandering atrial pacemaker (WAP) An arrhythmia originating in pacemakers that shift back and forth between the SA node and an ectopic pacemaker in the atria or AV junction. It is characterized by P waves varying in size, shape, and direction in any given lead.

Warning arrhythmias PVCs that are more prone than others to initiate life-threatening arrhythmias, particularly after an acute myocardial infarction or ischemic episode:

- PVCs falling on the T wave (the *R-on-T phenomenon*)
- Multiform and multifocal PVCs
- Frequent PVCs of more than five or six per minute
- Ventricular group beats with bursts or salvos of two, three, or more

Watt/seconds Units of electrical energy delivered by a source of energy, such as a defibrillator. One watt/second equals *1 joule*.

Waves Refers to various components of the ECG—the P, Q, R, S, T, and U waves. Waves may be large or small.

Wenckebach block See *Second-degree AV block type I AV block (Wenckebach)*

Wenckebach phenomenon A progressive prolongation of the conduction of electrical impulses through the AV node, most commonly until conduction is completely blocked, occurring in cycles. Conduction block may also occur infranodally.

Wide-QRS-complex tachycardia A tachycardia with abnormally wide QRS complexes (0.12 second or greater) that may be ventricular tachycardia or a supraventricular tachycardia with wide QRS complexes resulting from a preexisting bundle branch block, aberrant ventricular conduction, or ventricular preexcitation.

"Window" theory Refers to the popular theory of why Q waves occur over infarcted myocardium. According to this theory, the facing leads over electrically inert infarcted myocardium (or "window") view the endocardium of the opposite noninfarcted ventricular wall, and detect the R waves generated by the opposite wall as large Q waves.

"Zero" center of the heart Refers to the hypothetical reference point with an electrical potential of zero, located in the electrical center of the heart—left of the interventricular septum and below the AV junction. Formed by connecting the extremity electrodes together, the "indifferent," zero reference point is used as the central terminal for the unipolar leads. It also represents the central point for the hexaxial reference figure.

Zones of infarction (necrosis), injury, and ischemia A myocardial infarction at its height typically consists of a central area of dead, necrotic tissue—the *zone of infarction* (or *necrosis*), surrounded immediately by a layer of injured myocardial tissue—the *zone of injury*, and, lastly, by an outer layer of ischemic tissue—the *zone of ischemia*.

Index